Engineering 3D Tissue Test Systems

Engineering 3D Tissue Test Systems

Edited by
Karen J. L. Burg
Didier Dréau
Timothy Burg

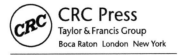
CRC Press
Taylor & Francis Group
Boca Raton London New York

CRC Press is an imprint of the
Taylor & Francis Group, an **informa** business

CRC Press
Taylor & Francis Group
6000 Broken Sound Parkway NW, Suite 300
Boca Raton, FL 33487-2742

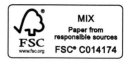

© 2018 by Taylor & Francis Group, LLC
CRC Press is an imprint of Taylor & Francis Group, an Informa business

No claim to original U.S. Government works

Printed on acid-free paper

International Standard Book Number-13: 978-1-1387-4567-4 (Paperback)
978-1-4822-3117-5 (Hardback)

This book contains information obtained from authentic and highly regarded sources. Reasonable efforts have been made to publish reliable data and information, but the author and publisher cannot assume responsibility for the validity of all materials or the consequences of their use. The authors and publishers have attempted to trace the copyright holders of all material reproduced in this publication and apologize to copyright holders if permission to publish in this form has not been obtained. If any copyright material has not been acknowledged please write and let us know so we may rectify in any future reprint.

Except as permitted under U.S. Copyright Law, no part of this book may be reprinted, reproduced, transmitted, or utilized in any form by any electronic, mechanical, or other means, now known or hereafter invented, including photocopying, microfilming, and recording, or in any information storage or retrieval system, without written permission from the publishers.

For permission to photocopy or use material electronically from this work, please access www.copyright.com (http://www.copyright.com/) or contact the Copyright Clearance Center, Inc. (CCC), 222 Rosewood Drive, Danvers, MA 01923, 978-750-8400. CCC is a not-for-profit organization that provides licenses and registration for a variety of users. For organizations that have been granted a photocopy license by the CCC, a separate system of payment has been arranged.

Trademark Notice: Product or corporate names may be trademarks or registered trademarks, and are used only for identification and explanation without intent to infringe.

Library of Congress Cataloging-in-Publication Data

Names: Burg, Karen J. L., editor. | Dréau, Didier, editor. | Burg, Timothy C., editor.
Title: Engineering 3D tissue test systems / editors, Karen J.L. Burg, Didier Dréau, and Timothy Burg.
Description: Boca Raton : Taylor & Francis, 2017. | "A CRC title, part of the Taylor & Francis imprint, a member of the Taylor & Francis Group, the academic division of T&F Informa plc." | Includes bibliographical references.
Identifiers: LCCN 2017006771| ISBN 9781482231175 (hardback : alk. paper) | ISBN 9781482231182 (ebook)
Subjects: LCSH: Tissue engineering. | Biomedical materials.
Classification: LCC R857.T55 E55 2017 | DDC 610.28/4--dc23
LC record available at https://lccn.loc.gov/2017006771

Visit the Taylor & Francis Web site at
http://www.taylorandfrancis.com

and the CRC Press Web site at
http://www.crcpress.com

Printed and bound in the United States of America by Sheridan

*This monograph is dedicated to Dr. Shalaby W. Shalaby,
who lived by the motto "everything is an opportunity"
and who inspired so many to learn, to teach, to innovate and,
most importantly, to be humble. His career was a blueprint
for how to, with focused dedication, move ideas from a lonely
landscape to a burgeoning field of research and translation.*

Contents

Preface xi
Acknowledgments xiii
Editors xv
Contributors xvii
Reviewers xxi

Chapter 1 Introduction to 3D Test Systems 1

Karen J. L. Burg, Didier Dréau, and Timothy Burg

SECTION I *Biofabrication Considerations*

Chapter 2 Biofabrication 9

Jordon Gilmore and Timothy Burg

Chapter 3 Bioreactor Instrumentation and Control for 3D Cellular and Tissue Systems 33

Steve Warren

Chapter 4 Control of 3D Environment: Redesign of the Flow Loop Bioreactor to Control Mitral Valve Regurgitation 61

Patrick S. Connell, Dragoslava P. Vekilov, and K. Jane Grande-Allen

Chapter 5 Nipple and Breast Construction: *In Vitro* and *In Vivo* Assessment 75

Maria Yanez, Scott Collins, and Thomas Boland

Chapter 6 3D Cancer Spheroid Biofabrication Using Thermal Inkjet-Based Bioprinting for Rapid Screening 91

Jorge I. Rodríguez-Dévora, Christopher Moody, Aesha Desai, Karen J. L. Burg, and Delphine Dean

SECTION II Materials Considerations

Chapter 7 Control Testing and Effect of Manufacturing Parameters on the Biocompatibility of Polypropylene Mesh Implants 107

Ahmed El-Ghannam

Chapter 8 Scaffolds for 3D Model Systems in Bone Regenerative Engineering 125

Keshia Ashe, Seth Malinowski, Yusuf Khan, and Cato T. Laurencin

Chapter 9 Engineered Composites for 3D Mammary Tissue Systems 141

Cheryl T. Gomillion, Chih-Chao Yang, Didier Dréau, and Karen J. L. Burg

Chapter 10 Mineralized 3D Culture Systems for Studying Bone Metastatic Breast Cancer 169

Frank He, Siyoung Choi, Lara A. Estroff, and Claudia Fischbach

Chapter 11 Design Considerations for 3D Cardiovascular Tissue Scaffolds 193

Scott Cooper, Christopher Moraes, and Richard L. Leask

SECTION III Biological Considerations

Chapter 12 Pro- and Anti-Inflammatory Cytokine Signaling within 3D Tissue Models 215

Stephen L. Rego, Tian McCann, and Didier Dréau

Chapter 13 Cell–Cell Communications through Gap Junctions and Cancer in 3D Systems 233

Stephanie Nicole Shishido and Thu Annelise Nguyen

Chapter 14 Advances in Breast Stem Cell Knowledge through 3D Systems 249

Kerri W. Kwist and Brian W. Booth

Chapter 15 Shape Matters: Understanding the Breast through 3D Tissue Culture Models 263

Lucia Speroni, Ana M. Soto, and Carlos Sonnenschein

Contents

Chapter 16 Cells and Tissue Structures in Cardiovascular 3D Tissue Systems 285

Justin McMahan, Rachel Hybart, and C. LaShan Simpson

Chapter 17 Signaling and Architectural Cues Necessary for 3D Diabetic Tissue Models 299

Rosalyn D. Abbott and David L. Kaplan

Chapter 18 Optimizing 3D Models of Engineered Skeletal Muscle 321

Megan E. Kondash, Brittany N. J. Davis, and George A. Truskey

Chapter 19 Recapitulating the Microenvironment of Glioblastoma Multiforme Using 3D Tissue Culture Models 351

Meghan Logun, Steven Stice, and Lohitash Karumbaiah

SECTION IV *Business Considerations*

Editor's Note on Business Considerations 377

Chapter 20 Bringing Regenerative Medicine to Patients: The Coverage, Coding, and Reimbursement Processes 381

Khin-Kyemon Aung, Scott Levy, and Sujata K. Bhatia

Index 401

Preface

When we first launched into this area of research in the early 2000s, the potential for engineered 3D tissue systems was uniformly regarded as science fiction. It is extremely satisfying to now see so many research groups focused on designing, building, and applying 3D tissues, to see conferences and sessions within conferences devoted to the topics, and to have been a part of translating initial tissue test system products to market. The focus of this monograph is the potential of 3D tissue systems. Current and future research responses are revealed, current and future diagnostic applications are examined, and a comprehensive overview is provided to foster innovation. The volume is divided into three major areas, each with supportive chapters. The first area focuses on instrumentation to build and house 3D systems, the second area focuses on issues surrounding biomaterials, and the last area speaks to the biological issues and overall system considerations. The final chapter, focused on coding and reimbursement issues, caps the three scientific areas and prompts us to consider the realities of translation. The underlying theme of this monograph is the soon-to-be realized potential of 3D tissue engineering.

Acknowledgments

We express our gratitude to the many contributing authors for taking the time to diligently compile the chapters of this monograph and we thank the many reviewers for thoughtfully and generously providing input. We are grateful to Allison Shatkin of CRC Press/Taylor & Francis and Jill Jurgensen (formerly of CRC Press/Taylor & Francis) and the CRC team members for their gracious persistence during the completion of this book.

Editors

Karen J. L. Burg earned a BS in chemical engineering with a minor in biochemical engineering from North Carolina State University, Raleigh, North Carolina, an MS in bioengineering from Clemson University, Clemson, South Carolina, and a PhD in bioengineering with a minor in experimental statistics from Clemson University. She completed a tissue engineering postdoctoral research fellowship at Carolinas Medical Center, Charlotte, North Carolina, later serving as Clemson University Interim Vice Provost for Research & Innovation, Clemson University Interim Vice Provost and Dean of the Graduate School, and Kansas State University Vice President for Research. She is currently Harbor Lights Endowed Chair of Small Animal Medicine and Surgery at the University of Georgia and Hunter Endowed Chair Emerita at Clemson University. Karen is a former President of the Society For Biomaterials and a former member of the Tissue Engineering and Regenerative Medicine International Society North American Council. She is currently serving as a member of the Board of Directors for the National Academy of Inventors as well as a member of the College of Fellows Executive Board for the American Council on Education. Honors to Dr. Burg include the 2001 National Science Foundation Faculty Early Career Award and 2001 Presidential Early Career Award for Scientists and Engineers; she is an American Council on Education Fellow, a Fellow of the American Institute for Medical and Biological Engineering, a Fellow of the Biomedical Engineering Society, a Fellow of the National Academy of Inventors, and a Fellow of the International Union of Societies for Biomaterials Science and Engineering. Among her research interests are the optimization of absorbable biomaterials processing for regenerative engineering applications and the development of 3D tissue engineered benchtop systems for diagnostic and discovery applications.

Didier Dréau earned a BS in physiology and cell biology from Rennes I University (Rennes, France), an MS in molecular and cell biology from Blaise Pascal University (Clermont-Ferrand, France), and a PhD in biochemistry, molecular and cell biology with emphasis on immunology from the Ecole Nationale Supérieure Agronomique (ENSA) de Rennes (France). Following his postdoctoral training in immunology and immunotherapy and serving as Research Scientist at Carolinas Medical Center, currently Dr. Dréau is an associate professor of biology at the University of North Carolina at Charlotte. Dr. Dréau also serves as the Honors in Biological Sciences Program director in the Department of Biological Sciences, and the area leader for the Applied Cancer Technology and Therapeutics in the Center for Biomedical Engineering and Science at the University of North Carolina at Charlotte. In addition to his teaching of cancer biology and physiology, Dr. Dréau, a member of the American Association for Cancer Research, serves on multiple granting agency review panels along with scientific journal editorial boards. The focus of the research developed in his laboratory is on angiogenesis, immune responses, and the physical and chemical tumor microenvironment in the promotion of metastasis. His research efforts include dedicated interests in the development of new approaches to prevention, early detection, monitoring, and treatment of cancers.

Timothy Burg earned a BS in electrical engineering from the University of Cincinnati, Cincinnati, Ohio and an MS and PhD in electrical engineering from Clemson University, Clemson, South Carolina. He is currently a professor of veterinary biosciences & diagnostic imaging in the University of Georgia College of Veterinary Medicine and director of the University of Georgia Office of Science, Technology, Engineering and Mathematics (STEM) Education. Dr. Burg has extensive experience in industrial applications of robotics and nonlinear control design tools and the academic investigation of the basis and future directions of these techniques. An intelligent system can be defined as the integration of hardware and software to create a new system that exceeds the capabilities of the hardware alone, for example, adding computer control to an electric motor. Current projects that capitalize on the promise of the intelligent systems approach include biofabrication, haptic trainers for laparoscopic surgery training, and force control algorithms for robots. The ongoing tissue engineering project centers on the application of controls and robotics tools to fabricate systems of living tissues. Dr. Burg is working with students and other collaborators to build a unique biofabrication system that assembles tissues in an assembly line fashion. One component of this system, a bioprinter that uses ink-jet printing to place living cells, was developed during an US National Science Foundation grant. Dr. Burg strives to connect the exciting research at the university level with K-12 students.

Contributors

Rosalyn D. Abbott
Biomedical Engineering
Tufts University
Medford, Massachusetts

Keshia Ashe
Department of Chemical &
 Biomolecular Engineering
University of Connecticut
Storrs, Connecticut

and

Institute for Regenerative Engineering
Raymond & Beverly Sackler Center for
 Biomedical, Biological, Physical &
 Engineering Sciences
UConn Health
Farmington, Connecticut

Khin-Kyemon Aung
Harvard Medical School
Boston, Massachusetts

Sujata K. Bhatia
Department of Biomedical
 Engineering
Harvard University
Cambridge, Massachusetts

Thomas Boland
Biomedical Engineering
University of Texas at El Paso
El Paso, Texas

Brian W. Booth
Department of Bioengineering
Institute for Biological Interfaces of
 Engineering
Clemson University
Clemson, South Carolina

Karen J. L. Burg
Department of Small Animal Medicine
 & Surgery
University of Georgia
Athens, Georgia

Timothy Burg
Department of Veterinary
 Biosciences & Diagnostic Imaging
College of Veterinary Medicine
University of Georgia
Athens, Georgia

Siyoung Choi
Nancy E. and Peter C. Meinig School of
 Biomedical Engineering
Cornell University
Ithaca, New York

Scott Collins
Tevido Biodevices LLC
University of Texas at El Paso
El Paso, Texas

Patrick S. Connell
Department of Bioengineering
Rice University
Houston, Texas

Scott Cooper
Department of Chemical
 Engineering
McGill University
Montreal, Quebec, Canada

Brittany N. J. Davis
Department of Biomedical
 Engineering
Duke University
Durham, North Carolina

Delphine Dean
Department of Bioengineering
Clemson University
Clemson, South Carolina

Aesha Desai
Department of Bioengineering
Clemson University
Clemson, South Carolina

Didier Dréau
Department of Biological Sciences
University of North Carolina at Charlotte
Charlotte, North Carolina

Lara A. Estroff
Department of Materials Science and Engineering
Kavli Institute at Cornell for Nanoscale Science
Cornell University
Ithaca, New York

Ahmed El-Ghannam
Department of Mechanical Engineering and Engineering Science
University of North Carolina
Charlotte, North Carolina

Claudia Fischbach
Nancy E. and Peter C. Meinig School of Biomedical Engineering
Kavli Institute at Cornell for Nanoscale Science
Cornell University
Ithaca, New York

Jordon Gilmore
Department of Mechanical Engineering
College of Engineering, Computing, and Applied Sciences
Clemson University
Clemson, South Carolina

Cheryl T. Gomillion
College of Engineering
University of Georgia
Athens, Georgia

K. Jane Grande-Allen
Department of Bioengineering
Rice University
Houston, Texas

Frank He
Nancy E. and Peter C. Meinig School of Biomedical Engineering
Cornell University
Ithaca, New York

Rachel Hybart
Agricultural and Biological Engineering
Mississippi State University
Mississippi State, Mississippi

David L. Kaplan
Biomedical Engineering
Tufts University
Medford, Massachusetts

Lohitash Karumbaiah
Regenerative Bioscience Center
University of Georgia
Athens, Georgia

Yusuf Khan
Department of Orthopaedic Surgery
Institute for Regenerative Engineering
Raymond & Beverly Sackler Center for Biomedical, Biological, Physical & Engineering Sciences
UConn Health
Farmington, Connecticut

and

Department of Material Science & Engineering; Department of Biomedical Engineering
University of Connecticut
Storrs, Connecticut

Contributors

Megan E. Kondash
Department of Biomedical
  Engineering
Duke University
Durham, North Carolina

Kerri W. Kwist
Institute for Biological Interfaces of
  Engineering
Clemson University
Clemson, South Carolina

Cato T. Laurencin
Department of Chemical &
  Biomolecular Engineering;
  Department of Biomedical
  Engineering; Department of
  Material Science & Engineering
Institute of Material Science
University of Connecticut
Storrs, Connecticut

and

Department of Orthopaedic Surgery
Institute for Regenerative Engineering
Raymond & Beverly Sackler Center for
  Biomedical, Biological, Physical &
  Engineering Sciences
UConn Health
Farmington, Connecticut

Richard L. Leask
Department of Chemical Engineering
McGill University
and
Montreal Heart Institute
Montreal, Quebec, Canada

Scott Levy
Yale Law School
New Haven, Connecticut

Meghan Logun
Regenerative Bioscience Center
University of Georgia
Athens, Georgia

Seth Malinowski
Department of Biomedical Engineering
University of Connecticut
Storrs, Connecticut

Tian McCann
Biomedical Engineering Department
University of Connecticut
Storrs, Connecticut

Justin McMahan
Agricultural and Biological Engineering
Mississippi State University
Mississippi State, Mississippi

Christopher Moody
Institute for Biological Interfaces of
  Engineering
Clemson University
Clemson, South Carolina

Christopher Moraes
Department of Chemical Engineering
McGill University
Montreal, Quebec, Canada

Thu Annelise Nguyen
Department of Diagnostic Medicine and
  Pathobiology
Kansas State University
Manhattan, Kansas

Stephen L. Rego
Department of Biochemistry
Wake Forest University
Winston Salem, North Carolina

Jorge I. Rodríguez-Dévora
Department of Mechanical Engineering
  and Bioengineering
Clemson University
Clemson, South Carolina

Stephanie Nicole Shishido
Department of Diagnostic Medicine and
  Pathobiology
Kansas State University
Manhattan, Kansas

C. LaShan Simpson
Agricultural and Biological Engineering
Mississippi State University
Mississippi State, Mississippi

Carlos Sonnenschein
Department of Integrative Physiology
  and Pathobiology
Tufts University School of Medicine
Boston, Massachusetts

and

Centre Cavaillès
École Normale Supérieure
Institut d'Etudes Avancées de Nantes
Paris, France

Ana M. Soto
Department of Integrative Physiology
  and Pathobiology
Tufts University School of Medicine
Boston, Massachusetts

and

Centre Cavaillès
République des Savoirs
Collège de France et Ecole Normale
  Supérieure
Paris, France

Lucia Speroni
Department of Integrative Physiology
  and Pathobiology
Tufts University School of Medicine
Boston, Massachusetts

Steven Stice
Regenerative Bioscience Center
University of Georgia
Athens, Georgia

George A. Truskey
Department of Biomedical Engineering
Duke University
Durham, North Carolina

Dragoslava P. Vekilov
Department of Bioengineering
Rice University
Houston, Texas

Steve Warren
Department of Electrical & Computer
  Engineering
Kansas State University
Manhattan, Kansas

Maria Yanez
Biomedical Engineering
University of Texas at El Paso
El Paso, Texas

Chih-Chao Yang
Research & Development Division
AMED Co., Ltd.
New Taipei City, Taiwan

Reviewers

Susan Arthur
Department of Kinesiology
University of North Carolina at Charlotte
Charlotte, North Carolina

Kris Biesinger
Office of Science Technology
   Engineering & Mathematics
   Education
University of Georgia
Athens, Georgia

Thomas Boland
Department of Metallurgical, Materials
   and Biomedical Engineering
University of Texas at El Paso
El Paso, Texas

Brian Booth
Department of Bioengineering
Institute for Biological Interfaces of
   Engineering
Clemson University
Clemson, South Carolina

Hansang Cho
Department of Mechanical Engineering
   and Engineering Science
University of North Carolina at Charlotte
Charlotte, North Carolina

Mark Clemens
Department of Biological Sciences
University of North Carolina at Charlotte
Charlotte, North Carolina

K. Jane Grande-Allen
Department of Bioengineering
Rice University
Houston, Texas

Yas Maghdouri-White
Department of Biomedical Engineering
Virginia Commonwealth University
Richmond, Virginia

Andrea Mastro
Department of Biochemistry and
   Molecular Biology
Pennsylvania State University
University Park, Pennsylvania

Gabriele Niederauer
Bluegrass Vascular Technologies
San Antonio, Texas

Annelise Nguyen
Department of Diagnostic Medicine &
   Pathobiology
Kansas State University
Manhattan, Kansas

Stephen Rego
Department of Biochemistry
Wake Forest University
Winston Salem, North Carolina

Suzanne Tabbaa
Department of Bioengineering
University of California
San Diego, California

1 Introduction to 3D Test Systems

Karen J. L. Burg, Didier Dréau, and Timothy Burg

Over the past two decades, we have been enthusiastically working to establish the field of three-dimensional (3D) tissue test systems and encouraging others to participate, building from what was a lonely ideas and research landscape to what is now a burgeoning field of research and translation. Given the remarkable progress and confluence of new, enabling technologies, we thought that it is an appropriate time to share a cross section of current perspectives as well as insights as to what might be realized over the next two decades.

Three-dimensional tissue test systems are biological models comprising cells and biomaterials that can be used to better understand normal and healthy processes to discover new drugs, vaccines, and therapies, and to assess new implant designs. To help visualize the potential, consider that traditional preclinical testing methods do not typically incorporate the complexities of the often diseased or subnormal *in vivo* state. For this reason, implants that initially appear, preclinically, to be adequate fail post implantation once exposed to a diseased environment. Three-dimensional test systems have the potential to revolutionize preclinical implant evaluation and provide significantly more relevant information than has ever been possible. To be successful, we must acknowledge at the outset that tissue test systems are models and hence only approximations of complex living systems. They do not fully replicate every mechanism or feature; yet, they can be powerful tools in translating new ideas to clinical practice. As long as we understand and respect the bounds and limitations of each model, we can extract enormously useful information to forward the field of biomedicine. By developing an array of models, we are building a toolbox from which we can select models (tools) most relevant to a particular question or objective.

It is technology that is driving our ability to produce the tissue test systems about which we could only once dream. In particular, biofabrication is a family of processes to precisely assemble cells and biomaterials into a 3D tissue with a desired form and function. To realize a diverse and useful set of tools in our toolbox, we must understand the technology behind the various 3D tissue system designs as well as the bounds and limitations in manufacturing these systems. The functionality of 3D test systems is affected by shape, chemistry, and mechanics. Defined by the biofabrication processes, these features significantly influence biological interactions and functions within 3D test systems. Since cell–material fabrication concepts are inextricably entwined, one cannot address the interaction from any one vantage point. Hence, we have divided this book into four sections—Biofabrication

Considerations, Materials Considerations, Biological Considerations, and Business Considerations. The concluding section draws on all aspects to speak to business issues and the concerns we must consider for clinical translation.

Section I comprises five chapters and begins with a review of biofabrication processes (Chapter 2 by Gilmore and Burg), with particular focus on issues, barriers, and opportunities. We are guilty as a research community of publishing the "wow" photos and accomplishments, and quietly ignoring or understating the many complex problems that necessitate a technical community to solve. Chapters 3 and 4 describe bioreactors as applied to biofabrication. The development of benchtop tissue models means building the structures and maintaining relevant environments as the structures change and develop over time. Of interest is the ability to monitor a wide variety of features of the tissue and the microenvironment and to apply feedback control to perturb the system; the two chapters overview these aspects. Chapter 3 by Warren overviews general bioreactor control and points to specific bioreactor types and control peculiarities. Chapter 4 by Connell and coworkers highlights bioreactor control for a specific application, i.e., endothelial cells and hemostatic mediators in the development of mitral valves. This application requires a bioreactor that supports tissue development under dynamic conditions that a valve might encounter *in vivo*. Chapters 5 and 6 follow with specific examples of biofabrication. Chapter 5 by Yanez and coworkers describes the path to fabricate an adipose implant, with particular focus on nipple or breast reconstruction. The long-term vision is to extract information from a printed benchtop tissue that will direct the design of an *in vivo* implant. Chapter 6 by Rodríguez-Dévora and coworkers details a biofabricated hanging drop model used for patterning mammalian cells with high speed and reproducibility, resulting in 3D cell spheroid formation. This work shows the versatility of biofabrication as well as the limitations, using a breast cancer cell—fibroblast model.

Beginning with sutures in early Egyptian times, materials for implantation application have been extensively studied. The current evolution of 3D tissue systems allows us the opportunity to study cellular implantable materials in more relevant and complex benchtop models. Moreover, those 3D systems permit investigations of cellular materials that can be used for prevention, diagnosis, as well as the study of basic processes in a tissue. Section II provides a broad view of biomaterial constructs and their use in soft and hard tissue applications in 3D test systems. Now that there are many efforts focused on cellular benchtop models, it is time to use these models to test implants under a range of relevant physiological conditions. We still rely on very basic *in vitro* testing—incorporation of implants in a 3D test system will allow an additional finer "screen" for new implants and will help eliminate clinical translation time and development costs of implants that are robust in standard two-dimensional (2D) cellular culture but which behave very differently in a 3D tissue environment. Chapter 7 by El-Ghannam describes hernia mesh fabrication and manufacturing-relevant properties linked to biocompatibility. The author postulates that significant manufacturing quality control tests, for example, that 3D tissue test systems could provide, must be considered for polymeric implants. This chapter supports new screens, perhaps first testing the mesh fibers that would reveal information otherwise invisible in existing preclinical screening. We are further inspired to consider other devices that might significantly benefit preclinically from relatively simple test system assessment. Most importantly, the chapter challenges us to think about how we might build tissue systems that represent different compromised or diseased states to further assess device failures prior to clinical translation. To build this array of test systems, we must consider foundational work in regenerative engineering on which we can build and extend to test systems. For example, a large emphasis has been placed on orthopedic tissue engineering and on scaffold development over the past years. These scaffolds can also be used in benchtop tissue systems. Ashe and colleagues describe, in Chapter 8, a diverse array of 3D "dual use" materials. Soft-tissue systems similarly benefit from historical work in tissue engineering, particularly the application of materials to 3D test systems. Normal and diseased breast tissues have been modeled and studied by cancer cell biology and bioengineering researchers, each one investigating the system through their own specific lenses, using concepts and approaches previously developed for reconstructing and assessing tissues. In Chapter 9, Gomillion and colleagues provide a bioengineering perspective of mammary models that have been used for studying basic cellular processes and for screening drugs. Their overview in this chapter reminds us that the biological-material interaction is indeed a handshake and each component (the cells and the materials) is an important part of this partnership. Tissue models allow the study of complex environments that are not readily studied *in vivo* and they allow the incorporation of relevant biological aspects that are not easily viewed in a petri dish. For example, tissue models can capture static and dynamic aspects of tumor progression, such as the role of microcalcifications in the tumor environment. Chapter 10 by He and coworkers describes various mineralized tumor models and their current and future capacities in the development of new therapies. The final chapter (Chapter 11) in Section II outlines the role of the 3D biomechanical environment in the development of meaningful 3D tissues. Although focused on cardiovascular, the concepts in this chapter may be transposed to many other clinical applications, reminding us that as we design new 3D systems, we must be as cognizant of mechanical features as we are of physicochemical and mechanical factors. Cooper and coworkers, in Chapter 11, describe how one can tune material elasticity, dynamic force application, and biochemical transport in order to effect the biomechanical environment of a 3D tissue system.

Section III comprises eight chapters that encompass biological issues of importance to 3D tissue test systems, as well as the integration of all factors into the biological application. The first two chapters detail underlying, fundamental cellular mechanisms that we take for granted in 2D culture but which warrant in-depth thought in 3D systems. Rego and colleagues (Chapter 12) discuss cellular behaviors in relation to cell signaling in 3D, that is, the importance of cytokines, especially inflammatory cytokines, in understanding the 3D system and *in vivo* mechanisms and behaviors. The chapter overviews the research geared toward pathophysiology as well as therapeutic discovery. Shishido and Nguyen (Chapter 13) make the point that cellular spatial arrangements strongly influence basic cellular processes. Lack of opportunity for cells to assemble in 3D results in massive oversimplifications of complex *in vivo* cellular behaviors and in significant physiological differences. The authors review the importance of 3D arrangements to gap junctions and cell–cell communication. The authors of the next two chapters (Chapters 14 and 15) examine specific cellular issues perturbed by materials selection. Kwist and Booth (Chapter 14) address stem cell behavioral changes with system selection, particularly in cancer systems. The authors compare and contrast hanging drop models with standing gel systems; their discussion emphasizes the underlying point that different models have different benefits and limitations and should be carefully selected in concert with the biological question of interest. Speroni and colleagues address the effect of biomaterial shape on cellular response in Chapter 15, using the mammary gland as an example. They provide an overview of the 3D culture models used to study the dynamics of normal and pathological breast development. A significant amount of work has showcased the stark differences between 2D and 3D testing of cardiovascular systems. McMahan and colleagues (Chapter 16) highlight a range of systems, both 2D and 3D, that have been used to better understand a plethora of diseased cardiovascular states. That is, we can use 3D tissue models to study variations of a disease or a range of diseases. The authors detail the cardiac system and genetic defects and present cellular sheets as "materials" of choice for studying contractile cardiac tissue. The second half of Section III is focused on systems as a whole, exemplified by four different clinical areas—glioblastoma, diabetes, bone, and cardiovascular. The underlying theme of these chapters is that, while the discussion is centered on the development of a 3D tissue system, the concepts are equally valuable to regenerative engineering. Diabetic cues, for example, may be built into a tissue model via biomaterial architecture in order to understand the diabetic response. Chapter 17 by Abbott and Kaplan contains an overview of diabetic tissue models and prompts us to consider multiple, integrated tissue models that interact and provide opportunity to discern features of *in vivo* feedback loops. The authors discuss the necessary variations between different organ types to achieve appropriate cell signaling cascades and diabetic cues. Models may be used to design optimal regenerative systems or to study healthy and diseased states. Kondash and colleagues (Chapter 18) provide an overview of skeletal tissue systems that can be used to screen drug responses and address basic science questions that are difficult to address *in vivo*. Current commonly used 3D glioblastoma models for brain tissue involve creating composites with tumor spheroids embedded into polymeric scaffolds as described in Chapter 19 by Logun and coworkers. The authors describe various extracellular matrices and enriched matrices used in glioblastoma models to better understand the interaction between the tumors and normal tissue. The chapter further describes models that address drug delivery and tumor response in specific environments.

The last section (Section IV) begins with a note from the editors and highlights the business issues associated with commercialization and clinical use of 3D tissue test systems. Chapter 20 by Aung and colleagues details the coding and reimbursement process for implantable tissue-engineered devices and provides a view of the, generally unconsidered, landscape that must be navigated to commercialize 3D tissue test systems.

The opportunities to use 3D tissue test systems for challenging new hypotheses about nature, developing innovative diagnostics, and creating novel treatments are tremendous. Experts with diverse technical backgrounds, including industrial and regulatory, will be instrumental to building and validating 3D tissue systems of clinical, scientific, and economic relevance. With the increased and open discussion of obstacles and challenges across and within our respective disciplines, we can accelerate the development and use of 3D tissue test systems for repair, diagnosis, and prevention. We are excited to have contributed to the establishment and evolution of this highly translatable research area and hope this book provides insights that similarly excite new participants with additional perspectives to contribute to this impactful field.

Section I

Biofabrication Considerations

2 Biofabrication

Jordon Gilmore and Timothy Burg

CONTENTS

2.1 Introduction 9
    2.1.1 Rapid Prototyping..9
    2.1.2 Fabrication Approaches 11
        2.1.2.1 Bulk Fabrication.. 11
        2.1.2.2 Single Layers Combination 12
        2.1.2.3 Layer-by-Layer Fabrication.. 14
    2.1.3 Fabrication Quality 15
2.2 3D Biofabrication... 16
    2.2.1 Biofabrication 16
    2.2.2 Design Considerations 17
        2.2.2.1 Self-Assembly 17
        2.2.2.2 Tissue Geometry... 18
        2.2.2.3 Permeability.. 19
        2.2.2.4 Promotion of Vascularity 19
        2.2.2.5 Mechanical Properties 19
        2.2.2.6 Substrate Biocompatibility...20
        2.2.2.7 Surface Modification..20
2.3 Technology Example 1: Single Layers Combination Using Woven Textiles 20
    2.3.1 Weaving 20
    2.3.2 Woven 3D Structures 23
    2.3.3 Challenges to Weaving 24
2.4 Technology Example 2: Layer-by-Layer Fabrication with Bioprinting 25
2.5 Conclusion and Perspective 27
References...28

2.1 INTRODUCTION

2.1.1 RAPID PROTOTYPING

Rapid prototyping (RP) fabrication (additive manufacturing) is the process of converting a computer model (think of this as an image created using computer software) into a three-dimensional (3D) physical object. We do this whenever we use a laser printer to transform an image from the computer onto a piece of paper. As shown in Figure 2.1 (top), the computerized version is sent to a laser printer where a colored polymer is selectively deposited onto the paper to create a physical representation (i.e., "hard copy"). When magnified, the side view of the print (right) shows a very thin layer of the polymer that forms the image. In this two-dimensional (2D)

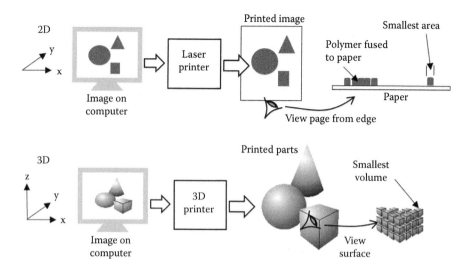

FIGURE 2.1 Office laser printers place a thin layer of polymer onto a piece of paper (a substrate) to produce a 2D image. Three-dimensional fabrication is visualized as stacking layers of small elements, for example, melted polymer drops, to produce a solid object.

process, the image spans the height and width of the paper with minimal thickness. Stacking layers of a 2D process allows the generation of 3D objects. As an example of a RP process (Figure 2.1, bottom), elements such as drops of melted polymer can be arranged to generate 3D objects such as a ball, cube, or cone.

The goal of RP fabrication is to build structures that meet certain small-scale requirements, such as material type or porosity, and large-scale requirements, such as features and dimensions. A successful fabrication approach will simultaneously fulfill both sets of requirements as illustrated in Figure 2.2. There are two possible approaches to generating the material structure: either deposit materials with the

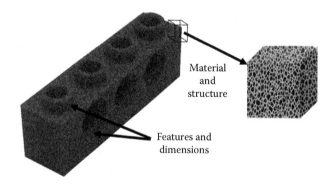

FIGURE 2.2 A fabricated part has large-scale features such as shape, length, and width and features such as holes. On the small scale, a fabricated part also has material properties such as type of material and porosity.

Biofabrication

desired intrinsic small-scale structure or use a deposition process that can directly build the small-scale structure. For example, the structure in Figure 2.2 could be generated by molding a foam material, or using a procedure that directly creates the walls of the foam-like structure. In parallel, the fabrication process must simultaneously generate structural features such as channels and overall size and shape. Note that the surface may comprise large-scale features such as undulating ridges, structure properties such as open cell porosity, and material properties such as surface chemistries.

2.1.2 Fabrication Approaches

Several design parameters are important to most substrates or tissue engineering scaffolds. Biofabricated scaffolds should (i) be three-dimensional and highly porous with an interconnected pore network for cell growth and flow transport of nutrients and metabolic waste; (ii) be biocompatible and bioabsorbable with a predictable degradation and absorption rate to match cell/tissue growth; (iii) have suitable surface chemistry for cell attachment, proliferation, and differentiation, and (iv) have mechanical properties to match those of the target tissue being modeled (Hutmacher 2000). Three-dimensional structures can be fabricated in a number of different ways as illustrated in Figure 2.3. An approach can be classified as bulk, single layers combination, or layer-by-layer according to the size and placement of the fabrication elements.

2.1.2.1 Bulk Fabrication

Bulk fabrication describes the family of processes that form objects in a single step, for example, a melted polymer cast into a mold (Figure 2.3, top). In such a fabrication approach, the structure and features of the object are defined by the parameters of the fabrication (i.e., casting, annealing, or heating). Small subvolumes within the part can vary as a result of the manufacturing process, for example, different subvolumes may have different porosity, or the surface may be affected by the interaction

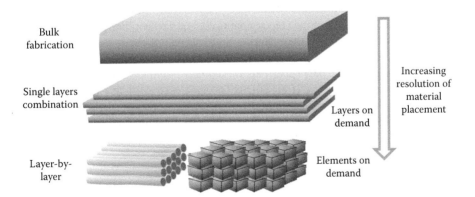

FIGURE 2.3 A 3D structure could be fabricated from a single process, assembled as a series of layers, or formed by placing discrete elements. Subvolumes within the final structure are affected, and can be manipulated, by the fabrication approach.

with the mold. Bulk fabrication is the approach that allows the least flexibility and control of subvolumes within the object; generally, this is considered the antithesis of RP fabrication. However, by manipulating variables such as the use/nonuse of solvents, heat, pressure, and pore-creating additives, researchers have been able to develop increasingly complex 3D structures for use as tissue scaffolds (Burg and Thomas 2006; Thavornyutikarn et al. 2014).

2.1.2.2 Single Layers Combination

The single layers combination (SLC) methods depicted in Figure 2.3 (middle) are based on stacking of thin, preassembled layers. The primary objective of SLC designed scaffolds is to combine individually fabricated layers of biocompatible material in ways that capitalize on both 2D and 3D characteristics. A number of recent developments in the area of biofabricated substrates have involved combining or configuring single layers of fabricated constructs to create complex 3D geometries (Hsu et al. 2012; Kang et al. 2012; Park et al. 2014). Researchers have worked to build SLC technologies that promote tissue generation within individual layers, but are greatly improved or provide some complementary function through addition of subsequent layers. The layers could be as simple as a homogeneous polymer sheet (resulting from a bulk process such as casting or extrusion) or could be a complex subassembly that is itself the output of a rapid fabrication process, for example, a layer of biomaterials and patterned cells. In the simplest form, all the layers are identical and homogenous; that is, all the elements are the same, and the only difference from the bulk approach is at the interface of the laminations. However, the SLC approach allows the possibility that each layer could be composed differently. An SLC approach increases the flexibility, beyond the bulk approach, to control structure and material types as each layer can be built from different materials, with different fabrication processes and have different geometry or patterning.

SLCs composed of paper-based layers have been proposed as the future of fabricated tissue scaffolds (Park et al. 2014). The primary advantages of these designs are the ability to create complexly shaped single layers, ease of stacking or other combination methods, favorable biocompatibility and surface characteristics, as well as the relatively low cost of the material. Single layers of paper were first targeted because they are inexpensive and easily altered by size and shape (Lee et al. 2008). Cell attachment to these paper scaffolds was demonstrated for a variety of cell types (Petersen et al. 2015; Wang et al. 2015). The long history of the manipulation of paper through art forms, such as origami, allowed researchers to quickly create complex structures (Kim et al. 2015). As an example application, stacking of single layers of paper was the proposed solution to generate 3D models for cell interactions during heart ischemia (Mosadegh et al. 2014).

In addition to paper fibers, the use of polymer fibers in the formation of layers for use in SLC scaffolds has also been explored (Chen et al. 2015). Electrospinning is one way to incorporate fibers. Electrospinning is the process by which polymer fibers are formed when the electric field applied at the surface of a polymer solution generates forces large enough to overcome the surface tension of the solution. The result is an electrically charged polymer stream, which solidifies into nanofibers as it is ejected (Reneker and Chun 1996). Modulation of electrospinning parameters through alternating electrical forces allows for variations in the shapes and constructs formed (Matthews et al. 2002). Once collected onto a surface or rotating mandrel, these fibers form a fiber mat. These fiber mats can be characterized as nonwoven scaffolds. One advantage of nonwoven scaffolds is the ability to combine complementary components (Liang et al. 2007). Indeed, electrospinning can be used to mesh polymers with various length degradation times, mechanical stiffness, or hydrophobicity and polymers that may improve overall scaffold properties (Agarwal et al. 2008; Bolgen et al. 2005; Kim et al. 2003). Additionally, when used in SLCs, individual layers can be alternated with fibers of different geometries or material types to generate complementary structures. Electrospinning results in a single layer of nonwoven nanoscale fibers in a random orientation that generates a pore structure of varying size and shape (Figure 2.4) favorable to cell attachment and growth (Lowery et al. 2010). Multiple single layers of electrospun nonwoven mesh could be combined through stacking, rolling, folding, sintering, or a variety of other methods (Pham et al. 2006; Xie et al. 2010). The result would be a complex 3D network of multiscale pores through nanoscale fibers.

The effects of a highly regulated fiber-based system with predictable pore sizes and porosities have also been explored. Using textile technology, standard textile weaving machineries (i.e., looms) have been modified to produce woven fiber-based tissue scaffolds. These small-scale looms allow for the design of textile scaffolds (i.e., meshes, fabrics, knits) for specific applications (Moutos et al. 2007; Moutos and Guilak 2010). Specificity is reached by altering a number of weaving parameters and material properties, including weft spacing, warp spacing, size of warp shed, fiber diameter, fiber compliance, and fiber strength (Gilmore et al. 2016). The resulting

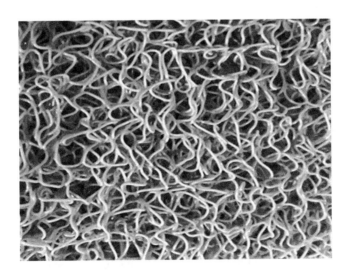

FIGURE 2.4 In a nonwoven mesh, the fibers are randomly oriented.

network of orthogonally or otherwise arranged fibers forms a regular pore structure that is the basis for a 3D microenvironment for cell growth (Wu et al. 2016). The pore size and porosity created through weave configuration designs could then be complemented through stacking, rolling, or otherwise adding successive layers to build a macroscale structure. These SLCs create a system for quickly iterated design and control of wide-ranging scaffold parameters on both the macro- and microscales.

2.1.2.3 Layer-by-Layer Fabrication

Layer-by-layer fabrication (bottom row of Figure 2.3) is one of the most versatile methods of scaffold development. In RP or solid free-form fabrication (SFF), a small element of material can be placed at specific locations to build the structure one element at a time. 3D objects are built using a layering technique in which a computer-aided design (CAD) system generates a series of cross-sections. Each cross-sectional layer of the scaffold is deposited onto the previous layer resulting in the completed design (Agrawal and Ray 2001; Liu and Ma 2004). The advantage of RP systems is the potential for fine control of the microstructure and macrostructure of the scaffold.

The umbrella of RP includes several specific technologies such as fused deposition modeling (FDM), selective laser sintering (SLS), and 3D printing (3DP) (Karande et al. 2004). FDM uses a moving nozzle to extrude a polymer bead in a horizontal pattern specified in the CAD file. Once that layer is complete, the platform is lowered so that the next layer can be deposited (Cao et al. 2003). In the simplest approach, in one layer, the material extruded is homogenous. However, the composition of the material extruded can be varied, leading to a more complex pattern. Further, smaller elements, for example, melted polymer droplets, as the building blocks can be used to increase pattern detail. SLS builds scaffolds by employing an infrared laser to selectively raise the local temperature between two powders (Rimell and Marquis 2000). The laser provides enough energy to raise the powder to its glass transition temperature where the particles can then fuse to each other and to adjacent layers (Yang et al. 2002). Three-dimensional printing is a method that prints a binder onto the surface of a ceramic, polymer, or composite powder surface (Curodeau et al. 2000; Giordano et al. 1996; Sachs et al. 1998). Dissolved by the binder, particles of the powder surface fuse together (Sachlos and Czernuszka 2003). Three-dimensional printing is currently limited by the resolution capability of the system, which is dependent on the size of the binder jet, making the design of small microstructures difficult (Yang et al. 2002).

Currently, deposition systems and material limitations make acheiving high resolution with SFF difficult (Yang et al. 2002). The means of depositing elements distinguishes deposition processes. In an on-demand process, single elements can be deposited (Figure 2.5, left) at any location. Thermal inkjet printing, used in many home/office color printers, is an on-demand process where a colored droplet of ink can be deposited at any location of the paper. This process contrasts with a continuous process, that is, one that cannot be stopped and started accurately. A pressurized spray from a nozzle could produce a continuous stream of droplets similar in size to the inkjet process; however, starting and stopping the spray stream remain difficult. Such a spray would be considered a continuous process.

Biofabrication

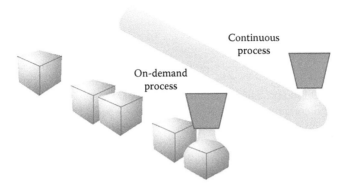

FIGURE 2.5 An on-demand process produces an element in any location, whereas a continuous process starts and stops at a larger time/distance scale.

2.1.3 Fabrication Quality

The quality of the output of a fabrication process is measured by the resolution and fabrication error. The resolution describes how well we expect to be able to control the fabrication process, the position, and element size (area in 2D and volume in 3D) as illustrated in Figure 2.6. The two sources of error in the fabrication process, formation and placement, dictate how well the output matches the expectations. First, the resolution is defined as a combination of the size of the smallest building block and how well that element can be placed when forming an object. For example, in a black-only 2D laser printer, a 300 dpi (dots per inch) resolution implies that the machine can place an element of sufficient size, with sufficient placement accuracy such that any 0.1 mm × 0.1 mm blank area on the page can be completely filled with black polymer. The resolution of 3D fabrication approaches includes the size of the elements. The resolution of a single layers combination fabrication process is limited by the thickness of the layers. The resolution of an extrusion includes the cross-section of the extrusion, the placement accuracy of each extrusion, and the degree to which the extrudant can be varied during deposition. The resolution of a droplet system includes the volume of drops. Second, the fabrication error encompasses how closely an element is placed in a pattern relative to a desired location and how closely the deposited element matches the expected element size and shape.

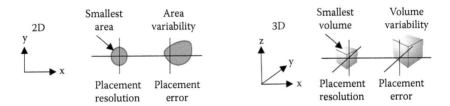

FIGURE 2.6 Expectations and errors in 2D (left) and 3D (right) fabrication processes. The 2D and 3D graphics define expectations including element size, shape, and location, and errors in location and size.

2.2 3D BIOFABRICATION

2.2.1 Biofabrication

The term "biofabrication" defines processes in which *biological* tissues are assembled using rapid prototyping *fabrication* techniques. Similar to 3D fabrication, rapid-prototyping 3D biofabrication uses materials that are assembled in small elements, layers, or solid components, including cellular components to build a tissue. Three fabrication approaches combine cellular components and biomaterials to generate a tissue structure (Figure 2.7). The traditional tissue engineering approach where a single scaffold, such as an open-cell foam, is seeded with cells to form a tissue (Figure 2.7, top) contrasts with the more complex biofabrication approaches (Figure 2.7, middle and bottom).

A *tissue voxel* represents a block of tissue substructure that may be repeated to build a larger structure. Though an abstraction, the voxel helps organize our thoughts about producing the local electrical, chemical, mechanical, and thermal environments that together form the structure and function of the tissue (Figure 2.8). Small tissue blocks could be repeated to build a skin patch. Various fabrication techniques are distinguished by the resolution that can be achieved with the tissue voxels comprising the resulting tissue structures. Three-dimensional biofabrication is an especially powerful technique to generate heterogeneous tissue. Indeed, while a bulk approach using a homogeneous material and structure is suitable to generate a mostly homogeneous tissue structure, a layer-by-layer method most appropriately will provide heterogeneous elements such as lesions within the skin tissue.

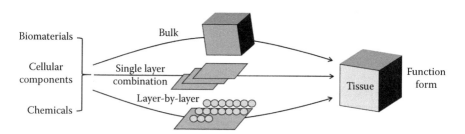

FIGURE 2.7 Three-dimensional biofabrication incorporates cellular components into a 3D fabrication process to produce a tissue of an appropriate form and function.

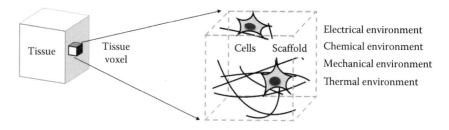

FIGURE 2.8 The smallest block of tissue (tissue voxel) repeated within the tissue.

Biofabrication

A 3D biofabrication method must generate tissue with the desired functions, dimensions, and properties so that the constructs can be employed as tissue test systems, or models for biomedical or scientific investigation.

2.2.2 Design Considerations

Biofabrication must accommodate many tissue constraints and requirements. In tissue engineering, biomaterial scaffolds are the foundation for the biological components that constitute a 3D tissue structure. The 3D scaffold provides biologically relevant support and cues to the developing tissue. Parameters favorable to 3D tissue systems include macro- and microscale geometry, mechanical properties, biocompatibility, promotion of vascularization, compatible surface features, support of cell proliferation and differentiation, promote the cell/tissue sustainment, and appropriate/normal tissue functions. Design considerations are highly linked to the method of 3D fabrication; therefore, the use of various 3D fabrication techniques along with material with different characteristics should be chosen to meet specific design considerations based on tissue requirements. Indeed, various 3D fabrication techniques lead to variable pore size, porosity, mechanical properties, and pore interconnectivity.

2.2.2.1 Self-Assembly

A functional 3D tissue model requires that cellular components be appropriately arranged. For example, 3D modeling of tumor angiogenesis requires that tumor cells interact with endothelial cells within an appropriate environment leading to angiogenesis. Regardless of the fabrication method, the cellular components need to connect and assemble into a tissue (Jakab et al. 2010). Cells (and potentially materials) autonomously organize into a biologically relevant pattern through self-assembly. The 3D fabrication considerations associated with self-assembly (Figure 2.9) include the initial cell density. Although debated, it seems logical that less self-assembly would be needed when the cells are initially placed closer to the final configuration. The review by Jakab and coworkers (Jakab et al. 2010) suggests that assemblies such as spheroids, already containing biologically oriented cells, could be used as building blocks that then serve to accelerate the self-assembly into a tissue. Thus, as

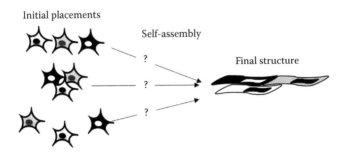

FIGURE 2.9 Self-assembly describes the degree to which cells must autonomously organize from an initial placement into the final structure.

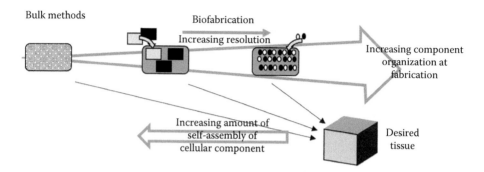

FIGURE 2.10 The resolution of the 3D biofabrication method defines the amount of cell self-assembly required.

different 3D fabrication methods can place cells with different accuracies, the self-assembly required distinguishes the fabrication methods.

As the resolution of the 3D printing process is increased, the closeness of the cell location to their location in the final tissue increases; thus, the self-assembly required is potentially reduced as the fabrication resolution is increased and cells are placed closer to their final position in the tissue. Thus, the resolution of the 3D biofabrication approach must be chosen to match the ability of the components to appropriately self-assemble as illustrated in Figure 2.10.

2.2.2.2 Tissue Geometry

Size and shape are the key tissue design parameters. Geometry also contributes to important characteristics such as mechanical properties or vascular in-growth (Chen et al. 1997). The generation of an interconnected macroporous structure yields volumes (e.g., triangles, hexagons, and pentagons), which equally distribute mechanical forces throughout the scaffold, that is, *tensegrity* (Chen et al. 1997; Ingber 1997). The porous structure and 3D design also contribute to the diffusion of nutrients into the scaffold, but the tissue geometry alone is not enough to independently promote cell viability in large scaffolds (Karande et al. 2004).

Porosity, the ratio of open pore volume to scaffold material volume (Karande et al. 2004), has been used as an indicator of mass transport ability, the ease with which cells access environmental factors such as oxygen, for tissue engineering scaffolds. Porosity could be as high as 90% to ensure the cell–material interaction (Yoon and Park 2001), while, when the primary focus is mechanical strength, porosities can be near 30% (Borden et al. 2003). Further, the tissue geometry is usually not uniform throughout a particular volume. Therefore, gradients of porosity that offer regions of varying mechanical strength, vascular, and tissue density have been investigated (Novak et al. 2016).

Specific cell types may react differently to the same pore size, thus pore size is also critically important (Burg et al. 2000). Furthermore, pore size also affects the amount of cell/tissue growth in a 3D construct. However, as mentioned earlier, pore size should vary throughout a scaffold. Both macro (>100 μm) and micro (<20 μm) pore structures are essential to the development of a tissue as illustrated in Figure 2.2

(Bose, Roy, and Bandyopadhyay 2012; Woodard et al. 2007). Macro-sized pores contribute to 3D tissue generation by facilitating cell and ion transport (Bignon et al. 2003), whereas micro-sized pores increase the surface area for protein adsorption and subsequent cell attachment (Hing et al. 2005).

2.2.2.3 Permeability

Permeability is a measure of the degree to which fluid flows through a structure and is related to fluid–biomaterial and fluid–cell interaction (Agrawal and Ray 2001). Along with porosity, permeability constrains tissue viability. Both porosity and permeability affect nutrient/waste transport, biomechanical cellular response, and material degradation. These two parameters are related through the degree of pore interconnectedness in a tissue (van Tienen et al. 2002). Indeed, two biofabricated tissues may have the same void space, but their measures of permeability may be different due to varying levels of pore interconnectivity and tortuosity (Karande et al. 2004). Passageways for nutrients and wastes for the seeded cells within 3D tissues are critical to the tissue viability. In a living tissue, vasculature supplies this function, directing both diffusive and convective transport. Currently, modeling a transport system capable of mimicking blood flow has proved to be difficult, with the most viable solutions being cumbersome and unstable leading to tissue death or uncharacteristic tissue behaviors (Karande et al. 2004).

2.2.2.4 Promotion of Vascularity

Optimal 3D engineered tissues should promote vascular in-growth for implanted constructs. Similarly, in 3D tissue test systems, the function of vasculature is highly clinically relevant and thus should be taken into account. Although an interconnected macroporous structure ranging from 200 to 500 µm may improve diffusion rates throughout the tissue, simple transport of nutrients and by-products is not sufficient for large biofabricated tissues (Hutmacher 2000). In the body, the distance between mesenchymal stem cells (MSC) and blood vessels is less than 100 µm. Because of this short distance, modeling nutrient/waste transport may be compromised without specific design consideration for vascularity. Embedding angiogenic factors into scaffold materials with the goal of controlling the rate and degree of vascularization in the tissue is one option. For example, vascular endothelial growth factor (VEGF) has been used to induce a vascular network in engineered tissues (Rouwkema et al. 2008).

2.2.2.5 Mechanical Properties

The mechanical properties of a tissue-engineered construct play a significant role in the effectiveness of a tissue-engineered design (Burg et al. 2000; Hutmacher 2000; Ingber 1997; Langer and Vacanti 1993; Vacanti 2006). The primary concern is that the scaffold accommodates the mechanical requirements of the tissue until the tissue itself can assume its proper functional role (Hutmacher 2000). Therefore, the 3D biofabricated tissue must at least be able to withstand the mechanical strength requirements of the modeled tissue until the cells, vasculature, and other tissue components have developed enough to retain the normal physiological function. Furthermore, dynamic mechanical loading may contribute to cell differentiation and the determination of cell phenotype (Burg et al. 2000; Ingber 1997). In 3D tissue test systems, mechanical properties and flow dynamics are a means to achieving the desired cell type or phenotypic expression of harvested MSCs.

2.2.2.6 Substrate Biocompatibility

As with any medical device coming in direct contact with the biological components such as cells, biocompatibility is also a major focus for biofabricated tissue substrates. The general challenge is that more reactive foreign material present may yield a larger impact on the cellular components. Indeed, with nonbiological substrate material (i.e., foreign material), the more contact there is with the biological components, the less favorable the 3D tissue outcome. On that basis, highly porous implants with large amounts of void space would be optimal (Yoon and Park 2001). However, mechanical strength must also be taken into account. Thus, the need for reactive material minimization and that for adequate mechanical strength should be balanced. This balance is application specific and the development of a standard ratio is difficult (Rose and Oreffo 2002). In that regard, the biocompatibility of several scaffold/substrate materials has been investigated. Upon the degradation of 3D scaffolds, the by-products may be basic or acidic leading to changes in local pH, thus promoting cell death and eventually, tissue degeneration (Vacanti 2006). This is especially true with bulk degrading materials (materials that do not degrade layer by layer from outside inward) that may exhibit a burst release of acidic by-product at a critical value (Burg et al. 2000). To better understand local pH variations, release profiles and degradation by-products have been investigated (Dee et al. 2003).

2.2.2.7 Surface Modification

Cell–biomaterial interactions are key variables in cell attachment, proliferation, and differentiation. Three-dimensional biofabricated substrates should include surface roughness and chemistries that are conducive to cell growth and development. Improvements of these interactions at the surface can be achieved by manipulating surface chemistry and topography (Liu et al. 2007). While both natural and synthetic materials have been used in engineering applications, synthetic materials lack biological recognition. Indeed, hydrophobic materials, specifically polymers, are not readily integrated due to incompatibility with the hydrophilic outer region of the phospholipid bilayer component of the cell membrane (Stevens and George 2005). Engineering the hydrophobicity/hydrophilicity of the material surface has been attempted to change cell interactions on the micro level. Further, improved hydrophilic surfaces have been successfully generated with an increasingly negative charge to accommodate the relative positive charge of the extracellular surface of the plasma membrane (Wei and Ma 2004).

2.3 TECHNOLOGY EXAMPLE 1: SINGLE LAYERS COMBINATION USING WOVEN TEXTILES

2.3.1 Weaving

While the modern meaning of the term "loom" began in the mid-1800s, the concept of using a machine to intersect longitudinal warp fibers with transverse weft

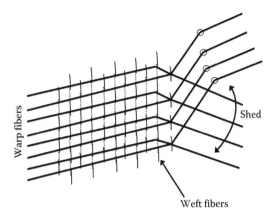

FIGURE 2.11 Basic weaving process schematic depicting weft fibers passing through the shed of the warp fibers. The friction at each interface of warp and weft fibers maintains the structure.

threads (Figure 2.11), or weaving, has been implemented since around 100 AD (Usher 2013). Customized looms (bio-looms) using this technology to generate new woven scaffolds for tissue engineering applications have been developed. They address the specific handling and features of the biologically focused threads and requirements on the resulting scaffolds. These looms are based on textile weaving technology such as shedding, picking, and battening, but have been designed to accommodate the special material qualifications for biologically relevant materials, for example, heat or moisture sensitivity and high cost per thread (Gilmore et al. 2016). Many current bio-looms are based on a dobby loom design in which a set of warp fibers is controlled to create a shed through which the weft fibers are inserted by a variety of methods, including air jets, water jets, and rapier systems (Collier 1970). Variations in the movement of the warp fibers relative to the weft fibers can be used to control weave properties, such as the shape of scaffold pores and strength of the scaffold, and may affect cell or protein attachment in some applications (Burg et al. 2000).

Woven substrates offer the opportunity to modulate scaffold parameters using the weft–warp structure. Some of the degrees of freedom within weave design (Figure 2.12) are the material type, weave configuration, fiber size, fiber geometry, and/or scaffold spacing of warp and/or weft fibers. This flexibility facilitates the customization of mechanical properties, fluid transport properties, cell behavior, and biocompatibility of the substrate.

The configuration or pattern with which a woven textile is fabricated plays a large role in the 2D layers and 3D structure of the scaffold. There are a number of traditional weave configurations that have been employed in biomedical applications (Figure 2.13). These configurations along with more specialized configurations have been studied due to their influence on pore size, pore shape, and the mechanical strength of the scaffold (Moutos et al. 2016; Younesi et al. 2014). Modifying weave configurations to affect pore size and pore shape can be used to modulate the characteristics of each layer in a single layers combination (SLC). On this lower level of

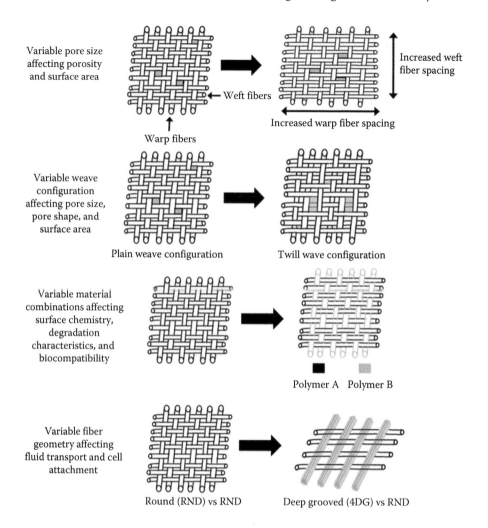

FIGURE 2.12 Potential bio-loom design degrees of freedom with woven scaffolds.

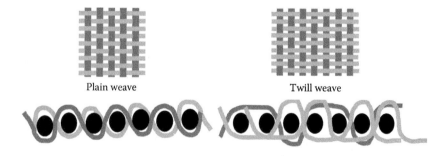

FIGURE 2.13 Comparison of standard and twill weave.

Biofabrication

structure, these properties can be engineered to affect cell behavior and small-scale transport. Given the surface characteristics or cross-sectional geometry of the fibers used, changing weave configuration can have a significant impact on cell attachment and proliferation.

Weave configuration can then be used to alter the large-scale 3D structure of a scaffold. In this case, properties such as the overall compliance of the material (important in clinical applications), the overall permeability of the construct, and its ability to interface with added layers are all affected. Intricate multiscale pore networks and shapes can be generated to add specific function to the overall construct.

2.3.2 Woven 3D Structures

3D biofabricated woven scaffolds may result in favorable tissue growth outcomes. For example, stacking 2D woven scaffolds to form 3D constructs of variable thickness in an *in vitro* culture environment may provide information regarding the effects of the 3D pore geometry with implications for nutrient/waste transport and cell attachment. Rolled scaffolds (Figure 2.14) provide an alternate means of generating 3D structures from 2D woven textiles. The ability to design modular models for specific biological conditions is the keystone to the woven scaffold approach.

In an SLC construction, a number of plain-woven scaffolds could be stacked on top of one another, either directly aligning or offsetting the adjacent scaffold by a predetermined angle. The result would be a scaffold with particular transport

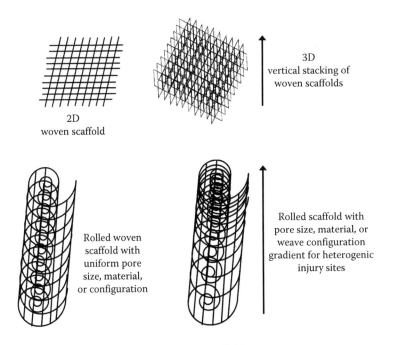

FIGURE 2.14 Potential applications of woven scaffolds.

properties based on weave configuration and proximity of warp and weft fibers. The same SLC would also have micro- and macroscale channels based on the orientation of the stacking.

Similarly, woven scaffolds can be rolled and/or folded to provide for the flexible accommodation of difficult applications. This rolling or folding also creates an additional dimension upon which more complex geometries can be achieved. A particularly interesting application is the development of a single-layer woven scaffold with a gradient of porosity or pore size. When folded or rolled, this 2D construct instantly gains a large network of interconnected pores, greatly multiplying scaffold transport properties. The gradient of the initial weave configuration design is also magnified by being placed in close proximity with regions of similar properties. The ability to create specific zones characterized by separate properties is a significant goal of biofabricated scaffold development.

2.3.3 Challenges to Weaving

Fibers created for the purpose of weaving scaffolds are generally formed through processes that enact a set of material characteristics on the resulting fiber. A typical extrusion and a drawing process are shown in Figure 2.15. Using heat or pressure to generate fibers can lead to residual effects on fiber compliance and strength. Electrical- and chemical-based processes may lead to altered surface electrostatic properties (Deitzel et al. 2001), sometimes rendering weaving difficult or impossible.

Compliance of the fibers plays a key role in the ability to successfully weave polymer fibers. Compliance relates to the flexibility or rigidity of a fiber and its tendency to maintain a particular shape when under a mechanical load. Fibers with a low degree of compliance generally resist deformation under an applied load. This can become problematic during the weave process, particularly during the shuttling step where the weft fiber is passed through the warp shed. In this case, fibers that are highly compliant can be straightened by the shuttling mechanism, where as

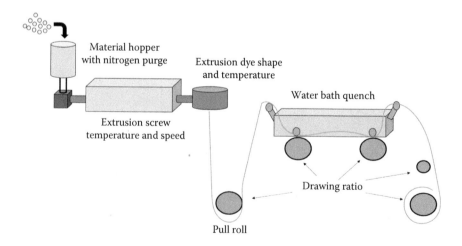

FIGURE 2.15 Illustration of typical extrusion and drawing process to improve strength.

Biofabrication

noncompliant fibers maintain the helical shape developed from being stored on a cylindrical spool. The resulting spiraling fibers do not cleanly pass through the warp shed, leading to missed picks by the loom. Compliance can also affect warp fibers in a similar fashion. Spiraling fibers that resist the tensile force applied to straighten them obstruct the warp shed, making shuttling difficult.

Fiber strength also must be optimized for weaving. The tensile strength of the warp fibers is of importance due to the constant strain placed on the fibers during the shedding and beating processes. These fibers must be able to maintain a constant level of tension under load to generate a clear warp shed.

The material type and fabrication method equally contribute to biocompatibility. The polymer selected for fiber production must first be compatible with the final application. Polymer degradation by-products must also be nontoxic and eliminated without disturbing the cell environment. Additionally, fiber size and configuration relate to the foreign body response (FBR) seen by the biofabricated scaffold. As the amount of fiber material implanted is increased, the FBR also increases (Saino et al. 2011).

Polymer fibers, particularly those manufactured by heat processing, are susceptible to oxidative degradation. Heat catalyzes this process, making necessary the use of a nitrogen-purging system during fiber manufacturing. In ambient temperatures, increased exposure of polymer fibers to air results in the breakdown of short polymer chains, weakening the overall structure of each fiber. This degradation leads to increasingly brittle fibers that are more difficult to weave. Fiber degradation can be limited by reducing materials exposure to air for long periods (>72 h).

As commonly fiber fabrication and weaving processes occur in nonsterile environments, post-sterilization of the scaffold is required. Scaffold sterilization can be achieved by exposure of scaffolds to ultraviolet light radiation for 15–30 min, ethylene-oxide gas sterilization, or cleaning in ethyl alcohol and buffer solutions.

2.4 TECHNOLOGY EXAMPLE 2: LAYER-BY-LAYER FABRICATION WITH BIOPRINTING

Bioprinting describes the adaptation of digital printing techniques, that is, processes used to print from a computer onto a piece of paper, to the problem of depositing cells and biomaterials onto a substrate. Bioprinting is a promising technique for creating layers in a 3D structure and supports a layer-by-layer fabrication process. The "bio" prefix indicates the hardware and software accommodations required to print living cells or special biomaterials, for example, replacing the ink, a dye solution, with a bio-ink, a mixture of cells and supporting media. There are two approaches to printing that have been demonstrated in bioprinting: continuous stream printers and drop-on-demand printers (Gudapati et al. 2016). The generic bioprinting process (Figure 2.16, left) identifies the two major challenges in the bioprinting process: forming consistent, appropriately sized droplets and formulating the mixture of materials and biological components that support a specific droplet formation process (Burg et al. 2010).

The three primary commercial technologies (Figure 2.16, right) developed for drop formation in printing applications have been used in bioprinting. The continuous jet

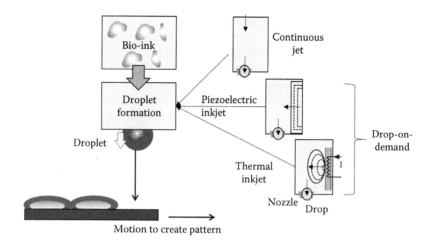

FIGURE 2.16 General components in a droplet deposition system are the bio-ink, a system to move the sample or drop depositor (or deflect the droplet stream), and the mechanism for forming droplets (left). The dashed lines represent the change in size of the piezo-material or the vapor bubble during droplet formation.

is a process where a pump pressurizes a vessel and droplets are created at a constant rate through a nozzle. The nozzle and the pressure system are designed to create a continuous stream of identical droplets. The nozzle or substrate can be moved to create a pattern, or the stream can be deflected with an electrostatic force as the means of creating a pattern. The advantage of the continuous jet system is that it can be used to quickly deposit a large amount of material. Since the stream is typically slow to start and stop, it is difficult to execute a pattern by just moving the stream alone; that is, the stream must be directed into a waste collection area during part of the printing. Both the piezoelectric inkjet and the thermal inkjet are drop-on-demand printers in that they both create and eject a single droplet from a control command. In the piezoelectric inkjet, a special material that changes shape or size when a voltage is applied acts to create pressure that ejects a single drop from the nozzle (Derby 2012); that is, a small, temporary displacement is used to extrude a single drop through the nozzle. The thermal inkjet works in a similar fashion, except that the displacement is generated by heating a small area to form a vapor bubble. The growing vapor bubble displacement is used to extrude a single drop through the nozzle. In both cases, the displacement is quickly removed after the drop is released so that the process can be repeated and the next drop can be printed. The pattern is formed by either moving the nozzle or the substrate below the nozzle; many printers move both the substrate (paper feed into the printer) and the nozzle (motion of the ink cartridge).

A significant advantage of inkjet printers is that they are inexpensive and widely available. One potential disadvantage of the drop-on-demand inkjet printers is the speed at which the process can be repeated to produce drops (compared to the continuous jet). A potential disadvantage of the thermal inkjet printers is the temperature effects on the bio-ink. The lineage of thermal inkjet printing of cells can be traced to the patent of Boland [US Patent # 7,051,654, 2003] where printing was done using

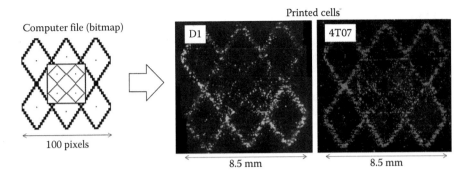

FIGURE 2.17 Two-dimensional printing of D1 murine MSCs (green fluorescent protein [GFP]) and 4T07 murine mammary tumor cells (red fluorescent protein [GFP]) in co-culture.

the proprietary drivers and embedded software of the Hewlett-Packard (Hewlett-Packard, Palo Alto, CA) HP 550 DeskJet family of inkjet printers (Burg and Boland 2003). This printing method has been shown to provide biological results where cells that are printed via the thermal ink jet process have been shown to retain 90% viability, or that the cells remain metabolically active (Xu et al. 2005). Therefore, the process has the potential to print patterns of cells and have them survive the process and proliferate. This is in part because the thermal process used to print the cells only raised the temperature of the surrounding liquid by 4°C (Xu et al. 2005). Different solutions have been used with the HP26 series cartridges as "bio-ink" (Parzel et al. 2009). A number of bio-inks have been demonstrated with this system, including water, serum-free cell media, ethanol, collagen, calcium chloride, laminin, alginate, and fibrin. However, the range in bio-ink density and viscosity is very limited (close to water); it cannot be changed far beyond the original ink. A sample output from an HP550-based printing system described by Pepper and coworkers (Pepper et al. 2009) is shown in Figure 2.17.

2.5 CONCLUSION AND PERSPECTIVE

Biofabrication will greatly benefit from the exponential growth in rapid prototyping fabrication techniques and machinery. Nearly every industry, from aircraft engines to consumer products, will see a huge benefit to quality, flexibility, and customization as rapid prototyping is integrated into development and production. The widespread use of these technologies will reduce costs and increase performance. The confluence of evolving fabrication tools with new biomaterials presents almost unlimited opportunities to build custom tissue structures. The ongoing challenge is to match the biomaterials to the right fabrication technology, so that biomaterials are not damaged by fabrication processes. Although fabrication tools are rapidly evolving, the trajectory of technologies that can deposit cellular components is more difficult to assess. Indeed, to date, few show promise for manipulating the cells directly. Importantly, to make best use of any given biofabrication tool, the biological potential and limitations of self-assembly must be fully characterized.

REFERENCES

Agrawal, C. M. and R. B. Ray. 2001. Biodegradable polymeric scaffolds for musculoskeletal tissue engineering. *J Biomed Mater Res* no. 55 (2):141–50.

Agarwal, S., J. H. Wendorff, and A. Greiner. 2008. Use of electrospinning technique for biomedical applications. *Polymer* no. 49 (26):5603–21.

Bignon, A., J. Chouteau, J. Chevalier, G. Fantozzi, J. P. Carret, P. Chavassieux, G. Boivin, M. Melin, and D. Hartmann. 2003. Effect of micro- and macroporosity of bone substitutes on their mechanical properties and cellular response. *J Mater Sci Mater Med* no. 14 (12):1089–97.

Bolgen, N., Y. Z. Menceloglu, K. Acatay, I. Vargel, and E. Piskin. 2005. *In vitro* and *in vivo* degradation of non-woven materials made of poly(epsilon-caprolactone) nanofibers prepared by electrospinning under different conditions. *J Biomater Sci Polym Ed* no. 16 (12):1537–55.

Borden, M., S. F. El-Amin, M. Attawia, and C. T. Laurencin. 2003. Structural and human cellular assessment of a novel microsphere-based tissue engineered scaffold for bone repair. *Biomaterials* no. 24 (4):597–609.

Bose, S., M. Roy, and A. Bandyopadhyay. 2012. Recent advances in bone tissue engineering scaffolds. *Trends Biotechnol* no. 30 (10):546–54.

Burg, K. and C. Thomas. 2006. Tissue engineering. In *Wiley Encyclopedia of Biomedical Engineering* Metin Akay (Editor). John Wiley & Sons, Hoboken, NJ, pp. 3510–3511.

Burg, K. J. and T. Boland. 2003. Minimally invasive tissue engineering composites and cell printing. *IEEE Eng Med Biol Mag* no. 22 (5):84–91.

Burg, K. J., S. Porter, and J. F. Kellam. 2000. Biomaterial developments for bone tissue engineering. *Biomaterials* no. 21 (23):2347–59.

Burg, T., C. A. Cass, R. Groff, M. Pepper, and K. J. Burg. 2010. Building off-the-shelf tissue-engineered composites. *Philos Trans A: Math Phys Eng Sci* no. 368 (1917): 1839–62.

Cao, T., K. H. Ho, and S. H. Teoh. 2003. Scaffold design and *in vitro* study of osteochondral coculture in a three-dimensional porous polycaprolactone scaffold fabricated by fused deposition modeling. *Tissue Eng* no. 9 (Suppl 1):S103–12.

Chen, C. S., M. Mrksich, S. Huang, G. M. Whitesides, and D. E. Ingber. 1997. Geometric control of cell life and death. *Science* no. 276 (5317):1425–28.

Chen, G., J. Chen, B. Yang, L. Li, X. Luo, X. Zhang, L. Feng, Z. Jiang, M. Yu, W. Guo, and W. Tian. 2015. Combination of aligned PLGA/Gelatin electrospun sheets, native dental pulp extracellular matrix and treated dentin matrix as substrates for tooth root regeneration. *Biomaterials* no. 52:56–70.

Collier, A. M. 1970. *A Handbook of Textiles, the Commonwealth and International Library*. Elsevier Science & Technology, Amsterdam, The Netherlands.

Curodeau, A., E. Sachs, and S. Caldarise. 2000. Design and fabrication of cast orthopedic implants with freeform surface textures from 3-D printed ceramic shell. *J Biomed Mater Res* no. 53 (5):525–35.

Dee, K. C., D. A. Puleo, and R. Bizios. 2003. *An Introduction to Tissue-Biomaterial Interactions*. John Wiley & Sons, Hoboken, NJ.

Deitzel, J. M., J. Kleinmeyer, D. Harris, and N. C. Beck Tan. 2001. The effect of processing variables on the morphology of electrospun nanofibers and textiles. *Polymer* no. 42 (1):261–72.

Derby, B. 2012. Printing and prototyping of tissues and scaffolds. *Science* no. 338 (6109):921–26.

Gilmore, J., T. Burg, R. E. Groff, and K. J. Burg. 2016. Design and optimization of a novel bioloom to weave melt-spun absorbable polymers for bone tissue engineering. *J Biomed Mater Res B: Appl Biomater,* doi: 10.1002/jbm.b.33700

Giordano, R. A., B. M. Wu, S. W. Borland, L. G. Cima, E. M. Sachs, and M. J. Cima. 1996. Mechanical properties of dense polylactic acid structures fabricated by three dimensional printing. *J Biomater Sci Polym Ed* no. 8 (1):63–75.

Gudapati, H., M. Dey, and I. Ozbolat. 2016. A comprehensive review on droplet-based bioprinting: Past, present and future. *Biomaterials* no. 102:20–42.

Hing, K. A., B. Annaz, S. Saeed, P. A. Revell, and T. Buckland. 2005. Microporosity enhances bioactivity of synthetic bone graft substitutes. *J Mater Sci Mater Med* no. 16 (5):467–75.

Hsu, S. H., C. H. Lin, and C. S. Tseng. 2012. Air plasma treated chitosan fibers-stacked scaffolds. *Biofabrication* no. 4 (1):015002.

Hutmacher, D. W. 2000. Scaffolds in tissue engineering bone and cartilage. *Biomaterials* no. 21 (24):2529–43.

Ingber, D. E. 1997. Tensegrity: The architectural basis of cellular mechanotransduction. *Annu Rev Physiol* no. 59:575–99.

Jakab, K., C. Norotte, F. Marga, K. Murphy, G. Vunjak-Novakovic, and G. Forgacs. 2010. Tissue engineering by self-assembly and bio-printing of living cells. *Biofabrication* no. 2 (2):022001.

Kang, H. W., J. H. Park, T. Y. Kang, Y. J. Seol, and D. W. Cho. 2012. Unit cell-based computer-aided manufacturing system for tissue engineering. *Biofabrication* no. 4 (1):015005.

Karande, T. S., J. L. Ong, and C. M. Agrawal. 2004. Diffusion in musculoskeletal tissue engineering scaffolds: Design issues related to porosity, permeability, architecture, and nutrient mixing. *Ann Biomed Eng* no. 32 (12):1728–43.

Kim, K., M. Yu, X. Zong, J. Chiu, D. Fang, Y. S. Seo, B. S. Hsiao, B. Chu, and M. Hadjiargyrou. 2003. Control of degradation rate and hydrophilicity in electrospun nonwoven poly(D, L-lactide) nanofiber scaffolds for biomedical applications. *Biomaterials* no. 24 (27):4977–85.

Kim, S. H., H. R. Lee, S. J. Yu, M. E. Han, D. Y. Lee, S. Y. Kim, H. J. Ahn, M. J. Han, T. I. Lee, T. S. Kim, S. K. Kwon, S. G. Im, and N. S. Hwang. 2015. Hydrogel-laden paper scaffold system for origami-based tissue engineering. *Proc Natl Acad Sci USA* no. 112 (50):15426–31.

Langer, R. and J. P. Vacanti. 1993. Tissue engineering. *Science* no. 260 (5110):920–26.

Lee, J., M. J. Cuddihy, and N. A. Kotov. 2008. Three-dimensional cell culture matrices: State of the art. *Tissue Eng B: Rev* no. 14 (1):61–86.

Liang, D., B. S. Hsiao, and B. Chu. 2007. Functional electrospun nanofibrous scaffolds for biomedical applications. *Adv Drug Deliv Rev* no. 59 (14):1392–412.

Liu, C., Z. Xia, and J. T. Czernuszka. 2007. Design and development of three-dimensional scaffolds for tissue engineering. *Chem Eng Res Design* no. 85 (7):1051–64.

Liu, X. and P. X. Ma. 2004. Polymeric scaffolds for bone tissue engineering. *Ann Biomed Eng* no. 32 (3):477–86.

Lowery, J. L., N. Datta, and G. C. Rutledge. 2010. Effect of fiber diameter, pore size and seeding method on growth of human dermal fibroblasts in electrospun poly(epsilon-caprolactone) fibrous mats. *Biomaterials* no. 31 (3):491–504.

Matthews, J. A., G. E. Wnek, D. G. Simpson, and G. L. Bowlin. 2002. Electrospinning of collagen nanofibers. *Biomacromolecules* no. 3 (2):232–38.

Mosadegh, B., B. E. Dabiri, M. R. Lockett, R. Derda, P. Campbell, K. K. Parker, and G. M. Whitesides. 2014. Three-dimensional paper-based model for cardiac ischemia. *Adv Healthc Mater* no. 3 (7):1036–43.

Moutos, F. T., L. E. Freed, and F. Guilak. 2007. A biomimetic three-dimensional woven composite scaffold for functional tissue engineering of cartilage. *Nat Mater* no. 6 (2):162–67.

Moutos, F. T., K. A. Glass, S. A. Compton, A. K. Ross, C. A. Gersbach, F. Guilak, and B. T. Estes. 2016. Anatomically shaped tissue-engineered cartilage with tunable and inducible anticytokine delivery for biological joint resurfacing. *Proc Natl Acad Sci USA* no. 113 (31):E4513–22.

Moutos, F. T. and F. Guilak. 2010. Functional properties of cell-seeded three-dimensionally woven poly(epsilon-caprolactone) scaffolds for cartilage tissue engineering. *Tissue Eng Part A* no. 16 (4):1291–301.

Novak, T., B. Seelbinder, C. M. Twitchell, C. C. van Donkelaar, S. L. Voytik-Harbin, and C. P. Neu. 2016. Mechanisms and microenvironment investigation of cellularized high density gradient collagen matrices via densification. *Adv Funct Mater* no. 26 (16):2617–28.

Park, H. J., S. J. Yu, K. Yang, Y. Jin, A. N. Cho, J. Kim, B. Lee, H. S. Yang, S. G. Im, and S. W. Cho. 2014. Paper-based bioactive scaffolds for stem cell-mediated bone tissue engineering. *Biomaterials* no. 35 (37):9811–23.

Park, J. H., J. W. Jung, H. W. Kang, and D. W. Cho. 2014. Indirect three-dimensional printing of synthetic polymer scaffold based on thermal molding process. *Biofabrication* no. 6 (2):025003.

Parzel, C. A., M. E. Pepper, T. Burg, R. E. Groff, and K. J. Burg. 2009. EDTA enhances high-throughput two-dimensional bioprinting by inhibiting salt scaling and cell aggregation at the nozzle surface. *J Tissue Eng Regen Med* no. 3 (4):260–68.

Pepper, M. E., C. A. Parzel, T. Burg, T. Boland, K. J. Burg, and R. E. Groff. 2009. Design and implementation of a two-dimensional inkjet bioprinter. *Conf Proc IEEE Eng Med Biol Soc* no. 2009:6001–05.

Petersen, G. F., B. J. Hilbert, G. D. Trope, W. H. Kalle, and P. M. Strappe. 2015. A paper-based scaffold for enhanced osteogenic differentiation of equine adipose-derived stem cells. *Biotechnol Lett* no. 37 (11):2321–31.

Pham, Q. P., U. Sharma, and A. G. Mikos. 2006. Electrospun poly(epsilon-caprolactone) microfiber and multilayer nanofiber/microfiber scaffolds: Characterization of scaffolds and measurement of cellular infiltration. *Biomacromolecules* no. 7 (10):2796–805.

Reneker, D. H. and I. Chun. 1996. Nanometre diameter fibres of polymer, produced by electrospinning. *Nanotechnology* no. 7 (3):216.

Rimell, J. T. and P. M. Marquis. 2000. Selective laser sintering of ultra high molecular weight polyethylene for clinical applications. *J Biomed Mater Res* no. 53 (4):414–20.

Rose, F. R. and R. O. Oreffo. 2002. Bone tissue engineering: Hope vs hype. *Biochem Biophys Res Commun* no. 292 (1):1–7.

Rouwkema, J., N. C. Rivron, and C. A. van Blitterswijk. 2008. Vascularization in tissue engineering. *Trends Biotechnol* no. 26 (8):434–41.

Sachlos, E. and J. T. Czernuszka. 2003. Making tissue engineering scaffolds work. Review: The application of solid freeform fabrication technology to the production of tissue engineering scaffolds. *Eur Cell Mater* no. 5:29–39.

Sachs, E., A. Curodeau, T. Fan, J. F. Bredt, M. Cima, and D. Brancazio. 1998. Three dimensional printing system. US Patent Office # US 08/596,707 to Massachusetts Institute of Technology.

Saino, E., M. L. Focarete, C. Gualandi, E. Emanuele, A. I. Cornaglia, M. Imbriani, and L. Visai. 2011. Effect of electrospun fiber diameter and alignment on macrophage activation and secretion of proinflammatory cytokines and chemokines. *Biomacromolecules* no. 12 (5):1900–11.

Stevens, M. M. and J. H. George. 2005. Exploring and engineering the cell surface interface. *Science* no. 310 (5751):1135–38.

Thavornyutikarn, B., N. Chantarapanich, K. Sitthiseripratip, G. A. Thouas, and Q. Chen. 2014. Bone tissue engineering scaffolding: Computer-aided scaffolding techniques. *Prog Biomater* no. 3:61–102.

Usher, A. P. 2013. *A History of Mechanical Inventions*. Revised Edition. Dover Publications, New York, NY.

Vacanti, C. A. 2006. History of tissue engineering and a glimpse into its future. *Tissue Eng* no. 12 (5):1137–42.

van Tienen, T. G., R. G. Heijkants, P. Buma, J. H. de Groot, A. J. Pennings, and R. P. Veth. 2002. Tissue ingrowth and degradation of two biodegradable porous polymers with different porosities and pore sizes. *Biomaterials* no. 23 (8):1731–38.

Wang, L., C. Xu, Y. Zhu, Y. Yu, N. Sun, X. Zhang, K. Feng, and J. Qin. 2015. Human induced pluripotent stem cell-derived beating cardiac tissues on paper. *Lab Chip* no. 15 (22):4283–90.

Wei, G. and P. X. Ma. 2004. Structure and properties of nano-hydroxyapatite/polymer composite scaffolds for bone tissue engineering. *Biomaterials* no. 25 (19):4749–57.

Woodard, J. R., A. J. Hilldore, S. K. Lan, C. J. Park, A. W. Morgan, J. A. Eurell, S. G. Clark, M. B. Wheeler, R. D. Jamison, and A. J. Wagoner Johnson. 2007. The mechanical properties and osteoconductivity of hydroxyapatite bone scaffolds with multi-scale porosity. *Biomaterials* no. 28 (1):45–54.

Wu, S., B. Duan, P. Liu, C. Zhang, X. Qin, and J. T. Butcher. 2016. Fabrication of aligned nanofiber polymer yarn networks for anisotropic soft tissue scaffolds. *ACS Appl Mater Interfaces* no. 8 (26):16950–60.

Xie, J., M. R. MacEwan, A. G. Schwartz, and Y. Xia. 2010. Electrospun nanofibers for neural tissue engineering. *Nanoscale* no. 2 (1):35–44.

Xu, T., J. Jin, C. Gregory, J. J. Hickman, and T. Boland. 2005. Inkjet printing of viable mammalian cells. *Biomaterials* no. 26 (1):93–99.

Yang, S., K. F. Leong, Z. Du, and C. K. Chua. 2002. The design of scaffolds for use in tissue engineering. Part II. Rapid prototyping techniques. *Tissue Eng* no. 8 (1):1–11.

Yoon, J. J. and T. G. Park. 2001. Degradation behaviors of biodegradable macroporous scaffolds prepared by gas foaming of effervescent salts. *J Biomed Mater Res* no. 55 (3):401–08.

Younesi, M., A. Islam, V. Kishore, J. M. Anderson, and O. Akkus. 2014. Tenogenic induction of human MSCs by anisotropically aligned collagen biotextiles. *Adv Funct Mater* no. 24 (36):5762–70.

3 Bioreactor Instrumentation and Control for 3D Cellular and Tissue Systems

Steve Warren

CONTENTS

3.1 Introduction 33
3.2 Bioreactor Embodiments 36
    3.2.1 Design Considerations 36
    3.2.2 Thematic Bioreactor Categories 37
        3.2.2.1 Stirred-Flask Bioreactors 37
        3.2.2.2 Rotating-Wall Bioreactors 38
        3.2.2.3 Perfusion Bioreactors 40
        3.2.2.4 Other Bioreactor Form Factors 40
3.3 Mechanical/Electrical Tissue Stimulation 41
    3.3.1 Mechanical Stimulation 41
    3.3.2 Electrical Stimulation 43
    3.3.3 Electromagnetic Stimulation 43
3.4 Aggregate Component Architecture for Bioreactor Systems 43
3.5 Sensing and Control in Bioreactor Systems 46
    3.5.1 Parameters and Sensing Methods 46
        3.5.1.1 Offline versus Online Measurement Modes 48
        3.5.1.2 Combined Parameter Assessments 48
    3.5.2 Controls 49
3.6 Conclusion and Perspective 51
Acknowledgments 53
References 53

3.1 INTRODUCTION

A tissue bioreactor embodies an artificial environment whose purpose is to maintain physicochemical conditions that promote tissue growth. Tissue bioreactors, also referred to as tissue incubators (Butler et al. 2009; Christen and Andreou 2007), have been used since the early 1980s to provide closed growth environments for human and animal cells (Eibl and Eibl 2009; Plunkett and O'Brien 2010). These active incubation apparatuses have promoted the growth of small quantities of tissue, such as cultured *skin cells* used for grafts and wound dressings applied to burn victims or patients with skin ulcers and cancers (Helmedag et al. 2015; Jeong et al. 2014; Prenosil and Kino-oka 1999). Bioreactors have also targeted tissue growth for *bone* (Bancroft et al. 2003; Carpentier et al. 2011; Cartmell et al. 2003; Gaspar et al. 2012; Rauh et al. 2011), *cartilage* (Darling and Athanasiou 2003; Popp et al. 2012; Sucosky et al. 2004; Wendt et al. 2005), *tendons/ligaments* (Ainsworth and Chaudhuri 2005; Laurent et al. 2014; Wang et al. 2013), *vessels* (Barron et al. 2003; Ferrechio et al. 2009; Niklason et al. 1999), *cardiac tissue* (Barron et al. 2003; Shachar and Cohen 2003), and *heart valves* (Amrollahi and Tayebi 2016; Barron et al. 2003).

A bioreactor simulates the physical environment required for the growth and maintenance of viable tissue (Martin and Vermette 2005). As such, a bioreactor should perform at least one of the following functions (Barron et al. 2003; Freed and Vunjak-Novakovic 2000; Partap et al. 2010; Plunkett and O'Brien 2010):

1. Promote cell proliferation and/or uniform tissue growth on a three-dimensional (3D) scaffold.
2. Maintain a culture medium with the correct concentrations of gases and nutrients.
3. Facilitate mass transfer to the tissue constructs.
4. Provide physical stimuli to growing tissue.
5. Offer data regarding the development of the tissue within the bioreactor.

The ideal responsibilities of a bioreactor would include real-time monitoring and control of dynamic physicochemical states and the concentrations of nutrients, metabolites, and cytokine concentrations germane to different kinds of cells (Christen and Andreou 2007; DeBusschere and Kovacs 2001; Xicai et al. 2007). Recent and ongoing bioreactor research themes address the following:

- *Cell/tissue scaling*: The production of tissue in large enough quantities for practical use (Buang et al. 2014; Wu et al. 2014).
- *Environmental management*: The creation of an environment that promotes growth for all cells either suspended in, or surrounded by, the bioreactor medium while minimizing the likelihood of tissue necrosis. This involves maintaining environmental parameters (e.g., pH, temperature, pressure, and osmolarity), nutrient delivery (e.g., oxygen), waste removal (e.g., urea and lactate), and flow in the culture medium (Barron et al. 2003; Carpentier et al. 2011; Martin and Vermette 2005; Pörtner and Giese 2006; Yeatts and Fisher 2011).
- *Mechanical stimuli*: Mechanical actuation to fabricate tissues such as blood vessels, cartilage, bone, tendons, and ligaments that can meet the mechanical rigors of their target environment or, in contrast, to minimize shear stress that cells experience during culture, which can have a detrimental effect on expansion (Barron et al. 2003; Butler et al. 2009; Darling and Athanasiou 2003; Elder and Athanasiou 2009; Laurent et al. 2014; Mauck et al. 2000; Popp et al. 2012; Rauh et al. 2011; Yeatts and Fisher 2011).

- *Electrical/electromagnetic (EM) stimuli*: The use of electromagnetic fields (EMFs) or direct electrical-current injection to stimulate artificial tissues for cardiac and nervous system applications (Dobson et al. 2006; Kim et al. 2011; Radisic et al. 2008; Tandon et al. 2008; Vunjak-Novakovic et al. 2011).
- *Real-time sensing*: Constant monitoring of (a) the constituents that affect the tissue growth process in the entire 3D space and (b) the size/number and viability of the tissue mass itself (Mazzei et al. 2008; Rolfe 2006; Xicai et al. 2008).
- *Real-time control*: Feedback-driven control systems that regulate the growth environment based upon input received from the sensors embedded in the bioreactor space (Christen and Andreou 2007; DeBusschere and Kovacs 2001; Mazzei et al. 2008; Rolfe 2006; Xiang et al. 2015; Xicai et al. 2008).
- *Alternative embodiments*: Portable bioreactors (DeBusschere and Kovacs 2001; Tandon et al. 2013), small complementary metal-oxide-semiconductor (CMOS)-scale, implantable bioreactors (Frantz et al. 2010; Kim et al. 2011), and various bioreactor geometries that support the growth of complex tissues (Atala et al. 2012; Mikos et al. 2006).

An array of bioreactor designs exists, and many of these are "one-off" designs, meaning that a given design is the only one in existence and is customized to the research group and application for which it was designed. Although these bioreactor manifestations offer different design goals in terms of basic operation, constituent concentrations of interest, and possibly the need for external mechanical/electrical stimulation, etc., they have similar needs in terms of (a) environment and medium management, (b) sensor-based instrumentation that can provide situational awareness regarding parameter levels and tissue viability, and (c) feedback-based control systems that continuously balance the incubation environment. This chapter addresses those general areas of need, with the realization that a specific bioreactor may deviate considerably from the base bioreactor designs, instrumentation, and control options presented here.

Note that the tissue bioreactor literature base is growing rapidly, more so in recent years. A number of excellent bioreactor reviews are available that address the following:

- *General bioreactor design* (Chen and Hu 2006; Eibl and Eibl 2009; Freed and Vunjak-Novakovic 2000; Freed et al. 2006; Georgiev et al. 2013; Korossis et al. 2005; Martin and Vermette 2005; Martin et al. 2004; Partap et al. 2010; Pörtner and Giese 2006; Portner et al. 2005; Salehi-Nik et al. 2013; Wendt et al. 2005).
- *Bioreactors for structural tissue growth* (e.g., bone, cartilage, tendons, ligaments) that often incorporate mechanical stimuli (Abousleiman and Sikavitsas 2006; Bancroft et al. 2003; Bilodeau 2004; Carpentier et al. 2011; Elder and Athanasiou 2009; Gardel et al. 2014; Gaspar et al. 2012; Rauh et al. 2011; Sladkova and de Peppo 2014; Wang et al. 2013; Wendt et al. 2005; Yeatts and Fisher 2011).

- *Bioreactors for cardiovascular tissue growth* (e.g., cardiac tissue, vessels, and valves) that may incorporate mechanical and/or electrical stimuli (Amrollahi and Tayebi 2016; Barron et al. 2003; Shachar and Cohen 2003; Vunjak-Novakovic et al. 2011).

Further, a collection of books is also available that addresses the engineering aspects of bioreactor design (Antolli and Liu 2011; Asnaghi et al. 2014; Blose et al. 2014; Chaudhuri and Al-Rubeai 2005; Eibl and Eibl 2009; Haycock 2011; Kasper et al. 2009, 2010; Partap et al. 2010; Wendt et al. 2008). Numerous technical papers speak to application- and tissue-dependent bioreactor design tradeoffs. A synopsis of instrumentation issues related to bioreactor system design, including thematic bioreactor categories, mechanical/electrical actuation, sensor-based monitoring, and environmental control is presented in this chapter.

3.2 BIOREACTOR EMBODIMENTS

3.2.1 Design Considerations

While each bioreactor implementation can be unique depending on the tissue type and application, the designer/user of a tissue bioreactor should consider a set of basic design criteria (Lyons and Pandit 2005; Partap et al. 2010; Portner et al. 2005). The bioreactor system should

- maintain a growth atmosphere at 37°C and 90%–100% humidity,
- properly control pH, pO_2, pCO_2, nutrient delivery, and waste removal,
- regulate steady versus pulsatile flow with a pump that can accurately apply small forces,
- control flow rate, volume, shear, pressure, resistance, and compliance,
- support mechanical or electrical stimulation,
- facilitate sampling of the medium, cells, and/or tissue construct,
- be constructed with biocompatible or bioinert materials (e.g., high-quality stainless steel, plastics, or other nonmetal materials),
- allow the user to easily affix the seeded scaffold,
- be easy to clean, sanitize, and maintain,
- incorporate disposable parts and/or reusable parts that are capable of being sterilized,
- offer a simple, robust design that is easy to assemble/disassemble, facilitating harvesting of cell or tissue products and minimizing tissue damage,
- utilize materials that minimize foam generation and allow the medium and tissue constructs to be visualized,
- incorporate flexible tubing and connectors to assist with assembly/disassembly, media exchanges, and microcarrier harvesting in an aseptic fashion,
- lack recesses which can harbor bacteria,
- accommodate multiple ports for various sensing devices employed during the growth phase,

- employ good fluid/gas seals and control headspace and gas exchange, and
- be scalable for the successful production of greater amounts of tissue while making efficient use of the medium.

Bioreactor designs support different types of mass-transfer flow (e.g., static versus turbulent versus laminar [Salehi-Nik et al. 2013]) depending on the cell types and the geometries of the aggregate physical tissues. Further, different physical mechanisms and bioreactor geometries can be used to accomplish a given type of mass transfer. In some cases, external mechanical/electrical stimulation may also be needed to tune the resulting tissues for their intended application environment.

Bioreactors that employ static cultures, meaning they incorporate no flow or mixing of the growth medium, have been useful for cell proliferation at a moderate scale (Georgiev et al. 2013; Martin et al. 2004). However, the resulting tissue structures can be heterogeneous, consisting of healthy cells that surround necrotic cores (Cartmell et al. 2003; Wendt et al. 2008) or poorly populated cores that result from chemotaxis—cell migration to regions of greater nutrient concentration (Goldstein et al. 2001). This is due to reliance on a diffusive mass-transfer mechanism that preferentially provides nutrients to outer cell layers while also harboring waste materials in central regions (Rolfe 2006). This chapter therefore focuses on bioreactor designs that utilize convective mass-transfer mechanisms, where continual mixing and/or flow of the culture medium helps to promote viable tissue growth in greater quantities due to improved nutrient delivery coupled with flow-induced stress. These bioreactors have various physical instantiations but a set of common thematic needs. The following subsections describe the primary categories of bioreactor form factors as well as the types of physical mechanisms that are commonly used to help stimulate tissue growth and enhance tissue viability.

3.2.2 THEMATIC BIOREACTOR CATEGORIES

3.2.2.1 Stirred-Flask Bioreactors

A stirred-flask (a.k.a., spinner flask or stirred suspension) bioreactor vessel design is a commonly used, active bioreactor which incorporates convective flow due to the continual mixing of the culture medium (Ismadi et al. 2014; Salehi-Nik et al. 2013; Sucosky et al. 2004). A representative solid model for a typical stirred-flask bioreactor is depicted in Figure 3.1a (after Martin and Vermette 2005; Partap et al. 2010; Rauh et al. 2011). In this arrangement, tissue scaffolds are attached to one or more suspension rods, or "needles," that hang from the top of the flask chamber. The surface of the medium is maintained at a level such that these scaffolds are constantly submerged. Input/output ports are provided at the top of the chamber to refresh the culture medium, sample its constituents, deliver oxygen, and remove carbon dioxide. A magnetic stirring rod constantly mixes the culture medium to provide nutrient delivery to, and waste removal from, cells that occupy the outer layers of the tissue constructs. For cells that occupy interior layers of the tissue constructs, nutrient delivery and waste removal occur primarily by diffusion. While the convective flow offered by this type of design is an improvement over static diffusive approaches, the shear forces generated on the tissue constructs by the eddy currents

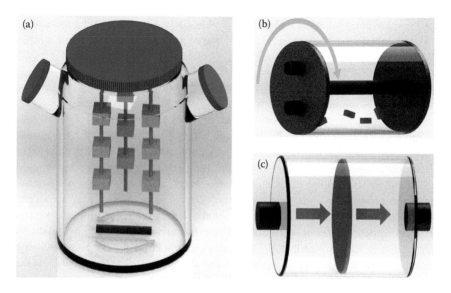

FIGURE 3.1 Representative depictions of three common classes of bioreactor vessel designs: (a) stirred-flask bioreactor, (b) rotating-wall bioreactor, and (c) perfusion bioreactor.

induced during the mixing process are heterogeneous, affecting the homogeneity of the resulting samples (Ismadi et al. 2014; Partap et al. 2010; Sucosky et al. 2004). Oxygen delivery provided at the gas–liquid interface (headspace aeration) or by a submerged sparger can be a challenge because of the low solubility of oxygen in the culture medium (Wu et al. 2014). Stirred-flask bioreactors have been useful for the assembly of artificial tissues that include cartilage (Freed and Vunjak-Novakovic 2000; Sucosky et al. 2004) and stem cell aggregates (Ismadi et al. 2014; Wu et al. 2014).

A commercial bioreactor assembly that utilizes the stirred-flask concept is depicted in Figure 3.2. The assembly consists of an Applikon Biotechnology ez-Control system (Biotechnology 2015) that monitors and regulates a 3 L, single-use Mobius bioreactor (Millipore 2016). The ez-Control unit adaptively controls pH, temperature, dissolved oxygen, foam/level, and agitation—parameters that can be managed via a touch screen interface. The 3 L, plastic, disposable Mobius bioreactor is pre-sterilized with gamma radiation and employs an impeller-like mechanism attached to a central shaft to stir the medium. It incorporates flexible tubing, vent/gas filters, ports for fluid addition/removal, and a drain port. This setup is suited for mammalian cell growth and allows samples to be acquired for offline analyses, for example, to evaluate microcarriers for cell density.

3.2.2.2 Rotating-Wall Bioreactors

A rotating-wall bioreactor vessel design (see the depiction in Figure 3.1b) promotes tissue growth in a laminar flow condition, keeping cellular constructs in a state of suspension, or continuous free-fall, by countering the force of gravity with rotational

Bioreactor Instrumentation and Control for 3D Cellular and Tissue Systems   39

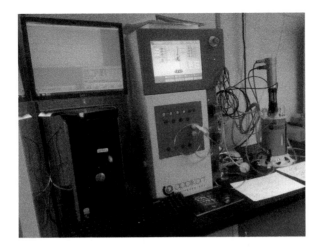

FIGURE 3.2 Three-liter, single-use Millipore Mobius bioreactor with an Applikon ez-Control host system housed in the Kansas State University Department of Anatomy and Physiology, Manhattan, KS, USA. Image courtesy Dr. Mark Weiss, Kansas State University.

forces exerted on the medium (Martin and Vermette 2005; Salehi-Nik et al. 2013; Sladkova and de Peppo 2014). This approach, intended to simulate microgravity, was originally developed by Schwarz and coworkers at Krug Life Sciences, Houston, TX (NASA, Johnson Space Center) to help protect cell cultures reserved for space shuttle experiments from the forces incurred during takeoff and landing (Schwarz, Goodwin, and Wolf 1992). The basic design, also known as a slow-turning lateral vessel (STLV), consists of two concentric cylinders that can be independently rotated (Begley and Kleis 2002). Input/output ports at the end of the cylindrical arrangement allow for the circulation of the growth medium, and oxygen is provided via a membrane that surrounds the inner cylinder. To grow tissue, mammalian cells are first seeded onto microcarrier beads (e.g., 100–200 μm polystyrene beads). As these beads accumulate cells, they group together to form larger constructs. On earth, the outer cylinder is rotated at speeds from 15 to 30 rpm. These speeds increase as the tissue structures get larger, in order to keep those constructs suspended, avoiding collisions with the cylindrical enclosure (Begley and Kleis 2002; Martin and Vermette 2005). An STLV variant referred to as a high aspect ratio vessel (HARV) reduces the rotation rate required to keep the tissue construct in suspension and also improves gas exchange. Refer to Freed et al. (1997), Martin and Vermette (2005), and Radtke and Herbst-Kralovetz (2012) for more detailed descriptions of the HARV design.

Rotating-wall bioreactors reduce shear stress levels in comparison to levels incurred in stirred-flask bioreactors. This results in tissue constructs with more homogeneous cell distributions (Goldstein et al. 2001). While arguably not well suited for the production of large tissue masses (Martin and Vermette 2005), rotating-wall bioreactors have shown promise for the growth of various types of tissue, including cartilage (Freed et al. 1997), bone (Granet et al. 1998), liver (Catapano and Gerlach 2007), neuron-like cells (Wang and Good 2001), aortic endothelial cells (Sanford et al. 2002), kidney cells (Xu et al. 2004), epithelial cells (Radtke and Herbst-Kralovetz 2012), stem cells (Lei et al. 2011), and skin (Lei et al. 2011).

3.2.2.3 Perfusion Bioreactors

A perfusion bioreactor vessel (refer to Figure 3.1c) is designed such that the culture medium must flow through a porous scaffold populated with seed cells (Gardel et al. 2014; Yeatts and Fisher 2011). This approach has dual benefit, improving mass transfer of nutrients to all areas of the cell construct while providing flow-dependent mechanical stimuli to the cells (Abousleiman and Sikavitsas 2006; Partap et al. 2010; Rauh et al. 2011; Sailon et al. 2009; Salehi-Nik et al. 2013; Yan et al. 2012). Flow is primarily convective in this context but is supplemented with nutrient diffusion to better maintain interior cell viability. Like rotating-wall bioreactors, perfusion reactors have shown promise for the growth of more homogeneous tissues with denser construct cores when compared to stirred-flask bioreactors (Goldstein et al. 2001; Sailon et al. 2009). Perfusion bioreactors have also offered improved cell proliferation and differentiation of osteoprogenitor cells, plus enhanced deposition of the extracellular matrix (ECM; Bjerre et al. 2008; Hofmann et al. 2003; Holtorf et al. 2005; Rauh et al. 2011).

One drawback of this design is the tendency for nutrient flow to follow the path of least resistance as determined by scaffold pore size and geometry. Flow rate optimization is a balance between nutrient delivery, metabolite transfer to/from cells, and shear stress applied to the cells (Wendt et al. 2008), for example, too much flow can result in cell "wash out," where the forces induced by the fluid remove the cells from the construct (Singh et al. 2007). The flow rate threshold is also influenced by the need for proper O_2 delivery to the tissue constructs given, as noted earlier, the poor solubility of O_2 in the culture medium. Further, cell harvesting can be difficult to manage and monitor with such a design.

Perfusion bioreactors have been successfully utilized to grow a number of tissue types, including bone (Bancroft et al. 2003; Cartmell et al. 2003; Gardel et al. 2014; Gaspar et al. 2012; Goldstein et al. 2001), cartilage grafts (Carver and Heath 1999; Nesic et al. 2006), cardiac tissue (Radisic et al. 2008; Tandon et al. 2013), intestinal tissue (Kim et al. 2007), vascular grafts (Hoenicka et al. 2010; Radisic et al. 2008; Williams 2003), and stem cells (Bjerre et al. 2008).

3.2.2.4 Other Bioreactor Form Factors

A number of creative bioreactor embodiments exist that are either variations on the themes noted above or are novel designs matched to a specific tissue need. A few selected examples follow:

- In a rocker platform, or wave bioreactor vessel, a flexible bag holding the culture medium is rocked back and forth. The tissue medium is aerated due to agitation from surface wave action, and nutrients are provided to the tissue construct through convective flow (Amrollahi and Tayebi 2016; Blose et al. 2014; Lyons and Pandit 2005; Yuk et al. 2011).
- A hollow fiber bioreactor vessel consists of a closed, medium-filled vessel filled with semipermeable hollow fibers. These fibers emulate blood vessels by providing nutrients and removing waste. Primarily intended for

mammalian cell growth, this design offers the advantage of better nutrient delivery to the center of the tissue, but oxygen delivery can be a challenge (Martin and Vermette 2005; Tharakan and Chau 1986). Monitoring cell growth and determining cell removal efficiency at harvest can also be a difficult.
- In an airlift reactor vessel, oxygen is supplied to the tissue through the delivery of air at the bottom of the vessel. A draft tube is needed to prevent sparging due to direct air contact with the developing tissue. Nutrient availability can be a challenge due to the lack of mixing of the glass spheres or polystyrene beads upon which cells are seeded, since they tend to settle on the bottom of the vessel (Al-Mashhadani et al. 2015; Martin and Vermette 2005).
- A double-chamber bioreactor vessel is employed for the growth of larger, more complex tissue constructs such as osteochondral grafts and tracheal allografts. Two chambers, for example, a chondral compartment and a bone compartment, each with their own mixing apparatus, are separated by a membrane, and the tissue scaffold spans the membrane so that it resides in both chambers (Chang et al. 2004; Haykal et al. 2014; Wendt et al. 2005).
- Microfluidic bioreactors based on the integration of electronics at, for example, the CMOS level are becoming available for portable and implantable applications (Christen and Andreou 2007; DeBusschere and Kovacs 2001; Kim et al. 2011).

3.3 MECHANICAL/ELECTRICAL TISSUE STIMULATION

Hydrodynamic forces such as the shear stress that fluid flow exerts on tissue constructs in stirred-flask, rotating-wall, and perfusion bioreactors can be healthy for tissue development by improving cell proliferation, expression of osteogenic marker genes, and ECM mineralization (Rauh et al. 2011). For musculoskeletal tissues (e.g., bone, cartilage, ligaments, and tendons) and cardiovascular tissues (e.g., cardiac tissue and vessels), additional pulsatile and steady-state mechanical forces created by bioreactor actuators can further improve the viability of those constructs. In the case of cardiovascular tissues, electrical/electromagnetic supplements provide additional improvements. This section addresses the tissue-stimulation role of bioreactor instrumentation as represented by mechanical actuation and electrical/electromagnetic excitation.

3.3.1 MECHANICAL STIMULATION

The incorporation of mechanical forces into tissue bioreactors is essential for the growth of viable load-bearing tissues, such as articular cartilage, which will atrophy in the absence of mechanical stimulation (Darling and Athanasiou 2003). External mechanical stimuli can also improve the homogeneity, structural viability, growth rate, and functionality of cultured tissue (Carver and Heath 1999; Mauck et al. 2000), in part because those stimuli encourage the production and mineralization of ECM, the noncellular tissue component that provides "not only essential physical scaffolding for the cellular constituents but also initiates crucial biochemical and biomechanical cues that are required for tissue morphogenesis, differentiation and homeostasis"

(Frantz et al. 2010; Hoffmann et al. 2015). Mechanical stimulation can also influence cell differentiation. One study illustrated that a combination of translational and rotational strain could differentiate mesenchymal progenitor cells from the bone marrow (embedded in a collagen gel) into aligned collagen fibers with a density indicative of ligament cells but with no cell markers indicative of bone or cartilage (Altman, Horan et al. 2002). As noted in Section 3.1, the types of engineered tissues that benefit from mechanical stimulation include bone, cartilage, tendons, ligaments, and vessels. (Refer to that section for citations associated with mechanical stimuli as well as citations for reviews that address structural tissue engineering.)

Bioreactors that incorporate mechanical stimulation take three primary forms:

1. *Compression bioreactor:* This type of bioreactor generally employs a computer-controlled linear actuator and a type of flat plate to deliver dynamic loading to the tissue scaffold(s), where the amplitude and rate of the displacement depend on the tissue type and size. For a tissue like cartilage, this compressive loading can help to improve fluid flow in the center of the scaffold and result in a more homogeneous construct with an elastic modulus that is close to that of native cartilage (Mauck et al. 2000). Load cells can be used to deliver real-time feedback regarding the force applied to the engineered tissue and scaffold (Popp et al. 2012). Compressive strains of 1–10% at a rate of 0.5–1 Hz over durations of several hours per day are typical for cell differentiation studies (Sladkova and de Peppo 2014).
2. *Tensile strain bioreactor:* The design of a strain bioreactor is similar to that of a compression bioreactor, but the scaffold is clamped in such a way that the linear actuator delivers a tensile strain instead of a compressive force. Rotational strains can also be applied (Altman, Horan et al. 2002). This type of bioreactor is a suitable match for tissues such as ligaments and tendons, which can exhibit a substantive increase in Young's modulus when compared to nonloaded control tissues (Garvin et al. 2003). Tensile strains of 0–30%, forces up to 200 N, and rates of 0–2 Hz are typical (Riehl et al. 2012).
3. *Hydrostatic pressure bioreactor:* A hydrostatic pressure chamber can be implemented with a medium-filled container and a piston driven by a computer-controlled linear actuator. Here, either the piston itself is sealed but in direct contact with the medium, or an impermeable membrane separates the two (Darling and Athanasiou 2003; Elder and Athanasiou 2009). Alternatively, the entire vessel containing the growth medium and tissue scaffold can be placed in a water-filled pressure chamber, where an impermeable membrane separates the two types of fluid media (Watanabe et al. 2005). Tissues subjected to hydrostatic forces are typically cultured separately and then placed in the hydrostatic chamber to be loaded for a predetermined treatment period using either constant or slowly varying pressure. For hydrostatic pressure systems applied to chondrocytes for cartilage tissue engineering, static pressures of 1–10 MPa have been applied for time intervals from a few hours to a few weeks. Dynamic systems have cycled at rates of 0.25–1 Hz using similar pressure ranges and time intervals. Refer to Tables 1 and 2 in Elder and Athanasiou (2009) for a good comparative

listing. Hydrostatic pressure benefits have included increased cell proliferation, improved cell differentiation, improved protein production, and enhanced biomechanical properties.

3.3.2 Electrical Stimulation

Electrical stimulation has been primarily employed in bioreactors designed for cardiac tissue growth, where the end goal is to replace tissue that has been destroyed by myocardial infarction: a "patch for a broken heart" (Vunjak-Novakovic et al. 2011). Pulsed electrical excitation (e.g., a 1 Hz square wave at 5 V/cm (Radisic et al. 2008); a 2 ms pulse at 3 Hz and 3 V/m (Tandon et al. 2011)) has been demonstrated to help induce contractile properties of engineered cardiac tissue, where the safe range of operation appears to be 0–8 V/cm (Tandon et al. 2008). The stimulation amplitude and frequency, as well as the electrode type, have a significant bearing on the quality of tissue produced (Tandon et al. 2011). Electrical stimulation can also be combined with mechanical stimulation in a hybrid bioreactor. Liao and coworkers illustrated that synchronized electromechanical stimulation (electrical stimulation coupled with mechanical cues) can improve the alignment and elongation of skeletal myoblasts as well as the upregulation of cardiac proteins (Liao et al. 2008).

3.3.3 Electromagnetic Stimulation

EMFs have long been known to assist with bone growth during fracture healing and bone stretching (Bassett et al. 1977; Eyres, Saleh, and Kanis 1996). In an EMF bioreactor, the tissue scaffold is placed in the electric field generated by a pair of Helmholtz coils. Typical flux densities in recent research are 0.3–2 mT, with pulse durations of 0.3–60 ms at pulse frequencies of 15–75 Hz (see Table 1E in (Rauh et al. 2011)). Field strengths can be verified with Hall-effect probes (Fassina et al. 2006). Benefits of EMF stimulation include improved osteogenic cell differentiation, enhanced osteoprogenitor cell proliferation, and increased mineralization of osteogenic cells (Rauh et al. 2011).

3.4 AGGREGATE COMPONENT ARCHITECTURE FOR BIOREACTOR SYSTEMS

Component architectures, or system block diagrams, have been presented in the literature for various types of tissue bioreactor systems, where the components employed depend on the type of bioreactor vessel, the fluid flow requirements, and the means for nutrient (e.g., oxygen) delivery and waste removal. This section presents an aggregate component architecture that lays out a superset of these system components, or building blocks, with a goal of identifying the sensing and control needs that are relevant within this overall design space. These needs drive the remaining discussion in this chapter.

The aggregate component architecture is depicted in Figure 3.3. This layout attempts to incorporate the collective components and functionality noted in the block diagrams and the accompanying text presented in a selected collection of

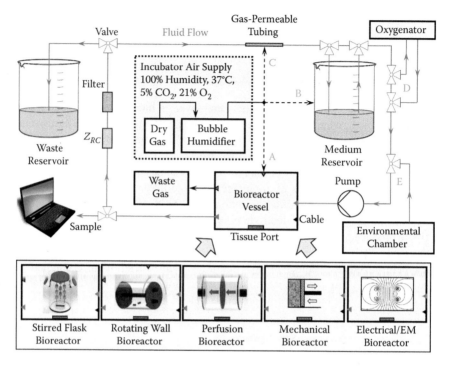

FIGURE 3.3 Aggregate component architecture representative of multiple classes of tissue bioreactor systems.

technical papers and reviews: Rauh et al. (2011, Figure 3), Singh et al. (2007, Figure 2), Kim et al. (2007, Figure 1), (Lyons and Pandit 2005, pp.18–19), Barron et al. (2003, Figures 1, 2, and 4), Wang et al. (2013, Figures 1, 4, and 5), Portner et al. (2005, Figure 1), Portner et al. (2005, Figures 2.2 and 2.3), Chen and Hu (2006, Figures 1 and 2), Bilodeau (2004, Figure 2.1), Bancroft et al. (2003, Figure 5), Yeatts and Fisher (2011, Figure 3), Gaspar et al. (2012, Figures 1 and 2), and Amrollahi and Tayebi (2016, Table 1 and Figure 3). Note that block diagrams for systems geared toward cell seeding will be different, as they have a short-term goal of populating a scaffold with cells just before that scaffold is removed and placed in a bioreactor growth chamber (Wendt et al. 2005).

The lower panel in Figure 3.3 displays five general embodiments of the *Bioreactor Vessel* component in the center of the diagram. Each of these was addressed in a prior section. In the flow diagram, blue lines with arrows denote the direction of fluid flow, and black lines denote gas flow. While the aggregate diagram appears complex, it may be helpful to note that several operational modes are depicted, labeled as green letters "A" through "E," where the modes depend on the type of bioreactor and the related nutrient delivery requirements. For modes A through D, the diagram makes the assumption that the collection of components (medium/waste reservoirs, bioreactor vessel, pump, valves, and tubing) all reside within a closed incubator space maintained at 100% humidity, 37°C, 5% CO_2, and 21% O_2 (Chen and Hu 2006; Christen and Andreou 2007; Wang et al. 2013). Prior to operation, all components to be operated within the incubator space are sterilized, for example, using an autoclave and ethylene glycol gas (Kim et al. 2007). These operational modes are characterized as follows:

- *Mode A*: Incubator air is fed directly to the bioreactor vessel for either headspace, airlift, or inner tubing aeration (Al-Mashhadani et al. 2015; Martin and Vermette 2005). Note in the lower panel of Figure 3.3 that only the stirred-flask and rotating-wall bioreactors depict an input port for that air (black, hashed triangle). The other bioreactors typically employ a flow perfusion model where the fluid is aerated externally prior to reaching the bioreactor vessel.
- *Mode B*: Incubator air is fed directly to the medium reservoir for headspace aeration.
- *Mode C*: Tubing is employed that is permeable to both carbon dioxide and oxygen, ensuring gas equilibrium with the incubator space (Bancroft et al. 2002).
- *Mode D*: An *Oxygenator* provides nutrients to the medium before it is pumped into the bioreactor vessel (Chen and Hu 2006), which is common when employing flow perfusion bioreactors that may have an added mechanical or electrical stimulation role (Janssen et al. 2006; Kim et al. 2007).
- *Mode E*: In this mode, the system components are not assumed to reside within an incubator. Rather, they reside in open air, and the environmental chamber heats the medium to 37°C and employs its own internal bubble humidifier and aeration scheme to provide dissolved oxygen to the medium (Wang et al. 2013).

With regard to other figure details:

- The *Pump* in many systems is, for example, a six-roller peristaltic pump capable of delivering fluid at various computer- or manually-controlled rates. Flow rates can vary, for example, from 1.5 mL/min up to 3 L/min depending on the vessel/tissue type and the number of pump channels (Kim et al. 2007; Lyons and Pandit 2005). Flow types can be steady state, oscillatory (less effective for bone), or pulsatile, where dynamic flow becomes less potent for tissue growth as frequency increases (Jacobs et al. 1998).
- The generic *Bioreactor Vessel* (container, single/dual chamber, or cartridge) offers input ports for incubator air, the fluid medium, and a cable that contains lines for mechanical and/or electrical stimulation (e.g., to drive the stirred-flask needle, the rotating-wall cylinders, linear actuators, etc.). It offers output ports for waste (exhaust) gases and the fluid medium. A tissue port offers a means to insert/extract the tissue scaffold(s) or to sample the cells within the medium.
- The lower left portion of the diagram depicts a means to sample the flow medium for offline analysis.
- A *Filter* offers a means to remove particles and other contaminants from the flow medium, and an impedance unit (Z_{RC}) provides the desired resistance and compliance for the flow "circuit" (Barron et al. 2003).

- The *Waste Reservoir* can function as a repository for a spent or contaminated medium, or it can be part of the active flow loop, occasionally offering a role as an exchange tank to refresh part of the medium while the system is in operation. Some systems do not incorporate this element, choosing instead to recirculate the medium from the bioreactor vessel back into the *Medium Reservoir*.

Note that computerized measurement and control connections are not specified in this connectivity diagram to avoid clutter. In many commercial systems (e.g., the Applikon system depicted in Figure 3.2), the incubation parameters, medium concentration/pH, pump, valves, and mechanical/electrical stimulation mechanisms are computer controlled.

The variety of needs met by the numerous instantiations of bioreactor systems is understandable, as each tissue construct is unique in terms of its cell distribution, nutrient, mechanical/electrical conditioning, and application requirements. In response to this reality, some investigators have moved toward the development and use of more modular, componentized systems, where interchangeable parts can be more rapidly combined to construct systems well matched to the needs of the target tissue, avoiding "one-off" designs that are typical in this research arena (Illa et al. 2014; Lovett et al. 2010; Mazzei et al. 2010; Orr and Burg 2008; Vinci et al. 2011).

3.5 SENSING AND CONTROL IN BIOREACTOR SYSTEMS

An "instrument" can be defined as any tool that helps one accomplish a task or measure its progress. To this point, this chapter has addressed bioreactor instrumentation issues that relate to bioreactor design requirements, chamber embodiments that address those needs, flow/medium management, actuators, and mechanical/electrical stimulation. The following sections complete that instrumentation overview with a summary of the sensing and control mechanisms that come into play when designing a bioreactor system. Here, the notion is that sensors are employed to measure (a) parameters that a researcher wishes to quantify, as a means to gauge the operational viability of the system and its resulting tissue products and (b) parameters that may also need to be controlled to maintain system viability.

3.5.1 Parameters and Sensing Methods

The number of bioreactor system parameters that warrant attention is potentially myriad. Parameters of interest for a given system (refer to Figure 3.3) depend on the type of tissue, the bioreactor vessel design, the approach to medium flow, the methods used to deliver nutrients to the medium/tissue, the presence of active components (e.g., mechanical actuators), the relative effects of waste/contamination, and the desire to track those parameters occasionally (e.g., manually) versus in real time. Table 3.1 lists the more common parameters tracked during bioreactor system operation, along with representative parameter ranges and sensing approaches. Some of these parameters are tracked offline versus online, and some are simply measured

TABLE 3.1
Selected Bioreactor Measurement Parameters and Approaches

Parameter	Typical Range or Value	Sensing Method(s)
Incubator/medium temperature	25–39°C	Thermistors or platinum resistance thermometers—see Section 4.4 in Najafpour (2015)
pH	6–8	Commercial blood gas analyzer (Ramaswamy et al. 2014) such as the NOVA Bioprofile 400 (Nova Biomedical), which can measure 14 different components in one pass; pH probes (e.g., AppliSens probes supported by the Applikon system in Figure 3.2); Fiberoptic sensors and variations on a standard hydrogen electrode—see Xu et al. (2006) Section 4.6 in Najafpour (2015); CMOS chip (Hammond et al. 2004)
pO_2	0%–20%	Commercial blood gas analyzer (Ramaswamy et al. 2014); Electrochemical sensor with polymeric membrane; optical fiber sensors (Rolfe 2006)
pCO_2	0%–8%	Commercial blood gas analyzer (Ramaswamy et al. 2014)
Dissolved oxygen	0–50,000 mg L/h	Tubing method, mass spectrometer probes, or electrochemical detectors—see Section 4.5 in Najafpour (2015); dissolved oxygen probes (e.g., AppliSens probes supported by the Applikon system in Figure 3.2)
O_2 transfer rate (volumetric mass transfer coefficient)	$0–0.5 \times 10^2\,s^{-1}$	Sulfite oxidation method and others—see Table 2 in Salehi-Nik et al. (2013); Table 1 in Garcia-Ochoa and Gomez (2009)
Flow rate (steady state, oscillating, or pulsatile)	1.5 mL–3 L/min	Particle image velocity and others—see Table 3 in Salehi-Nik et al. (2013); see also Janssen et al. (2006), Kim et al. (2007), and Lyons and Pandit (2005)
Flow profile	N/A	Particle image velocity and others (Salehi-Nik et al. 2013; Singh et al. 2007)
Compressive strain	1%–10% at 0.5–1 Hz over hours	Load cells, tomography, ultrasound, and others (Popp et al. 2012; Sladkova and de Peppo 2014; Wang et al. 2013)
Tensile strain/displacement	0%–30%; 0–200 N; 0–2 Hz	Actuator displacement and others (Popp et al. 2012; Rauh et al. 2011)
Surface shear stress	5×10^{-5} Pa	Particle image velocity (Rauh et al. 2011)
Hydrostatic pressure	1–10 MPa; hours to weeks; 0.25–1 Hz	Diaphragm-based commercial pressure sensors, load cells, and others—see Tables 1 and 2 in Elder and Athanasiou (2009) for studies
Tissue cell count	cells/mL; cells/cm^2	Upon cell removal from the bioreactor: hemocytometer, electronic cell counter, cell image analysis, or a metabolic activity assay (Divieto et al. 2013)

(Continued)

TABLE 3.1 (Continued)
Selected Bioreactor Measurement Parameters and Approaches

Parameter	Typical Range or Value	Sensing Method(s)
Electromagnetic flux density	0.3–2 mT; 0.3–60 ms; 15–75 Hz	Hall effect transverse Gaussmeter probe (Fassina et al. 2006; Rauh et al. 2011)
Valve position	On/Off	Contact voltage; Computer-controlled switch
Acetate	0–150 mM	Gas chromatography (Whiffin et al. 2004)
Glucose	0–35 mM	Enzymatic analysis (Whiffin et al. 2004; Xicai et al. 2007, 2008)
Lactate	0.25 mM	Enzymatic analysis (Whiffin et al. 2004; Xicai et al. 2007, 2008)

to quantify a process, whereas others play important roles for system control. These parameters are an aggregation of parameters noted in a number of bioreactor papers and reviews, some of which are cited in the table.

3.5.1.1 Offline versus Online Measurement Modes

Some parameters can be measured occasionally (e.g., every few hours or days) and are therefore often acquired manually, resulting in an *offline* measurement (e.g., refer to the *Sample* valve and the *Bioreactor Vessel Tissue Port* in Figure 3.3). Other parameters must be tracked more closely, or *online*, perhaps in real time, as a means to obtain continuous feedback regarding the viability of the tissue growth process and the surrounding support system. Such measurements are facilitated with computer analysis and control. As an example of an offline mode, a traditional method to track the viability of cell cultures is to incorporate flow injection analysis, where sensors are not in contact with the culture medium. Rather, a sample is removed from the bioreactor and analyzed offline, as is the case with the cell cultures related to the work depicted in Figure 3.2. These "spot checks" represent, at best, a time-averaged view of bioreactor activity and the viability of the physicochemical environment, even if the environmental variables themselves (e.g., temperature and flow) are continuously controlled. An active area of research and development relates to the real-time tracking of bioreactor parameters (e.g., tissue construct development) and continuous control of the bioreactor environment based upon these assessments (Christen and Andreou 2007; Popp et al. 2012; Xicai et al. 2008). This leads to the notion that one could optimally tweak processes such as tissue growth or cell differentiation based on immediate or just-in-time feedback.

3.5.1.2 Combined Parameter Assessments

Parameters are rarely monitored on their own. Rather, groups of parameters must often be assessed in order to obtain a sensible snapshot of the process of interest. For example, Xicai et al. note that the collection of pH, oxygen tension, carbon dioxide tension, and temperature are the most important physicochemical parameters, as they affect the cell expansion rate and therefore the cell population within the chamber medium (Xicai et al. 2008). They also note that cell growth, differentiation, and cell death are affected by four nutrient and metabolite parameters: glucose, glutamine, lactate, and ammonia. Likewise, Rauh and coworkers note that temperature, oxygen concentration, pH, nutrient concentration, and biochemical and mechanical stimuli all modulate bone growth in complex bioreactors (Rauh et al. 2011). Combined parameter assessments are also helpful in determining the status of components within the bioreactor system. For example, the functional viability of an oxygenation unit, as depicted in Figure 3.3, can be assessed by tracking the pH, pO_2, and pCO_2 of the culture medium over a range of incubator CO_2 concentrations (Bioprofile 400 Analyzer, NovaBiomed [Kim et al. 2007]).

3.5.2 Controls

The purpose of a control system is to regulate processes that might otherwise exhibit unsatisfactory static or dynamic behavior if left alone. The regulation process might entail parameter stabilization (i.e., keeping one or more parameters constant) or process implementation (i.e., allowing parameters to change according to a prescribed protocol). Consistent with other authors, Lyons and Pandit note several bioreactor parameters that warrant control (Lyons and Pandit 2005):

- *Biochemical parameters:* Temperature (37°C), humidity (100%), pH (7.2–7.4), nutrients (e.g., oxygen or glucose), partial pressures of dissolved gases (e.g., pO_2 at 21%, pCO_2 at 5%), and waste products.
- *Biomechanical parameters:* Flow rate, shear, pressure, volume, resistance, and compliance.

Note that these parameters can be interdependent on one another in a closed, fluid-filled system. In the context of controls, oxygen must be provided at the same rate it is consumed to avoid cell apoptosis; medium flow at a suitable rate must be present and often pulsatile to provide nutrients, shear stress, and proper mechanical loading to cell constructs; pH must be balanced in order to main cell homeostasis; heat must be maintained at a normal body temperature of ~37°C (the optimal growth temperature for most mammalian cells); humidity must be maintained at 100% to avoid water evaporation and related changes in medium concentration; and CO_2 concentrations can be heightened to help maintain the proper medium pH (Barron et al. 2003; Christen and Andreou 2007; Lyons and Pandit 2005).

Bioreactor control techniques have existed for a few decades, where early implementations were applied to fermentation bioreactors (Royce 1993; Sonnleitner et al. 1991). These techniques have been extended to tissue bioreactors (Couet and Mantovani 2012; Scutcher 2011), which in large part take advantage of control theory developed for a number of application domains. Bioreactor controls take multiple forms, from easy-to-implement manual/mechanical methods up to complex, adaptive, computer-controlled approaches that utilize real-time feedback. The paragraphs below briefly describe a few of these approaches.

As indicated by the bubble humidifier in Figure 3.3, *humidity control* within an incubator can be relatively straightforward to implement by allowing dry gas to rise through a fluid medium. This is a control system in its most basic form—a simple mechanical process. *Temperature control* as related to incubator/medium temperature is also well known in the bioreactor domain and is often implemented with a proportional-integral-derivative (PID) controller (Christen and Andreou 2007). This type of controller is well suited to parameters such as temperature and fluid level that are likely to change slowly and in small proportion. A PID controller, easily implemented on a microprocessor platform (DeBusschere and Kovacs 2001) or a personal computer (e.g., running LabVIEW [Xicai et al. 2007]), calculates the sum of the present (proportional) error, past (integral) error, and anticipated (derivative) error as they relate to a parameter value versus a targeted set point. The controller then adjusts a control variable (e.g., a heater position control) in an attempt to minimize the total error over time. Sources of information regarding this type of control are numerous. A reasonable summary is included in Astrom and Murray (2008). Other information regarding bioreactor temperature control can be found in Section 4.4 of Najafpour (2015).

Bioreactors employ *pH control* in an effort to maintain a medium pH between approximately 7.2 and 7.4. If the measured pH (see Table 3.1) falls below a prescribed value, the control system initiates the release of, for example, acetic acid, into the medium, whereas if pH is too high, an alkali pump engages—refer to Section 4.6 of Najafpour (2015). pH control can be implemented with an analog controller (Lee et al. 1987), PID controller, or first-order closed-loop control system (Griswold 2004), where the set point is the target pH and the controller drives the acid/base pumps.

Flow control and *mechanical stress/strain control* are a coupled problem. Medium flow can be important for both nutrient delivery and waste removal; yet, any type of flow results in surface shear stress, which can either be healthy for tissue development or result in surface-cell loss if flow rates or eddy currents are excessive. As noted earlier, tissue bioreactor systems also incorporate active flow profiles (steady state, oscillating, or pulsatile flow via a peristaltic pump) as a mean to induce mechanical stress/strain stimuli to tissue constructs and therefore increase their viability. Flow control systems must therefore specify the process for the physical flow profile (e.g., through voltage-level changes as input signals for the peristaltic pump) as well as confirm the amount of resulting flow (or applied stimulus, often via load cells [Popp et al. 2012]) and then offer the data as feedback to the computer that is driving the pump and/or actuator. Such systems can therefore incorporate relatively complicated control schema. For example, Xiang and coworkers designed a dual-frequency mechanical system that relied on the method of friction compensation to deliver linear mechanical loads to cartilage tissue (Xiang et al. 2015). Low-frequency pulsations (0–3 Hz) were designed to mimic human walking, whereas higher frequency pulsations (20–50 Hz) were designed to mimic muscle and ligament loading. This work employed a programmable multi-axis controller with a feed-forward closed loop. Translational controls can also be coupled with rotational controls, as demonstrated by Altman and colleagues in an effort geared toward engineered anterior cruciate ligament (Altman, Lu et al. 2002). Rotational controls are also traditional in the bioreactor domain for controlling the rate of rotating-wall vessels that must vary their rotation speed as a function of tissue construct size (Freed et al. 1997).

Dissolved oxygen control has also received attention in the bioreactor design community for over 20 years (Lee et al. 1991; Najafpour 2015), as this parameter is a direct indicator of nutrient availability to the engineered tissues. Variants of a linear PID controller have been used to regulate dissolved oxygen in stirred-tank bioreactors, where the stirrer speed was the actively controlled element (Akesson and Hagander 1997). Scutcher noted that such PID controllers are adequate when the assumption is that oxygen is the only contributing factor (Scutcher 2011). This tuning can be precise, as demonstrated by Whiffin and colleagues through the design of a "starvation-based" transient controller that tracked dissolved oxygen as a mean to control the delivery of glucose to fed-batch cultures of recombinant *Escherichia coli* (Whiffin, Cooney, and Cord-Ruwisch 2004).

3.6 CONCLUSION AND PERSPECTIVE

This chapter presented an overview and thematic description of various types of bioreactors and the engineered tissues they are designed to support. These systems employ active flow, possibly supplemented with mechanical and/or electrical stimuli to aid tissue growth and increase the viability of the resulting constructs for their intended application environments. This overview was followed by the presentation and description of an aggregate component diagram that can be a suitable means to compare different classes of bioreactor systems. Finally, the chapter provided an overview of the types of environmental and tissue parameters that are tracked with bioreactor-based sensors, followed by an overview of the types of control systems used to stabilize these parameters or drive tissue-development processes. A number of technical papers and reviews are cited in support of this overview.

While advancements in this domain are substantive, future work remains in various areas of bioreactor development. The first broad area of need relates to the real-time tracking and dynamic control of bioreactor parameters and components, including the ability to easily change nutrient delivery profiles and hardware component operations mid-experiment. This relates to what is measured and/or controlled at (1) the vessel (chamber) level (e.g., cell counts, differentiation status, and 3D structure development) using new sensing and imaging techniques, coupled with appropriate software and display support, as well as (2) the system level, which speaks to integrated online sensors for fluid flow/status, valve operation, etc., much the same way as a good vehicle dashboard allows one to view the system status, and ideally history, at a glance.

For example, as a driver for their own work, Xicai et al. note that, "there is no compact measurement system that records a variety of physicochemical parameters (such as pH, dissolved oxygen, tension, nutrient, and metabolite concentrations) simultaneously and in real-time" (Xicai et al. 2008). This is, in part, driven by the need for new types of sensors, as mentioned by Yan and coworkers: "it is also noted that the information (such as oxygen and glucose distribution) provided by model simulation may not be readily accessible using current experimental techniques" (Yan et al. 2012). Similarly, Martin and coworkers note that, "the presence of urea is rarely monitored in reactors, in part because on-line sensors are difficult to find" (Martin and Vermette 2005). Scutcher noted that the inability to monitor cell count online presented a significant obstacle in the ability to design the control system for a vascular bioreactor (Scutcher 2011).

These sensing needs are coupled with mid-experiment control needs in terms of how nutrients are delivered during different phases of the tissue-development process. Xicai et al. state this well when they note that, "in the future, the ability to supply cells with dynamic profiles of nutrients, oxygen and growth factors in an optimal manner" will alter the tissue engineering paradigm for the better (Xicai et al. 2008). Spatial and temporal information regarding the physicochemical well-being of the bioreactor system/medium, coupled with information regarding the development of the related tissue constructs, is an important step to this end. This is consistent with a statement by Scutcher, who noted that, "one key area is how process control can be designed to accommodate changes in cellular metabolic demand as immature cell types differentiate into more mature cell types" (Scutcher 2011).

These sensing and control needs supplement a more common statement of needs that is mentioned more often in the literature and is twofold: (1) the need for bioreactors that support the development of more complicated 3D tissue structures, possibly with layered or encapsulated tissues (Atala et al. 2012; Mikos et al. 2006), coupled with (2) the need for cell and tissue production at a much greater scale in order to create tissue constructs that are clinically useful (Garcia-Ochoa and Gomez 2009; Prenosil and Kino-oka 1999; Tharakan and Chau 1986). Some authors also note the need for portable, small-scale (even implantable) bioreactors that add the mobility goal to the desired set of bioreactor requirements (Christen and Andreou 2007; DeBusschere and Kovacs 2001; Kim et al. 2011).

From a system-design perspective, this research and development community can benefit from modular systems as improvements on current modular approaches (Illa et al. 2014; Lovett et al. 2010; Mazzei et al. 2010; Orr and Burg 2008; Vinci et al. 2011; Vorstius et al. 2011). The following system features apply:

- Interchangeable components designed for rapid system-level reconfiguration: plug-and-play components that can be rapidly reconfigured to create a bioreactor system well matched to the needs of the tissue constructs.
- Bioreactor system components that can be easily altered to support new tissue and sensing needs, including chambers with flexible insertion/extraction ports, adaptability for different types of scaffolds, and support for different types of mechanical or electrical stimuli.
- Proper software/app support, including customizable software interfaces for various component configurations (e.g., as an update to existing LabVIEW VI-based systems [Xicai et al. 2008]). This includes phone- and tablet-level support for personal apps that allow communication with wireless bioreactor components that may, for example, reside in sealed vessels where wired access can be difficult.
- Planning and assembly tools that offer intelligent advice to researchers based on lessons learned, in much the same way that existing board-layout tools aid electrical designers.

Such a toolset will promote the development and use of a variety of unique but robust bioreactor systems, each assembled in a "Lego-like" manner to support the growth and monitoring needs of an increasingly diverse array of cellular constructs.

ACKNOWLEDGMENTS

The author acknowledges Charles Carlson, Electrical Engineering doctoral student at Kansas State University, Manhattan, KS for the solid-model renderings of the bioreactor form factors in Figures 3.1 and 3.3. Appreciation is also offered to Dr. Mark Weiss, Professor, Kansas State University, Department of Anatomy and Physiology for his early feedback on the chapter content as well as the images depicting the commercial bioreactor in Figure 3.2.

REFERENCES

Abousleiman, R. I. and V. I. Sikavitsas. 2006. Bioreactors for tissues of the musculoskeletal system. *Adv Exp Med Biol* 585:243–59.

Ainsworth, B. J. and J. B. Chaudhuri. 2005. Bioreactors for ligament engineering. In *Bioreactors for Tissue Engineering: Principles, Design and Operation*, edited by J. B. Chaudhuri and M. Al-Rubeai, 221–33. Dordrecht, the Netherlands: Springer.

Akesson, M. and P. Hagander. 1997. Control of dissolved oxygen in stirred bioreactors. In. http://citeseerx.ist.psu.edu/index. CiteSeerX. http://citeseerx.ist.psu.edu/viewdoc/citations?doi=10.1.1.488.3657

Al-Mashhadani, M. K. H., S. J. Wilkinson, and W. B. Zimmerman. 2015. Airlift bioreactor for biological applications with microbubble mediated transport processes. *Chem Eng Sci* 137:243–53.

Altman, G. H., H. H. Lu, R. L. Horan, T. Calabro, D. Ryder, D. L. Kaplan, P. Stark, I. Martin, J. C. Richmond, and G. Vunjak-Novakovic. 2002. Advanced bioreactor with controlled application of multi-dimensional strain for tissue engineering. *J Biomech Eng* 124 (6):742–49.

Altman, G. H., R. L. Horan, I. Martin, J. Farhadi, P. R. Stark, V. Volloch, J. C. Richmond, G. Vunjak-Novakovic, and D. L. Kaplan. 2002. Cell differentiation by mechanical stress. *FASEB J* 16 (2):270–72.

Amrollahi, P. and L. Tayebi. 2016. Bioreactors for heart valve tissue engineering: A review. *J Chem Technol Biotechnol* 91 (4):847–56.

Antolli, P. G. and Z. Liu (eds.). 2011. *Bioreactors: Design, Properties and Applications*. https://www.novapublishers.com/catalog/product_info.php?products_id=28585&osCsid=. New York, NY: Nova Science Publishers.

Asnaghi, M. A., T. Smith, I. Martin, and D. Wendt. 2014. Bioreactors: Enabling technologies for research and manufacturing. In *Tissue Engineering*, edited by C. van Blitterswijk and J. De Boer, 393–425. Amsterdam, the Netherlands: Academic Press.

Astrom, K. J. and R. M. Murray. 2008. PID control. In *Feedback Systems: An Introduction for Scientists and Engineers*, edited by K. J. Astrom and R. M. Murray, 293–312. Princeton University Press.

Atala, A., F. K. Kasper, and A. G. Mikos. 2012. Engineering complex tissues. *Sci Transl Med* 4 (160):160rv12.

Bancroft, G. N., V. I. Sikavitsas, and A. G. Mikos. 2003. Design of a flow perfusion bioreactor system for bone tissue-engineering applications. *Tissue Eng* 9 (3):549–54.

Bancroft, G. N., V. I. Sikavitsas, J. van den Dolder, T. L. Sheffield, C. G. Ambrose, J. A. Jansen, and A. G. Mikos. 2002. Fluid flow increases mineralized matrix deposition in 3D perfusion culture of marrow stromal osteoblasts in a dose-dependent manner. *Proc Natl Acad Sci USA* 99 (20):12600–05.

Barron, V., E. Lyons, C. Stenson-Cox, P. E. McHugh, and A. Pandit. 2003. Bioreactors for cardiovascular cell and tissue growth: A review. *Ann Biomed Eng* 31 (9):1017–30.

Bassett, C. A., A. A. Pilla, and R. J. Pawluk. 1977. A non-operative salvage of surgically-resistant pseudarthroses and non-unions by pulsing electromagnetic fields. A preliminary report. *Clin Orthop Relat Res* (124):128–43.

Begley, C. M. and S. J. Kleis. 2002. RWPV bioreactor mass transport: Earth-based and in microgravity. *Biotechnol Bioeng* 80 (4):465–76.

Bilodeau, K. 2004. Bioreactors for tissue engineering: Focus on the mechanical constraints. A comparative review. In *Conception et validation d'un bioreacteur specificque a la regeneration du tissu arteriel sous contrantes mecaniques*, edited by K. Bilodeau, 16–38. Quebec: University of Laval.

Biotechnology, Applikon. 2015. *ez-Control, Total Control at Your Fingertips*. Available from http://www.applikonbio.com/en/products/controllers/ezcontrol

Bjerre, L., C. E. Bunger, M. Kassem, and T. Mygind. 2008. Flow perfusion culture of human mesenchymal stem cells on silicate-substituted tricalcium phosphate scaffolds. *Biomaterials* 29 (17):2616–27.

Blose, K. J., J. T. Krawiec, J. S. Weinbaum, and D. A. Vorp. 2014. Chapter 13—Bioreactors for tissue engineering purposes A2—Orlando, Giuseppe. In *Regenerative Medicine Applications in Organ Transplantation*, edited by J. Lerut, S. Soker and R. J. Stratta, 177–85. Boston, MA: Academic Press.

Buang, F., M. Z. M. Daud, and M. M. Shahimin. 2014. Scaling up adult stem cells for regenerative medicine. Paper presented at Biomedical Engineering and Sciences (IECBES), 2014 IEEE Conference on, Dec. 8–10, 2014, Miri, Malaysia.

Butler, D. L., S. A. Hunter, K. Chokalingam, M. J. Cordray, J. Shearn, N. Juncosa-Melvin, S. Nirmalanandhan, and A. Jain. 2009. Using functional tissue engineering and bioreactors to mechanically stimulate tissue-engineered constructs. *Tissue Eng Part A* 15 (4):741–49.

Carpentier, B., P. Layrolle, and C. Legallais. 2011. Bioreactors for bone tissue engineering. *Int J Artif Organs* 34 (3):259–70.

Cartmell, S. H., B. D. Porter, A. J. Garcia, and R. E. Guldberg. 2003. Effects of medium perfusion rate on cell-seeded three-dimensional bone constructs *in vitro*. *Tissue Eng* 9 (6):1197–203.

Carver, S. E. and C. A. Heath. 1999. Semi-continuous perfusion system for delivering intermittent physiological pressure to regenerating cartilage. *Tissue Eng* 5 (1):1–11.

Catapano, G. and J. C. Gerlach. 2007. Bioreactors for liver tissue engineering. In *Topics in Tissue Engineering*, edited by N. Ashammakhi, R. Reis and E. Chiellini. http://www.oulu.fi/spareparts/ebook_topics_in_t_e_vol3/

Chang, C. H., F. H. Lin, C. C. Lin, C. H. Chou, and H. C. Liu. 2004. Cartilage tissue engineering on the surface of a novel gelatin-calcium-phosphate biphasic scaffold in a double-chamber bioreactor. *J Biomed Mater Res B Appl Biomater* 71 (2):313–21.

Chaudhuri, J. B. and M. Al-Rubeai. 2005. *Bioreactors for Tissue Engineering: Principles, Design and Operation*. Berlin: Springer.

Chen, H. C. and Y. C. Hu. 2006. Bioreactors for tissue engineering. *Biotechnol Lett* 28 (18):1415–23.

Christen, J. B. and A. G. Andreou. 2007. Design, fabrication, and testing of a hybrid CMOS/PDMS microsystem for cell culture and incubation. *IEEE Trans Biomed Circuits Syst* 1 (1):3–18.

Couet, F. and D. Mantovani. 2012. Perspectives on the advanced control of bioreactors for functional vascular tissue engineering *in vitro*. *Expert Rev Med Devices* 9 (3):233–39.

Darling, E. M. and K. A. Athanasiou. 2003. Biomechanical strategies for articular cartilage regeneration. *Ann Biomed Eng* 31 (9):1114–24.

DeBusschere, B. D. and G. T. Kovacs. 2001. Portable cell-based biosensor system using integrated CMOS cell-cartridges. *Biosens Bioelectron* 16 (7–8):543–56.

Divieto, C., L. Revel, G. Sassi, and M. P. Sassi. 2013. Uncertainty analysis of cell counting by metabolic assays. *J Phys: Conf Series* 459 (1):012051.

Dobson, J., S. H. Cartmell, A. Keramane, and A. J. El Haj. 2006. Principles and design of a novel magnetic force mechanical conditioning bioreactor for tissue engineering, stem cell conditioning, and dynamic *in vitro* screening. *IEEE Trans Nanobioscience* 5 (3):173–77.

Eibl, D. and R. Eibl. 2009. Bioreactors for mammalian cells: General overview. In *Cell and Tissue Reaction Engineering*, edited by R. Eibl, D. Eibl, R. Pörtner, G. Catapano and P. Czermak, 55–82. Berlin: Springer-Verlag.

Elder, B. D. and K. A. Athanasiou. 2009. Hydrostatic pressure in articular cartilage tissue engineering: From chondrocytes to tissue regeneration. *Tissue Eng Part B: Rev* 15 (1):43–53.

Eyres, K. S., M. Saleh, and J. A. Kanis. 1996. Effect of pulsed electromagnetic fields on bone formation and bone loss during limb lengthening. *Bone* 18 (6):505–59.

Fassina, L., L. Visai, F. Benazzo, L. Benedetti, A. Calligaro, M. G. De Angelis, A. Farina, V. Maliardi, and G. Magenes. 2006. Effects of electromagnetic stimulation on calcified matrix production by SAOS-2 cells over a polyurethane porous scaffold. *Tissue Eng* 12 (7):1985–99.

Ferrechio, L., J. Skelly, A. Lopez, and J. Thompson. 2009. *Bioreactor Design for Vascular Tissue Engineering*. Worcester, MA: Engineering, Worcester Polytechnic Institute.

Frantz, C., K. M. Stewart, and V. M. Weaver. 2010. The extracellular matrix at a glance. *J Cell Sci* 123 (Pt 24):4195–200.

Freed, L. E., F. Guilak, X. E. Guo, M. L. Gray, R. Tranquillo, J. W. Holmes, M. Radisic, M. V. Sefton, D. Kaplan, and G. Vunjak-Novakovic. 2006. Advanced tools for tissue engineering: Scaffolds, bioreactors, and signaling. *Tissue Eng* 12 (12):3285–305.

Freed, L. E., R. Langer, I. Martin, N. R. Pellis, and G. Vunjak-Novakovic. 1997. Tissue engineering of cartilage in space. *Proc Natl Acad Sci USA* 94 (25):13885–90.

Freed, L. E. and G. Vunjak-Novakovic. 2000. Tissue engineering bioreactors. In *Principles of Tissue Engineering*. 2nd ed, edited by R. P. Lanza, R. Langer and J. Vacanti, 143–15656. San Diego, CA: Academic Press.

Garcia-Ochoa, F. and E. Gomez. 2009. Bioreactor scale-up and oxygen transfer rate in microbial processes: An overview. *Biotechnol Adv* 27 (2):153–76.

Gardel, L. S., L. A. Serra, R. L. Reis, and M. E. Gomes. 2014. Use of perfusion bioreactors and large animal models for long bone tissue engineering. *Tissue Eng Part B: Rev* 20 (2):126–46.

Garvin, J., J. Qi, M. Maloney, and A. J. Banes. 2003. Novel system for engineering bioartificial tendons and application of mechanical load. *Tissue Eng* 9 (5):967–79.

Gaspar, D. A., V. Gomide, and F. J. Monteiro. 2012. The role of perfusion bioreactors in bone tissue engineering. *Biomatter* 2 (4):167–75.

Georgiev, M. I., R. Eibl, and J. J. Zhong. 2013. Hosting the plant cells *in vitro*: Recent trends in bioreactors. *Appl Microbiol Biotechnol* 97 (9):3787–800.

Goldstein, A. S., T. M. Juarez, C. D. Helmke, M. C. Gustin, and A. G. Mikos. 2001. Effect of convection on osteoblastic cell growth and function in biodegradable polymer foam scaffolds. *Biomaterials* 22 (11):1279–88.

Granet, C., N. Laroche, L. Vico, C. Alexandre, and M. H. Lafage-Proust. 1998. Rotating-wall vessels, promising bioreactors for osteoblastic cell culture: Comparison with other 3D conditions. *Med Biol Eng Comput* 36 (4):513–19.

Griswold, A. A. 2004. *pH Control in a Miniaturized Bioreactor.* Cambridge, MA: Mechanical Engineering, Massachusetts Institute of Technology.

Hammond, P. A., D. Ali, and D. R. S. Cumming. 2004. Design of a single-chip pH sensor using a conventional 0.6-um CMOS process. *IEEE Sensors J* 4 (6):706–12.

Haycock, J. W. 2011. *3D Cell Culture: Methods and Protocols*, edited by J. W. Haycock. Humana Press.

Haykal, S., M. Salna, Y. Zhou, P. Marcus, M. Fatehi, G. Frost, T. Machuca, S. O. Hofer, and T. K. Waddell. 2014. Double-chamber rotating bioreactor for dynamic perfusion cell seeding of large-segment tracheal allografts: Comparison to conventional static methods. *Tissue Eng Part C: Methods* 20 (8):681–92.

Helmedag, M. J., S. Weinandy, Y. Marquardt, J. M. Baron, N. Pallua, C. V. Suschek, and S. Jockenhoevel. 2015. The effects of constant flow bioreactor cultivation and keratinocyte seeding densities on prevascularized organotypic skin grafts based on a fibrin scaffold. *Tissue Eng Part A* 21 (1–2):343–52.

Hoenicka, M., L. Wiedemann, T. Puehler, S. Hirt, D. E. Birnbaum, and C. Schmid. 2010. Effects of shear forces and pressure on blood vessel function and metabolism in a perfusion bioreactor. *Ann Biomed Eng* 38 (12):3706–23.

Hoffmann, W., S. Feliciano, I. Martin, M. de Wild, and D. Wendt. 2015. Novel perfused compression bioreactor system as an *in vitro* model to investigate fracture healing. *Front Bioeng Biotechnol* 3:10.

Hofmann, A., L. Konrad, L. Gotzen, H. Printz, A. Ramaswamy, and C. Hofmann. 2003. Bioengineered human bone tissue using autogenous osteoblasts cultured on different biomatrices. *J Biomed Mater Res A* 67 (1):191–9.

Holtorf, H. L., J. A. Jansen, and A. G. Mikos. 2005. Flow perfusion culture induces the osteoblastic differentiation of marrow stroma cell-scaffold constructs in the absence of dexamethasone. *J Biomed Mater Res A* 72 (3):326–34.

Illa, X., S. Vila, J. Yeste, C. Peralta, J. Gracia-Sancho, and R. Villa. 2014. A novel modular bioreactor to *in vitro* study the hepatic sinusoid. *PLoS One* 9 (11):e111864.

Ismadi, M. Z., P. Gupta, A. Fouras, P. Verma, S. Jadhav, J. Bellare, and K. Hourigan. 2014. Flow characterization of a spinner flask for induced pluripotent stem cell culture application. *PLoS One* 9 (10):e106493.

Jacobs, C. R., C. E. Yellowley, B. R. Davis, Z. Zhou, J. M. Cimbala, and H. J. Donahue. 1998. Differential effect of steady versus oscillating flow on bone cells. *J Biomech* 31 (11):969–76.

Janssen, F. W., J. Oostra, Av Oorschot, and C. A. van Blitterswijk. 2006. A perfusion bioreactor system capable of producing clinically relevant volumes of tissue-engineered bone: *In vivo* bone formation showing proof of concept. *Biomaterials* 27 (3):315–23.

Jeong, C., H. Y. Chung, H. J. Lim, J. W. Lee, K. Y. Choi, J. D. Yang, B. C. Cho, J. O. Lim, J. J. Yoo, S. J. Lee, and A. J. Atala. 2014. Applicability and safety of *in vitro* skin expansion using a skin bioreactor: A clinical trial. *Arch Plast Surg* 41 (6):661–7.

Kasper, C., M. van Griensven, and R. Portner. 2009. Bioreactor systems for tissue engineering. In *Advances in Biochemical Engineering/Biotechnology*, edited by T. Scheper, S. Belkin, T. Bley, J. Bohlmann, P. M. Doran, M. B. Gu, W.-S. Hu, B. Mattiasson, J. Nielsen, H. Seitz, R. Ulber, A.-P. Zeng, J.-J. Zhong and W. Zhou. Berlin: Springer-Verlag.

Kasper, C., M. van Griensven, and R. Portner. 2010. Bioreactor systems for tissue engineering II. In *Advances in Biochemical Engineering/Biotechnology*, edited by T. Scheper, S. Belkin, T. Bley, J. Bohlmann, P. M. Doran, M. B. Gu, W.-S. Hu et al. Vol. 123, Berlin: Springer-Verlag.

Kim, I. S., T. H. Lee, Y. M. Song, I. S. Kim, T. H. Cho, S. J. Hwang, and I. S. Kim. 2011. An implantable electrical bioreactor for enhancement of cell viability. Paper presented at 2011 Annual Intl Conf of the IEEE Engineering in Medicine and Biology Society, Aug 30, 2011–Sept. 3, 2011.

Kim, S. S., R. Penkala, and P. Abrahimi. 2007. A perfusion bioreactor for intestinal tissue engineering. *J Surg Res* 142 (2):327–31.

Korossis, S. A., F. Bolland, J. N. Kearney, J. Fisher, and E. Ingham. 2005. Bioreactors in tissue engineering. In *Topics in Tissue Engineering*, edited by N. Ashammakhi and R. L. Reis, 1–23. http://www.oulu.fi/spareparts/ebook_topics_in_t_e_vol2/

Laurent, P. C., C. Vaquette, C. Martin, E. Guedon, X. Wu, A. Delconte, D. Dumas, S. Hupont, D. N. Isla, R. Rahouadj, and X. Wang. 2014. Towards a tissue-engineered ligament: Design and preliminary evaluation of a dedicated multi-chamber tension-torsion bioreactor. *Processes* 2 (1):167–79.

Lee, S. C., Y. B. Hwang, H. N. Chang, and Y. K. Chang. 1991. Adaptive control of dissolved oxygen concentration in a bioreactor. *Biotechnol Bioeng* 37 (7):597–607.

Lee, Y. H., M. Takashima, and R. E. Speece. 1987. Microcomputer pH control of multiple bioreactors. *Biotechnol Bioeng* 30 (2):329–30.

Lei, X. H., L. N. Ning, Y. J. Cao, S. Liu, S. B. Zhang, Z. F. Qiu, H. M. Hu, H. S. Zhang, S. Liu, and E. K. Duan. 2011. NASA-approved rotary bioreactor enhances proliferation of human epidermal stem cells and supports formation of 3D epidermis-like structure. *PLoS One* 6 (11):e26603.

Liao, I. C., J. B. Liu, N. Bursac, and K. W. Leong. 2008. Effect of electromechanical stimulation on the maturation of myotubes on aligned electrospun fibers. *Cell Mol Bioeng* 1 (2–3):133–45.

Lovett, M., D. Rockwood, A. Baryshyan, and D. L. Kaplan. 2010. Simple modular bioreactors for tissue engineering: A system for characterization of oxygen gradients, human mesenchymal stem cell differentiation, and prevascularization. *Tissue Eng Part C: Methods* 16 (6):1565–73.

Lyons, E. J. and A. Pandit. 2005. Design of bioreactors for cardiovascular applications. In *Topics in Tissue Engineering*, edited by N. Ashammakhi and R. L. Reis. Galway, Ireland: Department of Mechanical and Biomedical Engineering, National Centre for Biomedical Engineering Science, National University of Ireland.

Martin, I., D. Wendt, and M. Heberer. 2004. The role of bioreactors in tissue engineering. *Trends Biotechnol* 22 (2):80–86.

Martin, Y. and P. Vermette. 2005. Bioreactors for tissue mass culture: Design, characterization, and recent advances. *Biomaterials* 26 (35):7481–503.

Mauck, R. L., M. A. Soltz, C. C. Wang, D. D. Wong, P. H. Chao, W. B. Valhmu, C. T. Hung, and G. A. Ateshian. 2000. Functional tissue engineering of articular cartilage through dynamic loading of chondrocyte-seeded agarose gels. *J Biomech Eng* 122 (3):252–60.

Mazzei, D., M. A. Guzzardi, S. Giusti, and A. Ahluwalia. 2010. A low shear stress modular bioreactor for connected cell culture under high flow rates. *Biotechnol Bioeng* 106 (1):127–37.

Mazzei, D., F. Vozzi, A. Cisternino, F. Vozzi, and A. Ahluwalia. 2008. A high-throughput bioreactor system for simulating physiological environments. *IEEE Trans Ind Electron* 55 (9):3273–80.

Mikos, A. G., S. W. Herring, P. Ochareon, J. Elisseeff, H. H. Lu, R. Kandel, F. J. Schoen, M. Toner, D. Mooney, A. Atala, M. E. Van Dyke, D. Kaplan, and G. Vunjak-Novakovic. 2006. Engineering complex tissues. *Tissue Eng* 12 (12):3307–39.

Millipore, EMD. 2016. *Mobius 3L Single-Use Bioreactor.* Available from https://www.emdmillipore.com/US/en/product/Mobius-3L-Single-use-Bioreactor,MM_NF-C84539

Najafpour, G. D. 2015. *Biochemical Engineering and Biotechnology.* 2nd ed. Amsterdam, the Netherlands: Elsevier.

Nesic, D., R. Whiteside, M. Brittberg, D. Wendt, I. Martin, and P. Mainil-Varlet. 2006. Cartilage tissue engineering for degenerative joint disease. *Adv Drug Deliv Rev* 58 (2):300–22.

Niklason, L. E., J. Gao, W. M. Abbott, K. K. Hirschi, S. Houser, R. Marini, and R. Langer. 1999. Functional arteries grown *in vitro*. *Science* 284 (5413):489–93.

Orr, D. E. and K. J. Burg. 2008. Design of a modular bioreactor to incorporate both perfusion flow and hydrostatic compression for tissue engineering applications. *Ann Biomed Eng* 36 (7):1228–41.

Partap, S., N. A. Plunkett, and F. J. O'Brien. 2010. Bioreactors in tissue engineering. In *Tissue Engineering*, edited by D. Eberli, http://www.intechopen.com/books/tissue-engineering/bioreactors-in-tissue-engineering

Plunkett, N. and F. J. O'Brien. 2010. Bioreactors in tissue engineering. *Stud Health Technol Inform* 152:214–30.

Popp, J. R., J. J. Roberts, D. V. Gallagher, K. S. Anseth, S. J. Bryant, and T. P. Quinn. 2012. An instrumented bioreactor for mechanical stimulation and real-time, nondestructive evaluation of engineered cartilage tissue. *J Med Devices* 6 (2):21006.

Pörtner, R. and C. Giese. 2006. An overview on bioreactor design, prototyping and process control for reproducible three-dimensional tissue culture. In *Drug Testing in Vitro*, 53–78. Berlin: Wiley-VCH Verlag GmbH & Co. KGaA.

Pörtner, R., S. Nagel-Heyer, C. Goepfert, P. Adamietz, and N. M. Meenen. 2005. Bioreactor design for tissue engineering. *J Biosci Bioeng* 100 (3):235–45.

Prenosil, J. E. and M. Kino-oka. 1999. Computer controlled bioreactor for large-scale production of cultured skin grafts. *Ann N Y Acad Sci* 875:386–97.

Radisic, M., A. Marsano, R. Maidhof, Y. Wang, and G. Vunjak-Novakovic. 2008. Cardiac tissue engineering using perfusion bioreactor systems. *Nat Protoc* 3 (4):719–38.

Radtke, A. L. and M. M. Herbst-Kralovetz. 2012. Culturing and applications of rotating wall vessel bioreactor derived 3D epithelial cell models. *J Vis Exp* 3 (62): pii 3868.

Ramaswamy, S., S. M. Boronyak, T. Le, A. Holmes, F. Sotiropoulos, and M. S. Sacks. 2014. A novel bioreactor for mechanobiological studies of engineered heart valve tissue formation under pulmonary arterial physiological flow conditions. *J Biomech Eng* 136 (12):121009.

Rauh, J., F. Milan, K. P. Gunther, and M. Stiehler. 2011. Bioreactor systems for bone tissue engineering. *Tissue Eng Part B: Rev* 17 (4):263–80.

Riehl, B. D., J. H. Park, I. K. Kwon, and J. Y. Lim. 2012. Mechanical stretching for tissue engineering: Two-dimensional and three-dimensional constructs. *Tissue Eng Part B: Rev* 18 (4):288–300.

Rolfe, P. 2006. Sensing in tissue bioreactors. *Measurement Sci. Technol* 17 (3):578.

Royce, P. N. 1993. A discussion of recent developments in fermentation monitoring and control from a practical perspective. *Crit Rev Biotechnol* 13 (2):117–49.

Sailon, A. M., A. C. Allori, E. H. Davidson, D. D. Reformat, R. J. Allen, and S. M. Warren. 2009. A novel flow-perfusion bioreactor supports 3D dynamic cell culture. *J Biomed Biotechnol* 2009:873816.

Salehi-Nik, N., G. Amoabediny, B. Pouran, H. Tabesh, M. A. Shokrgozar, N. Haghighipour, N. Khatibi, F. Anisi, K. Mottaghy, and B. Zandieh-Doulabi. 2013. Engineering parameters in bioreactor's design: A critical aspect in tissue engineering. *Biomed Res Int* 2013:762132.

Sanford, G. L., D. Ellerson, C. Melhado-Gardner, A. E. Sroufe, and S. Harris-Hooker. 2002. Three-dimensional growth of endothelial cells in the microgravity-based rotating wall vessel bioreactor. *In Vitro Cell Dev Biol Anim* 38 (9):493–504.

Schwarz, R. P., T. J. Goodwin, and D. A. Wolf. 1992. Cell culture for three-dimensional modeling in rotating-wall vessels: An application of simulated microgravity. *J Tissue Cult Methods* 14 (2):51–57.

Scutcher, M. W. 2011. *Modelling and development of process control for a vascular tissue engineering bioreactor.* PhD Thesis, University College London.

Shachar, M. and S. Cohen. 2003. Cardiac tissue engineering, ex-vivo: Design principles in biomaterials and bioreactors. *Heart Fail Rev* 8 (3):271–76.

Singh, H., E. S. Ang, T. T. Lim, and D. W. Hutmacher. 2007. Flow modeling in a novel non-perfusion conical bioreactor. *Biotechnol Bioeng* 97 (5):1291–99.

Sladkova, M. and M. G. de Peppo. 2014. Bioreactor systems for human bone tissue engineering. *Processes* 2 (2): 494–525.

Sonnleitner, B., G. Locher, and A. Fiechter. 1991. Automatic bioprocess control. 1. A general concept. *J Biotechnol* 19 (1):1–17.

Sucosky, P., D. F. Osorio, J. B. Brown, and G. P. Neitzel. 2004. Fluid mechanics of a spinner-flask bioreactor. *Biotechnol Bioeng* 85 (1):34–46.

Tandon, N., A. Marsano, C. Cannizzaro, J. Voldman, and G. Vunjak-Novakovic. 2008. Design of electrical stimulation bioreactors for cardiac tissue engineering. *Conf Proc IEEE Eng Med Biol Soc* 2008:3594–97.

Tandon, N., A. Marsano, R. Maidhof, L. Wan, H. Park, and G. Vunjak-Novakovic. 2011. Optimization of electrical stimulation parameters for cardiac tissue engineering. *J Tissue Eng Regen Med* 5 (6):e115–25.

Tandon, N., A. Taubman, E. Cimetta, L. Saccenti, and G. Vunjak-Novakovic. 2013. Portable bioreactor for perfusion and electrical stimulation of engineered cardiac tissue. *Conf Proc IEEE Eng Med Biol Soc* 2013:6219–23.

Tharakan, J. P. and P. C. Chau. 1986. A radial flow hollow fiber bioreactor for the large-scale culture of mammalian cells. *Biotechnol Bioeng* 28 (3):329–42.

Vinci, B., C. Duret, S. Klieber, S. Gerbal-Chaloin, A. Sa-Cunha, S. Laporte, B. Suc, P. Maurel, A. Ahluwalia, and M. Daujat-Chavanieu. 2011. Modular bioreactor for primary human hepatocyte culture: Medium flow stimulates expression and activity of detoxification genes. *Biotechnol J* 6 (5):554–64.

Vorstius, J. B., M. Kohlmann, R. Zhou, Y. Xu, and R. Keatch. 2011. Novel modular and perfused bioreactor for tissue engineering. Paper presented at 4th Intl Conf on Biomedical Engineering and Informatics (BMEI), Oct. 15–17, 2011, Shanghai, China.

Vunjak-Novakovic, G., K. O. Lui, N. Tandon, and K. R. Chien. 2011. Bioengineering heart muscle: A paradigm for regenerative medicine. *Annu Rev Biomed Eng* 13:245–67.

Wang, S. S. and T. A. Good. 2001. Effect of culture in a rotating wall bioreactor on the physiology of differentiated neuron-like PC12 and SH-SY5Y cells. *J Cell Biochem* 83 (4):574–84.

Wang, T., B. S. Gardiner, Z. Lin, J. Rubenson, T. B. Kirk, A. Wang, J. Xu, D. W. Smith, D. G. Lloyd, and M. H. Zheng. 2013. Bioreactor design for tendon/ligament engineering. *Tissue Eng Part B: Rev* 19 (2):133–46.

Watanabe, S., S. Inagaki, I. Kinouchi, H. Takai, Y. Masuda, and S. Mizuno. 2005. Hydrostatic pressure/perfusion culture system designed and validated for engineering tissue. *J Biosci Bioeng* 100 (1):105–11.

Wendt, D., M. Jakob, and I. Martin. 2005. Bioreactor-based engineering of osteochondral grafts: From model systems to tissue manufacturing. *J Biosci Bioeng* 100 (5):489–94.

Wendt, D., N. Timmins, J. Malda, F. Janssen, A. Ratcliffe, G. Vunjak-Novakovic, and I. Martin. 2008. Bioreactors for tissue engineering. In *Tissue Engineering*, 483–506. Burlington, VM: Academic Press.

Whiffin, V. S., M. J. Cooney, and R. Cord-Ruwisch. 2004. Online detection of feed demand in high cell density cultures of *Escherichia coli* by measurement of changes in dissolved oxygen transients in complex media. *Biotechnol Bioeng* 85 (4):422–33.

Williams, C. 2003. *Perfusion bioreactor for tissue-engineered blood vessels.* Tech Thesis, Bioengineering, Georgia Institute of Technology.

Wu, J., M. R. Rostami, D. P. Cadavid Olaya, and E. S. Tzanakakis. 2014. Oxygen transport and stem cell aggregation in stirred-suspension bioreactor cultures. *PLoS One* 9 (7):e102486.

Xiang, P. A., S. Wang, C. Zhang, X. Li, and J. Liu. 2015. Design of dual-frequency bioreactor control system. Paper presented at 2015 IEEE Intl Conf. on Mechatronics and Automation (ICMA), Aug. 2–5, 2015, Beijing, China.

Xicai, Y., E. M. Drakakis, M. Lim, A. Radomska, Ye Hua, A. Mantalaris, N. Panoskaltsis, and A. Cass. 2008. A real-time multi-channel monitoring system for stem cell culture process. *IEEE Trans Biomed Circuits Syst* 2 (2):66–77.

Xicai, Y., E. M. Drakakis, H. Ye, M. Lim, A. Mantalaris, N. Panoskaltsis, A. Radomska, C. Toumazou, and T. Cass. 2007. An on-line, multi-parametric, multi-channel physicochemical monitoring platform for stem cell culture bioprocessing. Paper presented at 2007 IEEE Intl Symp on Circuits and Systems, May 27–30, 2007, New Orleans, LA.

Xu, X., S. Smith, J. Urban, and Z. Cui. 2006. An in line non-invasive optical system to monitor pH in cell and tissue culture. *Med Eng Phys* 28 (5):468–74.

Xu, Y., J. Sun, G. Mathew, A. S. Jeevarajan, and M. M. Anderson. 2004. Continuous glucose monitoring and control in a rotating wall perfused bioreactor. *Biotechnol Bioeng* 87 (4):473–77.

Yan, X., D. J. Bergstrom, and X. B. Chen. 2012. Modeling of cell cultures in perfusion bioreactors. *IEEE Trans Biomed Eng* 59 (9):2568–75.

Yeatts, A. B. and J. P. Fisher. 2011. Bone tissue engineering bioreactors: Dynamic culture and the influence of shear stress. *Bone* 48 (2):171–81.

Yuk, I. H., D. Baskar, P. H. Duffy, J. Hsiung, S. Leung, and A. A. Lin. 2011. Overcoming challenges in WAVE Bioreactors without feedback controls for pH and dissolved oxygen. *Biotechnol Prog* 27 (5):1397–406.

4 Control of 3D Environment

Redesign of the Flow Loop Bioreactor to Control Mitral Valve Regurgitation

Patrick S. Connell, Dragoslava P. Vekilov, and K. Jane Grande-Allen

CONTENTS

4.1	Introduction	62
4.2	Original System and Need for Modification	62
	4.2.1 Creation of System	62
	4.2.2 Increasing Regurgitation Over Time	63
4.3	Nonsterile Systems to Control Papillary Muscle Geometry	64
4.4	RUFLS Redesign	66
	4.4.1 Original Papillary Muscle Geometric Control	66
	4.4.2 Success and Design Criteria	68
	4.4.2.1 Control Papillary Muscle Position	68
	4.4.2.2 Maintain Sterility	69
	4.4.2.3 Maximize Modularity	69
	4.4.2.4 Limit Changes to Mitral Valve Holder	69
	4.4.3 New Mitral Valve Holder	69
	4.4.3.1 Network of Holes Method	69
	4.4.3.2 Slot and Screw Method	70
	4.4.4 New Papillary Muscle Holders	71
	4.4.4.1 Sawtooth-Clamping System	71
	4.4.4.2 Platform System	71
4.5	Findings: Models and Consistent Regurgitation	72
4.6	Conclusion and Perspective	72
Acknowledgments		73
References		73

4.1 INTRODUCTION

The Rice University Flow Loop System (RUFLS) is a sterile flow loop bioreactor that is capable of long-term culture of intact porcine mitral valves (MVs). It is capable of physiologic pressures (up to 150 mmHg systolic pressure), physiologically relevant pressure waveforms (high pressure [120–150 mmHg] systole, low pressure [~20 mmHg] diastole, systole 1/3 length of total cardiac cycle), and near- physiological flow (3 L/min). This chapter will offer an insight into a particular modification of the design of RUFLS to incorporate three-dimensional (3D) control of the papillary muscles (PMs) of the MV within the system for the purposes of regulating the degree of mitral regurgitation, which was not possible with the original design.

4.2 ORIGINAL SYSTEM AND NEED FOR MODIFICATION

4.2.1 CREATION OF SYSTEM

The flow loop system consists of three main chambers (left ventricle, compliance, reservoir) connected by tubing (Figure 4.1). The compliance (CC) and reservoir chambers (RC) are positioned so that they are elevated above the left ventricular chamber (LVC). The LVC is divided into two compartments using a silicone rubber membrane. The air side of the membrane is connected to a piezoelectric pressure regulator, which produces a pressure waveform resulting in a high-pressure systolic pumping phase within the LVC, and to a pressure sensor used to measure pressure within the chamber. The medium side of the chamber houses the intact porcine MV within the MV holder and a mechanical aortic valve (AV) in the AV port. During systole, the medium flows out the AV port, prevented from backflow regurgitation by

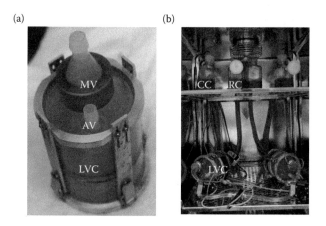

FIGURE 4.1 Rice University Flow Loop System (RUFLS). (a) The left ventricular chamber (LVC) consists of a fluid chamber (top) and an air chamber (bottom), which are separated by a membrane. The membrane moves in response to the pressure waveform produced by a piezoelectric pressure regulator to create a mock cardiac cycle. The LVC includes a mechanical aortic valve (AV) port and a mitral valve (MV) port. (b) RUFLS consists of three chambers: The LVC, the compliance chamber (CC), and the reservoir chamber (RC).

an intact, nonregurgitant MV, and through tubing up to the elevated CC. There, the pressure waveform is dampened, and then the medium flows to the RC that contains a filtered air port to facilitate air exchange. The medium then flows down, via gravity, from the RC through tubing into the LVC by way of the MV holder. To measure the bi-directional flow within the system, an ultrasonic flow probe is clamped onto the tube connecting the RC to the MV holder, just proximal to the MV holder.

The original bioreactor design concentrated on several design factors (Gheewala and Grande-Allen 2010). First, a sterile design was required, which necessitated that the system be self-contained with no media or air leaks. It also required that all materials be capable of repeated sterilization cycles, preferably using an autoclave. In order to minimize damage to the tissue and cell death in the harvesting process, the system was designed for quick assembly. Additionally, in order to facilitate long-term culture, the system was sized to fit within the confines of a standard tissue-culture incubator. Finally, the system was designed and modified to produce physiological pressures and flows, including a high-pressure systole and low-pressure diastole within the system. During preliminary studies of tissue culture within the system, sterility and pH of media were maintained throughout the culture period.

Valves cultured in the system for three weeks ($n = 5$) were compared to fresh tissue ($n = 7$) and static controls ($n = 7$). Static controls were valves grown submerged in media for three weeks without any mechanical stimulation. Statistical analysis was performed on leaflets from each culture condition using a two-way analysis of variances (ANOVA). Dynamic controls were statistically more similar to the fresh tissue than were static controls in terms of tissue hydration ($p < 0.03$ static vs. fresh and dynamic), DNA content ($p < 0.0001$ static vs. fresh and dynamic), and proliferating cell nuclear antigen staining ($p < 0.04$ static vs. fresh) (Gheewala et al. 2013). Although the groups did not show significant differences in their tensile modulus, the static controls trended toward lower moduli compared to the dynamically cultured valves ($p = 0.0976$). The ability to maintain cellularity and mechanical integrity of the dynamically cultured tissues provided evidence that organ culture studies of the MV were viable and that RUFLS had achieved its major design goals.

4.2.2 INCREASING REGURGITATION OVER TIME

One of the disappointing findings of the original RUFLS experiments was the gradual development of regurgitation over time within the system (Figure 4.2). Despite initial regurgitation values consistent with levels of regurgitation that would be considered low to insignificant in a clinical setting, the system would develop regurgitation consistent with moderate–to-severe clinical regurgitation over the three-week culture duration. There was a concern that the altered mechanics and hemodynamics induced by this increasing regurgitation were contributing to aberrant remodeling seen in the original studies of RUFLS, in which some differences were observed between fresh and dynamically cultured tissues. If this were the case, this regurgitation would have to be corrected to ensure that there were not inherent shortcomings to culturing valves in RUFLS. We hypothesized that this increased regurgitation was

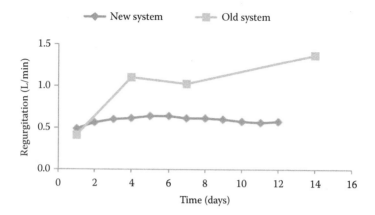

FIGURE 4.2 Representative trials showing the development of regurgitation over time in the old system vs. the new system. In the old system, regurgitation gradually increased over the two-week culture. The new system is able to successfully culture valves for up to two weeks while maintaining regurgitation below 600 mL/min.

the result of imprecise control of PM positioning. This hypothesis was supported by various literature reports that examined the effects of regurgitation on valve movement and forces experienced by the valve throughout the cardiac cycle, normally in the context of the altered PM geometry.

4.3 NONSTERILE SYSTEMS TO CONTROL PAPILLARY MUSCLE GEOMETRY

Pathologic conditions that alter the geometry of the left ventricle often result in changes in the PM positioning relative to the MV annulus. Altered displacement of the PM, either toward or away from the annulus, changes the tension experienced by the chordae tendineae, which in turn affects the leaflets' ability to coapt properly and leads to mitral regurgitation (Jimenez et al. 2005b). Because PM position plays such an important role in proper valve function, nonsterile bioreactors have been built to elucidate the effect of PM displacement on mitral disease progression. These *in vitro* studies allow the complex analysis of individual valvular components, as well as a comprehensive understanding of the MV structure and function in normal and diseased states. Published reports of these nonsterile bioreactors and their mechanisms of PM control were highly influential in guiding the development of an improved means of controlling PM position within RUFLS.

The research group of Dr. Ajit Yoganathan at the Georgia Institute of Technology has a long history of using such *in vitro* setups to study the MV geometry and function in a finely controlled environment. For example, they employed an *in vitro* left ventricle flexible bag model to demonstrate that mitral PM displacement and annular dilation can create moderate to severe mitral regurgitation by preventing proper leaflet coaptation (He et al. 2003). To create a system capable of manipulating these structures and elucidating the effects of these manipulations on the overall valve structure and function, they developed the Georgia Tech Left Heart Simulator that accurately mimics physiological and pathophysiological flow and pressure waveforms and allows control of annular size (normal, dilated) and shape (flat, saddle), along with PM position (Jimenez et al. 2003, 2005b). The Left Heart Simulator was constructed to allow measurements of various parameters, such as the force on chordae and valvular fluid flow, on a single valve (Nielsen et al. 1999; Rabbah et al. 2013). In addition, the system was designed to be compatible with multiple imaging modalities, including echocardiography, microcomputed tomography, and digital particle image velocimetry (Jimenez et al. 2003; Rabbah et al. 2013). These technologies enable the monitoring of hemodynamics and tissue deformation such that they can be correlated for in-depth biomechanical analyses. This nonsterile bioreactor has been used to elucidate MV mechanics and behavior, as well as to validate existing computational models of valve function and biomechanics.

The Left Heart Simulator contains an intricate system to allow precise PM positioning (Jimenez et al. 2003, 2005a). After dissecting the MV, chordae tendineae, and PMs from a porcine, ovine, or human heart, the PMs are wrapped in Dacron cloth and sutured onto holding disks (Jimenez et al. 2003). These holding disks are then attached to force rods that allow the total force applied to each PM to be measured in order to determine their appropriate position in physiological and pathophysiological states (Jensen et al. 2001; Jimenez et al. 2003). A series of alignments take place in order to ensure accurate PM positioning: first in the medial–lateral position, then in the anterior–posterior plane, and then in the basal–apical position (Jimenez et al. 2003, 2005a). This alignment recreates the native geometry of the valve so that there is neither slack nor tension in the chordae. The PM positioning can also be altered along any of the three axes in order to mimic pathological conditions and analyze the effects on other valve components. One study found that the apical displacement of the PM creates tension on the strut chordae and results in leaflet tenting, as is often seen in functional mitral regurgitation (MR) (Jimenez et al. 2005a). In addition, displacing the PM apically, laterally, and posteriorly and measuring the distribution of chordal force at different locations unveiled that strut and basal chordae that insert closer to the annulus show a greater response to PM displacement than marginal chordae that insert near the free edge. Another study revealed that PM displacement and annular dilation drastically increase regurgitant fraction (He et al. 1997). Decreasing transmitral pressure also contributes to greater regurgitation by altering the force exerted on the leaflets during ventricular contraction. The Left Heart Simulator has been vital in broadening our understanding of MV structure and mechanics.

Other research groups have also sought to engineer systems for the *in vitro* study of MV characteristics and disease. Dr. Stephen Little's team at Houston Methodist Hospital has created a nonsterile flow-loop model containing a main circulatory loop with variable compliance and resistance and a regurgitation limb branching off the circulatory loop that includes an ultrasound imaging chamber (Little et al. 2008; Quaini et al. 2011). The circulatory loop is capable of creating a physiologically-relevant hemodynamic environment that mimics that observed in clinical MR. The main feature of interest is the ultrasound imaging chamber that enables the acquisition of high-quality two-dimensional (2D) and three-dimensional (3D) Doppler echocardiography of the MV in order to assess regurgitant flow and volume. The Little group has used the flow loop system to validate the 3D color Doppler proximal isovelocity surface area (PISA) as a more precise method for estimating regurgitant volume, compared to 2D PISA (Little et al. 2007). In addition, it has been used to validate computational fluid dynamics models of MV regurgitation (Quaini et al. 2011). Together, these studies both confirm and add clarity to measurement and diagnosis tools used to analyze MV disease in clinical settings.

While these nonsterile systems have been critical in understanding MV mechanics and flow patterns in response to altered PM positioning, their greatest limitation is their inability to incorporate the analysis of biological parameters into their studies. The sterile environment of RUFLS offers a means by which to overcome this limitation.

4.4 RUFLS REDESIGN

In order to expand on the preliminary work conducted using RUFLS, we needed to improve the system in two major ways. First, we needed to establish a mechanism by which we could reliably create nonregurgitant organ cultured valves to serve as normal controls for future *in vitro* models of MV disease. Without a reliable means of controlling the PM position to ensure nonregurgitant hemodynamics, any result obtained through the manipulation of hemodynamics using RUFLS would be confounded by the effects of culturing control valves in regurgitant conditions. Second, we needed to achieve this through a mechanism conducive to further manipulation of valves within RUFLS. Such a mechanism would facilitate the types of manipulations on valves that would allow us to study the effects of different hemodynamic variations on valve remodeling.

By successfully achieving these two goals, RUFLS would be improved in a manner that would take advantage of the two most promising features of the system: First, the successful recreation of physiological pressures within a sterile valve culture system, and second, the ability to manipulate the system conditions in a highly controlled manner. Such a system would allow us to explore the response of valve cells and tissues to mechanical manipulations over a long time frame. This redesigned system would improve on the current *in vitro* culture technology in that it would incorporate elements of physiologic mechanical stimulation. Furthermore, this system would improve on current *in vitro* nonsterile flow loops by allowing the examination of the biological, in addition to mechanical, response of the valve to altered mechanics.

4.4.1 ORIGINAL PAPILLARY MUSCLE GEOMETRIC CONTROL

In the original version of RUFLS, the PMs were encased within metal coils that were restrained by metal wires within an MV holder (Figure 4.3a and b). The loosely constructed nature of the coil allowed the easy placement of the intact PM within its interior, whereas the metal rods enabled the placement of the PMs within various sets of holes drilled into the base of the MV holder to maintain the appropriate length of chordae within the culture system (Figure 4.4a). Despite the simplicity of this original

Control of 3D Environment

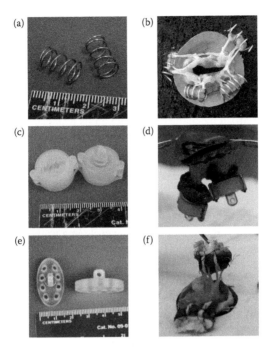

FIGURE 4.3 Evolution of papillary muscle holders. (a) The original RUFLS used metal coils to encase the PMs. (b) The PMs metal coils were wrapped around the PMs. (Reprinted from previous publication (Gheewala et al. 2013), Copyright © Biomedical Engineering Society 2010, with permission of Springer.) (c) A later iteration of the PM holders used a sawtooth-clamping system and introduced an eyehook to allow proper positioning within the MV holder. (d) The sawtooth system pierced the muscles to hold them in place. Suture on the anterior and posterior ends of the sawtooth helped keep the clamps in place. (e) The new PM holders consist of a platform with eight holes and an eyehook. (f) The PM holders are held in place using the umbilical tape and suture.

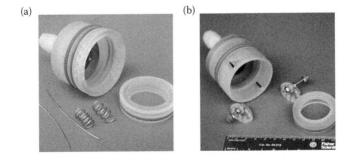

FIGURE 4.4 Evolution of the MV holder. (a) The original RUFLS encased PMs within a metal spring-like coil. The coil was then placed on metal rods and positioned in a set of discrete holes in the MV holder to maintain the appropriate geometry. (b) The new RUFLS held PMs in place with a system of screws and nuts. The discrete holes in the MV holder were replaced with long holes for the insertion of the screws to allow movement along the apical–basal axis. The screws and nuts allowed movement along the medial–lateral axis.

design, it had a number of flaws. First, the rods used to place the PMs were not stiff enough to prevent PM movement during systole. Due to PM contraction, the PMs normally change position relative to the native valve during the cardiac cycle. In healthy individuals, the tops of the PMs move away from the annulus, as opposed to the original culture system in which they moved toward the annulus. In lieu of an active contraction mechanism to oppose the forces of systole (which remains a challenge within a sterile system), a mechanism that maintains a stable position during systole would be preferable. In addition to allowing PM movement in the basal–apical direction through the cardiac cycle, the PM coils in the original design were not affixed to the metal rods that held the PMs in place. This arrangement allowed for the movement of the PMs in the medial–lateral direction as the rod would move freely within the coil, and in the anterior–posterior direction as the coil could slide freely along the rod. This lack of precise control of PM position made it difficult to recapitulate the natural valve geometry throughout the cardiac cycle in a way that mimicked the pre-dissection geometry within the heart in a reproducible manner.

Furthermore, the reliance on discrete holes in the side of the MV holder made it impossible to accommodate the continuous apical distances present throughout natural physiological variation of our valves. Correctly positioning the PMs in relation to the valve is vitally important to maintain nonregurgitant flow and normal forces on valve tissues. In addition, the range of apical distances available in the original design was inadequate for appropriate PM placement based on the PM distances measured in porcine hearts prior to valve dissection.

4.4.2 Success and Design Criteria

In order to address these limitations of the original system, several aspects of RUFLS were redesigned. The primary success criteria for the redesign was the ability to culture intact MVs for 2 weeks with less than 600 mL/min of regurgitation, a criterion that would serve as a control for future valve studies in RUFLS. This criterion is based on the regurgitant fraction of total volume considered to be the threshold between mild and moderate regurgitation clinically. Based on our observation of valves in the original RUFLS systems and the previous literature exploring the mechanical effects of PM manipulation on valve motion and forces (He et al. 1997), we hypothesized that the largest barrier to success for achieving this criterion was the relative lack of control of PM positioning within our system. We therefore considered four major design criteria in exploring the improvements to our bioreactor system.

The redesign of RUFLS was undertaken as a two-part process: the redesign of the MV holder to better secure the PM holder to the MV holder for control over the geometric position of the PMs in space, and the redesign of the PM holders to better secure the PM to the positioning mechanism without damaging the muscle.

4.4.2.1 Control Papillary Muscle Position

The redesigned system needed to be able to provide independent control of each PM in all three dimensions (apical–basal, medial–lateral, and anterior–posterior) in a continuous manner. This control was required so that both native healthy and diseased valve geometry could be reproduced within RUFLS.

Control of 3D Environment

4.4.2.2 Maintain Sterility

Any adjustments to RUFLS needed to maintain the consistent sterility of the existing system. This constraint necessitated avoiding any reliance on positioning mechanisms exterior to the existing LVC, which could potentially lead to media or air leaks and contamination. In addition, it mandated that all new components were autoclave, or otherwise sterilization, compatible.

4.4.2.3 Maximize Modularity

The constraints associated with the sterile conditions of RUFLS also made it difficult to visualize the valve motion within the system. Therefore, in order to confirm proper valve motion and hemodynamics within RUFLS, we used the imaging flow loop system (described above) of our collaborator, Dr. Stephen Little. This collaboration required that the design of the new PM control mechanism for RUFLS be simple enough and compatible with the nonsterile flow loop system in order to accurately reproduce the geometry of RUFLS.

4.4.2.4 Limit Changes to Mitral Valve Holder

In order to (1) limit the cost of the redesign, (2) maintain the advantages already present in the original design of RUFLS, and (3) focus the scope of the redesign, the final design criteria for the redesign was to limit changes to the MV holder and its components.

4.4.3 NEW MITRAL VALVE HOLDER

4.4.3.1 Network of Holes Method

The first iteration of the redesign involved the elongation of the "network of holes" approach used in the original RUFLS. There were two main design differences in this new system (Figure 4.4). The first difference was that, in the new system, in place of the metal rod threaded through the holes, a screw and nut would be placed through the hole in order to hold the PM in position. The second difference was a rotation of the holes 90 degrees so that they were placed on the medial–lateral axis of the holder as opposed to the anterior–posterior axis. The screws were selected to replace the metal bar because (1) their increased stiffness would halt the basal movement of the PMs during systole and (2) a series of nuts to be placed on the screw inside the MV holder around the new PM holder would allow for the control of the medial–lateral position within the holder (see the next section for how this nut setup was ultimately implemented). The rotation of the discrete holes was to accommodate the changes in the PM holders while allowing continuous manipulation of the medial–lateral position of the PMs. The original orientation would have allowed for continuous anterior–posterior positioning along the screw-nut setup, while leaving medial–lateral manipulation limited to discrete holes placed in the holder. As most valves require neutral placement along the anterior–posterior axis (directly apical to the commissures of the valve, which are placed in the midline of the MV holder in our system), it was decided that more flexible medial–lateral manipulation was a higher priority.

Although an improvement on the original design, this first iteration redesign had the drawback of allowing for only discrete manipulation of the basal–apical positioning of the PMs. This restriction would limit the precise position in the basal-apical direction, a vital component of PM position based on previous work. As a result, this first iteration redesign did not meet the criteria, and therefore was passed over for other redesign ideas.

4.4.3.2 Slot and Screw Method

The second (and final) MV holder redesign was based on a slot and screw method that allowed for continuous control of the basal–apical, medial–lateral, and anterior–posterior positioning (Figure 4.5). The design incorporated a slot cut into the side of the MV holder along the apical–basal axis at the anterior–posterior midline. The medial–lateral positioning of the PM is controlled by the positioning of nuts along the length of screws secured within these slots on either side. The anterior–posterior position of the valve is controlled by other elements of the system, including the positioning of the valve on the suture ring (placing the valve commissure more anterior on the suture ring has the practical effect of placing the PMs posterior on the PM holders). This positioning mechanism is technically difficult in the anterior–posterior direction, as it cannot be manipulated after the valve and PMs are sutured in place. However, it still allows for continuous anterior–posterior positioning. Additionally, under normal control circumstances, PMs are placed at the midline of the commissures, thus eliminating the need for anterior–posterior manipulation in most cases (Figure 4.5a).

This design successfully matched all of our established design criteria. It allowed for the precise continuous control of the PM position in all three cardinal directions. All parts used in this new design (metal screws and nuts, silicone washers) were autoclavable and remained contained within the confines of the bioreactor, making it an insignificant sterility risk. In addition, the simplicity of the design limited changes to the MV holder and PM holders, and made the system highly compatible with the imaging flow loop used by our collaborators, allowing us to accurately recreate the valve geometry in their system using easily obtained measurements.

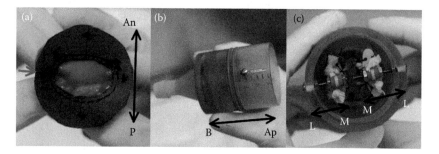

FIGURE 4.5 PM positioning in new RUFLS. (a) MV is sutured onto a ring with the commissures lined up with black lines on the ring (red arrow). These commissural lines are aligned with the holes in the MV holder to ensure proper PM positioning along the anterior–posterior axis (black axis). (b) The suture ring seen in A is inserted in the basal end of the MV holder. The elongated holes on the sides of the MV holder allow for proper PM positioning along the apical–basal axis (black axis). (c) The PM holder is sandwiched between nuts on the screws to allow proper PM positioning along the medial–lateral axis (black axis). An = Anterior, P = Posterior, B = Basal, Ap = Apical, L = Lateral, M = Medial.

Control of 3D Environment

The new system did, however, require a redesign of the PM holder attachment system, meaning the mechanism by which we attached the PMs to the MV holder. The iterative design process for the PM holders is described in detail in the following section.

4.4.4 NEW PAPILLARY MUSCLE HOLDERS

4.4.4.1 Sawtooth-Clamping System

The change of the MV holder system, with its transition from a metal rod to a screw-and-nut system in order to secure the PM holder, necessitated a move away from the metal coils used in the previous system. The PM holder system needed to directly connect to the MV holder system to maintain the tight control of position, but the screws could not constrain the muscle in the same manner as the old coil. Therefore, to secure the PM holders onto the MV holders, an eyehook was added to the PM holder design.

To secure the muscle within the PM holder, our initial proposed design revision took advantage of a sawtooth-clamping system (Figure 4.3c and d). Utilizing a simple hinge mechanism, this system would pierce the muscle with multiple sawtooth "spikes" to hold the muscle in place. Suture could then be added to the anterior and posterior edge of the muscle through holes at the end of the hinge mechanism. These holders were printed in an autoclave compatible resin using a 3D printer.

This sawtooth-clamping method had two major drawbacks when piloted in our system. First, the clamping mechanism resulted in fraying of the muscle during repeated cycles in RUFLS. Second, repeated autoclaving cycles resulted in a reduced mechanical strength of the resin material used in the 3D printing process. The need to make new sawtooth clamps again and again would result in the system becoming prohibitively expensive over the long term. Given the impracticality of this technique, another option compatible with the modified MV holder was sought.

4.4.4.2 Platform System

Given the limitations presented by the sawtooth-clamping system, we looked to make two major changes for the next iteration of the PM holder system. The first change was to simplify the design so that we could avoid the higher costs of 3D printing in lieu of machining a material that would have better long-term properties after repeated sterilization. The second change was to move away from a mechanism that depended on a solid material piercing and holding the muscle in place, as we felt that this would continue to lead to muscle fraying and the failure of the holder after repeated cycles. We, however, would maintain the use of an eyehook to connect our PM holder to our MV holder, as this contributed to the modular nature of our system, and its compatibility with our collaborator's imaging the flow loop system.

The new system would be comprised of a simple platform connected to an eyehook, constructed out of Delrin, an easily machined, strong, plastic material that could withstand repeated autoclaving (Figure 4.3f). The platform would then have a series of eight holes machined around its edge, which would be used to suture the muscle to the platform and hold it in place. After initial tests were conducted, we found that muscle fraying around the suture sites remained an issue. We hypothesized that this was the result of stress concentrations forming around the suture sites throughout the 600,000 mock cardiac cycles performed over the one-week time period. In order to reduce the stress concentrations on the tissue, a sterilized umbilical tape was looped around the muscle, through gaps in the chordae tendineae, and tied down to the platform in order to secure the PM to the holders. Suture was then used in this system to ensure that the muscle was well secured (Figure 4.3f). The new system, with the umbilical tape absorbing most of the force of systole and distributing it across a larger surface area, was successful in securing the PMs to the platform holders without muscle fraying for up to two weeks of culture.

4.5 FINDINGS: MODELS AND CONSISTENT REGURGITATION

Having successfully created a complete MV and PM holder system capable of securing the PM in a consistent manner capable of continuous manipulation in all three dimensions of the valve geometry, we then proceeded to test the hypothesis that such control would allow us to produce a nonregurgitant organ culture system capable of two-week valve culture. With the successful reproduction of the native valve geometry, we were able to culture valves for up to two weeks with regurgitation levels below 600 mL/min (Figure 4.2). In addition, by altering the position of the PM (5 mm basal displacement), we were able to create a moderate to severe model of MV prolapse, which produced an eccentric regurgitation jet on color Doppler echocardiography, consistent with clinical findings in MV prolapse patients. Then, by displacing the PMs 5 mm apically and laterally and dilating the MV annulus by 65%, we were able to create a moderate to severe model of functional mitral regurgitation, with a characteristic central jet confirmed on color Doppler echocardiography. The successful creation of a nonregurgitant control and two models of disease hemodynamics using manipulations of valve geometries validated the successful redesign of RUFLS (Connell et al. 2016).

4.6 CONCLUSION AND PERSPECTIVE

Having successfully redesigned the RUFLS system to allow for the precise geometry control of intact MVs within a sterile culture system, we are able to draw several important conclusions from our experience. First, in order to create a system that enables the ability to understand physiologic and pathophysiologic phenomenon, it is important to understand the form and function of the tissue under consideration. By understanding the importance of PM position on the MV function, for example, we were able to design the second generation of RUFLS accordingly, allowing us to overcome the deficiencies in the original RUFLS and to create controls that mimicked healthy valves *in vivo*. Second, it is essential to consider design criteria carefully in order to produce a system that is simple and compatible with future design iterations. By keeping the original RUFLS system as simple as the design requirements could allow, we were able to change a single major component, the MV holder and associated PM holders, in order to make a dramatic improvement to the system. Finally, in order to allow for component optimization, it is also important to keep costs low and, when viable, attempt to produce or buy components with quick turnaround time. Regardless of the sophistication of the initial design, unanticipated modifications to the system will likely be required, and budgeting both cost and time accordingly will increase the chances for success.

ACKNOWLEDGMENTS

The authors would like to acknowledge Dr. Stephen Little for his guidance throughout the redesign process and for the use of his imaging flow loop system during the hemodynamic validation of the system.

REFERENCES

Connell, P. S., A. F. Azimuddin, S. E. Kim, F. Ramirez, M. S. Jackson, S. H. Little, and K. J. Grande-Allen. 2016. Regurgitation hemodynamics alone cause mitral valve remodeling characteristic of clinical disease state *in vitro*. *Ann Biomed Eng* no. 44 (4):954–67, doi:10.1007/s10439-015-1398-0.

Gheewala, N. and K. J. Grande-Allen. 2010. Design and mechanical evaluation of a physiological mitral valve organ culture system. *Cardiovasc Eng Technol* no. 1 (2):123–31.

Gheewala, N., K. A. Schwarz, and K. J. Grande-Allen. 2013. Organ culture of porcine mitral valves as a novel experimental paradigm. *Cardiovasc Eng Technol* no. 4 (2):139–50.

He, S., A. A. Fontaine, E. Schwammenthal, A. P. Yoganathan, and R. A. Levine. 1997. Integrated mechanism for functional mitral regurgitation: Leaflet restriction versus coapting force: *In vitro* studies. *Circulation* no. 96 (6):1826–34.

He, S., J. Jimenez, Z. He, and A. P. Yoganathan. 2003. Mitral leaflet geometry perturbations with papillary muscle displacement and annular dilatation: An *in vitro* study of ischemic mitral regurgitation. *J Heart Valve Dis* no. 12 (3):300–07.

Jensen, M. O., A. A. Fontaine, and A. P. Yoganathan. 2001. Improved *in vitro* quantification of the force exerted by the papillary muscle on the left ventricular wall: Three-dimensional force vector measurement system. *Ann Biomed Eng* no. 29 (5):406–13.

Jimenez, J. H., D. D. Soerensen, Z. He, S. He, and A. P. Yoganathan. 2003. Effects of a saddle shaped annulus on mitral valve function and chordal force distribution: An *in vitro* study. *Ann Biomed Eng* no. 31 (10):1171–81.

Jimenez, J. H., D. D. Soerensen, Z. He, J. Ritchie, and A. P. Yoganathan. 2005a. Effects of papillary muscle position on chordal force distribution: An *in vitro* study. *J Heart Valve Dis* no. 14 (3):295–302.

Jimenez, J. H., D. D. Soerensen, Z. He, J. Ritchie, and A. P. Yoganathan. 2005b. Mitral valve function and chordal force distribution using a flexible annulus model: An *in vitro* study. *Ann Biomed Eng* no. 33 (5):557–66.

Little, S. H., S. R. Igo, M. McCulloch, C. J. Hartley, Y. Nose, and W. A. Zoghbi. 2008. Three-dimensional ultrasound imaging model of mitral valve regurgitation: Design and evaluation. *Ultrasound Med Biol* no. 34 (4):647–54, doi: 10.1016/j.ultrasmedbio.2007.08.009.

Little, S. H., S. R. Igo, B. Pirat, M. McCulloch, C. J. Hartley, Y. Nose, and W. A. Zoghbi. 2007. *In vitro* validation of real-time three-dimensional color Doppler echocardiography for direct measurement of proximal isovelocity surface area in mitral regurgitation. *Am J Cardiol* no. 99 (10):1440–47, doi: 10.1016/j.amjcard.2006.12.079.

Nielsen, S. L., H. Nygaard, A. A. Fontaine, J. M. Hasenkam, S. He, N. T. Andersen, and A. P. Yoganathan. 1999. Chordal force distribution determines systolic mitral leaflet configuration and severity of functional mitral regurgitation. *J Am Coll Cardiol* no. 33 (3):843–53.

Quaini, A., S. Canic, G. Guidoboni, R. Glowinski, S. R. Igo, C. J. Hartley, W. A. Zoghbi, and S. H. Little. 2011. A three-dimensional computational fluid dynamics model of regurgitant mitral valve flow: Validation against *in vitro* standards and 3D color Doppler methods. *Cardiovasc Eng Technol* no. 2 (2):77–89, doi: 10.1007/s13239-011-0038-6.

Rabbah, J. P., N. Saikrishnan, A. W. Siefert, A. Santhanakrishnan, and A. P. Yoganathan. 2013. Mechanics of healthy and functionally diseased mitral valves: A critical review. *J Biomech Eng* no. 135 (2):021007, doi: 10.1115/1.4023238.

5 Nipple and Breast Construction
In Vitro *and* In Vivo *Assessment*

Maria Yanez, Scott Collins, and Thomas Boland

CONTENTS

5.1	Introduction	75
5.2	Materials and Methods	76
	5.2.1 Cell Culture and Scaffold Fabrication	76
	5.2.2 A Nipple Areola Complex	78
	5.2.3 *In Vitro* Scaffold Assessment	78
	5.2.4 *In Vivo* Assessment	79
	5.2.5 Histological Analysis	80
5.3	Results and Discussion	81
	5.3.1 Adipocytes Incorporation in Fibrin	81
	5.3.2 Forming Thick Tissue-Engineered Constructs	81
	5.3.3 Formation of Endothelial Cell Channels in Constructs	81
	5.3.4 Molding Mass Customized Implants	83
	5.3.4.1 *In Vivo* Studies	84
	5.3.5 Vascular Anastomosis	85
5.4	Conclusion and Perspective	87
Acknowledgments		88
References		88

5.1 INTRODUCTION

Breast cancer is a malignant tumor that starts in breast cells (Miller et al. 2016). There are different types of breast cancers: ductal carcinoma *in situ*, invasive ductal carcinoma, invasive lobular carcinoma, and inflammatory breast cancer. According to the Centers for Disease Control and Prevention, breast cancer is one of the most common cancers among women in the United States. The American Cancer Society estimates that in 2017, invasive breast cancer will be diagnosed in about 252,710 women (www.cancer.org).

There are different surgical procedures to remove the malignant cells such as lumpectomy, partial mastectomy (quadrantectomy mastectomy), simple mastectomy, modified radical mastectomy, and radical mastectomy. Currently, women undergo different procedures for breast reconstruction, including tissue flap procedures, graft for tissue support, and cell suspension injection after a liposuction (Miller et al. 2016; Riccio et al. 2015). These procedures have different problems associated with hernia, limited to high donor site morbidity, cell damage during liposuction, necrosis postinjection, and often implants are avoided while undergoing radiation treatments. Besides breast reconstruction, the majority of mastectomy cases also require nipple/areola reconstruction. Nipple sparing mastectomies in small-to-moderate size breast typically render the best cosmetic outcomes, though there are not always good results due to the nature of breast cancer. Results of available nipple areola complex (NAC) reconstruction techniques can be unpredictable. There are many different techniques, including nipple sharing, free-composite grafts, and local "pull-out" flaps, all of which are vulnerable to an unpredictable degree of loss (shape and volume), and in most cases require a second procedure.

This study was focused on developing a three-dimensional (3D) printed engineered adipose tissue graft to apply, especially during breast reconstruction after a solid tumor removal for breast or NAC reconstruction. In addition, this engineered tissue could potentially fill voids created by congenital malformation, injury reconstruction, or for other cosmetic reconstruction. Regarding the NAC reconstruction, we developed a process to create the proper shape starting with a 3D image of the NAC building an acrylonitrile butadiene styrene prototype, and obtaining an agarose mold into which we could print the tissue graft.

Fibrin gel is formed by the enzymatic crosslink between thrombin and fibrinogen at room temperature in the presence of calcium ions. Fibrin gel was selected as the main material for the adipose tissue graft and NAC because fibrin plays an important role during wound healing, and it acts as a provisional matrix. It has been utilized in 3D printing applications to create bio-inks because it is highly compatible with cells, and it presents good degradation and low toxicity (Cui and Boland 2009; Janmey et al. 2009; Lee and Mooney 2001; Yanez et al. 2015). Three-dimensional printed fibrin gels can serve as a temporary scaffold, allowing cells to attach, migrate, and create their own extracellular matrix (Yanez et al. 2015).

Our laboratory has assessed different scaffolds, including an engineered bilayer skin graft that was constructed using fibrin gel and collagen as the main components, and a modified inkjet printer was utilized to create prevascularized channels lined with endothelial cells (ECs; Yanez et al. 2015). Previous data (*in vitro* and *in vivo* studies) helped us to assess graft integration with the host tissue, and the histological aspects of dermis and epidermis in a mouse model, and served as a guide in this study to assess an NAC and adipose graft.

5.2 MATERIALS AND METHODS

5.2.1 Cell Culture and Scaffold Fabrication

Human microvascular endothelial cells (HMVEC) were obtained from Lonza, maintained and subcultured according to manufacturer's procedures. HMVEC were cultured in endothelial cell basal media (EBM-2, Lonza CC-3156) supplemented with endothelial cell growth medium (EGM-2 BulletKit, Lonza CC-4176) containing 2% fetal bovine serum (FBS), hydrocortisone, vascular endothelial growth factor (VEGF), human epidermal growth factor (hEGF), R3-insulin-like growth factor-1 (R3-IGF-1), ascorbic acid, heparin, human epidermal growth factor (hEGF), gentamicin/amphoterecin (GA-1000), and human fibroblast growth factor (hFGF-β). Mesenchymal stem cells (MSC) and 3T3-L1 embryonic fibroblast mouse Pre-adipocytes (PA) were purchased from American Type Culture Collection (ATCC). MSC were subcultured in the MSC basal medium from ATCC (PCS-500-030) supplemented with the MSC growth kit (ATCC PCS-500-040), and PA were cultured in basal media I (BMI) containing Dulbecco's Modified Eagle's Medium (DMEM), 10% neonatal calf serum (NCS), and penicillin/streptomycin (100 U/mL–100 μg/mL) as recommended by ATCC.

Pre-adipocytes were cultured in BMI for one week before initiating differentiation to obtain high confluence in the cell culture flask. PA were differentiated to adipocytes as described by Zebisch et al. (2012) using the following differentiation medium I (DMI) containing DMEM 10% FBS, 1.0 μM dexamethasone, 0.5 mM methylisobutylxanthine, 1.0 μg/mL insulin, and 2 μM rosiglitazone for 48 h. Then, the medium was changed to differentiation media II (DMII) containing DMEM 10% FBS, and 1.0 μg/mL insulin, and finally, adipocytes were kept in culture for 14 days in basal media II (BMII) containing DMEM 10% FBS and penicillin/streptomycin (100 U/mL–100 μg/mL). This protocol allowed for approximately 85%–90% of cells to exhibit the adipocyte phenotype.

Adipocytes were collected by trypsinizing and gently scraping the surface of the flask, and then they were counted and resuspended in a fibrinogen solution (cell viability was assessed by live/dead assay) (14–20×10^6 cells/mL). MSCs and HMVECs were trypsinized and resuspended in EGM (HMVECs 4×10^5 cells/mL, and MSCs 4×10^4 cells/mL).

Fibrin gels were prepared as previously published by Cui and coworkers (Cui and Boland 2009) mixing 60 mg/mL of fibrinogen with 50 units/mL thrombin in 80 mM Ca^{2+} in Dulbecco's phosphate buffer saline solution (DPBS). Printed gels were prepared by printing the thrombin solution onto a thin film of the fibrinogen solution (Cui and Boland 2009; Yanez et al. 2015). Molded gels were prepared by pipetting the thrombin solution onto the fibrinogen film. Fibrin glue was prepared by mixing fibrinogen (60 mg/mL) with thrombin (50 units/mL). To create the fibrin glue, the ratio between fibrinogen and thrombin was 10:1.

In order to fabricate the microcapillary tubes, the thrombin solution was mixed with HMVECs or HMVECs/MSCs, and added as bio-ink into a modified cartridge, which was placed into a cell printer developed in our laboratory (Yanez et al. 2012, 2015). Adipocytes were mixed with the fibrinogen solution keeping a concentration of 14–20×10^6 cell/mL. The thrombin-cell solution of 250 μL was placed inside of a modified printer cartridge and 200 μL of the fibrinogen–adipocyte solution was pipetted onto a microscope slide. Then, the thrombin-cell solution was printed using a grid pattern designed in the Adobe Illustrator. The printing process was repeated for a total of 12 layers. Then, the samples were incubated for 10–20 min for fibrin gelation. Grafts were maintained in EGM for 24 h before animal implantation.

Molded samples were prepared in the same manner. But in this case, the fibrinogen and thrombin solutions were manually mixed utilizing a pipette (printer was not utilized). After the 24-h graft incubation, the samples were folded and glued with fibrin glue to achieve a thickness of approximately 1.2–1.5 mm (three layers).

5.2.2 A Nipple Areola Complex

Fused deposition modeling, a 3D printing technique, was utilized to create an areola nipple complex prototype made from ABS plastic. NX software was used to design the 3D rendering of the NAC prototype. The printed NAC prototype was used as a positive mold to develop a negative agarose mold. To create the agarose mold, agarose was dissolved in distilled water to obtain a final concentration of 2% agarose. Then, the agarose solution was sterilized in an autoclave. Agarose solution was allowed to cool to 50–60°C in a biosafety cabinet, and then it was poured into a sterile Petri dish that contained the NAC prototype previously sterilized in a 70% ethanol solution for 3 h. The agarose mold was cooled at room temperature in a biosafety cabinet to keep it sterile. The prototype was carefully removed, resulting in the NAC agarose mold. To obtain the NAC fibrin scaffold, thrombin, fibrinogen, and cells were mixed as previously described and poured into the agarose mold. After the fibrin gel crosslinked, it was carefully removed from the agarose mold. Then, samples were placed in a culture medium and incubated overnight. Several challenges had to be overcome to realize the custom implants, including how to maintain sterility, separation of the 3D part from the mold, and separation of the implant from the mold without damaging the fibrin structures.

5.2.3 In Vitro Scaffold Assessment

Cell viability of the encapsulated cells was assessed by live/dead assay (live/dead viability/Cytotoxicity kit) at 24 and 72 h. Briefly, an old medium was aspirated, and the samples were washed with PBS to remove remaining DMEM. Ethidium homodimer-1 (EthD-1) (red) of 20 µL and calcein of 1 µL were diluted in 10 mL of PBS (green). The samples were placed in a multiwell plate, and the EthD-1-calcein-PBS solution was added until the solution was 1 mm level above the scaffold. The samples were incubated at 37°C in a 5% CO_2 environment for 30 min. Three different samples were analyzed to assess graft cell viability. The samples were analyzed by confocal microscopy using 488 nm excitation for calcein and 530 nm excitation for EthD-1.

For *in vitro* experiments, the ECs were stained with PKH26 red fluorescence cell membrane labeling dye before the printing process to assess the cells and microchannel formation over time. The labeling protocol of the manufacturer was followed. Briefly, cells were suspended in diluent C, and PKH26 was diluted in diluent C at the final concentration of 4 mM. The PKH26 solution was mixed with the cell suspension and kept in the dark for 5 min to allow the dye to bind to the cell membrane, swirling gently to assure the dye distribution. The reaction was stopped by adding an equal amount of serum-supplemented media.

Gel degradation was assessed by immersion in PBS (pH 7.4), following which the gels were incubated in a control environment at 37°C and 5% CO_2. Gel dimensions were calculated at the beginning and end of the study.

5.2.4 IN VIVO ASSESSMENT

The animal protocol was approved by the Institutional Animal Care and Use Committee at the University of Texas at El Paso. Thirty female, athymic nude mice (homozygous nude *Foxn1^{nu}/Foxn1^{nu}*; strain name: J:NU) were purchased from The Jackson Laboratory and housed in the animal care facility under barrier conditions. Four different groups of animals were selected and different types of grafts were implanted in each group along with controls over 21 days. Group 1 contained grafts with printed microchannels with ECs with a cell concentration of 4×10^6 cells/mL and pipetted adipocytes (1×10^6 cells/mL). Group 2 in addition to the printed EC included MSC with a concentration of 4×10^6 cells/mL. Group 3 was an injected control containing the same components and volumes of Group 1, but in this case fibrin gels were polymerized *in situ* over a grid representing the *x*- and *y* dimensions of the implant. Group 4 contained a nonprinted control (manually created). This was similar to Group 3 except that the gel was formed *ex vivo* and handled just as the printed controls. It was surgically implanted as Groups 1 and 2.

On the day of the surgery, the mice were anesthetized with intraperitoneal injection using ketamine and xylazine, and maintained under isoflurane anesthesia. The animal had a preoperative injection of analgesic 20 min prior to the surgical procedure. Buprenorphine or carprofen was used as postoperative analgesic given to mice every 8 h for the first two days, and then as needed for pain relief.

The animals were surgically prepared, a 2 cm long incision was made on the dorsum, and a pocket was made under the skin. The grafts were sutured to the inner surface of the skin, and an adhesion barrier was inserted beneath the graft in order to assess vascular anastomoses only from the skin. For the injected control, an adhesion barrier was surgically implanted and sutured to the skin (as above) and cells were directly injected subcutaneously over injection sites, spanning the same area as the implant.

The animals were continuously monitored during the recovery period until they were fully ambulatory and foraging with no overt signs of pain/distress. The animals were monitored at a minimum twice daily for pain/distress, self-mutilation, infections, and adequate healing.

The animals were subjected multiple biopsies in order to analyze graft integration with the host as well as inflammation. The thickness of the implanted gels was evaluated at the time of the implantation, and then it was compared with the thickness of the different biopsies to assess the thick gel degradation. Figure 5.1 illustrations an implanted scaffold. The white square depicts the adhesion barrier (5 mm larger than the adipose tissue graft). The red box denotes the adipose tissue-engineered graft centered on the barrier with approximate dimensions of 1 cm × 1 cm. Sutures were paced at the four corners through the barrier and skin. The circles labeled 1–4 represent the biopsy sites and the chronological order in which they were taken. Biopsies were done using a 3 mm sterile biopsy punch at each corner of the adipose graft. The

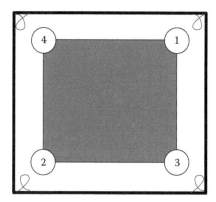

FIGURE 5.1 Illustration of the implant scaffold and the order of the biopsies. The white square depicts the adhesion barrier (5 mm larger than the adipose tissue graft). The red box denotes the adipose tissue-engineered graft centered on the barrier with approximate dimensions of 1 cm × 1 cm. Sutures were placed at the four corners through the barrier and skin. The circles labeled 1–4 represent the biopsy sites and the chronological order in which they were taken.

biopsies penetrated down through the skin and fascia but not into the muscular layer. Biopsies were taken at days 1, 3, 7, and 14 following the graft implant. The mice were placed under general inhalant (isoflurane) anesthesia for the biopsy and a single 4-0 monofilament suture was placed to close the biopsy defect. The mice were recovered and monitored postbiopsy until they were in sternal recumbency and ambulating normally to ensure no additional pain/distressed was observed. Additional analgesic was administered if the animal exhibited signs of pain/distressed.

The mice were followed until the completion of the specified experimental timeline, at which the animals were humanely euthanized and tissue samples were collected. The tissue was collected, washed with PBS, and fixed with the 10% formalin solution for 24 h. Other tissue samples were frozen in Tissue-Tek optimum cutting compound (OCT), and sliced in a cryotome.

5.2.5 Histological Analysis

Frozen tissues were placed on Leica cryocut 1800 maintained at −30°C and sectioned to 7–20 μm. The sections were collected on poly-L-Lysine-coated slides for improved adherence. Tissue samples were stained with hematoxylin and eosin (H&E) staining and Masson's trichrome staining. Tissue sections for immunohistochemistry were hydrated using successive concentrations of ethanol starting from 100%, 95%, 70%, 50% and finishing with distilled water. For antigen unmasking, the samples were boiled for 15 min in an antigen retrieval solution consisting of 10 mM sodium citrate, 0.05% Tween 20 at pH 6.0, cooled on a bench top for 30 min, and rinsed with 1× PBS. Cells were permeabilized with 100% methanol at −20°C for 6 min to provide access to the antibody. Tissue samples were blocked for 1 h at room temperature in 5% normal goat serum. Samples were incubated for 1 h at room temperature with FITC, labeled mouse monoclonal CD34 antibody in PBS (1:100).

Unbound antibodies were removed by washing the samples three times with PBS 10 min each. During the final rinse, the cells were incubated with DAPI. Samples were mounted with DAKO mounting media and covered with a coverslip. Imaging was performed with a Nikon Confocal microscope using a 10× objective.

5.3 RESULTS AND DISCUSSION

5.3.1 ADIPOCYTES INCORPORATION IN FIBRIN

Adipocytes have been successfully encapsulated into fibrin gels using a 60 mg/mL gel density (Cui et al. 2010; Yanez et al. 2015). *In vitro* as well as *in vivo* analysis of these gels showed they had little signs of degradation over the three weeks duration of the study. Adipocytes can be as large as 100 μm making printing of these cells difficult. Therefore, we did not print the adipocytes; they were added to the fibrinogen prior to EC printing. Previous studies have shown that adipocyte cells size is between 80 and 100 μm after computerized image processing, corroborating with our results (Bjornheden et al. 2004).

5.3.2 FORMING THICK TISSUE-ENGINEERED CONSTRUCTS

Live/dead assays showed that both the ECs and adipocytes remained alive until the time of implantation (24 h after the gels were printed). Figure 5.2a shows live adipocytes within the gel, while Figure 5.2b shows the printed ECs.

To obtained thicker tissues, it was necessary to print different layers (three times the dimension of the final scaffold). Each layer contained adipocytes and ECs, and optionally MSCs. The thickness of each layer was close to 0.5 mm. Prior to surgery, the constructs were cut in three different parts, and each part was glued to each other to obtain a thicker graft (final thickness = 1.5 mm) with three different layers of fibrin. Although the production of thicker grafts was achieved, the animals presented high inflammatory signals due to the fibrin glue. Mouse tissue was stained with Masson's trichrome, where inflammatory cells (Figure 5.3) were present. Polymorphonuclear neutrophils were found in tissue sections after 21D postimplantation (marked by the black arrow in Figure 5.3). This inflammation was attributed to the fibrin glue formulation (fibrinogen–thrombin ratio, 1:1). Then, it was necessary to lower this concentration to 10:1. Constructs were easily handled utilizing a combination of normal cell culture and surgical techniques.

5.3.3 FORMATION OF ENDOTHELIAL CELL CHANNELS IN CONSTRUCTS

Printed microvascular channels have been studied by Cui and coworkers; these studies found that a modified inkjet printer helped to develop a hollow structure where EC proliferated through the microchannel structure (Cui and Boland 2009). In this study, the process followed by Cui was slightly modified by printing different layers to create thicker constructs. Figure 5.4 shows the EC network with a tubular structure six days postprinting. This image shows ECs proliferating in the printed pattern. This type of structure has been seen before when ECs were dispersed in thrombin and printed on fibrinogen (Cui and Boland 2009).

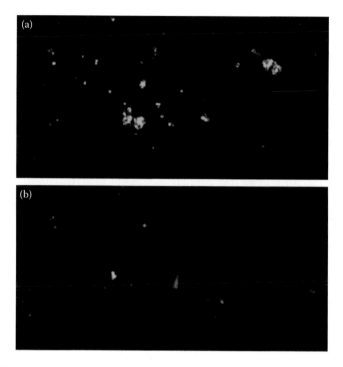

FIGURE 5.2 Live/dead assay performed in printed gels right after 24 h. (a) Live adipocyte cells in green, while (b) shows live endothelial cells.

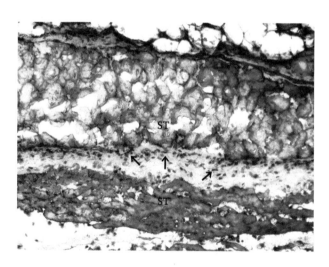

FIGURE 5.3 Masson's trichrome image shows the inflammatory response of the mouse at day 21 after graft implantation. Here, the presence of inflammatory cells with high proliferation is observed. Arrows indicate the subcutaneous tissue (ST) and the adipose tissue graft (TG).

Nipple and Breast Construction

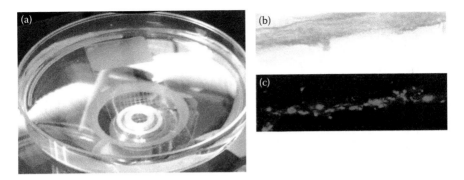

FIGURE 5.4 Images of endothelial networks printed with fibrin gels. The cells were stained with Sigma red dye prior to printing. (a) Gross anatomical view, (b) bright-field view at 20× six days postprinting, (c) confocal view of the same area as B.

The differentiation process took 3 weeks. This process started after PA cells were seeded in a cell culture flask. Figure 5.5 shows the differentiation process from pre-adipocytes to adipocytes obtaining 85%–90% of transformed cells. To assess adipocyte differentiation by assessing cell morphology and staining cells with Oil Red O (data not shown). Figure 5.5a shows pre-adipocytes when they were ready to start the differentiation process cultured in BMI, (b) shows pre-adipocytes 48 h after they began the differentiation process in the DMI medium, and finally (c) shows adipocytes 48 h after they were subjected to the second differentiation medium, DMII. These results are consistent with previous studies carried out by Zebisch and coworkers (Zebisch et al. 2012). They observed higher percentage of cell differentiation when they used rosiglitazone because early results obtained by Tontonoz and coworkers revealed that human liposarcoma cells can be induced to experiment adipose differentiation (Tontonoz et al. 1997).

5.3.4 Molding Mass Customized Implants

A procedure was developed to create an NAC. First, it was necessary to design a 3D image and print it using a conventional 3D printing. Then, the printed NAC

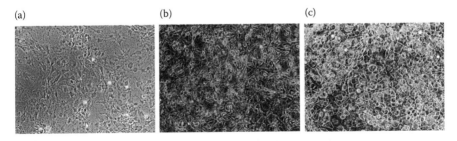

FIGURE 5.5 Differentiation process from pre-adipocytes to adipocytes. (a) Pre-adipocytes in BMI culture, ready to start the differentiation process, (b) pre-adipocytes 48 h after the differentiation process has begun, and cells were culture in DMI for 48 h, and (c) adipocytes 48 h after they were culture in DMII.

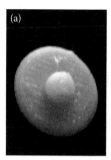 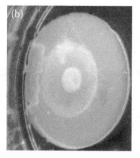 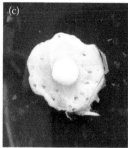

FIGURE 5.6 Customized nipple implant. (a) 3D printed implant, (b) mold, and (c) fibrin implant.

3D structure was introduced and a Petri dish and an agarose solution were poured into the Petri dish containing the NAC 3D structure. Figure 5.6 shows the NAC 3D printed structure (a), the agarose mold (b), and the final fibrin NAC implant (c).

5.3.4.1 *In Vivo* Studies

For *in vivo* analysis, four different groups of animals were selected and different types of grafts were implanted along with controls over twenty-one days. In Group 1, grafts with printed microchannels with ECs and adipocytes were implanted. In Group 2, the grafts with printed EC and MSC adipocytes were implanted. In Group 3 (Control #1), the animals received an injection containing the same components and volumes of Group 1, and the gel was polymerized *in situ* over a grid representing the x- and y-dimensions of the implant. Group 4 (Control #2) contained a nonprinted control where the gels were created *in vitro* and later implanted in animals.

The NAC graft was implanted to judge appearance and shape retention of the graft over the time. Figure 5.7a shows the appearance of the NAC graft before it was implanted, (b) shows the NAC graft on the day of implantation, (c) shows the NAC graft into the mouse at day 7, and (d) shows the explanted NAC graft at day 7. As can be seen from the figures, the appearance and shape of the graft are constant over a period of time (7 days). Currently, there are not many options for NAC reconstruction. Most of the options have been achieve grafting (from donor multiple areas), replantation, dermabrasion, and tattoo (Farhadi et al. 2006). This may be a good option, but some patients do not desire to have further surgery (Hyza et al. 2015; Riccio et al. 2015). Other studies suggest to utilize a dermal flap and Alloderm® (a decellularized human dermis which preserves the biological components and structure of the dermis [Garramone and Lam 2007; Riccio et al. 2015]) which maintained an average of 56% nipple projection up to 12 months (Garramone and Lam 2007; Riccio et al. 2015). Results presented here, although preliminary, support further assessment of time-extended adipose tissue graft.

All samples showed fibrous encapsulation after twenty-one days, but differed in the size of the capsule. Injected cells showed the thickest capsules as shown in Figure 5.8.

Capsule thickness was greatest to smallest in this order: Injected fibrin with cells, molded fibrin with cells, printed endothelial and MSCs with adipocytes, and printed ECs with adipocytes. In addition, fibrous encroachment at the glued layers was

Nipple and Breast Construction

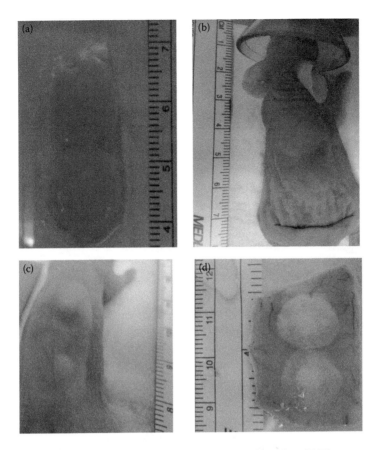

FIGURE 5.7 Nipple areola complex before and after implantation. (a) The appearance of the NAC graft before it was implanted, (b) shows the graft at time of implantation, (c) shows the graft at day 7, and (d) shows the explanted NAC.

observed, indicating an inflammatory response inside the gels. One possible reason of the observed inflammatory response could be the repeated injury of the animals at the implant site to retrieve punch biopsies. Thus, the use of improper formulated fibrin glue and the repeated injury to the animals may have contributed to some of the encapsulation observed in all samples. Nevertheless, judging by standard biomaterial performance criteria, the most biocompatible implants were those printed with ECs and printed with ECs and MSCs.

5.3.5 Vascular Anastomosis

Larger vessels were observed in the graft after tissue processing, immunohistochemical staining (Figure 5.9a [DAPI staining] and Figure 5.9b [CD34 marker]), and Masson's trichrome staining (Figure 5.9c). Clearly, different vessels can be seen throughout the explant, the smallest of which are tens of microns of diameter, the size of capillaries. Larger vessels are also seen. But as the sectioning could have

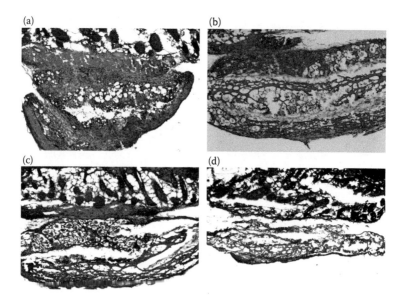

FIGURE 5.8 Extent of fibrous capsule formation as seen in H&E stains of adipocyte containing fibrin gels. (a) Injected cells, (b) molded samples, (c) printed ECs and MSCs, and (d) printed ECs.

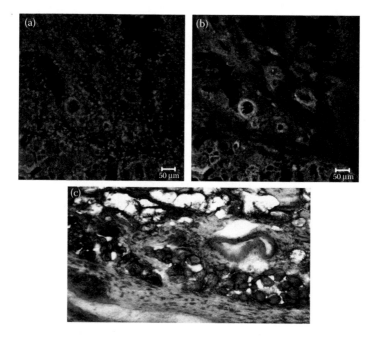

FIGURE 5.9 Immunohistochemistry staining of a mouse explant, with printed endothelial cells laden with adipocytes. (a) DAPI staining indicating cell nuclei, (b) CD34 staining indicating endothelial cells, and (c) Masson's trichrome staining of the sample.

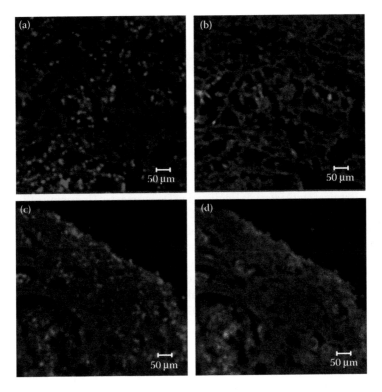

FIGURE 5.10 Immunohistochemistry staining of a mouse explant. (a) DAPI staining of a molded implant laden with adipocytes and endothelial cells, (b) CD34 staining of the molded implant, (c) DAPI staining of injected fibrin with adipocytes and endothelial cells, and (d) CD34 staining of the injected cells.

cut those at a glancing angle, we cannot conclude in a definite manner that larger vessels grew into the implant. Masson's trichrome and H&E staining confirmed the fibrous tissue encapsulation (blue) as well as fibrous infiltration within the implant. Adipocytes appeared in brown color Masson's trichrome staining. As before, the fibrous encapsulation is attributed to a slightly inflammatory glue formulation and the repeated injuries to the animals. However, the data taken together offer the first concrete evidence that printed microvasculature is integrating with the host upon implantation.

CD34 stains of molded or injected gels never showed any evidence of microvessels or capillaries, although positive CD 34 stains were observed as shown in Figure 5.10. This suggests that the phenotype was present, but incomplete, or leaky vessels may have formed, but were not functionally integrating with the host.

5.4 CONCLUSION AND PERSPECTIVE

In this study, adipocytes were successfully differentiated from 3T3-L1 pre-adipocytes to adipocytes. We were able to print and encapsulate human ECs in a fibrin matrix. Live/dead analysis showed living cell (adipocytes and EC) after the graft construction and/or printing process. The adipose tissue graft with the EC network was implanted in mouse, and after the tissue analysis, graft acceptance was observed. Immunohistochemistry analysis revealed that the new vessels formed. In addition, we successfully developed an NAC, and implant it in mice to analyze its appearance and shape retention overtime. After seven days of implantation, NAC shows good appearance and shape retention. However, more studies need to be performed in order to create a fully functional NAC graft.

ACKNOWLEDGMENTS

The Metallurgical and Materials Engineering Department at University of Texas at El Paso (UTEP) is acknowledged. The SBIR Award IIP-1248451 to Tevido Biodevices, LLC funded this research. The authors thank the staff of the Cell Culture and High Throughput Screening (HTS) Core Facility, Border Biomedical Research Center of the University of Texas at El Paso for services and facilities provided, especially to Dr. Armando Varela for his support during the immunohistochemical testing. This core facility is supported by National Institutes on Minority Health and Health Disparities (NIMHD grant # 8G12MD007592).

REFERENCES

Bjornheden, T., B. Jakubowicz, M. Levin, B. Oden, S. Eden, L. Sjostrom, and M. Lonn. 2004. Computerized determination of adipocyte size. *Obes Res* no. 12 (1):95–105.

Cui, X. and T. Boland. 2009. Human microvasculature fabrication using thermal inkjet printing technology. *Biomaterials* no. 30 (31):6221–27.

Cui, X., D. Dean, Z. M. Ruggeri, and T. Boland. 2010. Cell damage evaluation of thermal inkjet printed Chinese hamster ovary cells. *Biotechnol Bioeng* no. 106 (6):963–69.

Farhadi, J., G. K. Maksvytyte, D. J. Schaefer, G. Pierer, and O. Scheufler. 2006. Reconstruction of the nipple-areola complex: An update. *J Plast Reconstr Aesthet Surg* no. 59 (1):40–53.

Garramone, C. E. and B. Lam. 2007. Use of AlloDerm in primary nipple reconstruction to improve long-term nipple projection. *Plast Reconstr Surg* no. 119 (6):1663–68.

Hyza, P., L. Streit, J. Vesely, D. Stafova, and P. Sin. 2015. New technique of immediate nipple reconstruction during immediate autologous DIEP or MS-TRAM breast reconstruction. *Ann Plast Surg* no. 74 (6):645–51.

Janmey, P. A., J. P. Winer, and J. W. Weisel. 2009. Fibrin gels and their clinical and bioengineering applications. *J R Soc Interface* no. 6 (30):1–10.

Lee, K. Y. and D. J. Mooney. 2001. Hydrogels for tissue engineering. *Chem Rev* no. 101 (7):1869–79.

Miller, K. D., R. L. Siegel, C. C. Lin, A. B. Mariotto, J. L. Kramer, J. H. Rowland, K. D. Stein, R. Alteri, and A. Jemal. 2016. Cancer treatment and survivorship statistics, 2016. *CA Cancer J Clin* no. 66 (4):271–89.

Riccio, C. A., M. R. Zeiderman, S. Chowdhry, and B. J. Wilhelmi. 2015. Review of nipple reconstruction techniques and introduction of v to y technique in a bilateral wise pattern mastectomy or reduction mammaplasty. *Eplasty* no. 15:e11.

Tontonoz, P., S. Singer, B. M. Forman, P. Sarraf, J. A. Fletcher, C. D. Fletcher, R. P. Brun et al. 1997. Terminal differentiation of human liposarcoma cells induced by ligands for peroxisome proliferator-activated receptor gamma and the retinoid X receptor. *Proc Natl Acad Sci USA* no. 94 (1):237–41.

Yanez, M., J. Rincon, P. Cortez, N. Günther, T. Boland, and C. de Maria. 2012. Printable cellular scaffold using self-crosslinking agents. *J Imaging Sci Technol* no. 56 (4):40506.

Yanez, M., J. Rincon, A. Dones, C. De Maria, R. Gonzales, and T. Boland. 2015. In vivo assessment of printed microvasculature in a bilayer skin graft to treat full-thickness wounds. *Tissue Eng Part A* no. 21 (1–2):224–33.

Zebisch, K., V. Voigt, M. Wabitsch, and M. Brandsch. 2012. Protocol for effective differentiation of 3T3-L1 cells to adipocytes. *Anal Biochem* no. 425 (1):88–90.

6 3D Cancer Spheroid Biofabrication Using Thermal Inkjet-Based Bioprinting for Rapid Screening

Jorge I. Rodríguez-Dévora, Christopher Moody, Aesha Desai, Karen J. L. Burg, and Delphine Dean

CONTENTS

6.1 Introduction 91
6.2 Materials and Methods 93
    6.2.1 Bioprinting Printer Setup..93
    6.2.2 Bioprinting Process...95
    6.2.3 Cell Culture and Staining 95
    6.2.4 Aggregate Shape Factor and Growth..95
    6.2.5 Data Analysis..96
6.3 Results and Discussion 96
6.4 Conclusion and Perspective 100
Acknowledgments..100
References..100

6.1 INTRODUCTION

Spheroid/aggregate culture techniques have gained interest among regenerative medicine researchers because they provide an intermediate system, with biological complexity between the standard monolayer cell culture and animal models. A key challenge of spheroid/aggregate culture techniques is achieving increased biofabrication reproducibility (low variance) and throughput, thereby increasing quality control over future rapid screening platforms. Inkjet-based biofabricator for patterning mammalian cells in order to improve the speed and reproducibility of three-dimensional (3D) cell spheroid formation is a possible option. Inkjet technology is a promising approach to increase the throughput of rapid screening for personalized drug screening.

Collective evidence suggests that *in vitro* 3D culture reduces the biological information gap found between observations made from a standard monolayer culture and that from *in vivo* cellular response (Yamada and Cukierman 2007). A 3D biological disease model has the potential to serve as a more superior screening platform than a standard 2D culture system model since the 3D model may be capable of better resembling the complex cell–cell and cell–matrix spatial interactions, natural occurring extracellular matrix (ECM), and dimensionality of native tissues (Burg and Boland 2003; Pampaloni et al. 2007). The increasing number of compounds to screen in the drug discovery process makes animal models prohibitively expensive and time-consuming (McArthur and Borsini 2006; Remick 2013); in addition, animal models cannot always adequately replicate human diseases and drug interactions (McArthur and Borsini 2006). As an alternative, biofabrication techniques have been developed to create more physiologically relevant tissue and organ models (Burg et al. 2010). Many of these techniques rely on the use of small cell aggregate or spheroid building blocks (Mironov et al. 2009). These cell spheroids can be used to mimic simplified tissues, or multiple spheroids of varying compositions may be assembled precisely into larger structures to more closely resemble tissue complexity. These model systems can be made using multiple cellular spheroids of various cell types, including stem, cancer, liver, and others (LaBarbera et al. 2012; Lin and Chang 2008). Several groups have shown that *in vitro* 3D models are better able to mimic the *in vivo* cell–tissue state (Abbott 2003; Asghar et al. 2015; Edmondson et al. 2014). In particular, the focus of this chapter is the use of inkjet-based bioprinting for the formation of cancer spheroid cultures.

The main techniques explored in recapitulating a more physiological-relevant cell culture include hanging drop (Del Duca et al. 2004; Foty 2011; Timmins and Nielsen 2007; Tung et al. 2011), nonadhesive substrates (Landry et al. 1985; Tavana et al. 2010; Yuhas et al. 1977), simulated microgravity (Ingram et al. 1997; Khaoustov et al. 1999), pellet formation (Akiyama and Nakamura 2009; Qihao et al. 2007), microfluidic trapping (Dean et al. 2007; Wu et al. 2008), external force enhancement (Chen et al. 2015; Han et al. 2013), scaffold based approaches (Mosadegh et al. 2015; Yan et al. 2015), and magnetic levitation (Tseng et al. 2015). Comprehensive reviews of these techniques have recently been published (Lin and Chang 2008; Mehta et al. 2012). A key challenge with cell spheroid culture is the difficulty of increasing aggregate/spheroid formation reproducibility and throughput (Mehta et al. 2012). Several efforts have been pursued in this regard. In particular, bioprinting systems can be used to create high-throughput aggregates/spheroids that are based on several methods including: extrusion systems (Ouyang et al. 2015; Xu, Sridharan et al. 2011; Xu, Wu et al. 2011), valve-based printers (Faulkner-Jones et al. 2013), and laser direct writing printers (Odde and Renn 2000). Demirci and colleagues used a bioprinter to arrange embryonic stem cells, demonstrating improved reproducibility in terms of size, shape, and uniformity (Xu, Sridharan et al. 2011). Their system generated up to 160 cell droplets per second, which decreased patterning time by at least two orders of magnitude compared to manual pipetting. In addition, it resulted in cell spheroids with 57%–94% less variance in size compared to manual micropipetting techniques. In another approach, a valve-based bioprinter controlled volume down to 2 nL, or fewer than 5 cells per droplet, rapidly creating spheroid/aggregates of human embryonic stem cells (Faulkner-Jones et al. 2013). Valve-based bioprinters promise to significantly improve spheroid size control and provide lineage differentiation cues for 3D embryonic bodies. More recently, laser direct writing has been used to print cells, resulting in relatively uniform cell spheroid/embryonic bodies (Dias et al. 2014). However, laser direct writing has limited throughput, and multiple aggregates can be formed within cell colonies. The focus of our current study is the use of thermal inkjet technology. Thermal inkjet technology is readily customized for a desirable output and high speed can be achieved with the associated multi-nozzle cartridges. Inkjet technology holds potential for improving the speed at which cell clusters are dispensed to create 3D spheroid cultures that may be used in rapid screening applications.

Thermal inkjet technology was introduced to biological applications in the early 2000s (Roth et al. 2004; Xu et al. 2004, 2005). Using this technology, live cells may be patterned in arrays at high speed, 100 spots per cm^2 at high throughput (Rodriguez-Devora et al. 2012; Roth et al. 2004). Inkjet technology is growing in the modern at-home printing industry due to printer affordability, ease of set up, and high speed; however, further development is required to bring those benefits to the bioengineering realm. A thermal inkjet cartridge includes hundreds of small orifices called nozzles that, with the assistance of a heating element, are activated to fire droplets from the cartridge. Current systems can fire all nozzles at once or in sequence as required to deliver as many droplets as the printing pattern requires. Challenges remain, however, in fully introducing inkjet technology into the drug-screening applications; problems include nozzle clogging, shear forces, and thermal shock which can compromise cell integrity, limited range of viscosity, and surface tension properties on bio-ink (Parzel et al. 2009). We present the use of a thermal inkjet-based biofabricator and that of the hanging-drop culture technique to improve the speed and reproducibility of 3D cell aggregate/spheroid formation.

6.2 MATERIALS AND METHODS

6.2.1 BIOPRINTING PRINTER SETUP

A custom bioprinting system was used with commercially available HP 26 inkjet cartridges (Hewlett-Packard; Figure 6.1). Details of the bioprinter design have been previously published (Pepper et al. 2009). Briefly, the printer includes three main components: the cell delivery system, including inkjet cartridges, the motion system, consisting of a two-axis positioning stage, and control hardware and software residing in a personal computer.

To prepare the cartridges for printing, all of the ink was removed and the cartridges were cleaned prior to use with cells. The cartridges were cut open to allow access to the deposit cylinder. The cartridges were cleaned in ethanol before and after each experiment. Before each experiment, approximately 10 cartridges were prepared by loading each cartridge cylinder with the original black ink and printing a validation pattern. This pattern comprises 50 horizontal lines, each printed one at a time for each nozzle. Completion of the pattern shows which nozzles are firing

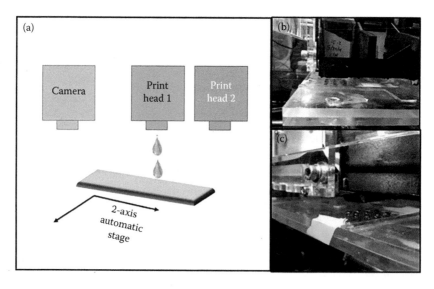

FIGURE 6.1 Thermal inkjet-based biofabricator. (a) Schematic of the biofabricator showing the two-axis positioning stage and thermal inkjet heads dispensing droplets over a glass slides. (b) Frontal view of an inkjet head. (c) Angled view of inkjet while printing.

and which may be clogged or damaged. Subsequently, all of the cartridges were washed with warm water to remove the ink and any other residue in the nozzles. The cartridges were then cleaned with distilled water and flushed with ethanol. Specifically, the cartridges were semisubmerged in ethanol for 10–15 s and then ethanol was pulled through the nozzles with vacuum. The cartridges were then dried in a hood. Only one nozzle was used for this experiment. The cartridges were loaded with 150 μL of cell bio-ink and the nozzle head was wiped to promote the flow of ink through the nozzles. The cartridges were then loaded into the slot on the bioprinter for use.

Glass slides were loaded on the biofabricator stage. Each slide had an array of 3 × 4 30-μL droplets of medium supplemented with methylcellulose. The first drop was moved under the camera based on an estimated value. With slight adjustment, a program was used that allowed the selection of a location on a captured image and the conversion of that location to the coordinates of the drop's location. This process was repeated for each drop by inputting the layout (number of columns and rows) and an estimated distance (in mm) between each drop. The 32-bit MATLAB® with the XPC Target code was programmed so that each row would increase the number of drops printed in multiples of a desired value. In this test, multiples of 100 and 150 were used, as noted. Thus, the number of printed drops on each drop was equal to the "inputted value" × "the row" (e.g., 100 × 3rd row = 300 drops). Once all the drops were selected using the image processing program, the cartridge was filled with 150 μL of the bio-ink and loaded into the biofabricator slot. The printer ejected each drop based on the coordinates and printed the desired number of drops on each. This was done in relatively quick time of 5 min and repeated for each sample.

6.2.2 BIOPRINTING PROCESS

Using the inkjet-based biofabricator (Figure 6.1), mouse fibroblasts (NIH-3T3) and human breast cancer (MCF-7) cells were patterned on top of a glass slide. Cells were ejected by a single nozzle in a gradient consisting of 100, 200, 300, and 400 droplets. Immediately following printing, both cell types were cultured using the standard hanging-drop conditions to promote the formation of cell aggregates/spheroids. Dulbecco's Modified Eagle's Medium supplemented with methylcellulose (0.04% w/v in DMEM) was used as the culture substrate, while the printed bio-ink consisted of the cell suspension at a cell density ranging from 6 to 8 × 10^6 cells/mL. Cellular aggregates/spheroids were monitored for 10 days. Viability and growth were monitored via live/dead assay (Invitrogen) and bright light images, respectively. Image J was used to analyze the aggregate/spheroid growth over time.

6.2.3 CELL CULTURE AND STAINING

NIH 3T3 fibroblasts and MCF-7 breast cancer cells were cultured, using the aseptic technique, in DMEM supplemented with fetal bovine serum (FBS). Cells were collected by trypsinization prior to their use as bio-ink for cell bioprinting. Prior to printing, cell suspensions were passed through a 70 μm cell strainer to decrease aggregates and mitigate nozzle clogging; cells were suspended in phosphate buffered saline (PBS) supplemented with ethylenediaminetetraacetic acid (EDTA) and cell concentration determined. This bio-ink formulation was previously found to print well and minimize nozzle clogging issues (Pepper et al. 2012). After the cells were printed, the culture dish was inverted to promote culture using a hanging-drop technique. The hanging drops were suspended over a medium bath to avoid evaporation. For live/dead assay staining, spheroids were exposed to calcein AM and ethidium homodimer 1, and washed up to five times with PBS, to stain live cells (fluorescent green) and dead cells (fluorescent red) over the time periods of the study. Fluorescent color was quantified using Image J, using 8-bit images with a threshold range of 8–25. Data was normalized to the total number of pixels that represent 100% of each image.

6.2.4 AGGREGATE SHAPE FACTOR AND GROWTH

Bright field images for size and shape distribution analysis were obtained at Days 1, 3, 5, and 10 using a prior scientific microscope fitted with a Motic video camera. Both cell lines images were analyzed to measure the projected cell spheroid area, A, and perimeter, P using Image J version 1.47v. Data was exported to MS Excel to calculate a spherical shape factor, Φ, based on the following formula (Kelm et al. 2003). The spherical shape factor ranged from 0 to 1, with 1 being the closest to a perfect spheroid shape.

$$\Phi = \frac{\pi \times \sqrt{4A/\pi}}{P}$$

6.2.5 Data Analysis

All data was reported as mean ± standard deviation. Statistical analysis was performed using a two-way analysis of variance (ANOVA) in conjugation with Student's *t*-test. Statistical significance was defined as $p < 0.05$. The nonparametric Spearman's rank correlation test was used to compare the relationship between the nozzle firing times and the number of cells expelled from the cartridge.

6.3 RESULTS AND DISCUSSION

The bioprinting system used in this study allowed the control of the cells dispensed through manipulation of the droplet firing times. NIH 3T3 fibroblasts were printed consistently throughout the range of firing times (Figure 6.2). The number of printed cells is equivalent to 0.7473 times the firing time, as shown in the linear regression in Figure 6.2a, which had an R^2 value of 91.7%. This value indicates a high correlation

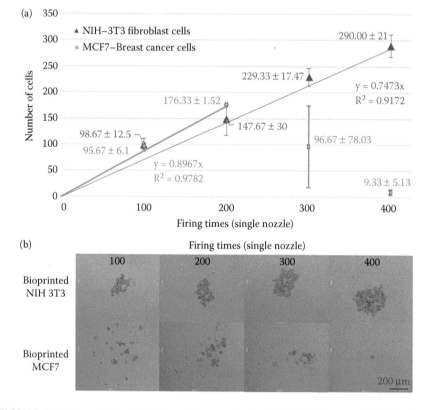

FIGURE 6.2 Bioprinted cells' plots and representative bright field images. (a) Firing times with the corresponding cells dispensed per spot. Linear relation and R^2 (including the origin) values shown, n = 3. (b) Representative bright light images of bioprinted cells when printed 100, 200, 300, and 400 times. Scale bar = 200 μm.

between the printing firing times and the cells dispensed. Nozzle clogging was not observed for the range of fibroblast cell densities used in this study. In comparison, there did not appear to be a linear relationship between MCF7 firing times and cell number; rather, the cell number reached a maximum when the firing times reached 200. Comparing MCF7 behavior to 3T3 behavior, similar printability was observed in the first two printing periods; however, at higher times, the number of MCF7 cells ejected decreased considerably until clogging occurred at 400 firing times. The results suggest that the MCF7 cells tend to decrease the continuous printability of the bio-ink by clogging the inkjet nozzle. This observation can be explained by the tendency of MCF7 cells to self-aggregate in smaller colonies. Figure 6.2c depicts representative images taken 2 h after cells were bioprinted. Interestingly, at this point of time, the fibroblasts had aggregated into single large aggregates more rapidly within a drop than had the MCF7 cells. In comparison to the fibroblast cultures, the MCF7 cultures comprised small clusters of cancerous cells, which quickly formed but remained scattered after 2 h. The images are further confirmation of the clogging issues noted earlier that occurred during printing in the 300 firing times period. The nonparametric Spearman rank correlation test was used to compare the single nozzle firing time to the number of cells expelled by the system. Numbers of cells in NIH 3T3 fibroblast cell cultures were strongly correlated with the firing times, with a Spearman correlation coefficient of above 0.9. MCF-7 breast cancer cell cultures were moderately correlated with a Spearman correlation coefficient of above 0.65, at firing times of 100 and 200; however, there was a negative coefficient of −0.51 when considering all firing times, due to the decreased number of cells expelled in the 300 and 400 times test groups.

Bioprinted cells aggregated immediately following 24 h of culture and grew over the 10-day period in approximate spherical shapes. NIH 3T3 fibroblasts were printed consistently throughout the range of nozzle firing times as depicted in Figure 6.3. During the period of 10 days, fibroblast aggregates grew up to 4–5 times fold the projected area of the spheroids, which translates to 16–25 times in three dimensionality. The maximum spherical shape factor (calculated from the projected area) was

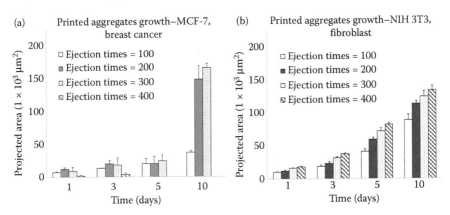

FIGURE 6.3 Proliferation plots of bioprinted mammalian cells. (a) MCF7 breast cancer cells. (b) NIH 3T3 mouse fibroblasts.

0.89 ± 0.03 and 0.9 ± 0.01 for 3T3 fibroblasts (at day 5) and MCF7 cells (at day 3) respectively. In addition, it was observed that 100% of spheroids formed reproducible shapes and no satellite aggregates occurred. This finding is in contrast to results from most other common bioprinting technologies, particularly for wells with lower cell numbers (Faulkner-Jones et al. 2013; Odde and Renn 2000). At a firing time of 400, MCF7 breast cancer cells had different growth behaviors than the 3T3 fibroblasts due to the MCF7 cell printability issues. No spheroids were formed by the 400 time nozzle firing group after day 5, suggesting that viable aggregates require more cells than those numbering this group. Figure 6.3b shows that MCF7s took more time to proliferate, up to day 5. Nevertheless, although MCF7 cells proliferated more slowly than 3T3 fibroblasts, by day 10 the MCF7 spheroids reached similar size (diameter) as the fibroblast spheroids.

Spheroids/aggregates have been shown to elicit a typical biphasic growth pattern of solid tumors *in vivo* (Figure 6.3), with exponential growth, independent of an external factor, followed by size-limited proliferation followed by plateau (Sutherland 1988). Growth in this *in vitro* study was decayed after day 10 in concordance with previously reported results (Kelm et al. 2003). This result could be due to the degradation of glutamine, photodegradation of some vitamins and amino acids, and increased osmolarity due to evaporation. While thermal inkjet printing was combined in this study with the hanging-drop technique, it can also be used in combination with microfluidic- or well-based techniques to ease the manipulation of spheroids along the process and extend the viability of cultures. Figure 6.4 shows representative images of the progression of tumor growth throughout the study, from day 1 to 10, when the inkjet nozzle was activated 200 times.

Manual micropipetting is a labor-intensive and time-consuming process that can suffer from human error and inhomogeneous droplets. The creation of more uniform spheroids/aggregates can be improved by the use of automated approaches, such as extrusion, laser, and inkjet. Thermal inkjet printing provides an economical system with the potential to create another breakthrough in the high-throughput-screening field. The available robotic systems in the market can indeed dispense hundreds of thousands of screening assays per day but they come with a healthy price tag.

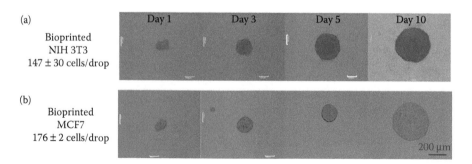

FIGURE 6.4 Representative images of bioprinted mammalian cells at 200 firing times through culture time. (a) NIH 3T3 mouse fibroblasts. (b) MCF7 breast cancer cells. Scale bar = 200 μm.

The high-throughput robotic systems require a high investment, which renders them unsuitable for many academic labs and small and medium companies. This accessibility limits the scientific discovery that can be potentially achieved by the scientific community.

The live/dead assay revealed that cells remained viable up to 10 days; after that time, aggregates start to deteriorate and lose their spherical shapes. This change is likely due to the lack of media change in the hanging-drop technique. However, dynamic systems incorporated into the screening platform will extend the viability of cells. There was a concern regarding the prolonged firing times that can increase the level of shear stress and thermal shock experience by cells. However, viability results (Figure 6.5) indicate that the viability of spheroids in either cell line was not significantly affected by the number of firing times. NIH 3T3 fibroblast cells remained viable up to 80% until day 11, and even by day 17 the viability was reasonable for some groups. A single spheroid was analyzed at day 25 to confirm that by that time span, most cells were dead. MCF-7 human breast cancer cells maintained a viability rate of 50%–80% on days 5 and 11. By day 19, the MCF7 cells deteriorated in the same fashion as the fibroblasts.

This study provides evidence that 3D biological models can be biomanufactured with improved control of size and shape. These characteristics are the key in quality control for any future 3D cell culture model, in particular for cancer models that resemble physiological tissue characteristics and structure. Our custom biofabricator uses commercially available inkjet printing heads (from HP systems) that have been previously reported as high throughput (Ouyang et al. 2015), a feature that will be beneficial for the mass production of more physiological relevant

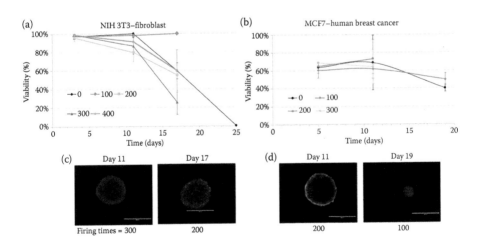

FIGURE 6.5 Viability plots over time of printed spheroids. Micropipetted control samples are plotted as series name "0" and the rest of the series corresponds to the number of times the inkjet nozzle was activated. (a) NIH 3T3 mouse fibroblasts, n = 3. (b) MCF-7 human breast cancer cells, n = 3. (c, d) Representative images of aggregates/spheroids labeled with calcein AM (green, live cells) and ethidium homodimer-1 (red, dead cells). Scale bar = 400 μm.

cell aggregates/spheroids. Inkjet technology speed can be translated into a high-throughput field when translated into the drug discovery realm. The past studies have shown that inkjet bioprinting models can array 213 distinct assays per second (Rodriguez-Devora et al. 2012). Current commercial paper printing systems can print up to 12 pages per minute tested under ISO/IEC 24734, while the maximum print speed (draft quality) can reach up to 33 pages per second (Epson Inc. 2016). This output can translate into up to 42,240 droplets per second. In addition to the current speed of inkjet systems, these printers use print heads that contain hundreds of nozzles, which increases the promising capacity of such technology (Epson Inc. 2012). This technology offers a rapid automated system that has the potential to accelerate the pace of drug screening assays in upcoming years.

The development of a cartridge/system that can continuously print cell bodies without incurring clogging is still required. Future studies are expected to improve nozzle coatings with materials that improve cell printability properties. The creation of a more physiologically relevant tumor model requires the development of enabling technologies to conquer this biomanufacturing challenge. While the effect on metastatic behavior remains to be shown, tumorous spheroids/aggregates can be engineered to a desired size by inkjet-based biofabrication, which can be incorporated into the design of future rapid screening platforms. These biofabrication techniques can enable future technologies to accelerate drug identification for precise and personalized medicine.

6.4 CONCLUSION AND PERSPECTIVE

This study offers an assessment of the capabilities of an inkjet-based printing system for printing 3D cell spheroid aggregates. These aggregates could have potential applications such as tissue engineering, high-throughput screening, diagnostics, stem cell research, and more. Inkjet-based bioprinting systems offer a great potential for reproducible and high-throughput dispensing of cellular aggregates/spheroids. This work confirms that inkjet-based technology is well suited to accommodate miniature (pico-, nano-, submicroliter) volumes required for controlled, reproducible, and rapid cell spheroid aggregate culture. These highly reproducible spheroid models hold a great potential to become a fundamental tool for drug discovery, clinical research, and precise and personalized medicine.

ACKNOWLEDGMENTS

This research was conducted with support from the IDeA Networks of Biomedical Research Excellence grant, NIH 5 P20 RR-016461, 8 P20 GM-103499, and the Institute for Biological Interfaces of Engineering.

REFERENCES

Abbott, A. 2003. Cell culture: Biology's new dimension. *Nature* no. 424 (6951):870–72.
Akiyama, M. and M. Nakamura. 2009. Bone regeneration and neovascularization processes in a pellet culture system for periosteal cells. *Cell Transplant* no. 18 (4):443–52.

Asghar, W., R. El Assal, H. Shafiee, S. Pitteri, R. Paulmurugan, and U. Demirci. 2015. Engineering cancer microenvironments for *in vitro* 3-D tumor models. *Mater Today* no. 18 (10):539–53.

Burg, K. J. and T. Boland. 2003. Minimally invasive tissue engineering composites and cell printing. *IEEE Eng Med Biol Mag* no. 22 (5):84–91.

Burg, T., C. A. Cass, R. Groff, M. Pepper, and K. J. Burg. 2010. Building off-the-shelf tissue-engineered composites. *Philos Trans A: Math Phys Eng Sci* no. 368 (1917):1839–62.

Chen, P., S. Guven, O. B. Usta, M. L. Yarmush, and U. Demirci. 2015. Biotunable acoustic node assembly of organoids. *Adv Healthc Mater* no. 4 (13):1937–43.

Dean, D. M., A. P. Napolitano, J. Youssef, and J. R. Morgan. 2007. Rods, tori, and honeycombs: the directed self-assembly of microtissues with prescribed microscale geometries. *FASEB J* no. 21 (14):4005–12.

Del Duca, D., T. Werbowetski, and R. F. Del Maestro. 2004. Spheroid preparation from hanging drops: Characterization of a model of brain tumor invasion. *J Neurooncol* no. 67 (3):295–303.

Dias, A. D., A. M. Unser, Y. Xie, D. B. Chrisey, and D. T. Corr. 2014. Generating size-controlled embryoid bodies using laser direct-write. *Biofabrication* no. 6 (2):025007.

Edmondson, R., J. J. Broglie, A. F. Adcock, and L. Yang. 2014. Three-dimensional cell culture systems and their applications in drug discovery and cell-based biosensors. *Assay Drug Dev Technol* no. 12 (4):207–18.

Epson Inc. 2012. HP PageWide technology: Breakthrough speed, professional quality. In, Epson Inc. http://h20195.www2.hp.com/v2/GetPDF.aspx/4aa4-3489eeci.pdf

Epson Inc. 2016. Laser quality print speeds (ISO/IEC 24734). In, Epson Inc. http://www.epson.com/cgi-bin/Store/Landing/PrintSpeedISO.jsp

Faulkner-Jones, A., S. Greenhough, J. A. King, J. Gardner, A. Courtney, and W. Shu. 2013. Development of a valve-based cell printer for the formation of human embryonic stem cell spheroid aggregates. *Biofabrication* no. 5 (1):015013.

Foty, R. 2011. A simple hanging drop cell culture protocol for generation of 3D spheroids. *J Vis Exp* no. 6 (51):2720.

Han, Y. L., Y. Yang, S. Liu, J. Wu, Y. Chen, T. J. Lu, and F. Xu. 2013. Directed self-assembly of microscale hydrogels by electrostatic interaction. *Biofabrication* no. 5 (3):035004.

Ingram, M., G. B. Techy, R. Saroufeem, O. Yazan, K. S. Narayan, T. J. Goodwin, and G. F. Spaulding. 1997. Three-dimensional growth patterns of various human tumor cell lines in simulated microgravity of a NASA bioreactor. *In Vitro Cell Dev Biol Anim* no. 33 (6):459–66.

Kelm, J. M., N. E. Timmins, C. J. Brown, M. Fussenegger, and L. K. Nielsen. 2003. Method for generation of homogeneous multicellular tumor spheroids applicable to a wide variety of cell types. *Biotechnol Bioeng* no. 83 (2):173–80.

Khaoustov, V. I., G. J. Darlington, H. E. Soriano, B. Krishnan, D. Risin, N. R. Pellis, and B. Yoffe. 1999. Induction of three-dimensional assembly of human liver cells by simulated microgravity. *In Vitro Cell Dev Biol Anim* no. 35 (9):501–09.

LaBarbera, D. V., B. G. Reid, and B. H. Yoo. 2012. The multicellular tumor spheroid model for high-throughput cancer drug discovery. *Expert Opin Drug Discov* no. 7 (9):819–30.

Landry, J., D. Bernier, C. Ouellet, R. Goyette, and N. Marceau. 1985. Spheroidal aggregate culture of rat liver cells: Histotypic reorganization, biomatrix deposition, and maintenance of functional activities. *J Cell Biol* no. 101 (3):914–23.

Lin, R. Z. and H. Y. Chang. 2008. Recent advances in three-dimensional multicellular spheroid culture for biomedical research. *Biotechnol J* no. 3 (9–10):1172–84.

McArthur, R. and F. Borsini. 2006. Animal models of depression in drug discovery: A historical perspective. *Pharmacol Biochem Behav* no. 84 (3):436–52.

Mehta, G., A. Y. Hsiao, M. Ingram, G. D. Luker, and S. Takayama. 2012. Opportunities and challenges for use of tumor spheroids as models to test drug delivery and efficacy. *J Control Release* no. 164 (2):192–204.

Mironov, V., R. P. Visconti, V. Kasyanov, G. Forgacs, C. J. Drake, and R. R. Markwald. 2009. Organ printing: Tissue spheroids as building blocks. *Biomaterials* no. 30 (12):2164–74.

Mosadegh, B., M. R. Lockett, K. T. Minn, K. A. Simon, K. Gilbert, S. Hillier, D. Newsome. et al. 2015. A paper-based invasion assay: Assessing chemotaxis of cancer cells in gradients of oxygen. *Biomaterials* no. 52:262–71.

Odde, D. J. and M. J. Renn. 2000. Laser-guided direct writing of living cells. *Biotechnol Bioeng* no. 67 (3):312–18.

Ouyang, L., R. Yao, S. Mao, X. Chen, J. Na, and W. Sun. 2015. Three-dimensional bioprinting of embryonic stem cells directs highly uniform embryoid body formation. *Biofabrication* no. 7 (4):044101.

Pampaloni, F., E. G. Reynaud, and E. H. Stelzer. 2007. The third dimension bridges the gap between cell culture and live tissue. *Nat Rev Mol Cell Biol* no. 8 (10):839–45.

Parzel, C. A., M. E. Pepper, T. Burg, R. E. Groff, and K. J. Burg. 2009. EDTA enhances high-throughput two-dimensional bioprinting by inhibiting salt scaling and cell aggregation at the nozzle surface. *J Tissue Eng Regen Med* no. 3 (4):260–68.

Pepper, M. E., C. A. Parzel, T. Burg, T. Boland, K. J. Burg, and R. E. Groff. 2009. Design and implementation of a two-dimensional inkjet bioprinter. *Conf Proc IEEE Eng Med Biol Soc* no. 2009:6001–05.

Pepper, M. E., V. Seshadri, T. C. Burg, K. J. Burg, and R. E. Groff. 2012. Characterizing the effects of cell settling on bioprinter output. *Biofabrication* no. 4 (1):011001.

Qihao, Z., C. Xigu, C. Guanghui, and Z. Weiwei. 2007. Spheroid formation and differentiation into hepatocyte-like cells of rat mesenchymal stem cell induced by co-culture with liver cells. *DNA Cell Biol* no. 26 (7):497–503.

Remick, D. 2013. Use of animal models for the study of human disease—a shock society debate. *Shock* no. 40 (4):345–46.

Rodriguez-Devora, J. I., B. Zhang, D. Reyna, Z. D. Shi, and T. Xu. 2012. High throughput miniature drug-screening platform using bioprinting technology. *Biofabrication* no. 4 (3):035001.

Roth, E. A., T. Xu, M. Das, C. Gregory, J. J. Hickman, and T. Boland. 2004. Inkjet printing for high-throughput cell patterning. *Biomaterials* no. 25 (17):3707–15.

Sutherland, R. M. 1988. Cell and environment interactions in tumor microregions: The multicell spheroid model. *Science* no. 240 (4849):177–84.

Tavana, H., B. Mosadegh, and S. Takayama. 2010. Polymeric aqueous biphasic systems for non-contact cell printing on cells: Engineering heterocellular embryonic stem cell niches. *Adv Mater* no. 22 (24):2628–31.

Timmins, N. E. and L. K. Nielsen. 2007. Generation of multicellular tumor spheroids by the hanging-drop method. *Methods Mol Med* no. 140:141–51.

Tseng, H., J. A. Gage, T. Shen, W. L. Haisler, S. K. Neeley, S. Shiao, J. Chen. et al. 2015. A spheroid toxicity assay using magnetic 3D bioprinting and real-time mobile device-based imaging. *Sci Rep* no. 5:13987.

Tung, Y. C., A. Y. Hsiao, S. G. Allen, Y. S. Torisawa, M. Ho, and S. Takayama. 2011. High-throughput 3D spheroid culture and drug testing using a 384 hanging drop array. *Analyst* no. 136 (3):473–78.

Wu, L. Y., D. Di Carlo, and L. P. Lee. 2008. Microfluidic self-assembly of tumor spheroids for anticancer drug discovery. *Biomed Microdevices* no. 10 (2):197–202.

Xu, F., B. Sridharan, S. Wang, U. A. Gurkan, B. Syverud, and U. Demirci. 2011. Embryonic stem cell bioprinting for uniform and controlled size embryoid body formation. *Biomicrofluidics* no. 5 (2):22207.

Xu, F., J. Wu, S. Wang, N. G. Durmus, U. A. Gurkan, and U. Demirci. 2011. Microengineering methods for cell-based microarrays and high-throughput drug-screening applications. *Biofabrication* no. 3 (3):034101.

Xu, T., J. Jin, C. Gregory, J. J. Hickman, and T. Boland. 2005. Inkjet printing of viable mammalian cells. *Biomaterials* no. 26 (1):93–9.

Xu, T., S. Petridou, E. H. Lee, E. A. Roth, N. R. Vyavahare, J. J. Hickman, and T. Boland. 2004. Construction of high-density bacterial colony arrays and patterns by the ink-jet method. *Biotechnol Bioeng* no. 85 (1):29–33.

Yamada, K. M. and E. Cukierman. 2007. Modeling tissue morphogenesis and cancer in 3D. *Cell* no. 130 (4):601–10.

Yan, S., J. Wei, Y. Liu, H. Zhang, J. Chen, and X. Li. 2015. Hepatocyte spheroid culture on fibrous scaffolds with grafted functional ligands as an *in vitro* model for predicting drug metabolism and hepatotoxicity. *Acta Biomater* no. 28:138–48.

Yuhas, J. M., A. P. Li, A. O. Martinez, and A. J. Ladman. 1977. A simplified method for production and growth of multicellular tumor spheroids. *Cancer Res* no. 37 (10):3639–43.

Section II

Materials Considerations

7 Control Testing and Effect of Manufacturing Parameters on the Biocompatibility of Polypropylene Mesh Implants

Ahmed El-Ghannam

CONTENTS

7.1 Introduction 107
7.2 Materials-Science Triad 108
    7.2.1 Mesh Manufacturing 109
    7.2.2 FTIR Analysis of Oxidation Degradation of Polypropylene 112
    7.2.3 Differential Scanning Calorimetry of Degradation of Polypropylene 113
7.3 Molecular Weight Analyses of Failed Implants 116
7.4 Recent Approaches for Pelvic Organ Prolapse (POP) Implant Design 119
7.5 Conclusion and Perspective 121
References 121

7.1 INTRODUCTION

Polypropylene (PP) mesh is widely used for the treatment of pelvic organ prolapse. The whole theory of transvaginal PP mesh for prolapse and stress urinary incontinence is to augment tissue and support the vaginal wall (Altman et al. 2005; Chaliha and Khullar 2006). The mesh has to be inert (nondegradable), has appropriate mechanical properties, and has the stability of the chemical and mechanical properties after implantation. The pores of the mesh are usually in the range of several hundred micrometers to millimeters scale, which are supposed to facilitate rapid tissue ingrowth and implant fixation. However, more than 4000 reports of complications related to the insertion of the transvaginal PP mesh, in the period 2005–2010, have been conveyed to the US Food and Drug Administration (FDA 2008; Skoczylas et al. 2014). Many clinical complications including dyspareunia, infection, and erosion or extrusion of the mesh after short and long implantation periods have been reported (Iglesia et al. 2010; Liang et al. 2011; Nazemi and Kobashi 2007; Rzepka et al. 2010). The failure of the mesh implant to integrate with the host tissue points to the influence of the physicochemical characteristics of the implant on stimulating inflammatory cells to trigger a destructive chronic inflammation that leads to implant failure (Anderson et al. 2008; Mikos et al. 1998). Although PP is classified as an inert material, manufacturing procedures during mesh fabrication can introduce major damage to the integrity of the structure and composition of the material. Analyses of pristine (unused before implantation) as well as failed PP mesh implants showed the deterioration of the mechanochemical stability, which led to implant failure. This chapter discusses the effect of manufacturing parameters on the stability of the PP mesh. Moreover, it sheds light on significant quality control tests that need to be considered for polymeric implants. Recent trends in polymer fiber production and mesh implant design are also discussed.

7.2 MATERIALS-SCIENCE TRIAD

PP mesh has been widely used as a permanent implant to repair hernia and to augment the vaginal wall for patients with urination incontinence. The biocompatibility of the mesh device is determined by the microstructure of PP that induces chemical inertness at the interface with the biological system. The microstructure is defined by the composition, the molecular weight, the molecular weight distribution, and the crystallinity parameters, including crystallization percent, crystal kind, size, and morphology. Processing parameters such as temperature, mechanical stresses, and environmental conditions can affect the microstructure, chemical stability, and hence the biocompatibility of PP. The interrelationship among processing, structure, and properties is explained by the materials-science triad (Figure 7.1). Therefore, it is essential to employ processing techniques that maintain the microstructure during mesh manufacturing in order to maintain inertness and biocompatibility for an implant that is supposed to be permanent in the body.

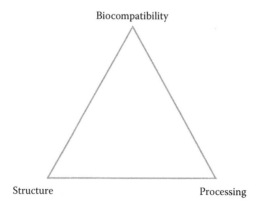

FIGURE 7.1 The materials-science triad represents the interrelationship among processing, structure, and biocompatibility of a biomaterial implant.

7.2.1 MESH MANUFACTURING

Knitting PP fibers of different diameters into mesh is the most common manufacturing method for the vaginal and hernia implants. The advantage of knitting over weaving is that the former prevents the ends of the mesh from unraveling when cut (Usher 1963). During knitting, fibers are mechanically stressed by stretching and bending forces parallel and perpendicular to the fiber axis. These mechanical stresses cause alteration in the geometrical shape of the fiber, including change in the diameter and occasional flattening deformation (Figure 7.2).

After knitting, the PP mesh is subjected to setting treatment to straighten it up and make it flat. For setting treatment, the PP mesh is heated under stress cycles with an applied force. The applied force values significantly exceed the load needed to fail the fibers of the PP mesh. However, because heat is applied, the PP mesh acquires viscoelastic behavior where the strain (deformation) increases with time (viscoelastic creep). While PP fibers between the knits of the mesh experience an increase in length and decrease in diameter, other fibers bended at the knit will be flattened. These deformations are associated with major alterations in the molecular structure and create new interspaces between the molecules that facilitate the diffusion of oxygen, leading to the well-known oxidative degradation mechanism of PP. During the heat cycle, the stress decreases with time causing viscoelastic relaxation that flattens the mesh. The relaxation modulus is a time-dependent elastic modulus for viscoelastic polymers. As the temperature increases, the modulus drops abruptly by about a factor of 10^3 within a 20°C temperature span, enhancing time-dependent deformation that is not recoverable on the release of the applied force. The deformation of the fibers is nonrecoverable because the original bonds between the molecules were

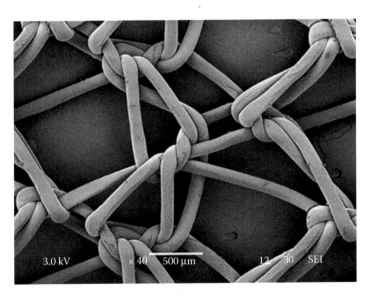

FIGURE 7.2 Scanning electron microscopic image of a pristine-knitted polypropylene mesh showing the deformation of the fibers due to the excessive multimode stresses applied during knitting.

broken, causing the molecular fragments to change their locations and environment. The sudden cooling of the hot mesh in air after each heat cycle provides a thermal shock that preserves the shape of the mesh flat, however with significant stored stress energy in the fibers. The release of the stored stress energy and the cross-linking between degraded molecules could be responsible for the significant changes in pore size reported in the literature when PP meshes were immersed in various biological solutions (Coda et al. 2003).

The sensitivity of the mechanical properties of PP to temperature and the strain rate is expected since it is a thermoplastic polymer. Figure 7.3 demonstrates the stress–strain behavior of PP at different temperatures (Zhou and Mallick 2002). Both elastic modulus and yield strength decreased with increasing temperature. At the same strain rate, the overall stress level decreased with increasing temperature. For example, as the temperature increases from 21.5°C to 100°C, the yield strength of PP decreased from 35.16 to 14.77 MPa at a strain rate of 0.05 min^{-1}. The yield strength decreases when the entangled polymer molecules break bonds, unwind, and separate from each other.

The setting temperature of the mesh (under mechanical stress) falls within the melting temperature range of PP as has been confirmed by differential scanning calorimetry (DSC) analysis performed on the pristine mesh. The application of a high load at elevated temperature will have a strong synergizing effect on facilitating the breakdown of bonds and the deterioration of the molecular and crystalline structures. These permanent structural defects cause permanent alterations to the mechanical properties, enhance the oxidation degradation, and deteriorate the biocompatibility

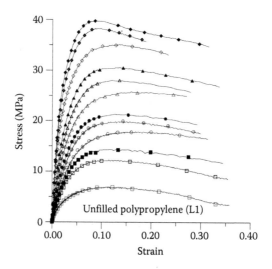

FIGURE 7.3 Stress–strain curves of unfilled polypropylene in the flow (L) direction at various strain rates and temperature: + 21.5°C, 0.05 min^{-1}; × 2.15°C, 0.5 min^{-1}; * 21.5°C, 5 min^{-1}; Δ 50°C, 0.05 min^{-1}; ▶ 50°C, 0.5 min^{-1}; ▲ 50°C, 5 min^{-1}; ○ 75°C, 0.05 min^{-1}; ⊕ 75°C, 0.5 min^{-1}; ● 75°C, 5 min^{-1}; □ 100°C, 0.05 min^{-1}; 100°C, 0.5 min^{-1}; ■ 100°C, 0.5 min^{-1}. (Zhou, Y. and P. K. Mallick: *Polym Eng Sci. 2002.* 42. 2449–2460. Copyright Wiley-VCH Verlag GmbH & Co. KGaA. Reproduced with permission.)

Control Testing and Effect of Manufacturing Parameters

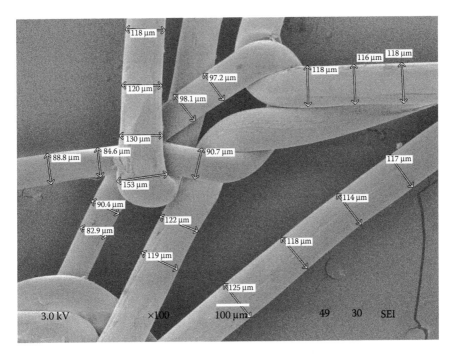

FIGURE 7.4 Scanning electron microscopic image of pristine polypropylene mesh showing significant variability in the diameters of the fibers.

of the material. Similar alterations to the microstructure of the polymer are also expected during knitting where the fibers are stretched, heated, and deformed, especially at the knit, as confirmed by scanning electron microscopy (SEM) analyses.

SEM analyses of a pristine mesh (Figure 7.4) showed significant variability in the diameters of the fibers ranging from 82.9 to 125 μm. Due to this variability, thin fibers will experience more stress, in response to the applied forces during setting, and hence more alteration in the molecular structure and degradation than thick fibers. The variation in the extent of the deformation and degradation does not exist just among individual fibers but it also exists within the same fiber. The left fiber in the SEM image (arrow) shows more than 30% increase in width near the folded area (knit). SEM analyses of the failed implants repeatedly showed the significant deformation of the fibers due to fabrication (Figure 7.5). The flattening of the fibers at the knit is due to compressive stresses perpendicular to the drawing direction of the fiber. At this stress direction, the strength of the fiber is reduced one-third to one-half of its strength value registered when the fiber is stretched in a tensile mode or a direction parallel to the drawing direction.

The consequence of the molecular degradation and movement of the polymer chains at high temperature is an increase in the permeability of the polymer toward the diffusion of small foreign molecules (e.g., O_2, H_2O, CO_2, etc.) present in air. Penetration of these molecules enhances the swelling and degradation of the materials' mechanical and physical properties (Callister Jr. and Rethwisch 2009). The

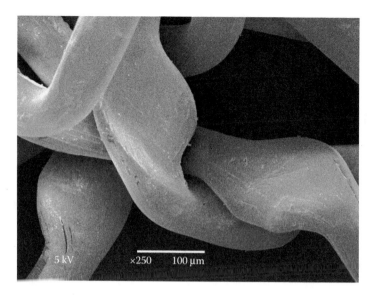

FIGURE 7.5 Scanning electron microscopic image of a failed polypropylene vaginal mesh implant showing significant fiber deformation created during manufacturing.

molecular diffusion of foreign molecules (e.g., oxygen) in a polymer is a strong function of temperature, polymer molecular weight, and polymer morphology. The diffusion coefficient **D** is a property of the material that measures how easily the diffusion of foreign molecules inside the polymer can occur. The diffusion coefficient **D** is exponentially dependent on the temperature. The diffusion of oxygen, nitrogen, carbon dioxide, and/or water vapor present in air through the PP fiber that is under elevated temperature and stresses is facilitated.

7.2.2 FTIR ANALYSIS OF OXIDATION DEGRADATION OF POLYPROPYLENE

Fourier transform infrared spectrometry (FTIR) analyses (Figure 7.6) of a pristine mesh confirmed the oxidation and showed characteristic bands for carbonyl groups, indicating the oxidation of the pristine implant materials.

The FTIR bands between the two dotted blue lines (Figure 7.6) show the bands for the carbonyl (C=O) stretching vibrations groups in the wave number range 1640–1850 cm^{-1}. The carbonyl bands in this wave number range are corresponding to ketones, aldehydes, and carboxylic acids. These degradation products are common for PP that is thermally oxidized (Bernstein et al. 2007). The FTIR analysis of a medical-grade PP three-dimensional (3D) block did not show the carbonyl band characteristic of degradation. This indicated that the thermo-mechanical stresses the fibers exposed to during mesh manufacturing are responsible for the deterioration of the integrity of the molecular structure and oxidation degradation.

The oxidation of the pristine PP mesh is maximized by the high surface area of the fibers. The fibers of the mesh showed longitudinal cracks along the axis of the fiber that enhances the diffusion of the oxygen into the bulk of the fiber. The wide

Control Testing and Effect of Manufacturing Parameters

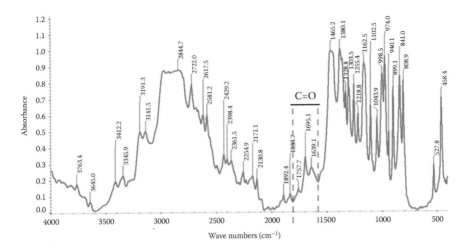

FIGURE 7.6 FTIR spectrum of a pristine polypropylene vaginal mesh showing the numerous carbonyl bands characteristics for ketone, aldehyde, and ester thermal oxidation degradation products.

distribution of polymeric debris and the torn thin sheets partially attached to the fibers would have a similar effect on increasing the oxidative degradation of the polymer.

Therefore, the deformation of the fibers of the pristine mesh seen by SEM is not just a defect in the geometrical shape or symmetry, rather it is a strong indicator of the degradation of the molecular structure, chemical stability, and biocompatibility. Such degradation evidence was confirmed by the thermal analysis (DSC) of pristine PP mesh implant.

7.2.3 Differential Scanning Calorimetry of Degradation of Polypropylene

Differential scanning calorimetry (DSC) is an important analysis method that measures the heat absorbed or liberated during the various transitions (e.g., melting and crystallization) in the material as it is heated up. The temperature of the sample is raised at a controlled rate and the amount of heat absorbed or rejected is recorded in the thermogram as endothermic or exothermic peaks. Thus, the DSC analysis defines the polymer melting and crystallization temperatures. Both the melting point and the crystallization temperature are controlled by the molecular weight and characteristics of the crystalline phase of the PP. The higher the molecular weight, the higher the melting temperature. In addition, the width of the melting band reflects the homogeneity and purity of the crystalline structure of the polymer. A narrow melting band indicates a homogenous narrow crystal size range. The appearance of more than one melting band is indicative of the presence of impurities, degradation compounds, and defective crystalline structure. The DSC analysis of the pristine (unused) PP mesh is shown in Figure 7.7a.

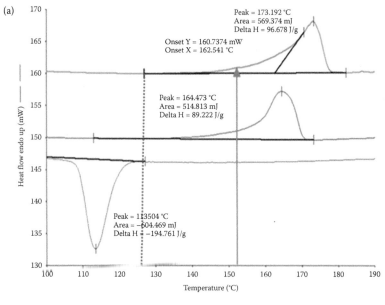

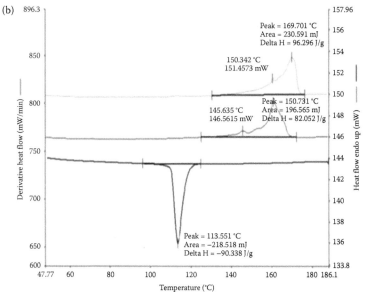

FIGURE 7.7 (a) DSC analysis of the pristine polypropylene mesh implant. (b) DSC analysis of a different pristine polypropylene mesh showing two melting points.

The first melt curve, in green, is for the received pristine mesh. The second melt curve, in red, is shown, as per ASTM, to remove the processing phenomenon. The recrystallization curve is shown in blue. DSC data show the sample to have a broad melting peak with a melting point at 173°C (first melt) and a recrystallization peak at 113.6°C. The first melt curve shows an onset of melting at 126°C and most importantly it shows the presence of a melting shoulder at about 153°C. The broadness of the melting peak is indicative of the presence of contaminants in the PP from manufacturing. Data in the literature indicated that the presence of contaminants in PP broadens the melting band during DSC analysis. Plato and coworkers reported that the melting peak width is a valuable measure of purity (Plato and Glasgow 1969). The less pure and nonperfect crystals melt first followed by purer larger crystals. It should be emphasized that according to the basics of Materials Science and Engineering, imperfection and defects in the crystals raise the overall energy of the material and, therefore, enhance the chemical reactivity and degradation of the PP mesh.

The DSC plot (Figure 7.7) shows that the PP melting process starts at about 126°C (left dotted red line). This is the temperature at which the polymer chains (molecules) within the fiber start to move and slide over each other in the beginning of the melting. The chains (molecules) within the crystals inside the fiber move because the bonds that connect them are broken by the energy delivered by heat. Thus, during the melting of the polymer, there will be a rearrangement of the molecules in the transformation from an ordered (crystalline) to a disordered (amorphous) molecular state. The melting of a polymer takes place over a range of temperatures (not just one specific temperature, from 126°C to 180°C) because the polymer is composed of molecules having a variety of molecular weights. Within the PP fiber, the short molecules separate from each other at lower temperature than long chain molecules. Thus, there will be a temperature range through which the melting process is complete. The melting temperature of the polymer is usually taken as the one near the high ends of the melting temperature range (i.e., 173°C).

The DSC analysis does not apply any forces to stretch the mesh fibers during analysis. However, if mechanical stress is applied in the temperature range 126–180°C, the movement of chains will be further facilitated and the deterioration of the integrity of the structure will be enhanced. Heat by itself (without mechanical stress) breaks the bonds between the molecules and makes them move to new positions in the material. This damages the molecular structure and properties of the material. Mechanical stress by itself (without heat) separates the molecules away from each other and damages the structure and properties of the material. Combining both heat and mechanical stress will synergize the destruction of the structural integrity of the material due to the breakdown of the bonds between molecules as well as within the same molecule and thus deteriorate the chemical and mechanical stabilities of PP fibers of the mesh.

The DSC thermogram in Figure 7.7b is for a different pristine mesh showing two melting points at 160.3°C and at 169.7°C. The appearance of multiple melting points is due to the degradation and collapsed lamella (crystals) of the PP crystals due to subjecting the material to heat and mechanical stresses (in the processing conditions described above). Zhu and coworkers investigated the double-melting endotherms of isotactic PP and reported that when the crystallization temperature is lower than 117°C, a spontaneous crystallization occurs in which the Lamellae formed is imperfect (Zhu et al. 2000). At a lower heating rate, the recrystallization or reorganization of these imperfect lamellae lead to double endotherms. Paukkeri and coworkers studied the thermal behavior of PP fractions as it relates to the multiple peaks (Paukkeri and Lehtinen 1993). The double peaks were detected for low molecular weight, nonisotactic fractions, as well as for low molecular weight fractions with isotacticity around 90%. Fractions consisted of a pure crystal form and those showing double-melting endotherms have low average isotactic sequence, generally below 80 PP units. The occurrence of double-peak shapes was attributed to two different processes: one is characteristic of highly stereo-regular material and probably constituted by melting of two different crystalline species, and the other consists of the reorganization of less ordered domains of crystalline material taking place during the melting scan. Another explanation for the two melting points is that there are two different α-forms corresponding to the folded chain crystal and the extended chain crystal in the system. Thus, alterations in the structure of the PP occur together with the degradation of the molecular weight.

Since the DSC main melting point of PP appeared at 173°C, the appearance of second melting points at significantly lower temperatures 149°C, 150°C, and/or 160°C is a strong evidence of the degradation of the material into a lower molecular weight polymer. Runt and Harrison in the book *Crystal Structure and Morphology* mentioned, "the annealing temperature range within which double melting peaks may be obtained on subsequent melting is dependent on molecular weight and molecular weight distribution" (Runt and Harrison 1980). Elvira and coworkers showed that the crystalline phase of isotactic PP is highly metastable, as it is obtained from the polymerization reaction, and also that the higher the melting temperature T_m of the associations, the more liable they are to be affected by oxidation (Elvira et al. 2004). The endotherm's shape can be strongly modified, shifting the melting peak toward lower temperatures, if longer degradation times are run. Many reports in the literature have correlated the alteration in the structure of PP mesh with the processing conditions. Afonso and coworkers analyzed the structure and thermal properties of PP mesh used in the treatment of stress urinary incontinence (Afonso et al. 2009). It has been reported that the PP polymers used in mesh fabrication, although (hypothetically) chemically identical, may present differences in fiber morphology and thermal history due to industrial processing. Moreover, chemical differences of molecular mass and polymeric structure are also possible (Chu et al. 1993; Maier and Calafut 1998).

7.3 MOLECULAR WEIGHT ANALYSES OF FAILED IMPLANTS

The molecular weights of the failed vaginal PP mesh from five different patients were analyzed through high-temperature tetra detection gel permeation chromatography (HT-GPC). Parallel analyses of three pristine meshes (unused, brand new from the boxes) were performed for comparison. The percent decrease in the average molecular weight (M_{wt}) of the explants compared to that of the original pristine implant (Figure 7.8) was calculated using the following equation:

$$\% \text{ decrease in } M_{wt} = \frac{(M_{wt} \text{ of the explant} - M_{wt} \text{ of the original implant})}{M_{wt} \text{ of the original implant}} \times 100$$

Four explants out of five showed a significant decrease in the average molecular weight compared to the original pristine meshes. The one explant that showed the

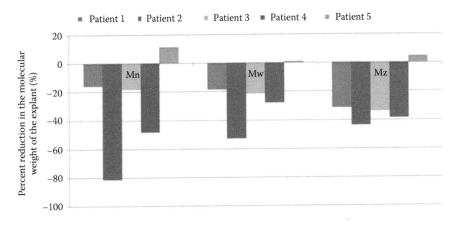

FIGURE 7.8 Percent decrease in the average molecular weight (M_{wt}) of the explants compared to that of the original pristine implant.

increase in the molecular weight can be attributed to the termination reaction during the degradation mechanism. Data in the literature indicate that, during degradation, termination reactions can take place in a way that results in an increase in the molecular weight (Bertin et al. 2010). The effect of the termination reaction at this stage of degradation can overweigh the effect of fragmentation of the molecules during the free radical degradation mechanism. In regard to the other four explants, the percent decrease in number average molecular weight (M_n) of the explants ranged from 16% to 81%. The percent decrease in the weight average molecular weight (M_w) of the explants ranged from 18% to 52%. The percent decrease in the Z average molecular weight (M_z) ranged from 31% to 39%. M_n is related to the flexibility and tackiness of a polymer and is a function of the amount of low molecular weight material. M_w is related to the strength of the polymer as well as the content of high molecular weight chains in the polymer. M_z is related to the brittleness and the amount of very high molecular weight material (Mori and Barth 2013). The decrease in the molecular weight of the explants is due to the degradation of PP inside the patient. SEM confirmed the results of the (HT-GPC) molecular weight analyses and showed severe cracking and roughening of the surface of the PP fibers of the failed implants (Figure 7.9).

Failed implants retrieved from patients are no longer flexible as they were at the time of implantation; rather, they are found to be stiff and cracked. The cracks have sharp edges and flat fracture surface indicating brittleness. The stiffness and cracking indicate that the mesh material is not chemically stable and hence is not biocompatible. Similar cracking observation was reported in the literature for highly cross-linked ultra-high molecular weight polyethylene acetabular liners that were retrieved from patients at an average of 10 months after implantation (Bradford et al. 2004). Both PP and polyethylene are olefins, so they belong to the same polymer family. Like cracking in degraded PP, the cracking of degraded polyethylene is perpendicular to the machining marks. Similar observation was also reported by Mary and coworkers (Mary et al. 1998) for PP sutures explanted after one and two years

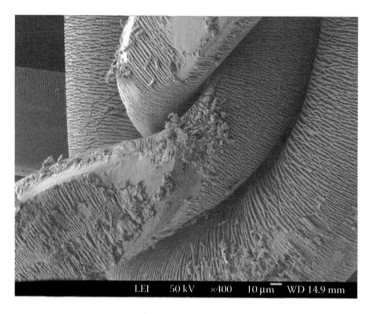

FIGURE 7.9 Scanning electron micrograph of the failed mesh implant retrieved from a patient showing severe cracking and roughening of the surface of the polypropylene fibers.

of implantation where the deterioration of the outermost surface layer was associated with uniformly spaced circumferential cracking and peeling and flaking of the polymer material. One consequence of the cracking and degradation of the fibers is the loss of the mechanical strength and the ability of the mesh to augment tissue. Laroche and colleagues reported that PP monofilament lost strength more rapidly than the polyvinylidene fluoride (PVDF) material with residual tensile strength values of the two sutures after seven years being 53.4% and 92.5%, respectively (Laroche et al. 1995). Clave and coworkers and Costello and colleagues all reported seeing degradations in PP fibers from explanted meshes, which were in the form of transverse cracks (Clave et al. 2010; Costello et al. 2007). The combination of stresses and environmental conditions at the implantation site can act synergistically to cause environmental stress crazing, cracking, and rupture (Ratner 2004). The sequence of these events occurs at low stress levels for polymers sensitive to these effects when they are in contact with aggressive environments, such as tissue fluids and hostile chemicals produced by irritated macrophages.

Degradation of PP is associated with severe immune response, acute inflammation, and thickening of the fibrous capsule. In addition, a major consequence of the degradation is the instability of the PP mesh inside the implantation bed due to poor or absence of tissue integration through the pore structure. The progress of the degradation mechanism is expected to escalate the rate of degradation as more cracks are formed due to the change in the stiffness of the material. Toxic effects of the degradation products and the loss of the mechanical strength are obvious adverse effects of the degradation of a polymeric implant that is supposed to have chemical and mechanical stabilities to be able to serve as a permanent implant. Data in the literature indicated that tissue response to prosthetic meshes depends on the material used and its structure. The PP mesh contact of fibroblasts led to a major decrease of matrix metalloproteinase activity and mRNA expression (Jain et al. 2009; Rosch et al. 2006). Moreover, other studies have reported a decrease in the ratio of collagen type I/collagen type III in the scar tissue in patients treated with mesh implant. The alteration in the extracellular matrix, especially the quality and quantity of collagen, is thought to compromise the normal wound-healing mechanism. For example, the decrease in the ratio of collagen I to collagen III in the scar tissue results in a reduced tensile strength which may be a major reason for hernia recurrence. In the case of transvaginal implants, it may be responsible for the extrusion of the implant.

7.4 RECENT APPROACHES FOR PELVIC ORGAN PROLAPSE (POP) IMPLANT DESIGN

The significant damage introduced by traditional mesh-weaving manufacturing procedures to the PP structure and biocompatibility highlights the importance of developing new processing technology using a 3D benchtop tissue system. Moreover, there is an urgent need for the development of new materials for mesh fabrication. Klinge and colleagues reported the PVDF woven mesh (DynaMesh) as a new potential material for POP applications (Klinge et al. 2002). Although PVDF exhibited improved biocompatibility and better issue ingrowth compared to PP mesh (Klinge et al. 2007), mesh erosion and exposure still occurred (Fortelny et al. 2010; Sommer and Friis-Andersen 2013). These problems are similar to those reported for the PP-woven mesh and related to the structure damage due to the weaving procedures.

Electrospinning provides a simple approach to fabricate nanofibers and porous scaffolds that mimics many aspects of the extracellular matrix, including large specific surface area available for cell adhesion and 3D growth. In addition, the nanofibrous scaffold can serve as a delivery vehicle for therapeutic agents (Chen et al. 2011; Ge et al. 2015; Ingavle and Leach 2014; Mohamed and Xing 2012). The nanofibrous PVDF biomimetic mesh was introduced by Medprin Biotech BmbH (Frankfurt, Germany) as chemically stable and nonabsorbable *in vivo*. To construct the mesh, PVDF was dissolved and sprayed by electronically controlled jets, layer by layer to form a fibrous structure similar to the extracellular matrix. The relatively high surface area of the mesh may facilitate its use as a cell carrier for a stem cell-based therapy for POP that can result in an improved tissue regeneration (Ding et al. 2016). On the other hand, measurements of the mechanical properties showed that the nanofibrous biomimetic mesh has a relatively high stiffness that would compromise conformability with the surrounding tissue. The mismatch between the stiffness of the implanted material and host tissue is known to contribute to tissue degeneration and loss of mechanical integrity (Deprest et al. 2006; Gamble et al. 1984).

Ge and coworkers reported on the core–sheath polystyrene/gelatin electrospun nanofiber mesh (Ge et al. 2015). The goal of coating polystyrene fibers with gelatin is to create a hydrophilic surface that enhances tissue integration. The 20% gelatin solution and 20% PS solution were used to produce the shell and core of nanofibers using coaxial electrospinning (Figure 7.10).

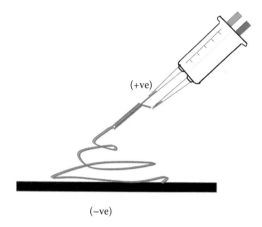

FIGURE 7.10 Schematic diagram of an electrospinning setup for the core–sheath polystyrene/gelatin nanofibrous membrane.

Young's modulus of the gelatin/PS scaffold was 12.42 ± 2.92 MPa, similar to that of the corresponding native tissues (Chaliha and Khullar 2006). Histological and pathological examinations as well as real-time PCR analyses showed mesh graft accommodation in the pelvic submucosa, two-week post-implantation in rats. Hematoxylin and eosin (H&E) staining showed that a prominent host tissue response occurred in the first and second weeks, and then decreased with time, and only minimal inflammatory responses were observed in the sixth week, with the evidence of the presence of multinucleated giant cells adjacent to materials. The detection of multinucleated giant cells on the implant surface after six weeks of implantation is indicative of the irritation of the immune system by the implant. Polymer degradation may go through an initial incubation period characterized by a relatively slow rate of degradation followed by an exponential increase in the degradation rate. A long-term evaluation of the biological performance of the gelatin/polystyrene implant is needed.

Tissue engineering approaches for POP have included the use of stem cells cultured on natural and synthetic meshes (Dolce et al. 2010; Ho et al. 2009). Polyamide 6 (PA6) polymers are stronger than PP and are biocompatible, permitting cell attachment and proliferation (Edwards et al. 2013). Su and colleagues coated a PA6 mesh with porcine gelatin under various gelation conditions (Su et al. 2014). The nylon mesh was warp knitted from 100 μm monofilament, giving a mass/area of 85 g m^{-2} and a large pore diameter of 1.3 mm. Endometrial mesenchymal stem cells (eMSCs) attached to the coated mesh and differentiated into smooth muscle cells and fibroblasts, essential for generating new-tissues, which could confer the necessary tissue elasticity and strength for the effective repair of the damaged fascial tissue in POP. Long-term animal studies are needed for the assessment of this approach. Moreover, the use of absorbable biomaterials as well as material that can signal cells may be a promising regenerative medicine approach.

7.5 CONCLUSION AND PERSPECTIVE

The processing condition of the polypropylene mesh resulted in the alteration of the microstructure, deterioration of the crystalline phase, and oxidative degradation of polypropylene fibers as confirmed by FTIR, DSC, SEM analyses of pristine fibers. Under these conditions of heat, set temperature, and applied stress, major alterations of the polypropylene structure, including lowering the molecular weight, increasing molecular polydispersity and deterioration of the crystalline structure, are expected to take place. All these expectations came to be proven true when the material was subjected to tests using various analysis methods as discussed above. Analysis of the failed polypropylene mesh explants confirmed the degradation. These results highlight the need to put standards for the polypropylene to be used for medical devices. These standards should include molecular weight, molecular weight distribution, crystallization percentage, and crystalline parameters. Moreover, the quality control tests performed by industry for polypropylene mesh require major revision. New methods for manufacturing polypropylene that do not include stretching the fibers or subjecting them to heat need to be developed. Alternatively, an absorbable bioactive ceramic or drug delivery system can be used to stimulate cells to regenerate tissue and strengthen the muscle.

REFERENCES

Afonso, J. S., R. M. Jorge, P. S. Martins, S. Soldi Mda, O. L. Alves, B. Patricio, T. Mascarenhas, M. G. Sartori, and M. J. Girao. 2009. Structural and thermal properties of polypropylene mesh used in treatment of stress urinary incontinence. *Acta Bioeng Biomech* no. 11 (3):27–33.

Altman, D., A. Lopez, C. Gustafsson, C. Falconer, J. Nordenstam, and J. Zetterstrom. 2005. Anatomical outcome and quality of life following posterior vaginal wall prolapse repair using collagen xenograft. *Int Urogynecol J Pelvic Floor Dysfunct* no. 16 (4):298–303.

Anderson, J. M., A. Rodriguez, and D. T. Chang. 2008. Foreign body reaction to biomaterials. *Semin Immunol* no. 20 (2):86–100.

Bernstein, R., S. M. Thornberg, R. A. Assink, A. N. Irwin, J. M. Hochrein, J. R. Brown, D. K. Derzon, S. B. Klamo, and R. L. Clough. 2007. The origins of volatile oxidation products in the thermal degradation of polypropylene, identified by selective isotopic labeling. *Polym Degrad Stab* no. 92 (11):2076–94.

Bertin, D., M. Leblanc, S. R. A. Marque, and D. Siri. 2010. Polypropylene degradation: Theoretical and experimental investigations. *Polym Degrad Stab* no. 95 (5):782–91.

Bradford, L., D. A. Baker, J. Graham, A. Chawan, M. D. Ries, and L. A. Pruitt. 2004. Wear and surface cracking in early retrieved highly cross-linked polyethylene acetabular liners. *J Bone Joint Surg Am* no. 86-A (6):1271–82.

Callister Jr., W. D. and D. G. Rethwisch. 2009. Diffusion in polymeric materials. In *Materials Science and Engineering: An Introduction*, edited by W. D. Callister Jr. and D. G. Rethwisch. New York: Wiley & Sons. pp. 559–60.

Chaliha, C. and V. Khullar. 2006. Surgical repair of vaginal prolapse: A gynaecological hernia. *Int J Surg* no. 4 (4):242–50.

Chen, J., B. Zhou, Q. Li, J. Ouyang, J. Kong, W. Zhong, and M. M. Xing. 2011. PLLA-PEG-TCH-labeled bioactive molecule nanofibers for tissue engineering. *Int J Nanomedicine* no. 6:2533–42.

Chu, C. C., L. Pratt, L. Zhang, A. Hsu, and A. Chu. 1993. A comparison of a new polypropylene suture with Prolene. *J Appl Biomater* no. 4 (2):169–81.

Clave, A., H. Yahi, J. C. Hammou, S. Montanari, P. Gounon, and H. Clave. 2010. Polypropylene as a reinforcement in pelvic surgery is not inert: Comparative analysis of 100 explants. *Int Urogynecol J* no. 21 (3):261–70.

Coda, A., R. Bendavid, F. Botto-Micca, M. Bossotti, and A. Bona. 2003. Structural alterations of prosthetic meshes in humans. *Hernia* no. 7 (1):29–34.

Costello, C. R., S. L. Bachman, B. J. Ramshaw, and S. A. Grant. 2007. Materials characterization of explanted polypropylene hernia meshes. *J Biomed Mater Res B: Appl Biomater* no. 83 (1):44–9.

Deprest, J., F. Zheng, M. Konstantinovic, F. Spelzini, F. Claerhout, A. Steensma, Y. Ozog, and D. De Ridder. 2006. The biology behind fascial defects and the use of implants in pelvic organ prolapse repair. *Int Urogynecol J Pelvic Floor Dysfunct* no. 17 (Suppl 1):S16–S25.

Ding, J., M. Deng, X. C. Song, C. Chen, K. L. Lai, G. S. Wang, Y. Y. Yuan, T. Xu, and L. Zhu. 2016. Nanofibrous biomimetic mesh can be used for pelvic reconstructive surgery: A randomized study. *J Mech Behav Biomed Mater* no. 61:26–35.

Dolce, C. J., D. Stefanidis, J. E. Keller, K. C. Walters, W. L. Newcomb, J. J. Heath, H. J. Norton, A. E. Lincourt, K. W. Kercher, and B. T. Heniford. 2010. Pushing the envelope in biomaterial research: Initial results of prosthetic coating with stem cells in a rat model. *Surg Endosc* no. 24 (11):2687–93.

Edwards, S. L., J. A. Werkmeister, A. Rosamilia, J. A. Ramshaw, J. F. White, and C. E. Gargett. 2013. Characterisation of clinical and newly fabricated meshes for pelvic organ prolapse repair. *J Mech Behav Biomed Mater* no. 23(July):53–61.

Elvira, M., P. Tiemblo, and J. M. Gomez-Elvira. 2004. Changes in the crystalline phase during the thermo-oxidation of a metallocene isotactic polypropylene. A DSC study. *Polym Degrad Stab* no. 83 (3):509–18.

Food and Drug Administration. 2008. *Serious Complications Associated with Transvaginal Placement of Surgical Mesh in Repair of Pelvic Organ Prolapse and Stress Urinary Incontinence.* Food and Drug Administration 2008. Available from http://www.fda.gov/MedicalDevices/Safety/AlertsandNotices/PublicHealthNotifications/ucm061976.htm.

Fortelny, R. H., A. H. Petter-Puchner, K. S. Glaser, F. Offner, T. Benesch, and M. Rohr. 2010. Adverse effects of polyvinylidene fluoride-coated polypropylene mesh used for laparoscopic intraperitoneal onlay repair of incisional hernia. *Br J Surg* no. 97 (7):1140–45.

Gamble, J. G., C. C. Edwards, and S. R. Max. 1984. Enzymatic adaptation in ligaments during immobilization. *Am J Sports Med* no. 12 (3):221–28.

Ge, L., Q. Li, J. Jiang, X. You, Z. Liu, W. Zhong, Y. Huang, and M. M. Xing. 2015. Integration of nondegradable polystyrene and degradable gelatin in a core-sheath nanofibrous patch for pelvic reconstruction. *Int J Nanomedicine* no. 10(April):3193–201.

Ho, M. H., S. Heydarkhan, D. Vernet, I. Kovanecz, M. G. Ferrini, N. N. Bhatia, and N. F. Gonzalez-Cadavid. 2009. Stimulating vaginal repair in rats through skeletal muscle-derived stem cells seeded on small intestinal submucosal scaffolds. *Obstet Gynecol* no. 114 (2 Pt 1):300–09.

Iglesia, C. B., A. I. Sokol, E. R. Sokol, B. I. Kudish, R. E. Gutman, J. L. Peterson, and S. Shott. 2010. Vaginal mesh for prolapse: A randomized controlled trial. *Obstet Gynecol* no. 116 (2 Pt 1):293–303.

Ingavle, G. C. and J. K. Leach. 2014. Advancements in electrospinning of polymeric nanofibrous scaffolds for tissue engineering. *Tissue Eng Part B: Rev* no. 20 (4):277–93.

Jain, V., R. Srivastava, S. Jha, S. Misra, N. S. Rawat, and D. V. Amla. 2009. Study of matrix metalloproteinase-2 in inguinal hernia. *J Clin Med Res* no. 1 (5):285–89.

Klinge, U., M. Binneboesel, S. Kuschel, and B. Schuessler. 2007. Demands and properties of alloplastic implants for the treatment of stress urinary incontinence. *Expert Rev Med Devices* no. 4 (3):349–59.

Klinge, U., B. Klosterhalfen, A. P. Ottinger, K. Junge, and V. Schumpelick. 2002. PVDF as a new polymer for the construction of surgical meshes. *Biomaterials* no. 23 (16):3487–93.

Laroche, G., Y. Marois, R. Guidoin, M. W. King, L. Martin, T. How, and Y. Douville. 1995. Polyvinylidene fluoride (PVDF) as a biomaterial: From polymeric raw material to monofilament vascular suture. *J Biomed Mater Res* no. 29 (12):1525–36.

Liang, C. C., Y. H. Lin, Y. L. Chang, and S. D. Chang. 2011. Urodynamic and clinical effects of transvaginal mesh repair for severe cystocele with and without urinary incontinence. *Int J Gynaecol Obstet* no. 112 (3):182–86.

Maier, C. and T. Calafut. 1998. Chemistry. In *Polypropylene: The Definitive User's Guide and Databook*, edited by C. Maier and T. Calafut. Norwich, NY: William Andrew Inc., pp. 3–10.

Mary, C., Y. Marois, M. W. King, G. Laroche, Y. Douville, L. Martin, and R. Guidoin. 1998. Comparison of the *in vivo* behavior of polyvinylidene fluoride and polypropylene sutures used in vascular surgery. *ASAIO J* no. 44 (3):199–206.

Mikos, A. G., L. V. McIntire, J. M. Anderson, and J. E. Babensee. 1998. Host response to tissue engineered devices. *Adv Drug Deliv Rev* no. 33 (1–2):111–39.

Mohamed, A. and M. M. Xing. 2012. Nanomaterials and nanotechnology for skin tissue engineering. *Int J Burns Trauma* no. 2 (1):29–41.

Mori, S. and H. G. Barth. 2013. Molecular weight average and distribution. In *Size Exclusion Chromatography*, edited by S. Mori and H.G. Barth, Berlin: Springer Science. pp. 77–94.

Nazemi, T. M. and K. C. Kobashi. 2007. Complications of grafts used in female pelvic floor reconstruction: Mesh erosion and extrusion. *Indian J Urol* no. 23 (2):153–60.

Paukkeri, R. and A. Lehtinen. 1993. Thermal behaviour of polypropylene fractions: 2. The multiple melting peaks. *Polymer* no. 34 (19):4083–88.

Plato, C. and A. R. Glasgow Jr. 1969. Differential scanning calorimetry as a general method for determining the purity and heat of fusion of high-purity organic chemicals. Application to 95 compounds. *Anal Chem* no. 41 (2):330–36.

Ratner, B.D. 2004. Introduction: Degradation of materials in biological environment. In *Biomaterials Science: An Introduction to Materials in Medicine*, edited by B. D. Ratner, A. S. Hoffman, F. J. Schoen and J. E. Lemons. New York, NY: Academic Press. p. 411.

Rosch, R., P. Lynen-Jansen, K. Junge, M. Knops, B. Klosterhalfen, U. Klinge, P. R. Mertens, and V. Schumpelick. 2006. Biomaterial-dependent MMP-2 expression in fibroblasts from patients with recurrent incisional hernias. *Hernia* no. 10 (2):125–30.

Runt, J. and I. R. Harrison. 1980. Thermal analysis of polymers. In *Methods in Experimental Physics*, edited by R. A. Fava. New York, NY: Academic Press. pp. 287–337.

Rzepka, J., K. Brocker, C. Alt, C. Corteville, C. Sohn, and F. Lenz. 2010. Pelvic organ prolapse: Does the postoperative course of mesh-repair surgery differ in elderly women when compared with younger patients? *J Obstet Gynaecol* no. 30 (8):852–56.

Skoczylas, L. C., L. C. Turner, L. Wang, D. G. Winger, and J. P. Shepherd. 2014. Changes in prolapse surgery trends relative to FDA notifications regarding vaginal mesh. *Int Urogynecol J* no. 25 (4):471–77.

Sommer, T. and H. Friis-Andersen. 2013. DynaMesh(R) in the repair of laparoscopic ventral hernia: A prospective trial. *Hernia* no. 17 (5):613–18.

Su, K., S. L. Edwards, K. S. Tan, J. F. White, S. Kandel, J. A. Ramshaw, C. E. Gargett, and J. A. Werkmeister. 2014. Induction of endometrial mesenchymal stem cells into tissue-forming cells suitable for fascial repair. *Acta Biomater* no. 10 (12):5012–20.

Usher, F. C. 1963. Hernia repair with knitted polypropylene mesh. *Surg Gynecol Obstet* no. 117:239–40.

Zhou, Y. and P. K. Mallick. 2002. Effects of temperature and strain rate on the tensile behavior of unfilled and talc-filled polypropylene. Part I: Experiments. *Polym Eng Sci* no. 42 (12):2449–60.

Zhu, X., D. Yan, S. Tan, T. Wang, D. Yan, and E. Zhou. 2000. Further study on double-melting endotherms of isotactic polypropylene. *J Appl Polym Sci* no. 77 (1):163–70.

8 Scaffolds for 3D Model Systems in Bone Regenerative Engineering

*Keshia Ashe, Seth Malinowski,
Yusuf Khan, and Cato T. Laurencin*

CONTENTS

8.1 Introduction 125
8.2 Bone Grafts and Bone Graft Substitutes 126
    8.2.1 Current Bone Graft Options 126
    8.2.2 Relevance to 3D Model Systems 127
8.3 Regenerative Engineering 127
8.4 Scaffold Design and Fabrication 129
    8.4.1 Porogen Leaching in Bone Engineering 129
    8.4.2 Microsphere Based Scaffold Development 131
    8.4.3 Electrospinning Nanofiber Structures for Bone Tissue Engineering 131
    8.4.4 Thermally Induced Phase Separation to Form 3D
          Nanofiber Structures 133
    8.4.5 3D Printing Bone Scaffolds 135
    8.4.6 Degradable and Nondegradable Hydrogels in Bone
          Tissue Engineering 135
8.5 Conclusion and Perspective 137
References 137

8.1 INTRODUCTION

Bone tissue regeneration and repair is an inherent capability of the human body. In the event of a bony fracture, the body is able to fully restore the damaged tissue through a complex set of steps that can vary depending on the location of the fracture, extent of the damage, and the type of bone that is damaged, but it generally follows a similar path. Fracture of cortical bone, found along the length of our long bones, is typically repaired by a callus formation mechanism, in which new bone (callus) composed of fibrous tissue, blood vessels, cartilage, and bone, forms in order to bridge the gap between the two fractured bone fragments and secure it mechanically. This process may be described in four stages that overlap temporally (Schultz 1990). The first stage is inflammation, which is stimulated immediately following the disruption of the endosteum, periosteum, soft tissue, and blood vessels that occur in the event of an injury. The second stage of cortical bone healing is soft (or primary) callus formation, which includes the formation and organization of extracellular matrix and fibrous granulation tissue at the ends of the fractured bones. The third stage of fracture healing is the formation of the hard (or secondary) callus, in which hard woven bone replaces the soft callus. The fourth and final stage of fracture healing is when the callus is removed by osteoclast-mediated resorption and the new bone gradually undergoes a remodeling process that is mechanosensitive to applied physiological stresses. The timeline for bone regeneration and repair varies from several months to years, depending on the individual's genetic and environmental factors as well as the severity of the injury (Schultz 1990).

There are, however, instances when bone damage exceeds a simple fracture. As the extent of this damage increases it eventually exceeds the body's ability to heal itself. In these cases different approaches are necessary to regain bone integrity, some requiring surgical intervention and implantation of a bone graft or a bone graft substitute.

0.2 BONE GRAFTS AND BONE GRAFT SUBSTITUTES

Bone graft implantation is a surgical procedure that is performed to provide mechanical support, enhance tissue repair, and fill voids in skeletal defects that may result from traumatic injury or after tumor resection. Ideally, a bone graft should impart appropriate mechanical strength to support the defect site while providing an osteoconductive surface that facilitates cellular attachment, migration, and tissue remodeling for the eventual replacement of the implanted graft by host tissue. While autografts, allografts, and bone graft substitutes are clinical tools currently used to treat patients suffering from bone loss, advanced grafting materials are under constant development and now include a wider variety of materials and applications. Increased demands for grafting procedures, improvements in associated technologies, and advancements in biological understanding of bone formation and repair continue to fuel the investigation of ever more improved grafting methods.

8.2.1 CURRENT BONE GRAFT OPTIONS

The autograft, in which the donor tissue is harvested from the patient's own body, is currently considered the clinical gold standard of bone grafting. As autografts intrinsically possess optimal biocompatibility, three-dimensional (3D) pore structure, and biological components necessary for complete bone repair, they represent the most ideal bone grafting option and boast an 80%–90% success rate (Cook et al. 1994). There are relatively few bones in the human body that both satisfy these criteria and are available for harvest without incurring significant morbidity that would outweigh the overall benefit. Examples include the iliac crest, rib, and fibula (Fleming et al. 2000). However, the harvest of these bones provides limited quantities of tissue and still carries a threat of donor-site morbidity, limiting autograft procedures in their clinical utility.

Allografting, in which the graft tissue is harvested from a cadaver, is a common alternative to autografts. While allografts similarly provide a porous 3D template for bone tissue remodeling, it is challenging to ensure allograft safety while also maintaining appropriate biologic and biomechanical properties to the defect because donor tissue must be processed with treatment solutions and/or radiation methods in order to produce disease-free bone grafts that will not elicit an immune response in the host. However, this process also removes vital cellular and molecular components that are otherwise valuable to the bone regeneration process and are typically left intact in autografts.

8.2.2 RELEVANCE TO 3D MODEL SYSTEMS

The success of autografts and allografts has proven critical in the development of bone graft substitutes. The benefits and drawbacks of each, coupled with the details of how bone heals at the cellular level, have governed many of the approaches taken to try to develop alternatives to current strategies. A number of bone graft substitutes have been approved or cleared by the U.S. Food and Drug Administration and are currently available for clinical use, and many more are currently under investigation and development. Materials used to construct *synthetic* bone grafts range from natural and synthetic polymers, to ceramics, to composites of one or more materials. Although synthetic bone grafts can circumvent current limitations like supply constraints (autograft) and risk of disease transmission (allograft), many that are clinically available fail to fully recapitulate the autograft's ability to heal. In attempts to match the autograft's ability to heal bony defects researchers have been designing natural and synthetic scaffolds based on the hierarchical structure of bone and functionalizing them based on what is known about how bone heals. In using bone as the template for the ideal bone graft substitute and by mimicking its molecular, cellular, and structural cues at the nano-, micro-, and macroscale, respectively, researchers have by default developed extensive model systems. Here we summarize several strategies to scaffold-based bone repair in which several elements of the tissue's native structure and known molecular cues have been used as a template for design, and we discuss these approaches within the context of a new approach to tissue regeneration, termed regenerative engineering.

8.3 REGENERATIVE ENGINEERING

The goal of bone regeneration is to design a methodology that facilitates the regrowth of bone tissue in a specific skeletal area. Regenerative engineering presents a novel approach to this task, wherein it is defined as convergence of advanced materials sciences, stem cell sciences, physics, developmental biology, and clinical translation for the regeneration of complex tissues and organ systems (Laurencin and Nair 2015). Regenerative engineering has been put forth as a paradigm shift in tissue regeneration by emphasizing the multipronged approach needed to address the significant grand challenges foreseen on the clinical horizon. This encompasses the combination of various components from traditional scaffold-based tissue regeneration (biomaterials, cells, and growth factors) and expanding this to incorporate the physical stimulation of tissues, lessons learned from developmental biology, and knowledge from the growing body of stem cell science. Here, we focus on the development of

3D material-based scaffold systems, specifically those used for next-generation bone regeneration, and discuss them as model systems of bone regeneration. Ideally, the perfect bone scaffold should mimic the body's own bone tissue by encompassing the following properties:

Biocompatibility—Biocompatible grafts do not elicit an immune response and therefore minimize the body's natural tendency to eliminate the foreign species.

3D, Interconnected Pore Structure—An interconnected pore structure provides conduits for cellular migration and a means to transfer nutrients and waste between the cells on the scaffold and the surrounding environment. Without proper transfer, cells become starved of required nutrients and poisoned with generated toxins.

Osteoconductivity—This property refers to a graft's ability to support the attachment, proliferation, and migration of cells throughout the structure.

Osteointegrity—An osteointegrative graft can bond to the surrounding tissues through new tissue growth and/or mineral formation. A graft stably fixed in position is necessary to direct the proper localized bone formation while accepting the required mechanical responsibilities.

Osteoinductivity—This property describes the ability of a graft to stimulate the differentiation of osteoprogenitors down the osteoblastic lineage. A graft usually possesses this capability via the addition of growth factors or other osteoinductive agents.

Osteogenicity—An osteogenic graft is cellularized with osteoblast-lineage cells, and furthermore supports the mineralization of the cells' collagen-based extracellular matrices.

Biodegradability—Biodegradable scaffolds gradually decompose so that newly formed tissue may appropriately fill in the defect site, thereby eliminating the need for a second surgery to remove the original graft.

Appropriate mechanical properties—A graft should have mechanical properties that are similar to those of the native bone. A weak graft may not have sufficient load-bearing capabilities, while an overly strong graft may result in stress shielding that could lead to the resorption of the newly forming bone.

Interestingly, these parameters also provide important design criteria for a 3D model system. Designing the structural support, or scaffold, onto which new tissue may grow is a critical step. Although some tissue regeneration approaches simply involve the injection of viscous materials and/or growth factors into the defect site, many bone defects require strategies that provide mechanical support to develop a physical foundation during the healing process. Moreover, the incorporation of osteoinductive growth factors (such as bone morphogenetic protein-2 and transforming growth factor β-1) into the scaffold both mimics an endogenously healing bony fracture and enhances osteoinductivity and can stimulate the differentiation of osteoblastic precursors into mature bone forming cells and increase the rate of healing. To this are often added osteoprogenitor cells in order to accelerate the initial process of cell migration and therefore expedite the overall tissue formation process.

Following graft implantation, seeded and migratory preosteoblasts adhere, spread, and proliferate throughout the scaffold, and then eventually differentiate into osteoblasts in response to physiochemical cues. Upon differentiation, osteoblasts secrete type I collagen to form an extracellular matrix, the foundation of the new bony matrix. This maturation and mineralization process allows for the osteointegration of the graft with the host bone, during which stress is transferred to the graft site. As is seen in normal bone tissue metabolism, once osteoblastic tissue is formed on the surface of the graft, it begins to undergo remodeling through resorption and reprecipitation of the mineral phase. Ideally, the scaffold is made of either absorbable material that can be remodeled by endogenous cells or biodegradable material that degrades in accordance with the new bone formation. Clinically, the goal is that by the end of the healing process, the implanted scaffold is completely replaced by the patient's own regenerated tissue, as would occur during the remodeling phase of typical fracture repair. By designing the degradation process to match that of new bone formation the transition between the two is ideally seamless, and also approximates the body's ability to remodel newly formed bone into mature bone, although the time scale is not always the same.

8.4 SCAFFOLD DESIGN AND FABRICATION

Several strategies have been employed to develop suitable bone graft substitutes that are osteoinductive, osteoconductive, biocompatible, absorbable, easy to use, and cost effective to restore, maintain, or improve bone tissue function. Biodegradable scaffolds are highly porous, biocompatible, 3D structures capable of providing a temporal and spatial environment for cellular growth and tissue in-growth (Mulari et al. 2003; Otsuru et al. 2008; Pittenger et al. 1999). Such scaffolds also provide an elegant way for the short-term delivery of cells and/or growth factors, proteins, or drugs that have been bound to or encapsulated within the scaffold construct to stimulate bone repair. Over time the implanted matrix degrades and releases its payload and is gradually replaced by viable, regenerated host tissue. Polymeric scaffolds are prime candidates because of the associated ease of processability and tailorability toward specific chemical and physical properties (Glowacki 1998). Many candidate materials have been evaluated for biocompatibility and cell–material interactions, but to fully understand how cells will participate in bone healing they must be placed into 3D model systems. The behavior of cells seeded within 3D structures can be markedly different from those same cells seeded on two-dimensional (2D) substrates of similar materials. The 3D environment also provides a more realistic *in vivo* parallel and, for certain tissues like bone, is necessary to accurately mimic endogenous tissue. Below we summarize the literature around several methods of 3D scaffold fabrication for both the study of cells in 3D environments and actual bone scaffold synthesis.

8.4.1 POROGEN LEACHING IN BONE ENGINEERING

A wide range of synthetic and natural polymers can be used to fabricate 3D scaffold designs; however, porosity, which allows for cellular migration and proliferation, and also more accurately mimics the macroscale of trabecular bone, remains a mandatory parameter regardless of material choice. Pores can be created in scaffolds either during the synthesis process (as detailed in following sections) or post-synthesis using a technique known as porogen leaching. Porogen leaching involves mixing small sacrificial particles, often salt or sugar, with the polymer solution and then dissolving them out of the scaffold leaving behind voids, or pores, in their place. These pores allow for host cellular infiltration into the implant leading to increased osteoconductivity. Furthermore, porous, interconnected structures permit increases in vascularization and dynamic exchanges of nutrients and oxygen with waste products, both known to increase osteogenesis.

In one example of porogen leaching, polycaprolactone (PCL), a widely used synthetic polymer in bone tissue engineering applications, and fluoridated hydroxyapatite (HA) scaffolds were generated using sodium chloride (NaCl) as the porogen, which was leached out of the scaffold using deionized water (Johari et al. 2012). It was observed that an increase in porosity resulted in an increase in degradation time, suggesting that the amount of NaCl added directly modulated scaffold degradation time, an essential property to ensure that the rate of scaffold degradation corresponds to the rate of new tissue formation, which, as mentioned above, can approximate the remodeling phase of bone repair when the hard callus that has formed as protection for the healing defect is restored to the original bone dimensions. However, as porosity increased, the mechanical properties of the scaffold were eventually compromised (Sadiasa et al. 2014) necessitating an optimization of the two parameters. Scanning electron microscop (SEM) imaging confirmed that as opposed to mere surface adhesion, increased porosity facilitated osteoblasts migration into the scaffold (Johari et al. 2012). A similar study fabricated PCL scaffolds with salt alone as a porogen and a salt–polyethylene glycol (PEG) compound as a secondary porogen. The study demonstrated that pore formation using the salt–PEG compound led to extensive cellular proliferation of preosteoblasts due to increased porosity, pore volume, pore size, and scaffold interconnectivity, which allowed cells to spread throughout the scaffold. Moreover, the salt–PEG porogen increased the mineral deposition in comparison to the salt porogen-only scaffolds (Thadavirul et al. 2014). Although NaCl is the most commonly used porogen, others have demonstrated the usefulness of other compounds. For instance, Park and coworkers fabricated scaffolds composed of silk fibroin and HA particles using both salt and sucrose as porogens (Park et al. 2015). While the HA-containing scaffolds showed an increase in osteoconductivity as compared to the silk fibroin only scaffolds, the addition of sucrose as a porogen led to increases in scaffold porosity, swelling, and water uptake as compared to scaffolds fabricated with the salt porogen. This also resulted in increased calcium deposition and higher bone density (Park et al. 2015).

While porogen leaching has been demonstrated as an effective method to synthesize bone scaffolds with a porous network, there are some notable disadvantages to the technique. One significant issue is the need for microchannels to facilitate porogen leaching. Given that porogens are oftentimes completely encapsulated within the polymer during fabrication, leaching can be ineffective without microchannels that extend from the scaffold exterior to the scaffold interior. As this can lead to particular regions that do not contribute to the porous network, care must be taken to ensure that the porogen is added in sufficient concentration to result in an interconnected pore structure. The lack of an interconnected pore structure will not only prevent cells from migrating and fully occupying the scaffold, but more alarmingly, improperly leached porogens will eventually be released during polymer degradation and may prove toxic to migrating cells. While there are several instances in the literature where care was taken to avoid these pitfalls (Park et al. 2015; Thadavirul et al. 2014), these issues nevertheless necessitate the investigation of other techniques that focus on alternative approaches to build porous, interconnected 3D structures.

8.4.2 Microsphere Based Scaffold Development

The sintered microsphere scaffold methodology presents an excellent approach for bone graft applications due to its proven mechanical integrity and load-bearing capability, as well as ease of processing and versatility (Dvorak et al. 2004; Schmid et al. 1998). Further, microsphere scaffolds inherently possess design flexibility due to the "bottom-up" fabrication method wherein desired degradation rates, size, and morphology can be achieved by adjusting processing and fabrication parameters (Michigami 2013). These 3D structures are capable of mechanically and structurally supporting cellular activity such as cell adhesion, proliferation, migration, and differentiation (Beck et al. 2003; Bilezikian et al. 2008).

Microsphere scaffolds were first fabricated in 1998 by Laurencin and coworkers (Borden et al. 2002; Laurencin et al. 1998) and have since been studied extensively. Using the single emulsion technique, a solution of organic poly(lactide-*co*-glycolide) (PLAGA) in methylene chloride ($MeCl_2$) is usually added to an aqueous polyvinyl alcohol (PVA) surfactant. Under constant mixing, the $MeCl_2$ evaporates from the emulsion to produce solid PLAGA microspheres. After their synthesis, microspheres are collected, rinsed, lyophilized, and sieved to the desired diameter size range. To construct scaffolds, the microspheres within a narrow size range are poured into a cylindrical stainless steel mold and heated above the glass transition temperature of the PLAGA (Tg~57°C) such that microspheres become thermally fused in the desired 3D shape. In comparison to other techniques to bind microspheres, such as microsphere-aggregation and gel microsphere techniques, it has been shown that sintered scaffolds to possess physical properties most like trabecular autografts (Borden et al. 2003). Furthermore, microsphere scaffolds provide an excellent method for the controlled and sustained release of bioactive agents, such as growth factors, into the local cellular environment. Several types of natural and synthetic polymers have been used to construct 3D microsphere-based scaffolds for various applications in bone regenerative engineering as well as in the wider biomedical industry (Prajapati et al. 2015). While studies consistently demonstrate advantages of these micro-sized constructs, greater understanding of cellular biology has led to interest in scaffolds with nanoscale features.

8.4.3 Electrospinning Nanofiber Structures for Bone Tissue Engineering

Electrospinning is a process that produces thin, polymeric nanofibers that can be collected in random or aligned orientations. Typically, a polymeric solution is placed in a syringe with an appropriately sized needle opening, and the syringe is placed in a pump apparatus that slowly expels the solution. An electrical field is applied between the polymer solution within the needle and a metal collection plate, and at a certain critical voltage, this electrical field causes the polymer solution to extrude as a charged jet, thereby forming polymeric fibers that deposit on the collection substrate (Tuzlakoglu et al. 2005). The goal of electrospinning is to create a biomimetic scaffold that resembles the natural extracellular matrix (ECM), a network of interwoven fibers that provides a microenvironment for cells. The ECM provides a physical surface onto which cells can adhere, supports mechanical stresses and compressive forces, as well as contains a porous network, which allows for cellular migration and signaling. Electrospun nanofibers presents a facile strategy to mimic the ECM's mechanical properties, and thus recapitulate the nanoscale of newly forming, unmineralized bone, while providing an opportunity to endow biological functionality through the encapsulation or surface binding of growth factors, small molecules, and other bioactive agents that are also found within the intact extracellular matrix of newly forming bone. These design parameters have been shown to enhance cellular attachment, infiltration, and differentiation, resulting in desired outcomes for bone regeneration.

The application of synthetic polymeric nanofibers for biomedical use was first demonstrated by our group in studies using poly(lactide-*co*-glycolide) fibers (Li et al. 2002) and has continued to expand to other tissues (Katti et al. 2004; Kumbar et al. 2006). Since then the use of electrospinning as a template for tissue repair has grown given the ability to adjust the size of nanofibers to match the ECM of various tissue types and the ease with which different materials can be electrospun.

PCL, for instance, is a widely used synthetic polymer in electrospinning and bone engineering due to its biodegradability, compatibility, mechanical strength, and tailorability of overall properties based on processing conditions (Liao et al. 2016). However, it is often used as a composite due its shortcomings in biological settings, including lower cellular adhesion, proliferation, and differentiation in comparison to other commonly used degradable polymers (Ghasemi-Mobarakeh et al. 2008; Kim et al. 2006; Liao et al. 2016). In fact, studies have compared starch and PCL (SPCL) composite microfiber meshes with SPCL microfiber meshes containing SPCL nanofibers embedded within the scaffold. The study demonstrated that the inclusion of SPCL electrospun nanofibers in the porous scaffolds increased osteoblast metabolic activity, proliferation, mineralization, and vascularization throughout the composite nanofibrous matrix relative to SPCL scaffolds without electrospun fibers (Tuzlakoglu et al. 2005). SEM imaging showed nanofiber bridges between microfibers, mimicking physiological ECM and allowing cells to also bridge between the microfiber layers and attach to the nanofibers, due to the increased surface area. Cells were evenly distributed throughout the matrix and exhibited an elongated morphology, which was thought to enhance receptor activation and gene expression. This notion was corroborated by measured increases in mineralization markers *in vitro* (Tuzlakoglu et al. 2005). The investigators then cross-linked type I collagen nanofibers with the SPCL fibers to increase the scaffolds overall mechanical properties and induce vascularization (Tuzlakoglu et al. 2011). Vascularization is a key step in the bone healing process because blood vessels will provide oxygen, nutrients, and waste removal at the wound site, while also supporting the migration of bone forming progenitor cells to the defect site. The SPCL scaffolds supported endothelial cell attachment *in vitro*, and the authors noted that the formation of circular structures on the nanofiber mesh resembled capillary structure during angiogenesis (Tuzlakoglu et al. 2011). This suggests that the scaffold would have the ability to promote angiogenesis *in vivo*, ultimately leading to enhanced bone growth due to the formation of vessels transporting nutrients and waste to and from the defect site. Liao and coworkers likewise sought to overcome disadvantages of PCL alone by creating composite nanofibers as with calcium L-lactate (CL). Given the immiscibility of the different solvent systems, the nanofibers were synthesized using a two-nozzle approach. The resulting nanofibrous construct enhanced mineralization as demonstrated by increased improved cellular attachment, osteoblast proliferation, and differentiation in comparison to the control of a pure PCL scaffold (Liao et al. 2016).

In addition to PCL, investigators have electrospun matrices using conductive materials as well as utilized various techniques to endow osteoinductivity. Conductive materials have been used in an effort to replicate the natural ability of propagating electrical signals to increase and regulate cellular adhesion, proliferation, and differentiation (Liu et al. 2014). In a recent study, poly(L-lactide) (PLLA) and conductive analine pentamer–graft–gelatin (AP-g-GA) composites were synthesized at various ratios of PLLA: AP-g-GA to modulate the overall scaffold degradability and conductivity. Under electrical stimulation, the resulting scaffolds increased *in vitro* proliferation and differentiation of preosteoblasts after 14 days compared to pure, nonconductive PLLA (Liu et al. 2014). Alternatively, others have explored how the technique of incorporating osteoinductive materials can affect the overall efficacy of the scaffold system. For instance, Ramier and coworkers coated electrospun poly(3-hydroxybutyrate) nanofibers with nanoscale hydroxyapatite via electrospraying, a technique that forms nanoparticles rather than nanofibers. In comparison to electrospun polymeric nanofibers with nanohydroxyapatite embedded within the fibers, it was shown that embedded nanoparticles exhibited better mechanical properties, but electrosprayed nanohydroxyapatite resulted in superior biological properties (Ramier et al. 2014).

Although nanofibrous scaffolds are porous 3D networks with large surface areas, there are inherent challenges in creating constructs that have substantial volumes to fill defect voids, making it difficult to truly generate 3D tissue mimics from electrospinning alone. However, thermally induced phase separation has recently emerged as a technique that allows for the development of nanofiber structures while retaining larger overall volumes than those allowed by electrospinning.

8.4.4 THERMALLY INDUCED PHASE SEPARATION TO FORM 3D NANOFIBER STRUCTURES

Thermally induced phase separation (TIPS) for musculoskeletal tissue engineering utilizes thermal energy-driven material phase separation to create porous structures, such as nanofibrous matrices, with high porosity and interconnected channels, and provides a more realistic nanoscale 3D environment than electrospinning. While electrospinning can mimic the nanoscale environment of newly forming bone, the technique does not lend itself to making 3D models of any significant depth. TIPS, however, allows for a similar nanoscale ECM mimic but also has the ability to create 3D environments of larger dimensions, particularly in depth, such that cells can reside completely encased within nanofibers. This technique is commonly accomplished by freeze-drying a polymer solution, such as by submersion in liquid nitrogen. Once thermal equilibrium is established, the polymer solution solidifies and crystallizes, and the solvent is subsequently evaporated. The resulting crystallized, porous, polymer structure is composed of a nanofibers network, which can be generated into a variety of shapes and sizes depending on the specific synthesis parameters. Interestingly, Zhang and coworkers demonstrated the possibilities of forming hollow microspheres with walls composed of nanofibers which, in comparison to an intact solid microsphere, increased the available surface area and permitted drug loading within the fibers itself (Zhang and Ma 2015). To accomplish this, microspheres were synthesized using the double emulsion method, which involved water/oil/water (W/O/W) phases of both PLLA and glycerol. The obtained microspheres were quenched in liquid nitrogen, and then solvent and glycerol were extracted to obtain nanofibrous hollow microspheres. The researchers experimented with adding varying levels of Diacetin, a biocompatible glycerol derivative widely used in food and pharmaceutical formulations, to the PLLA solution in an effort to stabilize the emulsion process and generate spheres or disks depending on the concentration of Diacetin (Zhang and Ma 2015). While bone regeneration applications were not specifically tested in this instance, other work details similar microspheres tested as substrates for cartilage regeneration (Liu et al. 2011). Results indicated that the nanofibrous hollow microspheres induced higher chondrocyte proliferation and attachment, as well as enhanced cartilage regeneration and viability compared to solid-interior microspheres with a smooth surface (Liu et al. 2011).

Other groups have explored how 3D scaffolds with micro- and nano-sized features could be advantageous for bone regeneration by mimicking native bone on two scales. Nelson and coworkers fabricated 17% HA/PLLA composite microspheres using a single oil in water (O/W) emulsion system in PVA (Nelson et al. 2014). The microspheres were initially sintered to create a porous structure, then PLLA was added to the pore space and the TIPS method was used to synthesize a nanofiber mesh network within the pore spaces. The resulting design combined the controllability of synthetic polymers, the bioactivity of calcium phosphate ceramics, and the generation of a synthetic nanofibrous ECM into one single construct (Nelson et al. 2014). PLLA fibers were designed to heighten cell attachment and migration, while the microsphere scaffold served to support load due to comparable mechanical properties to trabecular bone (Nelson et al. 2014). The scaffolds were shown to support osteoblast adhesion throughout the entire scaffold, as compared to strictly surface attachment noted on control microspheres with no nanofiber network within the pores. These scaffolds can mimic bone in mechanical integrity, interconnected porosity, and nanoscale precision simultaneously, providing a 3D system of considerable complexity.

8.4.5 3D Printing Bone Scaffolds

While much advancement has been made in the development of 3D scaffolds, there are still many existing limitations related to the specificity of pore location, size, and overall pore volume, regardless of the proficiency of design. 3D printing of bone scaffolds is a relatively new technology that uses computer-aided design to provide precise specificity of geometric details such as pore size, connectivity, and beyond, allowing the shape and architecture of a scaffold to be tailor-made to a patient's needs, such as exact size of the defect site, using additional information like tomography scans (Arealis and Nikolaou 2015). For example, Temple and coworkers printed 3D scaffolds with varying porosities to determine the optimal conditions for the *in vitro* development of vascular networks by human adipose-derived stem cells (Temple et al. 2014). 3D printed scaffolds can also consist of components aimed at enhancing overall scaffold bioactivity. Although synthetic polymers such as poly(lactic acid) (PLA), poly(glycolic acid) (PGA), and PCL exhibit controllable degradation, oftentimes these constructs lack biological activity (Mozafari et al. 2015). The addition of functional groups can increase the amount of available binding sites for cells, and increasing surface roughness can increase the surface area onto which cells can adhere (Mozafari et al. 2015). However, as previously mentioned, these polymers are also sometimes created as a composite with calcium phosphate to provide a balance of osteoconductivity and strength.

Wang and coworkers sought to increase the bioactivity of 3D printed scaffolds by developing a composite scaffold comprised of HA and tricalcium phosphate, as well as an Arg-Gly-Asp (RGD) peptide sequence, wherein RGD has been proven to increase cell attachment and activate endothelial cells for vascularization (Wang et al. 2014). The RGD peptide sequence was fused with a nanofiber-like virus, or phage nanofiber, and bonded to the composite scaffolds. The composite, 3D printed nanofibrous scaffolds were shown to increase bone formation and density when compared to scaffolds with no nanofibers and scaffolds with a "wild-type" phage—nanofibers without fused RGD peptides (Wang et al. 2014). Wang and coworkers also loaded vascular endothelial growth factor (VEGF), a growth factor that mediates angiogenesis, onto the 3D scaffolds and observed an even further increase of vascularized bone tissue and bone formation (Wang et al. 2014). Lee and coworkers also incorporated growth factors onto a 3D scaffold by coating a printed PCL scaffold with dopamine hydrochloride to bind recombinant human bone morphogenetic protein-2 (rhBMP-2), which is well established to play a role in new bone formation by mediating bone cell proliferation and differentiation while promoting osteogenesis (Lee et al. 2016). Immunostaining and polymerase chain reaction (PCR) confirmed that culturing preosteoblasts on 3D printed PCL/rhBMP-2 scaffolds showed increases in bone cell differentiation and calcium deposition, key indicators of osteogenesis (Lee et al. 2016).

8.4.6 Degradable and Nondegradable Hydrogels in Bone Tissue Engineering

As previously mentioned, growth factors are excellent therapeutic agents that are endogenously produced during bone repair and therefore when delivered *in vivo,* can initiate cellular signaling at the wound site to direct bone formation and vascularization, as happens in normal bone healing. However, to elicit a functional effect, these molecules often need to be delivered in supraphysiological doses, which is expensive and can moreover result in cellular toxicity. To address this concern, researchers are currently exploring the use of hydrogels for bioactive agent delivery due their well-controlled delivery kinetics, which lowers the drug load requirement to be closer to those noted physiologically, and provides a form of 3D model system of therapeutic molecules versus 3D structure for study. This maintains functional, yet nontoxic, levels of drug in the body. Hydrogels are typically cross-linked polymer networks with water—in fact, over 90% water—as the swelling agent. Biodegradable hydrogels can deliver growth factors or other molecules as their polymeric network breaks down via degradation, whereas nondegradable hydrogels can deliver factors through passive diffusion or osmotic pressure, forcing the drugs to be expelled. Hydrogels can also be used as delivery vehicles for cell therapy approaches in tissue regeneration (Agarwal and Garcia 2015). For instance, Olabisi and coworkers demonstrated that a nondegradable hydrogel comprised of poly(ethylene glycol) diacrylate (PEGDA) was bioinert, mimicked soft tissue properties, and actively regulated waste and nutrient transmission (Olabisi et al. 2010). Thus, the PEGDA hydrogels were loaded with bone morphogenetic protein-2 (BMP-2)-producing cell lines and shown to promote rapid bone formation *in vitro*, up to 93% the strength and stiffness of healthy bone (Olabisi et al. 2010). While the bone formed was irregularly shaped, perhaps due to the nondegradability of the hydrogel, the gel itself was found to be nontoxic to the environment (Olabisi et al. 2010).

Another use of nondegradable hydrogels is to provide extended drug release. Alginate is often used for this purpose, as Perez and coworkers showed by the development of a nondegradable, multilayered hydrogel. Collagen was placed in the inner core to benefit from its ability to enhance cell loading and overall material biocompatibility, while the outer alginate hydrogel layer, which does not disintegrate in aqueous solutions, served to overcome collagen's mechanical instability over time (Perez et al. 2014). An increase of alginate concentration increased the mechanical properties of the hydrogel, which supported cell proliferation and viability throughout the study. Cellular elongation of mesenchymal stem cells was observed, and increased bone healing and enhanced osteogenic properties were detected in the composite hydrogels in comparison to collagen hydrogels alone (Perez et al. 2014).

Hydrogels are often developed using natural polymers, however synthetic polymers such as PEG are also typically used. Recently, PEG hydrogels have been functionalized with the collagen peptide sequence GFOGER, a sequence that is specific to integrins that interact with collagen I (Shekaran et al. 2014). Shekaran and coworkers encapsulated BMP-2 within PEG hydrogels, providing sustained release at an overall lower dose, lowering cell toxicity and increasing cost efficiency. BMP-2 bioactivity was indicated by the enhanced recruitment of osteoprogenitor cells to the defect site *in vitro*, and additionally the ability *in vivo* to bridge critical size defects and display improved bone repair when compared to collagen only carriers (Shekaran et al. 2014). Furthermore, the degradability of the PEG hydrogel, an important feature for all bone scaffolds, was shown *in vivo*. The PEG hydrogel has strong implications for the use of a 3D scaffold, due to its ability to controllably deliver osteogenic growth factors that are essential for bone healing, as well as matching the scaffold degradation rate to the rate of bone formation, providing the backbone for the regeneration of new bone tissue in its place.

8.5 CONCLUSION AND PERSPECTIVE

Bone is an intriguing tissue to study because its repair and regeneration requires the inclusion of a vast array of expertise, from developmental biology to stem cell science, materials science, physics, and beyond. Bone is unique in that it has both mechanical and physiological responsibilities within the human body, and as such requires the consideration of each when developing regeneration strategies or when developing 3D model systems to study its repair. The field of regenerative engineering has emerged as in important tool in this task to encompass each of these aspects. When considering a scaffold-based approach to bone repair or regeneration, one must consider the development of a 3D structure onto which cells can attach, migrate, proliferate, differentiate, and ultimately mineralize and many of the adopted techniques and designs have arisen from the inherent biological structure of bone itself. Indeed many of the regenerative strategies used for bone involve the development of 3D systems of bone repair. Here, we have summarized some of the techniques that have been used to synthesize this 3D environment, along with some of the successes realized with each approach. While not a comprehensive list of all available approaches, the methods listed provide a starting point for the regenerative engineer choosing to model healing bone or to take a scaffold-based approach to bone repair and regeneration.

REFERENCES

Agarwal, R. and A. J. Garcia. 2015. Biomaterial strategies for engineering implants for enhanced osseointegration and bone repair. *Adv Drug Deliv Rev* no. 94:53–62.

Arealis, G. and V. S. Nikolaou. 2015. Bone printing: New frontiers in the treatment of bone defects. *Injury* no. 46 (Suppl 8):S20–2.

Beck, G. R. Jr., E. Moran, and N. Knecht. 2003. Inorganic phosphate regulates multiple genes during osteoblast differentiation, including Nrf2. *Exp Cell Res* no. 288 (2):288–300.

Bilezikian, J. P., L. G. Raisz, and T. J. Martin. 2008. *Principles of Bone Biology*. 3rd ed. New York: Academic Press.

Borden, M., M. Attawia, Y. Khan, and C. T. Laurencin. 2002. Tissue engineered microsphere-based matrices for bone repair: Design and evaluation. *Biomaterials* no. 23 (2):551–9.

Borden, M., S. F. El-Amin, M. Attawia, and C. T. Laurencin. 2003. Structural and human cellular assessment of a novel microsphere-based tissue engineered scaffold for bone repair. *Biomaterials* no. 24 (4):597–609.

Cook, S. D., G. C. Baffes, M. W. Wolfe, T. K. Sampath, D. C. Rueger, and T. S. Whitecloud, 3rd. 1994. The effect of recombinant human osteogenic protein-1 on healing of large segmental bone defects. *J Bone Joint Surg Am* no. 76 (6):827–38.

Dvorak, M. M., A. Siddiqua, D. T. Ward, D. H. Carter, S. L. Dallas, E. F. Nemeth, and D. Riccardi. 2004. Physiological changes in extracellular calcium concentration directly control osteoblast function in the absence of calciotropic hormones. *Proc Natl Acad Sci* no. 101 (14):5140–5.

Fleming, J. E. Jr., C. N. Cornell, and G. F. Muschler. 2000. Bone cells and matrices in orthopedic tissue engineering. *Orthop Clin North Am* no. 31 (3):357–74.

Ghasemi-Mobarakeh, L., M. P. Prabhakaran, M. Morshed, M. H. Nasr-Esfahani, and S. Ramakrishna. 2008. Electrospun poly(epsilon-caprolactone)/gelatin nanofibrous scaffolds for nerve tissue engineering. *Biomaterials* no. 29 (34):4532–9.

Glowacki, J. 1998. Angiogenesis in fracture repair. *Clin Orthop Relat Res October* (355 Suppl):S82–9.

Johari, N., M. H. Fathi, M. A. Golozar, E. Erfani, and A. Samadikuchaksaraei. 2012. Poly(epsilon-caprolactone)/nano fluoridated hydroxyapatite scaffolds for bone tissue engineering: *In vitro* degradation and biocompatibility study. *J Mater Sci Mater Med* no. 23 (3):763–70.

Katti, D. S., K. W. Robinson, F. K. Ko, and C. T. Laurencin. 2004. Bioresorbable nanofiber-based systems for wound healing and drug delivery: Optimization of fabrication parameters. *J Biomed Mater Res B Appl Biomater* no. 70 (2):286–96.

Kim, C. H., M. S. Khil, H. Y. Kim, H. U. Lee, and K. Y. Jahng. 2006. An improved hydrophilicity via electrospinning for enhanced cell attachment and proliferation. *J Biomed Mater Res B Appl Biomater* no. 78 (2):283–90.

Kumbar, S. G., L. S. Nair, S. Bhattacharyya, and C. T. Laurencin. 2006. Polymeric nanofibers as novel carriers for the delivery of therapeutic molecules. *J Nanosci Nanotechnol* no. 6 (9–10):2591–607.

Laurencin, C. T., F. K. Ko, M. A. Attawia, and M. D. Borden. 1998. Studies on the development of a tissue engineered matrix for bone regeneration. *Cells Mater* no. 8:175–81.

Laurencin, C. T. and L. S. Nair. 2015. Regenerative engineering: Approaches to limb regeneration and other grand challenges. *Regen Eng Transl Med* no. 1 (1):1–3.

Lee, S. J., D. Lee, T. R. Yoon, H. K. Kim, H. H. Jo, J. S. Park, J. H. Lee, W. D. Kim, I. K. Kwon, and S. A. Park. 2016. Surface modification of 3D-printed porous scaffolds via mussel-inspired polydopamine and effective immobilization of rhBMP-2 to promote osteogenic differentiation for bone tissue engineering. *Acta Biomater* no. 40:182–91.

Li, W. J., C. T. Laurencin, E. J. Caterson, R. S. Tuan, and F. K. Ko. 2002. Electrospun nanofibrous structure: A novel scaffold for tissue engineering. *J Biomed Mater Res* no. 60 (4):613–21.

Liao, N., M. K. Joshi, A. P. Tiwari, C. H. Park, and C. S. Kim. 2016. Fabrication, characterization and biomedical application of two-nozzle electrospun polycaprolactone/zein-calcium lactate composite nonwoven mat. *J Mech Behav Biomed Mater* no. 60:312–23.

Liu, X., X. Jin, and P. X. Ma. 2011. Nanofibrous hollow microspheres self-assembled from star-shaped polymers as injectable cell carriers for knee repair. *Nat Mater* no. 10 (5):398–406.

Liu, Y., H. Cui, X. Zhuang, Y. Wei, and X. Chen. 2014. Electrospinning of aniline pentamer-graft-gelatin/PLLA nanofibers for bone tissue engineering. *Acta Biomater* no. 10 (12):5074–80.

Michigami, T. 2013. Extracellular phosphate as a signaling molecule. *Contrib Nephrol* no. 180:14–24.

Mozafari, M., M. Gholipourmalekabadi, N. P. Chauhan, N. Jalali, S. Asgari, J. C. Caicedoa, A. Hamlekhan, and A. M. Urbanska. 2015. Synthesis and characterization of nanocrystalline forsterite coated poly(L-lactide-co-beta-malic acid) scaffolds for bone tissue engineering applications. *Mater Sci Eng C Mater Biol Appl* no. 50:117–23.

Mulari, M. T., H. Zhao, P. T. Lakkakorpi, and H. K. Vaananen. 2003. Osteoclast ruffled border has distinct subdomains for secretion and degraded matrix uptake. *Traffic* no. 4 (2):113–25.

Nelson, C., Y. Khan, and C. T. Laurencin. 2014. Nanofiber-microsphere (nano-micro) matrices for bone regenerative engineering: A convergence approach toward matrix design. *Regen Biomater* no. 1 (1):3–9.

Olabisi, R. M., Z. W. Lazard, C. L. Franco, M. A. Hall, S. K. Kwon, E. M. Sevick-Muraca, J. A. Hipp, A. R. Davis, E. A. Olmsted-Davis, and J. L. West. 2010. Hydrogel microsphere encapsulation of a cell-based gene therapy system increases cell survival of injected cells, transgene expression, and bone volume in a model of heterotopic ossification. *Tissue Eng Part A* no. 16 (12):3727–36.

Otsuru, S., K. Tamai, T. Yamazaki, H. Yoshikawa, and Y. Kaneda. 2008. Circulating bone marrow-derived osteoblast progenitor cells are recruited to the bone-forming site by the CXCR4/stromal cell-derived factor-1 pathway. *Stem Cells* no. 26 (1):223–34.

Park, H. J., O. J. Lee, M. C. Lee, B. M. Moon, H. W. Ju, Jm Lee, J. H. Kim, D. W. Kim, and C. H. Park. 2015. Fabrication of 3D porous silk scaffolds by particulate (salt/sucrose) leaching for bone tissue reconstruction. *Int J Biol Macromol* no. 78:215–23.

Perez, R. A., M. Kim, T. H. Kim, J. H. Kim, J. H. Lee, J. H. Park, J. C. Knowles, and H. W. Kim. 2014. Utilizing core-shell fibrous collagen-alginate hydrogel cell delivery system for bone tissue engineering. *Tissue Eng Part A* no. 20 (1–2):103–14.

Pittenger, M. F., A. M. Mackay, S. C. Beck, R. K. Jaiswal, R. Douglas, J. D. Mosca, M. A. Moorman, D. W. Simonetti, S. Craig, and D. R. Marshak. 1999. Multilineage potential of adult human mesenchymal stem cells. *Science* no. 284 (5411):143–7.

Prajapati, V. D., G. K. Jani, and J. R. Kapadia. 2015. Current knowledge on biodegradable microspheres in drug delivery. *Expert Opin Drug Deliv* no. 12 (8):1283–99.

Ramier, J., T. Bouderlique, O. Stoilova, N. Manolova, I. Rashkov, V. Langlois, E. Renard, P. Albanese, and D. Grande. 2014. Biocomposite scaffolds based on electrospun poly(3-hydroxybutyrate) nanofibers and electrosprayed hydroxyapatite nanoparticles for bone tissue engineering applications. *Mater Sci Eng C Mater Biol Appl* no. 38:161–9.

Sadiasa, A., T. H. Nguyen, and B. T. Lee. 2014. In vitro and in vivo evaluation of porous PCL-PLLA 3D polymer scaffolds fabricated via salt leaching method for bone tissue engineering applications. *J Biomater Sci Polym Ed* no. 25 (2):150–67.

Schmid, C., C. Keller, I. Schlapfer, C. Veldman, and J. Zapf. 1998. Calcium and insulin-like growth factor I stimulation of sodium-dependent phosphate transport and proliferation of cultured rat osteoblasts. *Biochem Biophys Res Commun* 245 (1):220–5.

Schultz, R. J. 1990. *The Language of Fractures*. Baltimore, MD: Williams & Wilkins.

Shekaran, A., J. R. Garcia, A. Y. Clark, T. E. Kavanaugh, A. S. Lin, R. E. Guldberg, and A. J. Garcia. 2014. Bone regeneration using an alpha 2 beta 1 integrin-specific hydrogel as a BMP-2 delivery vehicle. *Biomaterials* 35 (21):5453–61.

Temple, J. P., D. L. Hutton, B. P. Hung, P. Y. Huri, C. A. Cook, R. Kondragunta, X. Jia, and W. L. Grayson. 2014. Engineering anatomically shaped vascularized bone grafts with hASCs and 3D-printed PCL scaffolds. *J Biomed Mater Res A* 102 (12):4317–25.

Thadavirul, N., P. Pavasant, and P. Supaphol. 2014. Development of polycaprolactone porous scaffolds by combining solvent casting, particulate leaching, and polymer leaching techniques for bone tissue engineering. *J Biomed Mater Res A* 102 (10):3379–92.

Tuzlakoglu, K., N. Bolgen, A. J. Salgado, M. E. Gomes, E. Piskin, and R. L. Reis. 2005. Nano- and micro-fiber combined scaffolds: A new architecture for bone tissue engineering. *J Mater Sci Mater Med* 16 (12):1099–104.

Tuzlakoglu, K., M. I. Santos, N. Neves, and R. L. Reis. 2011. Design of nano- and microfiber combined scaffolds by electrospinning of collagen onto starch-based fiber meshes: A man-made equivalent of natural extracellular matrix. *Tissue Eng Part A* 17 (3–4):463–73.

Wang, J., M. Yang, Y. Zhu, L. Wang, A. P. Tomsia, and C. Mao. 2014. Phage nanofibers induce vascularized osteogenesis in 3D printed bone scaffolds. *Adv Mater* 26 (29):4961–6.

Zhang, Z. and P. X. Ma. 2015. From nanofibrous hollow microspheres to nanofibrous hollow discs and nanofibrous shells. *Macromol Rapid Commun* 36 (19):1735–41.

9 Engineered Composites for 3D Mammary Tissue Systems

*Cheryl T. Gomillion, Chih-Chao Yang,
Didier Dréau, and Karen J. L. Burg*

CONTENTS

9.1 Introduction 141
9.2 The Human Breast 142
    9.2.1 Mammary Development and Anatomy 142
    9.2.2 Cancer Development and Tumor Progression 143
9.3 Native Mammary Tissue Properties to Consider for Engineered Systems 145
    9.3.1 Mechanical Properties 145
    9.3.2 Breast Microenvironment: Cell–Cell Interactions, Extracellular Matrix, and Tissue Composition 146
9.4 Engineered Mammary Tissue Systems 148
    9.4.1 Tissue Development and Morphogenesis 149
    9.4.2 Tumor Formation and Vascularization 153
    9.4.3 Tumor Cell Metastasis and Invasion 154
    9.4.4 Drug Evaluation 155
9.5 Technical Example: Evaluating Breast Cancer Cell Response within a Composite 3D System 156
    9.5.1 Composite System Fabrication and Characterization 157
    9.5.2 Three-Dimensional Cell Culture 159
9.6 Conclusion and Perspective 160
References 161

9.1 INTRODUCTION

In vitro model systems have long been used in biomedical research for evaluating factors affecting cell behavior, identifying key mechanisms regulating cell processes, such as proliferation, differentiation, and tumor formation, and screening drug compounds for disease treatment. Specifically, models of mammary or breast tissue have been developed and investigated in an attempt to better understand the underlying mechanisms for both normal and disease mammary tissue states, which include processes of normal tissue morphogenesis and tumorigenesis (i.e., breast cancer formation, tumor angiogenesis, and metastasis) (Hebner et al. 2008).

Two-dimensional (2D) monolayer cultures of breast cells are the simplest form of *in vitro* models; however, as with most systems of the body, three-dimensional (3D) breast tissue models are more appropriate as 3D systems provide key architectural cues from cell–cell and cell–matrix interactions that 2D models lack (Bissell et al. 2003). Thus, a large body of work aims to engineer and characterize optimal *in vitro* 3D mammary tissue systems.

The human mammary gland is one of the most complex systems within the body with its intricate structure and highly regulated function. The multiple cellular and tissue components of the breast, specific mechanical properties, and various other microenvironmental cues affect physiological tissue processes in the breast, and as such, these significant parameters should be considered in the design of engineered 3D mammary tissue systems. The goal of this chapter is to provide an overview of key properties of native mammary tissue influencing engineered 3D mammary systems, discuss existing 3D breast models, and highlight a new composite 3D system.

9.2 THE HUMAN BREAST

9.2.1 Mammary Development and Anatomy

The female mammary gland, or breast, is a dynamic organ that undergoes morphological and developmental changes throughout the stages of a woman's lifetime (Howard and Gusterson 2000; Parmar and Cunha 2004). Changes in the size, shape, and function of the breast occur in response to puberty, pregnancy, lactation, and menopause. The most significant changes in growth of the breast, however, occur following puberty (Osborne and Boolbol 2014). Following birth, the mammary gland is composed primarily of adipose tissue with small ductal structures present forming breast tissue that remains immature until the onset of puberty. At puberty, growth of the breast, that is, increased cellular growth of the epithelial ducts, is stimulated by the hormones estrogen and growth hormone produced by the ovaries and pituitary gland, respectively (Lanigan et al. 2007). In addition to increased deposition of adipose tissue in the breasts, the ducts stretch, elongate, and become more branched creating a more defined ductal network (Fridriksdottir et al. 2005; Geddes 2007; Russo and Russo 2004; Villadsen 2005; Zangani et al. 1999). The formation of lobules at the end of the ducts also occurs. As the female ages, during the course of menstruation, the growth of a mature network of ducts and lobules is formed, with slight growth apparent until approximately age 35 years when the growth of the breast reaches its maximum.

While a mature network of ductal and lobular structures is formed over time, complete development of the breast tissue does not occur unless pregnancy and childbirth are experienced (Geddes 2007; Wiseman and Werb 2002). Growth of the mammary gland is stimulated by production of progesterone hormones during pregnancy. During pregnancy, significant extension and branching of the breasts ductal system, accompanied by growth of glandular tissue, leads to maximal development of the breast whereby the lobules increase in both size and number. Systemic reproductive hormones, specifically progesterone and prolactin, stimulate the expansion and differentiation of the mammary epithelium into milk-producing cells (Lanigan et al.

2007). Lactation, or the production of milk, is the point where the breast reaches its fully functional capacity due to these functional changes of the glands, which now secrete milk. Following lactation, the breast undergoes involution, a regression of the tissue most notably caused by a collapse or folding of lobular structures and a narrowing of the ducts, which is accompanied by apoptosis and alveolar cell detachment (Macias and Hinck 2012). A similar type of tissue remodeling is observed following menopause when hormones levels, particularly estrogen levels, decrease and glandular tissue atrophies, leaving larger proportions of fat tissue, stromal connective tissue, and skin (Fridriksdottir et al. 2005; Geddes 2007; Gefen and Dilmoney 2007; Parmar and Cunha 2004; Russo and Russo 2004; Villadsen 2005; Wiseman and Werb 2002).

Structurally, the breast is divided into 15–20 lobes. The extremities of each of these lobes include lobules with multiple acini in which epithelial cells that produce milk following hormonal cues during lactation lie. Acini are interconnected by thin ducts, whose primary function is to transport the secreted milk from the lobules to the nipple of the breast. The spaces between the functional structures of the breast (lobules and ducts) are filled with stromal tissue providing the structural framework and support (Ackers 2002; Gray and Lewis 1918; Hirshaut et al. 2009; Jorstad and Payne 1964; Parmar and Cunha 2004; Snell 2004). The breasts receive nutrients and signals, including hormones, and dispose of waste through a complex associated vascular network and lymphatic system (Osborne and Boolbol 2014). The blood supply to the breast includes the internal mammary artery and the mammary branch of the thoracic artery that account for ~60% and 30%, respectively, of the blood flow to the breast (Geddes 2007). The primary vein that facilitates blood flow from the breast is the internal mammary vein (Geddes 2007). In addition, the lymphatic vessels carry in lymph fluid cell and cellular waste away from the breast. The network of lymphatic vessels in the breast converge to the axillary nodes, with the lymph fluid draining from the breast to the axillary nodes first and second to the internal mammary nodes located within the chest, and the supraclavicular or infraclavicular nodes located around the collar bone. This connection of the breasts to the lymphatic system is critical in the spreading of breast cancer cells to secondary sites in the body in the case of metastatic tumors (Rahman and Mohammed 2015; Shayan et al. 2006).

9.2.2 Cancer Development and Tumor Progression

Breast cancer is the form of cancer where cells in the breast tissue, typically epithelial cells of the breast, divide and grow abnormally (Sims et al. 2007). The origin of breast cancer cells is unclear and likely to be multifactorial, resulting in the presence of epithelial cells with spontaneous or hereditary DNA damage that promote oncogenes (genes that initiate cell proliferation and differentiation) and/or concomitantly suppress tumor suppressor genes (genes that inhibit growth and progression in the cell cycle). The initiation of breast cancer is thought to result from uncontrolled cell proliferation and/or an error in the apoptotic events of breast cells, often the result of genetic damages or alterations (Hanahan and Weinberg 2000, 2011; Polyak 2007). The net result is an uncontrolled growth or hyperplasia of the breast cancer cells with an unstable genome. Tumor formation, or tumorigenesis, occurs when the growing cells form a cluster or a tumor mass, which may or may not be malignant depending on its ability to vascularize and shed tumor cells in either the lymphatics or blood vessels (Hanahan and Weinberg 2011; Polyak 2007). Under certain microenvironmental constraints, that is, lack of oxygen or physical limitations, tumor growth may be limited; however, additional mutations in conjunction with these physical restraints may result in a larger vascularized tumor mass from which tumor cells may be able to intravasate and spread to other tissues. Malignant forms of breast cancers that develop metastases are associated with a poor prognosis and currently there is no efficient treatment for breast cancer patients with metastatic disease.

Numerous risk factors are associated with breast cancers, including gender, age, weight, family history, child-bearing history, environmental factors, such as smoking or radiation, and genetic predisposition, which affects the chances of a person developing breast cancer (Russo and Russo 2004; Tozeren et al. 2005). Genetic mutations inherited from a parent affect 10%–20% of breast cancer cases (Osborne and Boolbol 2014; Rice et al. 2000). The most commonly inherited mutations predisposing women to breast cancer are those of two tumor suppressor genes involved in DNA repair BRCA1 (Breast Cancer 1) and BRCA2, respectively. BRCA1 and BRCA2 are located on chromosome #17 and #13, respectively. The presence of an altered or mutated copy of either the BRCA1 or BRCA2 gene carries a 36%–85% lifetime risk for developing breast cancer (Yalcin 2013). The presence of these mutations and their associated risk for breast cancer is usually followed by either more careful monitoring of patient breast health, or in some rare, but high risk cases, by preventive radical mastectomy.

The majority of breast cancers originate in the ducts of the breast (85%), whereas others typically originate in the lobules (Korkola et al. 2003). The progression of breast cell growth from a normal to cancerous state is a spontaneous, multistep process. The progression of breast cancer begins with a hyperproliferation of cells or hyperplasia. The epithelial cells still appear normal in structure; however, they begin to divide uncontrollably and more cells are present within the duct. In the atypia stage, the epithelial cells look "atypical" or slightly abnormal upon microscopic examination. This condition is often diagnosed as benign; however, the patient may still be diagnosed as precancerous, indicating that they may have a high likelihood of developing cancer later (Habal 2006; Polyak 2007). Breast cancer can progress to ductal carcinoma *in situ* (DCIS). In DCIS, the epithelial cells have an abnormal appearance and are fast growing beginning to form clusters within the lining of the duct. When the *in situ* carcinomas occur in the lobule, it is designated as lobular carcinoma *in situ* (LCIS) (Habal 2006; Parmar and Cunha 2004; Polyak 2007). In invasive cancer, the abnormal cells of the duct have begun to infiltrate into the surrounding normal breast tissue. The invasive phenotype that is associated with the tumor cell secretion of enzymes is able to degrade the extracellular matrix (ECM) of the ductal basement membrane. These secretions also play a key role in allowing breast cancer cells to intravasate and extravasate the blood vessels or the lymphatic vessels in distant organs (Polyak 2007; Schedin and Keely 2011). The homing of breast cancer cells primarily occur in the lung, the liver, the bones, and the brain, and as the metastases grow in these organs, it negatively affects the entire physiology of the individual.

9.3 NATIVE MAMMARY TISSUE PROPERTIES TO CONSIDER FOR ENGINEERED SYSTEMS

9.3.1 MECHANICAL PROPERTIES

The normal mammary gland can be assimilated to a soft tissue with mechanical properties characterized as nonlinear, anisotropic, and viscoelastic. Breast tissue is characterized as nonlinear because its viscosity exhibits a nonconstant response to strain (nonconstant coefficient of viscosity). Further, breast tissue is described as anisotropic, because its stiffness depends on the direction of load application, and as viscoelastic because the differences in stiffness are a function of the rate of strain application (Fung 2013; Gefen and Dilmoney 2007). In addition, normal mammary tissue has been characterized as rubber-like due to its almost incompressible nature (Fung 2013; Gefen and Dilmoney 2007; Wellman and Howe 1998). These characteristics of mammary tissue may vary depending on age, water content, lipid content, temperature, and disease-state of the tissue specimen used for analysis (Gefen and Dilmoney 2007). The precise makeup of the tissue components, that is, distribution of ductal structures within the stromal network, will also influence the specific mechanical properties of mammary tissue (Fung 2013; Samani et al. 2007).

The mechanical properties of the mammary tissue have been further characterized through the analyses of the three main tissues that compose the breasts: skin, glandular tissue, and adipose tissue. The elastic modulus and the strength of selected tissues of the breast have been determined and can be used to model tissue dynamics and image breast tissue to detect malignancies (Krouskop et al. 1998; Samani and Plewes 2004; Sarvazyan et al. 1998; Wellman and Howe 1998). The elastic modulus of skin has been shown to be between 200 and 3000 kPa with an ultimate tensile strength of ~20 MPa (Gefen and Dilmoney 2007). For normal glandular tissue and mammary adipose tissue, the elastic moduli have been measured to be between 2 and 66 kPa (Krouskop et al. 1998; McKnight et al. 2002) and 0.5 and 25 kPa (Kruse et al. 2000; McKnight et al. 2002; Samani et al. 2007; Sinkus et al. 2000; Van Houten et al. 2003), respectively. Normal glandular tissue has been estimated to be 5–50 times stiffer than adipose tissue partly because of the higher lipid and water weight of the adipose tissue (Duck 2013; Gefen and Dilmoney 2007).

When considering the mechanical properties of the mammary gland, it is also important to account for the diseased state of tissue. Cancerous breast tissues have been shown to have an increased stiffness when compared to normal tissue samples, where increased stiffness is denoted as an indicator of the presence of tumorigenic tissue and of the cancer stage. Fibroadenomas (noncancerous breast lumps) have been found to be four times stiffer than normal tissue, whereas breast cancerous tissue was up to seven times stiffer than normal mammary tissue (Sarvazyan et al. 1998; Wellman and Howe 1998). Other researchers have reported up to 90-fold differences between the stiffness in surrounding tissues and breast cancer masses (Greenleaf et al. 2003; Sarvazyan et al. 1998). Such drastic stiffness variations may be associated with the intrinsic variations of the breast tumors. Nevertheless, the breast tissue stiffness may allow monitoring of the presence of a cancer mass.

9.3.2 BREAST MICROENVIRONMENT: CELL–CELL INTERACTIONS, EXTRACELLULAR MATRIX, AND TISSUE COMPOSITION

In addition to the mechanical and physical properties of the breast, the breast's normal microenvironment has to be considered when developing engineered breast tissue systems as the tissue mechanical, physical, and chemical cues are responsible for regulating mammary cell behavior (McCave et al. 2010; Weaver et al. 1995; Weigelt et al. 2014). The female mammary gland is composed of two primary cell categories: epithelial and stromal cells. A normal duct of the breast epithelium is composed of epithelial cells (a bilayer of inner luminal epithelial cells for milk production and an outer layer of myoepithelial cells for milk ejection) along the fully intact basement membrane of the duct (Sims et al. 2007). The epithelial cells along with myoepithelial cells form the glandular tissue that plays a role in lactation and milk production. The stromal tissue of the breast consists primarily of adipose cells and is associated with a complex vascular network that irrigates both the stromal and epithelial components of the breast.

The most prevalent cell types present within the breast tissue, epithelial cells, adipocytes, and fibroblasts, interact through physical contacts but mainly through paracrine signaling. In particular, the interactions between the epithelial cells and the stromal (fibroblast, adipocytes mostly) cells within the normal mammary microenvironment modulate the effects of hormones during mammary gland development, such as cell differentiation, ductal elongation, and ductal branching morphogenesis, where these processes are dependent on the cooperative interaction of epithelial and stromal cells of the breast (Howard and Gusterson 2000; Shekhar et al. 2001; Sternlicht 2006; Sternlicht et al. 2006; Xie and Haslam 1997).

Structurally, the cross-section of the human mammary gland, as shown in Figure 9.1, reveals a bilayered epithelium consisting of the innermost luminal epithelial cells and the outermost myoepithelial cells (Alcaraz et al. 2004; Sternlicht 2006; Sternlicht et al. 2006). The glandular epithelium lies directly on a basement membrane. The basement membrane functions primarily as a mechanical barrier separating the epithelium from the surrounding stroma and as a support structure anchoring the epithelium to its underlying connective tissue. The normal glandular basement membrane is a thin acellular layer of ECM composed primarily of collagen type IV, entactin, perlecan (heparin sulfate proteoglycan), and laminin (Kleinman et al. 1986; Krause et al. 2008; Schittny and Yurchenco 1989). In contrast, the predominant structural component of the fibroblastic connective tissue forming the stroma around the basement membrane is collagen type I (Krause et al. 2008; Schittny and Yurchenco 1989).

Adipose tissue is an endocrine organ that comprises a significant proportion of the breast volume (Wang et al. 2014) and secretes hormones and factors that significantly influence epithelial cell behavior and the mammary environment (Fonseca-Alaniz et al. 2007; Iyengar et al. 2003; Wang et al. 2009; Zangani et al. 1999). The white adipose tissue found within the mammary glands is a highly specialized connective tissue, which functions as an energy storage source within the body (Fonseca-Alaniz et al. 2007). White adipose tissue is primarily a collection of lipid-filled cells or adipocytes held together by collagen fibers. Adipose tissue also includes preadipocytes, which account for one-to two-thirds of adipose tissue composition. Dense blood

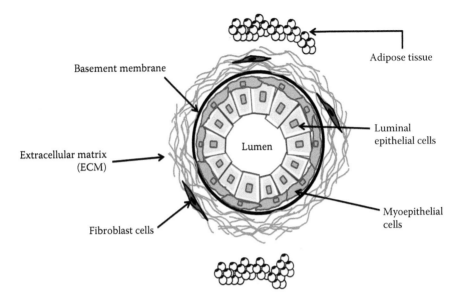

FIGURE 9.1 Structural components observed in the cross-section of the human mammary gland (Note: cell sizes are not to scale) (Heber, D., J.Ashley, and D. Bagga. 1996. *Adv Exp Med Biol* 399:41–51; Hebner, C., V. M. Weaver, and J. Debnath. 2008. *Annu Rev Pathol* 3:313-39; Sternlicht, M. D. 2006. *Breast Cancer Res* 8 (1):201; Sternlicht, M. D. et al. 2006. *Differentiation* 74 (7):365–81.)

vessels constituted of endothelial, smooth muscle, and red and white blood cells and fibroblasts are also an integral part of adipose tissue (Ailhaud et al. 1992; Albright and Stern 1998; Lanza et al. 2013; Sorisky 1999; Stillaert et al. 2006).

In addition to its energy storage metabolic role, adipocyte cells also secrete multiple proteins and cytokines, or adipokines, which influence other cells within the breast and other tissues of the body (Halberg et al. 2008; Hauner 2005; Karnoub and Weinberg 2006; Masaki and Yoshimatsu 2008; Miner 2004). Adipocyte factors influence numerous processes including ECM development, cell metabolism, and immunological functions (Halberg et al. 2008). The evaluation of the mammary extracellular and intracellular components of mammary adipose tissue yielded an extensive list of factors with potential influence on mammary epithelial cells (Celis et al. 2005). For example, stromal cells have been shown to modulate hormones that regulate ductal morphogenesis and branching, and adipose cells have been shown to promote functional differentiation of mammary epithelial cells synthesizing milk proteins (Levine and Stockdale 1985; Trujillo and Scherer 2006). Many sources have listed factors secreted by adipose cells in general (Halberg et al. 2008). Adipocyte-secreted factors that have been shown to influence epithelial cell behaviors are summarized in Table 9.1. Furthermore, adipocyte-secreted factors including matrix metalloproteinases (MMPs) also have key roles in breast tumor progression (Bouloumie et al. 2001; Chavey et al. 2003). These factors and their influence on epithelial cells must be taken into account when developing engineered model systems.

TABLE 9.1
Key Adipocyte-Secreted Factors that Influence Epithelial Cell Behavior

Factor	References
Estrogen	Heber et al. 1996, Fonseca-Alaniz et al. 2007
Glucocorticoids	Heber et al. 1996, Celis et al. 2005; Fonseca-Alaniz et al. 2007
Insulin-like growth factor-1	Hovey et al. 1999
Transforming growth factor	Heber et al. 1996, Barcellos-Hoff and Ewan 2000, Fonseca-Alaniz et al. 2007
Fibroblast growth factor	Hovey et al. 1999, Celis et al. 2005
Epidermal growth factor	Heber et al. 1996, Celis et al. 2005

The adipose tissue influence on the mammary microenvironment is also directly associated with fatty acids stored and trafficked within the breast. Fatty acids present within mammary tissue are useful biomarkers of dietary fatty acid intake (Arab 2003; Kohlmeier and Mendez 1997; London et al. 1991; Saadatian-Elahi et al. 2004; Simonsen et al. 1998). However, the influence of dietary fatty acids on the behavior of breast cancer cells remains controversial, with documented anti-cancer (eicosapentaenoic acid [EPA] and docosahexaenoic acid [DHA]) and cancer-promoting (linoleic acid and arachidonic acid) fatty acid molecules (Bagga et al. 1997; Hankin and Rawlings 1978; Klein et al. 2000; Kohlmeier 1997; Maggiora et al. 2004; Maillard et al. 2002; Pauwels and Kairemo 2008; Welsch 1992; Wendel and Heller 2009). The relationships between dietary fatty acids and breast cancer risk have been extensively studied (Bakker et al. 1997; Bougnoux et al. 2005; Godley 1995; Howe 1994; Lee and Lin 2000; Simonsen et al. 1998; Simonsen et al. 1998; Welsch 1994; Zhu et al. 1995). Comparative analyses of normal and breast cancer samples demonstrated a correlation between increased levels of linoleic acid and arachidonic acid and increased risk of breast cancer (Bagga et al. 1997; Maillard et al. 2002; Sakai et al. 1992). In contrast, the presence of increased levels of α-linolenic acid, EPA, DHA, and conjugated linoleic acid was associated with decreased risk of breast cancer occurrence (Bagga et al. 1997; Klein et al. 2000; Larsson et al. 2004; Maillard et al. 2002).

9.4 ENGINEERED MAMMARY TISSUE SYSTEMS

The most commonly used systems for evaluating breast cell behavior, as shown in Figure 9.2a, consist of 2D monolayer cultures and cocultures (direct or indirect with transwell inserts), of varying cell types, including mammary fibroblasts, adipocytes, mammary epithelial cells, and tumor cells (Padron et al. 2000). While providing a convenient and cost-efficient platform for studying cellular behavior, the lack of physiological architecture and cell–stroma interactions in 2D systems necessitates 3D models that recapitulate these vital tissue characteristics (Debnath and Brugge 2005; Kim et al. 2004). Mammary spheroids, consisting of one or more type of normal or cancerous cell, may be fabricated using various methods (Figure 9.2b) and are one option for evaluating cells in a more physiologically relevant environment. As such, mammospheres and tumor spheroids are widely used for studies of breast

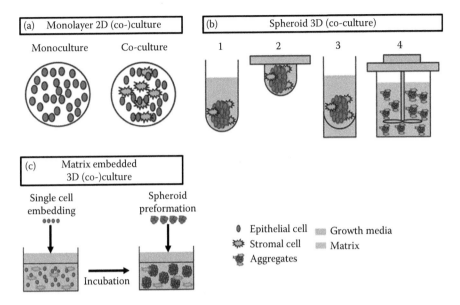

FIGURE 9.2 Two- and three-dimensional cell culture systems. (a) Conventional 2D monolayer (co-)culture. (b) Forced floating spheroid (co-)cultures, 1 = nonadhesive coating; poly(hema), ultra-low attachment or agarose, 2 = hanging drop method, 3 = agitation-based spinner culture. (c) Matrix-embedded 3D (co-)cultures either derived from single cells or preformed spheroids. (Hickman, J. A. et al. Three-dimensional models of cancer for pharmacology and cancer cell biology: Capturing tumor complexity *in vitro/ex vivo*. *Biotechnol J.* 2014. 9 (9):1115–28. Copyright Wiley-VCH Verlag GmbH & Co. KGaA. Reproduced with permission.)

morphogenesis and tumorigenesis. Further, with the importance of the stromal tissue and the basement membrane, which surround the structural components of the breast realized, additional forms of 3D tissue systems have evolved to include cells or spheroids embedded within biomaterial matrices (Figure 9.2c) made of synthetic polymers or hydrogels, in addition to biomimetic matrices made of materials such as fibrin, collagen, and the popularly used laminin-rich Matrigel® (Corning, Corning, NY) which provide important cues and stimuli from ECM-specific proteins. Specific types of models and methods used earlier for fabricating 3D systems have been reviewed (Kim 2005; Yamada and Cukierman 2007). More recent reviews have also described, at length, specific scaffold materials and matrices used for 3D breast models (Maghdouri-White et al. 2016; Rijal and Li 2016). Here, we highlight selected application-specific models (summarized in Table 9.2) for breast-related research.

9.4.1 Tissue Development and Morphogenesis

Mammary tissue models can be categorized as systems purposed for evaluating (1) tissue development and/or morphogenesis; (2) tumor formation and vascularization; (3) tumor cell metastasis and invasion; and (4) tumor cell responses to drugs. The stromal cell–epithelial cell relationship within the mammary gland has been proven

TABLE 9.2
Summary of Selected Existing Three-Dimensional *In Vitro* Mammary Models

Model Type	Model Basis	ECM/Matrix Material(s)	Mechanical Properties	Cell Type(s)	Chemotherapeutics Tested	References
Tissue development and/or morpho-genesis	3D matrix coculture	Matrigel® + collagen I	Not tested	MCF10A + primary human mammary fibroblasts	N/A	Krause et al. (2008)
	3D matrix coculture	Matrigel® + collagen on porous silk	Not tested	MCF10A + hADSCs	N/A	Wang et al. (2009)
	3D matrix tri-culture	Matrigel® + collagen on silk scaffold	Not tested	MCF10A + mammary fibroblasts + hADSCs	N/A	Wang et al. (2010)
	3D matrix culture	Matrigel® + collagen of varying density	Modulus ~50–6000 Pa	MCF10A	N/A	Lance et al. (2016)
Tumor formation and vascular-ization	3D porous microparticles	poly(D,L-lactide-*co*-glycolide)/polylactide	Not tested	MCF-7	N/A	Sahoo, Panda, and Labhasetwar (2005)
	3D matrix coculture	Culturex® or Matrigel®	Not tested	MCF-7, MDA-MB-231, MDA-MB-468, T47D, BT474, ZR-75 1 + hBMSCs	N/A	Sasser et al. (2007)
	3D cell spheroids	N/A	Not tested	MCF-7	N/A	do Amaral et al. (2011)
	3D matrix culture	Rat tail collagen I + hormones (estradiol, promegestone, or prolactin)	Not tested	T47D	N/A	Speroni et al. (2014)

(*Continued*)

TABLE 9.2 (Continued)
Summary of Selected Existing Three-Dimensional *In Vitro* Mammary Models

Model Type	Model Basis	ECM/Matrix Material(s)	Mechanical Properties	Cell Type(s)	Chemotherapeutics Tested	References
	3D matrix tri-culture	Rat tail collagen I	Not tested	HB2 (normal or overexpressing Her2/3) + Myo1089 + primary mammary fibroblasts	N/A	Nash et al. (2015)
	3D microencapsulated cell aggregates	Alginate	Not tested	MCF-7 + human dermal fibroblasts	N/A	Estrada et al. (2016)
	3D matrix culture	Poly(*N*-acryloyl L-lysine)/hyaluronic acid hydrogel	11.4 ± 0.8 kPa 31.5 ± 1.5 kPa 46.3 ± 3.2 kPa	MCF7	N/A	Xu et al. (2016)
Tumor cell metastasis and invasion	3D matrices for bone metastasis	PLG–hydroxyapatite	Non-mineralized: 0.5 MPa Mineralized: 1.1 MPa	MCF-7, MDA-MB-231	N/A	Pathi et al. (2010)
	3D matrix for cell invasiveness	Matrigel®	Not tested	MCF10A, MDA-MB-231	N/A	Cvetkovic, Goertzen, and Bhattacharya (2014)
	3D matrix for lung metastasis	Porous poly(caprolactone)	7 ± 0.5 kPa	MDA-MB-231	N/A	Balachander et al. (2015)
	3D matrix for bone metastasis	Porous chitosan–hydroxyapatite	Not tested	MCF-7, MDA-MB-231 + hMSCs	N/A	Zhu et al. (2015)
	3D spheroids in matrix for cell invasiveness	Basement membrane extract + collagen I	Not tested	MCF-7, MDA-MB-231 + hUVECs + hADSCs	Fluororuacil 100 μM Paclitaxel 1 μM	Benton et al. (2015)

(*Continued*)

TABLE 9.2 (Continued)
Summary of Selected Existing Three-Dimensional *In Vitro* Mammary Models

Model Type	Model Basis	ECM/Matrix Material(s)	Mechanical Properties	Cell Type(s)	Chemotherapeutics Tested	References
Drug evaluation	3D matrix culture	Chitosan	Not tested	MCF-7	Tamoxifen 10^{-5}–10^{-8} M	Dhiman, Ray, and Panda (2005)
	3D tumor spheroids	Growth factor reduced Matrigel®	Not tested	MCF-7, MDA-MB-231, BT474	Doxirubicin Cinorelbine Gemcitabine Docetaxel Paclitaxel 5-Fluorouracil Epirubicin (all at 0.0001–100 μM)	Lovitt, Shelper, and Avery (2013)
	3D matrix tri-culture	Star-shaped poly(ethylene glycol)–heparin hydrogels	500–3000 Pa	MCF-7 or MDA-MB-231 + hUVECs +hMSCs	Epirubicin 0–400 ng/mL Paclitaxel 0–500 nM	Bray et al. (2015)
	3D tumor spheroids	Growth factor reduced Matrigel®	Not tested	MCF-7, MDA-MB-231, BT-474	Epirubicin Paclitaxel Vinorelbine (all at 0.0002–200 μM)	Lovitt, Shelper, and Avery (2015)
	3D tumor spheroids	InSphero culture GravityPLUS™ plates	Not tested	T47D, JIMT-1	Trastuzumab 10 μg/mL	Falkenberg et al. (2016)
	3D matrix culture	Col-T gel (101Bio, Palo Alto, CA; commercially available transglutaminase crosslinked collagen-based gel characterized as soft, medium, and stiff)	0.8–50 kPa	MDA-MB-231	Gemcitabine 12.5 μM Paclitaxel 2.5 μM	Fang et al. (2016)

Note: ECM, extracellular matrix; hADSCs, human adipose-derived stem cells; hBMCs, human bone marrow stromal osteoprogenitor cells; hMSCs, mesenchymal stem cells; hUVECs, human umbilical vein endothelial cells; PLG, poly(D,L-lactide-*co*-glycolide).

essential for epithelial cell differentiation and ductal morphogenesis *in vivo*, and model systems for evaluating this phenomenon are important for better understanding these processes (Borellini and Oka 1989; Haslam and Woodward 2003; Howard and Gusterson 2000; Nelson and Bissell 2005). Indeed, only epithelial cells cocultured *in vitro* with either stromal fibroblast cells, or within laminin-rich Matrigel® or collagen gels, were associated with the development of 3D models that possess organized ductal and acinar structures similar in morphology to native mammary tissue, demonstrating the importance of stromal cell- and ECM-related stimuli (Chrenek et al. 2001; Cunha and Hom 1996; Hebner et al. 2008; Iyengar et al. 2005; Kleinman et al. 1986; Krause et al. 2008; Wiseman and Werb 2002). When the mechanical properties of the surrounding matrix were considered, however, the capacity of MCF10A cells alone to form breast cell acini in 3D was affected by the surrounding ECM density and stiffness (Lance et al. 2016), indicating the importance of mechanical properties, as well as the cellular presence in morphogenesis models.

As one of the primary stromal cell types within breast tissue, the inclusion of adipose cells within 3D morphogenesis models is also of interest. Coculture of mammary epithelial cells and adipocytes within a collagen gel yielded cellular clusters including breast ductal-like structures of the breast (Huss and Kratz 2001). Similarly, cocultures of pre-adipocytes with MCF10A mammary epithelial cells on 3D silk scaffold generated cellular structures appearing to undergo ductal morphogenesis (Wang et al. 2009). In these two cases, no analysis of milk proteins was presented, so it is unclear whether the generated breast-like structures were functional (Huss and Kratz 2001; Wang et al. 2009). Evaluation of a 3D tri-culture consisting of MCF10A cells, human adipose-derived stem cells, and mammary fibroblasts yielded a system more closely resembling native mammary tissue as evidenced by tissue organization into highly differentiated breast structures and expression of functional proteins. Kaplan and coworkers previously reviewed adipose tissue models for studying mammary gland development (Wang et al. 2010); however, precise understanding of the physical and chemical interactions between mammary epithelial cells and adipocytes in the generation of 3D *in vitro* breast-like structures remains limited.

9.4.2 TUMOR FORMATION AND VASCULARIZATION

As important as 3D models mimicking tissue morphogenesis and development are for breast-related research, it is probably of greater importance to have tumor models that aid in understanding how cancerous tumors form, develop vascular networks that mediate their survival and spreading, and how these tumors can be eradicated. As such, there are a significant number of mammary tissue models aimed at mimicking the diseased breast tissue state for these purposes. Similar to morphogenesis models, previously developed systems are largely biomaterial based and range from single-cell to tri-culture systems. Early application of biomaterials was observed in the form of porous microparticles that were shown to simply support MCF-7 tumor cell growth (Sahoo et al. 2005). In subsequent tumor cell models of single cell types as 3D tumor spheroids or within single-cell matrix systems, more attention was paid to the organization and arrangement of resulting tissue structures, where matrices, largely made of Matrigel® or collagen, were shown to support tumor assembly (do Amaral et al. 2011). Observed changes to epithelial cell organization and the density of ECM formed within a model of T47D tumor cells were shown to be influenced by regulation of hormones including estradiol, promegestone, and prolactin and the presence of hormonal gradients (Speroni et al. 2014).

The presence of stromal cells has been shown to also influence tumor cell behavior ad organization, as noted with normal mammary epithelial cells. In coculture and tri-culture systems of tumor cells with bone marrow stromal cells, culturing of various breast cancer cell types in the 3D system showed that the presence of the stromal cells enhanced the growth rates of specific tumor subtypes, estrogen receptor alpha-positive (ERα+) cell, which included MCF-7, T47D, BT474, and ZR-75-1 cells. Meanwhile, the growth rate of ERα-negative (ERα−) cells was not affected or only mildly affected in a similar coculture system (Sasser et al. 2007). In this case, as in many others (Nash et al. 2015), testing of these very different tumor types within a controlled model environment yielded a greater understanding of what modulates tumor cell organization and aids in delineating the differences that exist between tumor subtypes or genetically altered tumor cells (Nash et al. 2015).

The importance of the cues provided by the surrounding matrix materials is evident, as the processes of normal and tumor development and organization are largely dependent on an appropriate surrounding matrix. The formation of a tumor-associated vascular network is a key to tumor survival *in vivo*, and an appropriate environment is required *in vitro* for modeling tumor vascularization (Song et al. 2014). Further, the application of materials, such as alginate, which lacks the ECM protein content of collagen or Matrigel®, has also been investigated for tumor formation models. Microencapsulated aggregates of MCF-7 cells and human dermal fibroblasts were shown to support a long-term tumor model in which cell–cell interactions within a suitable matrix were key regulators of tumor formation (Estrada et al. 2016). In addition, the recent design of tunable poly(L-lysine)/hyaluronic acid hydrogels were shown to support the formation of 3D MCF-7 tumors, which was affected by matrix stiffness (Xu et al. 2016). The application of specific matrix modeling parameters may be an instrumental tool for evaluating other processes associated with tumor formation and spreading, such as epithelial to mesenchymal transitions (EMT), which may be linked to modulation of matrix properties.

9.4.3 Tumor Cell Metastasis and Invasion

While the majority of breast cancer deaths (~90%) are attributed to the metastasis, or spread, of cancerous tumors to other parts of the body outside of the breast, it is still not known how to permanently eradicate tumor metastasis or what role certain factors of the mammary microenvironment and alterations in the surrounding tissue mechanical properties specifically play in developing metastases. Tumor cell metastasis also relies on specific stroma cell types, that is, fibroblasts, immune cells, and endothelial cells, which are associated with ECM changes (fibrotic tissue formation), inflammation, and vasculogenesis, respectively (Cheung and Ewald 2014). These cells and their associated processes notably play some role in cancer induction and progression, and 3D model mammary systems provide a platform for systematically studying the causes of tumor spreading and invasion *in vitro* (Bersini et al. 2014).

Metastatic cell lines, such as MDA-MB-231 breast cancer cells, are often used in tumor metastasis and invasion models. Cultures of these cells in comparison to normal mammary epithelial cells led to development of methods to quantify cell invasiveness using 3D Matrigel®-based models (Cvetkovic et al. 2014). In addition, evaluation of tri-culture cellular spheroids comprised of MDA-MB-231 cells, endothelial cells, and adipose-derived stem cells within a 3D matrix yielded a physiologically relevant microtumor system useful for screening cancer therapeutics that would be more effective for treating highly invasive tumors (Benton et al. 2015).

Other applications of 3D metastasis models are aimed at creating model platforms for evaluating tumor spreading and migration to specific tissue types. Breast cancer cells have been observed to spread to various secondary sites in the body including the brain, liver, and lungs. A porous polycaprolactone matrix, with mechanical properties mimicking breast tumor tissue, was used in a model to study breast cancer cell behavior, and further evaluation of cells primed in this matrix demonstrated preferential lung metastasis *in vivo* (Balachander et al. 2015). While tumors spread to a number of different sites in the body, breast cancer cells metastasize most preferentially to patient bone. The American Cancer Society reports that 2 out of 3 cases of metastatic breast cancer will metastasize to patient bone, leading to a life expectancy of only 20 months after diagnosis (Society 2016). The manipulation of matrix mechanical properties is often used when studying breast cancer bone metastasis in an effort to recapitulate properties associated with bone tissue (Taubenberger 2014). By incorporating hydroxyapatite, a bioactive inorganic bone matrix molecule, into polymer matrices, the mechanical properties of model systems can be altered, yielding a platform to study how breast cells respond to significantly increased matrix stiffness (Pathi et al. 2010). The addition of stromal cells differentiated into bone cells within a model system with the increased matrix stiffness further increases the physiological relevance of the bone-like model, and when breast cancer cells were cultured in the system, increased expression of metastasis-associated genes was observed (Zhu et al. 2015), thus demonstrating the significant impact of matrix cues on cell behavior.

9.4.4 DRUG EVALUATION

2D monolayer and cocultures of breast cancer cells have been instrumental in the development of chemotherapeutic drugs, as they allow for cost-efficient preliminary baseline screening of novel drug compounds. For more rigorous testing, before reaching animal models, 3D mammary model systems are an appropriate platform for systematically evaluating cell response to therapies under controlled conditions. Early investigations of single cell cultures within 3D matrices demonstrated that simply changing from monolayer to 3D culture affected cancer cell response to drugs such as tamoxifen (Dhiman et al. 2004, 2005). With systems today that include multicell cultures and other microenviromental cues, researchers are better able to evaluate how chemotherapeutics affect various tumor types in response to systematically implemented model variations (Bray et al. 2015).

Stromal cell presence and matrix mechanical properties have been shown to affect normal mammary processes and tumor cell development; thus, mimicking these properties in drug-testing platforms is essential to elucidate tumor-cell response at those specified conditions. Cultures of different breast cancer cell types within similar matrices have been used successfully as a high-throughput screening platform to test different concentrations of multiple different drugs quickly, which is important for drug development (Lovitt et al. 2013). This particular system and others like it (Falkenberg et al. 2016; Lovitt et al. 2015), however, did not take into account any contribution that surrounding matrix properties, such as the stiffness, would have on the cancer cell drug responses. Culturing of metastatic MDA-MB-231 in commercially available matrices of varying defined stiffness (0.8–50 kPa) showed that the changes in matrix stiffness indeed affected tumor cell sensitivity to chemotherapeutics (Fang et al. 2016). Further, recently developed model systems consisting of tunable poly(ethylene glycol)-heparin gels, ranging in stiffness from 500 to 3000 Pa, and a tri-culture of breast cancer cells with endothelial cells and mesenchymal stem cells demonstrated the effects of multiparameter systems on tumor angiogenesis and the efficacy of treating those cells with chemotherapeutics (Bray et al. 2015). These advanced 3D drug screening models, in combination with metastasis models, will contribute greatly to identifying cures for treating breast cancer and determining how to best prevent it from spreading.

9.5 TECHNICAL EXAMPLE: EVALUATING BREAST CANCER CELL RESPONSE WITHIN A COMPOSITE 3D SYSTEM

Research within our group focused on the development of an injectable composite system for breast reconstruction, which uses injectable microcarrier beads as support scaffolds for cellular growth. *In vitro* and *in vivo* studies of this system showed that the polymeric microcarriers not only support cellular attachment, but also facilitate proliferation and differentiation of adipose cells, and yield biocompatible tissue response in an *in vivo* host (Cavin 2005; Gomillion 2005). We also showed that, in addition to serving as cellular supports, microcarrier beads fabricated from synthetic polymers such as poly-L-lactide or hydrogels such as chitosan (or a blend of chitosan and gelatin), as shown in Figure 9.3, could serve multiple purposes within *in vitro*

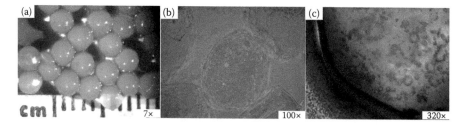

FIGURE 9.3 (a) Representative stereomicroscopic image of chitosan–gelatin beads. (b) Preadipocytes seeded on chitosan–gelatin beads. (c) Oil Red O staining of differentiated adipose cells, on the surface of chitosan–gelatin beads, showed the presence of intracellular lipid droplets characteristic of mature adipocytes following differentiation for 21 days. (Reprinted from *Comprehensive Biomaterials*, Gomillion, C. T., and K. J. L. Burg, Adipose tissue engineering, 529–539, Copyright 2011 with permission from Elsevier.)

model systems. In particular, we demonstrated the capacity of chitosan microcarriers to function also as delivery vehicles for growth factors, drugs, bioactive molecules, and media supplements, such as fatty acids, which effectively resulted in increased lipid production within adipose cells (Gomillion and Burg 2011b; Gray and Lewis 1918).

Based on these findings, we aimed to fabricate a composite 3D system designed to yield a novel platform for testing breast cancer cell response to drug therapies in an environment simultaneously presenting multiple parameters known to influence cell behavior–microenvironmental cues in the form of secreted factors and mechanical properties resembling that of native mammary tissue from a surrounding hydrogel matrix. Specifically, in a preliminary proof-of-concept study, the behavior of MCF-7 cells treated with tamoxifen was evaluated within a 3D system consisting of multiple biomaterial-based components in the form of chitosan–gelatin beads loaded with fatty acid embedded within a collagen–agarose hydrogel matrix.

9.5.1 Composite System Fabrication and Characterization

A 1% v/v glacial acetic acid was prepared with distilled water and filter sterilized with a 0.22 μm polyethylsulfone (PES) filter. Chitosan (MW: 100,000–300,000, Acros Organics, Morris Plains, NJ) and gelatin (Type A from porcine skin; Bloom Number: ~300, Sigma) powders were autoclaved at 124°C for 25 minutes to sterilize. Following sterilization, all subsequent steps in the bead fabrication process were carried out in a laminar flow biological safety cabinet to maintain sterility. A 3% w/v chitosan–gelatin solution was prepared by dissolving the chitosan and gelatin powders in 1% v/v glacial acetic acid and stirring at low heat until completely dissolved. A 0.5 N solution of sodium hydroxide (NaOH) was prepared by dissolving NaOH salt (Fisher Chemicals, Fair Lawn, NJ) in 1 L of distilled water, stirring at room temperature, and filter sterilizing.

The fatty acid-loaded chitosan–gelatin beads (FA-Beads) were formed using an electrostatic bead generator (Nisco, Zürich, Switzerland). Immediately before preparation, 10 mL of the chitosan–gelatin solution was mixed with 5 mL of sterile linoleic acid–albumin solution (Sigma) in a sterile 50-mL centrifuge tube (Fisher Scientific, Fair Lawn, NJ). The solution was pipetted up and down several times to ensure complete mixing and then drawn into a 20 cc syringe (BD, Franklin Lakes, NJ) using a 16-gauge needle (BD, Franklin Lakes, NJ). The syringe was secured in place on top of a syringe pump (kdScientific, New Hope, PA) set to eject the solution at a rate of 15 mL/h. The chitosan–gelatin solution was ejected from the syringe and guided through plastic tubing attached to the end of the syringe, into a metal needle ~4 cm above the surface of the NaOH solution below. The NaOH was pipetted into a glass 80 × 40 mm dish (Pyrex®, Corning, Corning, NY) until just overflowing (>180 mL) into a 100 × 20 mm glass collection dish (Pyrex) beneath. The NaOH was continuously stirred at an agitation rate of 25%. The applied voltage potential was set at 6.5 kV to obtain beads. The fabricated beads were collected in the 80 × 40 cm dish and stirred for an additional 30 minutes post formation in the NaOH solution at the same agitation rate. The NaOH was drained from the beads and the resulting beads were washed three times with sterile phosphate buffered saline (PBS; Sigma). The beads were then placed in sterile Dulbecco's Modified Eagle Medium (DMEM) until used for cell culturing. Beads without fatty acid were prepared in the same manner, with PBS included in the chitosan–gelatin solution instead of fatty acid.

For the hydrogel matrix, a volume of 1 mL of collagen–agarose solution was prepared by mixing 450 µL of 3 mg/mL PureCol® Purified Bovine Collagen (Advanced Biomatrix, San Diego, CA) with 450 µL of 1% agarose solution (Type VII-A, Sigma, St. Louis, MO) and 100 µL of collagen reconstitution buffer. The collagen reconstitution buffer consisted of 0.22 g sodium bicarbonate (Fisher, Fair Lawn, NJ) and 0.48 g N-2-hydroxyethylpiperazine-N-2-ethane sulfonic acid (Fisher) in 10 mL deionized water (Millipore, Billerica, MA). The collagen–agarose gels were cast in silicone molds. Specifically, two high-density silicone sheets (each sheet 6.5 cm L × 2.5 cm W, thickness per sheet = 1 mm) were punched to create three 1.4 cm circular "wells" in each sheet. The silicone sheets were placed on top of a polystyrene slide and the collagen–agarose gel solution was distributed evenly to each circular well.

The properties of the matrix-bead system were characterized using atomic force microscopy (AFM), as shown in Figure 9.4a. The stiffness of the following samples (Figure 9.4b) were evaluated: plain collagen–agarose gel, collagen–agarose gel-containing chitosan–gelatin bead, and collagen–agarose gel-containing fatty acid-loaded chitosan–gelatin bead. Because measurements were acquired at single points within the system, only one individual chitosan–gelatin bead or fatty acid-loaded chitosan–gelatin bead was placed into the center of an individual circular well such that the gels completely surrounded the beads. The solutions were gelled on the slides for 10 minutes at 4°C. The elastic modulus was tested immediately using AFM.

The MFD-3D-BIO™ AFM (Asylum Research, Santa Barbara, CA) and borosilicate AFM tips of radius 2.5 µm and spring constant 0.093 N/m were used. For AFM testing, the AFM tip approached the gel surface at a speed of 5 µm/s and the contact

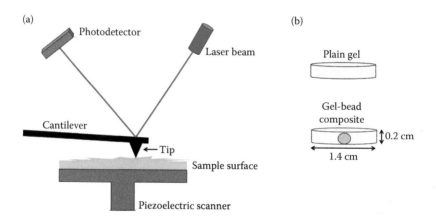

FIGURE 9.4 (a) Schematic of atomic force microscopy setup for measuring matrix mechanical properties. (b) Schematic of fabricated samples evaluated for mechanical testing (not to scale).

force was measured until an indentation depth of 10 μm. Each gel was tested at three random points in the central area of the gel and measured three times. The gel sample containing the chitosan–gelatin bead was tested at the interface of the gel and bead. The gel elastic modulus was estimated by fitting a Hertz model to indentation depths from 800 to 1000 nm using the following equation:

$$F = \frac{4E}{3(1-\upsilon^2)} R^{1/2} \delta^{3/2}$$

where F = measured force, υ = Poisson's ratio (0.5 for hydrogel), δ = indentation depth, and R = AFM tip radius. After applying the Hertz model equation to the resulting AFM data, the estimated elastic modulus for the plain collagen–agarose gel was determined to be 22.71 ± 1.76 kPa. Inclusion of the plain chitosan–gelatin bead and the fatty acid-loaded chitosan–gelatin bead to the gel resulted in a significant increase in the gel stiffness to 33.93 ± 3.7 and 28.86 ± 3.84 kPa, respectively ($p < 0.05$). While the inclusion of beads within the gel matrix significantly increased the elastic modulus, the values determined for each condition were each found to be within the range of values referenced for mammary tissues, which range from 0.5 to 25 and 2 to 66 kPa for adipose tissue and normal glandular tissue, respectively (Krouskop et al. 1998; Kruse et al. 2000; McKnight et al. 2002; Samani et al. 2007; Sinkus et al. 2000; Van Houten et al. 2003).

9.5.2 THREE-DIMENSIONAL CELL CULTURE

For evaluation in the 3D system, MCF-7 cells were cultured within a plain collagen–agarose gel or cocultured with either chitosan–gelatin beads (denoted as Beads) or fatty acid-loaded chitosan–gelatin beads (denoted as FA-Beads) encapsulated within a collagen–agarose gel. Samples containing beads were prepared by combining 20 beads with 1 mL of collagen–agarose gelation solution and 4×10^6 MCF-7 cells in individual wells of 12-well plates. Samples without beads were prepared using the same volume of gelation solution and quantity of MCF-7 cells per well. The cellular gelation solution was maintained at 4°C for 10 minutes to allow the collagen–agarose gels to solidify thoroughly. A volume of 2 mL of DMEM culture medium was then added to the gel. Plates were incubated at standard culturing conditions of 37°C and 5% CO_2. At Day 6, 10 μM of tamoxifen was added to each group and the samples were cultured until Day 9 when samples were harvested for evaluation.

Representative images (Figure 9.5a–c) of histological samples stained with Diff Quik stain showed MCF-7 cells (stained bluish-purple in color) distributed within the 3D matrices at Day 9 of culture. Properties of 3D matrices, such as their stiffness, have been associated with regulating many cellular functions including intracellular signaling and cell proliferation (Yamada and Cukierman 2007). MCF-7 cell aggregates were larger in size, most noticeably for the samples containing beads, indicative of continued cell growth, which is likely attributed to the increase in matrix stiffness observed due to the inclusion of beads. Staining of the cells cultured in 3D with the Alexa Fluor® 488 Annexin V/Dead Cell Apoptosis Kit (Molecular Probes, Invitrogen, Eugene, OR) showed the presence of apoptotic and necrotic cells stained

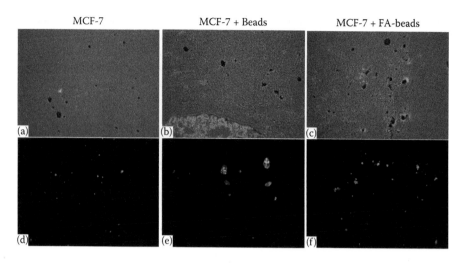

FIGURE 9.5 (a–c) Representative images of MCF-7 cell aggregates (stained bluish-purple) within the 3D culture systems at Day 9. (d–f) Staining of the cells cultured in 3D with the Alexa Fluor 488 Annexin V/Dead Cell Apoptosis Kit at Day 9 indicates the presence of apoptotic and necrotic cells stained green and red, respectively, following treatment with tamoxifen. Areas that appear yellow in color are indicative of overlapping red and green cells. Total magnification for all images is 100×.

green and red, respectively (Figure 9.5d–f), following treatment with tamoxifen, with more apoptotic and necrotic cells for the conditions cultured with plain or fatty acid-loaded beads than were seen in the control condition.

The preliminary evaluation of this composite system demonstrated several key findings. First, the hydrogel matrix stiffness is affected by the inclusion of microcarrier beads. This, along with the inclusion of biomolecules within the microcarrier beads, allows for a tunable system that could be specifically designed for mimicking certain properties of the mammary environment. Second, this composite system supports the growth and proliferation of breast cancer cells, which are responsive to treatment with cancer drug therapeutics. With microcarrier beads that can also support cell growth, it is then possible to also evaluate multiple cell types, such as adipocytes or fibroblasts, within this composite system to determine the effects of these cell–cell interactions on tumor cell behavior within defined microenvironments. Further investigation of this composite system could yield a novel tunable platform for testing cancer cell therapies.

9.6 CONCLUSION AND PERSPECTIVE

With the continued development and advancement of 3D mammary tissue systems, there is great promise for the knowledge attained from these highly optimized, physiologically relevant systems to significantly impact breast-related research. However, while the sophistication of existing models is growing, there is still a void that multiparameter composite systems could fill. For example, most traditional models recapitulate cell–cell, cell–molecule, or cell–matrix interactions independently, but as identified in summary (Table 9.2), matrix mechanical properties have not always been considered in the experimental design for application of these systems, and have only recently become more commonly included in 3D system characterization. Engineering strategies employing advanced fabrication techniques, such as 3D printing, bioprinting, microfluidics, and micropatterning, have already been applied to the development of mammary tissue systems for creating tumor microarray systems, miniaturized model platforms for studying drug therapeutics, precisely designed nanocomposite bone metastasis systems, and other applications (Bersini et al. 2014; Hakanson et al. 2014; Hirt et al. 2014; Peela et al. 2016; Sabhachandani et al. 2016; Sodunke et al. 2007; Zhu et al. 2016). Continued growth in these multidisciplinary approaches will drive the development of composite systems essential for designing more optimal mammary tissue systems.

Further, while not specifically overviewed in this chapter, 3D mammary systems are equally important for breast tissue engineering and regenerative medicine applications aimed at developing suitable autologous tissue options for breast reconstruction procedures. As the fabrication methods and designs of these systems continue to progress, it is foreseeable that the application of these 3D mammary systems could expand to include not only engineering breast tissue for aesthetic reconstruction purposes, but also to include functional tissue restorations, which will be particularly useful as reproductive concerns for breast cancer patients come to the forefront of research problems that need to be addressed to improve the quality of life for these patients.

REFERENCES

Ackers, R. M. 2002. *Lactation and the Mammary Gland*. Ames, IA: Iowa State Press.

Ailhaud, G., P. Grimaldi, and R. Negrel. 1992. Cellular and molecular aspects of adipose tissue development. *Annu Rev Nutr* 12:207–33.

Albright, A. L. and J. S. Stern. 1998. Adipose tissue. *Encyclopedia of Sports Medicine and Science 2016*, http://www.sportsci.org/encycl.

Alcaraz, J., C. M. Nelson, and M. J. Bissell. 2004. Biomechanical approaches for studying integration of tissue structure and function in mammary epithelia. *J Mammary Gland Biol Neoplasia* 9 (4):361–74.

American Cancer Society. 2016. *Cancer Facts & Figures 2016*. Atlanta, GA: American Cancer Society.

Arab, L. 2003. Biomarkers of fat and fatty acid intake. *J Nutr* 133(Suppl 3):925s–32s.

Bagga, D., S. Capone, H. J. Wang, D. Heber, M. Lill, L. Chap, and J. A. Glaspy. 1997. Dietary modulation of omega-3/omega-6 polyunsaturated fatty acid ratios in patients with breast cancer. *J Natl Cancer Inst* 89 (15):1123–31.

Bakker, N., P. Van't Veer, and P. L. Zock. 1997. Adipose fatty acids and cancers of the breast, prostate and colon: An ecological study. EURAMIC Study Group. *Int J Cancer* 72 (4):587–91.

Balachander, G. M., S. A. Balaji, A. Rangarajan, and K. Chatterjee. 2015. Enhanced metastatic potential in a 3D tissue scaffold toward a comprehensive *in vitro* model for breast cancer metastasis. *ACS Appl Mater Interfaces* 7 (50):27810–22.

Barcellos-Hoff, M. H. and K. B. Ewan. 2000. Transforming growth factor-beta and breast cancer: Mammary gland development. *Breast Cancer Res* 2 (2):92–9.

Benton, G., G. DeGray, H. K. Kleinman, J. George, and I. Arnaoutova. 2015. *In vitro* microtumors provide a physiologically predictive tool for breast cancer therapeutic screening. *PLoS One* 10 (4):e0123312.

Bersini, S., J. S. Jeon, G. Dubini, C. Arrigoni, S. Chung, J. L. Charest, M. Moretti, and R. D. Kamm. 2014. A microfluidic 3D *in vitro* model for specificity of breast cancer metastasis to bone. *Biomaterials* 35 (8):2454–61.

Bersini, S., J. S. Jeon, M. Moretti, and R. D. Kamm. 2014. *In vitro* models of the metastatic cascade: From local invasion to extravasation. *Drug Discov Today* 19 (6):735–42.

Bissell, M. J., A. Rizki, and I. S. Mian. 2003. Tissue architecture: The ultimate regulator of breast epithelial function. *Curr Opin Cell Biol* 15 (6):753–62.

Borellini, F. and T. Oka. 1989. Growth control and differentiation in mammary epithelial cells. *Environ Health Perspect* 80:85–99.

Bougnoux, P., V. Maillard, and V. Chajes. 2005. Omega-6/omega-3 polyunsaturated fatty acids ratio and breast cancer. *World Rev Nutr Diet* 94:158–65.

Bouloumie, A., C. Sengenes, G. Portolan, J. Galitzky, and M. Lafontan. 2001. Adipocyte produces matrix metalloproteinases 2 and 9: Involvement in adipose differentiation. *Diabetes* 50 (9):2080–6.

Bray, L. J., M. Binner, A. Holzheu, J. Friedrichs, U. Freudenberg, D. W. Hutmacher, and C. Werner. 2015. Multi-parametric hydrogels support 3D *in vitro* bioengineered microenvironment models of tumour angiogenesis. *Biomaterials* 53:609–20.

Cavin, A. N. M. 2005. *Adipocyte Response to Injectable Breast Tissue Engineering Scaffolds*. Clemson, SC: Department of Bioengineering, Clemson University.

Celis, J. E., J. M. Moreira, T. Cabezon, P. Gromov, E. Friis, F. Rank, and I. Gromova. 2005. Identification of extracellular and intracellular signaling components of the mammary adipose tissue and its interstitial fluid in high risk breast cancer patients: Toward dissecting the molecular circuitry of epithelial–adipocyte stromal cell interactions. *Mol Cell Proteomics* 4 (4):492–522.

Chavey, C., B. Mari, M. N. Monthouel, S. Bonnafous, P. Anglard, E. Van Obberghen, and S. Tartare-Deckert. 2003. Matrix metalloproteinases are differentially expressed in adipose tissue during obesity and modulate adipocyte differentiation. *J Biol Chem* 278 (14):11888–96.

Cheung, K. J. and A. J. Ewald. 2014. Illuminating breast cancer invasion: Diverse roles for cell–cell interactions. *Curr Opin Cell Biol* 30:99–111.

Chrenek, M. A., P. Wong, and V. M. Weaver. 2001. Tumour–stromal interactions. Integrins and cell adhesions as modulators of mammary cell survival and transformation. *Breast Cancer Res* 3 (4):224–9.

Cunha, G. R. and Y. K. Hom. 1996. Role of mesenchymal–epithelial interactions in mammary gland development. *J Mammary Gland Biol Neoplasia* 1 (1):21–35.

Cvetkovic, D., C. G. Goertzen, and M. Bhattacharya. 2014. Quantification of breast cancer cell invasiveness using a three-dimensional (3D) model. *J Vis Exp* 88:1–9.

Debnath, J. and J. S. Brugge. 2005. Modelling glandular epithelial cancers in three-dimensional cultures. *Nat Rev Cancer* 5 (9):675–88.

Dhiman, H. K., A. R. Ray, and A. K. Panda. 2004. Characterization and evaluation of chitosan matrix for *in vitro* growth of MCF-7 breast cancer cell lines. *Biomaterials* 25 (21):5147–54.

Dhiman, H. K., A. R. Ray, and A. K. Panda. 2005. Three-dimensional chitosan scaffold-based MCF-7 cell culture for the determination of the cytotoxicity of tamoxifen. *Biomaterials* 26 (9):979–86.

do Amaral, J. B., P. Rezende-Teixeira, V. M. Freitas, and G. M. Machado-Santelli. 2011. MCF-7 cells as a three-dimensional model for the study of human breast cancer. *Tissue Eng Part C Methods* 17 (11):1097–107.

Duck, F. A. 2013. *Physical Properties of Tissues: A Comprehensive Reference Book*. San Diego, CA: Elsevier Science.

Estrada, M. F., S. P. Rebelo, E. J. Davies, M. T. Pinto, H. Pereira, V. E. Santo, M. J. Smalley et al. 2016. Modelling the tumour microenvironment in long-term microencapsulated 3D co-cultures recapitulates phenotypic features of disease progression. *Biomaterials* 78:50–61.

Falkenberg, N., I. Hofig, M. Rosemann, J. Szumielewski, S. Richter, K. Schorpp, K. Hadian, M. Aubele, M. J. Atkinson, and N. Anastasov. 2016. Three-dimensional microtissues essentially contribute to preclinical validations of therapeutic targets in breast cancer. *Cancer Med* 5 (4):703–10.

Fang, J. Y., S. J. Tan, Y. C. Wu, Z. Yang, B. X. Hoang, and B. Han. 2016. From competency to dormancy: A 3D model to study cancer cells and drug responsiveness. *J Transl Med* 14:38.

Fonseca-Alaniz, M. H., J. Takada, M. I. Alonso-Vale, and F. B. Lima. 2007. Adipose tissue as an endocrine organ: From theory to practice. *J Pediatr (Rio J)* 83 (5 Suppl):S192–203.

Fridriksdottir, A. J., R. Villadsen, T. Gudjonsson, and O. W. Petersen. 2005. Maintenance of cell type diversification in the human breast. *J Mammary Gland Biol Neoplasia* 10 (1):61–74.

Fung, Y. C. 2013. *Biomechanics: Mechanical Properties of Living Tissues*. New York, NY: Springer.

Geddes, D. T. 2007. Inside the lactating breast: The latest anatomy research. *J Midwifery Womens Health* 52 (6):556–63.

Gefen, A. and B. Dilmoney. 2007. Mechanics of the normal woman's breast. *Technol Health Care* 15 (4):259–71.

Godley, P. A. 1995. Essential fatty acid consumption and risk of breast cancer. *Breast Cancer Res Treat* 35 (1):91–5.

Gomillion, C. T. 2005. *Evaluation of Tissue Engineered Injectable Devices for Breast Tissue Engineering*. Clemson, SC: Department of Bioengineering, Clemson University.

Gomillion, C. T. and K. J. L. Burg. 2011a. Adipose tissue engineering. In *Comprehensive Biomaterials*, edited by P. Ducheyne, K. Healy, D. E. Hutmacher, D. W. Grainger and C. J. Kirkpatrick, 529–39. Oxford, UK. Elsevier.

Gomillion, C. T. and K. J. L. Burg. 2011b. Fatty acid loaded chitosan gelatin beads for adipose tissue engineering. In 2011 Annual Meeting of the Society for Biomaterials. Orlando, FL.

Gray, H. and W. H. Lewis. 1918. *Anatomy of the Human Body*. 20th Ed. Philadelphia, PA: Lea & Febiger.

Greenleaf, J. F., M. Fatemi, and M. Insana. 2003. Selected methods for imaging elastic properties of biological tissues. *Annu Rev Biomed Eng* 5:57–78.

Habal, N. 2006. *Carolina Breast & Oncologic Surgery—Breast Cancer Information Booklet*. Greenville, SC: Greenville Hospital.

Hakanson, M., E. Cukierman, and M. Charnley. 2014. Miniaturized pre-clinical cancer models as research and diagnostic tools. *Adv Drug Deliv Rev* 69–70:52–66.

Halberg, N., I. Wernstedt-Asterholm, and P. E. Scherer. 2008. The adipocyte as an endocrine cell. *Endocrinol Metab Clin North Am* 37 (3):753–68, x–xi.

Hanahan, D. and R. A. Weinberg. 2000. The hallmarks of cancer. *Cell* 100 (1):57–70.

Hanahan, D. and R. A. Weinberg. 2011. Hallmarks of cancer: The next generation. *Cell* 144 (5):646–74.

Hankin, J. H. and V. Rawlings. 1978. Diet and breast cancer: A review. *Am J Clin Nutr* 31 (11):2005–16.

Haslam, S. Z. and T. L. Woodward. 2003. Host microenvironment in breast cancer development: Epithelial-cell–stromal–cell interactions and steroid hormone action in normal and cancerous mammary gland. *Breast Cancer Res* 5 (4):208–15.

Hauner, H. 2005. Secretory factors from human adipose tissue and their functional role. *Proc Nutr Soc* 64 (2):163–9.

Heber, D., J. Ashley, and D. Bagga. 1996. Stromal-epithelial cell interactions in breast cancer. *Adv Exp Med Biol* 399:41–51.

Hebner, C., V. M. Weaver, and J. Debnath. 2008. Modeling morphogenesis and oncogenesis in three-dimensional breast epithelial cultures. *Annu Rev Pathol* 3:313–39.

Hickman, J. A., R. Graeser, R. de Hoogt, S. Vidic, C. Brito, M. Gutekunst, and H. van der Kuip. 2014. Three-dimensional models of cancer for pharmacology and cancer cell biology: Capturing tumor complexity *in vitro/ex vivo*. *Biotechnol J* 9 (9):1115–28.

Hirshaut, Y., P. Pressman, and J. Brody. 2009. *Breast Cancer: The Complete Guide*. 5th Ed. New York, NY: Random House Publishing Group.

Hirt, C., A. Papadimitropoulos, V. Mele, M. G. Muraro, C. Mengus, G. Iezzi, L. Terracciano, I. Martin, and G. C. Spagnoli. 2014. "*In vitro*" 3D models of tumor-immune system interaction. *Adv Drug Deliv Rev* 79–80:145–54.

Hovey, R. C., T. B. McFadden, and R. M. Akers. 1999. Regulation of mammary gland growth and morphogenesis by the mammary fat pad: A species comparison. *J Mammary Gland Biol Neoplasia* 4 (1):53–68.

Howard, B. A. and B. A. Gusterson. 2000. Human breast development. *J Mammary Gland Biol Neoplasia* 5 (2):119–37.

Howe, G. R. 1994. Dietary fat and breast cancer risks. An epidemiologic perspective. *Cancer* 74 (3 Suppl):1078–84.

Huss, F. R. and G. Kratz. 2001. Mammary epithelial cell and adipocyte co-culture in a 3-D matrix: The first step towards tissue-engineered human breast tissue. *Cells Tissues Organs* 169 (4):361–7. doi: 47903.

Iyengar, P., T. P. Combs, S. J. Shah, V. Gouon-Evans, J. W. Pollard, C. Albanese, L. Flanagan et al. 2003. Adipocyte-secreted factors synergistically promote mammary tumorigenesis through induction of anti-apoptotic transcriptional programs and proto-oncogene stabilization. *Oncogene* 22 (41):6408–23.

Iyengar, P., V. Espina, T. W. Williams, Y. Lin, D. Berry, L. A. Jelicks, H. Lee et al. 2005. Adipocyte-derived collagen VI affects early mammary tumor progression *in vivo*, demonstrating a critical interaction in the tumor/stroma microenvironment. *J Clin Invest* 115 (5):1163–76.

Jorstad, L. H. and M. J. Payne. 1964. *Surgery of the Breast*. St. Louis, MO: Mosby.

Karnoub, A. E. and R. A. Weinberg. 2006. Chemokine networks and breast cancer metastasis. *Breast Dis* 26:75–85.

Kim, J. B. 2005. Three-dimensional tissue culture models in cancer biology. *Semin Cancer Biol* 15 (5):365–77.

Kim, J. B., R. Stein, and M. J. O'Hare. 2004. Three-dimensional *in vitro* tissue culture models of breast cancer-- a review. *Breast Cancer Res Treat* 85 (3):281–91.

Klein, V., V. Chajes, E. Germain, G. Schulgen, M. Pinault, D. Malvy, T. Lefrancq et al. 2000. Low alpha-linolenic acid content of adipose breast tissue is associated with an increased risk of breast cancer. *Eur J Cancer* 36 (3):335–40.

Kleinman, H. K., M. L. McGarvey, J. R. Hassell, V. L. Star, F. B. Cannon, G. W. Laurie, and G. R. Martin. 1986. Basement membrane complexes with biological activity. *Biochemistry* 25 (2):312–8.

Kohlmeier, L. 1997. Biomarkers of fatty acid exposure and breast cancer risk. *Am J Clin Nutr* 66 (6 Suppl):1548s–56s.

Kohlmeier, L. and M. Mendez. 1997. Controversies surrounding diet and breast cancer. *Proc Nutr Soc* 56 (1b):369–82.

Korkola, J. E., S. DeVries, J. Fridlyand, E. S. Hwang, A. L. Estep, Y. Y. Chen, K. L. Chew, S. H. Dairkee, R. M. Jensen, and F. M. Waldman. 2003. Differentiation of lobular versus ductal breast carcinomas by expression microarray analysis. *Cancer Res* 63 (21):7167–75.

Krause, S., M. V. Maffini, A. M. Soto, and C. Sonnenschein. 2008. A novel 3D *in vitro* culture model to study stromal–epithelial interactions in the mammary gland. *Tissue Eng Part C Methods* 14 (3):261–71.

Krouskop, T. A., T. M. Wheeler, F. Kallel, B. S. Garra, and T. Hall. 1998. Elastic moduli of breast and prostate tissues under compression. *Ultrason Imaging* 20 (4):260–74.

Kruse, S. A., J. A. Smith, A. J. Lawrence, M. A. Dresner, A. Manduca, J. F. Greenleaf, and R. L. Ehman. 2000. Tissue characterization using magnetic resonance elastography: Preliminary results. *Phys Med Biol* 45 (6):1579–90.

Lance, A., C. C. Yang, M. Swamydas, D. Dean, S. Deitch, K. J. Burg, and D. Dreau. 2016. Increased extracellular matrix density decreases MCF10A breast cell acinus formation in 3D culture conditions. *J Tissue Eng Regen Med* 10 (1):71–80.

Lanigan, F., D. O'Connor, F. Martin, and W. M. Gallagher. 2007. Molecular links between mammary gland development and breast cancer. *Cell Mol Life Sci* 64 (24):3159–84.

Lanza, R., R. Langer, and J. P. Vacanti. 2013. *Principles of Tissue Engineering, Tissue Engineering Intelligence Unit*. San Diego, CA: Elsevier Science.

Larsson, S. C., M. Kumlin, M. Ingelman-Sundberg, and A. Wolk. 2004. Dietary long-chain n-3 fatty acids for the prevention of cancer: A review of potential mechanisms. *Am J Clin Nutr* 79 (6):935–45.

Lee, M. M. and S. S. Lin. 2000. Dietary fat and breast cancer. *Annu Rev Nutr* 20:221–48.

Levine, J. F. and F. E. Stockdale. 1985. Cell–cell interactions promote mammary epithelial cell differentiation. *J Cell Biol* 100 (5):1415–22.

London, S. J., F. M. Sacks, J. Caesar, M. J. Stampfer, E. Siguel, and W. C. Willett. 1991. Fatty acid composition of subcutaneous adipose tissue and diet in postmenopausal US women. *Am J Clin Nutr* 54 (2):340–5.

Lovitt, C. J., T. B. Shelper, and V. M. Avery. 2013. Miniaturized three-dimensional cancer model for drug evaluation. *Assay Drug Dev Technol* 11 (7):435–48.

Lovitt, C. J., T. B. Shelper, and V. M. Avery. 2015. Evaluation of chemotherapeutics in a three-dimensional breast cancer model. *J Cancer Res Clin Oncol* 141 (5):951–9.

Macias, H. and L. Hinck. 2012. Mammary gland development. *Wiley Interdiscip Rev Dev Biol* 1 (4):533–57.

Maggiora, M., M. Bologna, M. P. Ceru, L. Possati, A. Angelucci, A. Cimini, A. Miglietta et al. 2004. An overview of the effect of linoleic and conjugated-linoleic acids on the growth of several human tumor cell lines. *Int J Cancer* 112 (6):909–19.

Maghdouri-White, Y., G. L. Bowlin, C. A. Lemmon, and D. Dreau. 2016. Bioengineered silk scaffolds in 3D tissue modeling with focus on mammary tissues. *Mater Sci Eng C Mater Biol Appl* 59:1168–80.

Maillard, V., P. Bougnoux, P. Ferrari, M. L. Jourdan, M. Pinault, F. Lavillonniere, G. Body, O. Le Floch, and V. Chajes. 2002. N-3 and N-6 fatty acids in breast adipose tissue and relative risk of breast cancer in a case-control study in Tours, France. *Int J Cancer* 98 (1):78–83.

Masaki, T. and H. Yoshimatsu. 2008. Obesity, adipocytokines and cancer. *Transl Oncogenomics* 3:45–52.

McCave, E. J., C. A. Cass, K. J. Burg, and B. W. Booth. 2010. The normal microenvironment directs mammary gland development. *J Mammary Gland Biol Neoplasia* 15 (3):291–9.

McKnight, A. L., J. L. Kugel, P. J. Rossman, A. Manduca, L. C. Hartmann, and R. L. Ehman. 2002. MR elastography of breast cancer: Preliminary results. *AJR Am J Roentgenol* 178 (6):1411–7.

Miner, J. L. 2004. The adipocyte as an endocrine cell. *J Anim Sci* 82 (3):935–41.

Nash, C. E., G. Mavria, E. W. Baxter, D. L. Holliday, D. C. Tomlinson, D. Treanor, V. Novitskaya, F. Berditchevski, A. M. Hanby, and V. Speirs. 2015. Development and characterisation of a 3D multi-cellular *in vitro* model of normal human breast: A tool for cancer initiation studies. *Oncotarget* 6 (15):13731–41.

Nelson, C. M. and M. J. Bissell. 2005. Modeling dynamic reciprocity: Engineering three-dimensional culture models of breast architecture, function, and neoplastic transformation. *Semin Cancer Biol* 15 (5):342–52.

Osborne, M. P. and S. K. Boolbol. 2014. Breast anatomy and development. In *Diseases of the Breast*, edited by J. R. Harris, M. E. Lippman, M. Morrow and C. K. Osborne. Philadelphia, PA: Lippincott Williams & Wilkins.

Padron, J. M., C. L. van der Wilt, K. Smid, E. Smitskamp-Wilms, H. H. Backus, P. E. Pizao, G. Giaccone, and G. J. Peters. 2000. The multilayered postconfluent cell culture as a model for drug screening. *Crit Rev Oncol Hematol* 36 (2–3):141–57.

Parmar, H. and G. R. Cunha. 2004. Epithelial-stromal interactions in the mouse and human mammary gland *in vivo*. *Endocr Relat Cancer* 11 (3):437–58.

Pathi, S. P., C. Kowalczewski, R. Tadipatri, and C. Fischbach. 2010. A novel 3-D mineralized tumor model to study breast cancer bone metastasis. *PLoS One* 5 (1):e8849.

Pauwels, E. K. and K. Kairemo. 2008. Fatty acid facts, part II: Role in the prevention of carcinogenesis, or, more fish on the dish? *Drug News Perspect* 21 (9):504–10.

Peela, N., F. S. Sam, W. Christenson, D. Truong, A. W. Watson, G. Mouneimne, R. Ros, and M. Nikkhah. 2016. A three dimensional micropatterned tumor model for breast cancer cell migration studies. *Biomaterials* 81:72–83.

Polyak, K. 2007. Breast cancer: Origins and evolution. *J Clin Invest* 117 (11):3155–63.

Rahman, M. and S. Mohammed. 2015. Breast cancer metastasis and the lymphatic system. *Oncol Lett* 10 (3):1233–9.

Rice, D. P., T. Aberg, Y. Chan, Z. Tang, P. J. Kettunen, L. Pakarinen, R. E. Maxson, and I. Thesleff. 2000. Integration of FGF and TWIST in calvarial bone and suture development. *Development* 127 (9):1845–55.

Rijal, G. and W. Li. 2016. 3D scaffolds in breast cancer research. *Biomaterials* 81:135–56.

Russo, J. and I. H. Russo. 2004. Development of the human breast. *Maturitas* 49 (1):2–15.

Saadatian-Elahi, M., T. Norat, J. Goudable, and E. Riboli. 2004. Biomarkers of dietary fatty acid intake and the risk of breast cancer: A meta-analysis. *Int J Cancer* 111 (4):584–91.

Sabhachandani, P., V. Motwani, N. Cohen, S. Sarkar, V. Torchilin, and T. Konry. 2016. Generation and functional assessment of 3D multicellular spheroids in droplet based microfluidics platform. *Lab Chip* 16 (3):497–505.

Sahoo, S. K., A. K. Panda, and V. Labhasetwar. 2005. Characterization of porous PLGA/PLA microparticles as a scaffold for three dimensional growth of breast cancer cells. *Biomacromolecules* 6 (2):1132–9.

Sakai, K., H. Okuyama, J. Yura, H. Takeyama, N. Shinagawa, N. Tsuruga, K. Kato et al. 1992. Composition and turnover of phospholipids and neutral lipids in human breast cancer and reference tissues. *Carcinogenesis* 13 (4):579–84.

Samani, A. and D. Plewes. 2004. A method to measure the hyperelastic parameters of *ex vivo* breast tissue samples. *Phys Med Biol* 49 (18):4395–405.

Samani, A., J. Zubovits, and D. Plewes. 2007. Elastic moduli of normal and pathological human breast tissues: An inversion-technique-based investigation of 169 samples. *Phys Med Biol* 52 (6):1565–76.

Sarvazyan, A. P., O. V. Rudenko, S. D. Swanson, J. B. Fowlkes, and S. Y. Emelianov. 1998. Shear wave elasticity imaging: A new ultrasonic technology of medical diagnostics. *Ultrasound Med Biol* 24 (9):1419–35.

Sasser, A. K., B. L. Mundy, K. M. Smith, A. W. Studebaker, A. E. Axel, A. M. Haidet, S. A. Fernandez, and B. M. Hall. 2007. Human bone marrow stromal cells enhance breast cancer cell growth rates in a cell line-dependent manner when evaluated in 3D tumor environments. *Cancer Lett* 254 (2):255–64.

Schedin, P. and P. J. Keely. 2011. Mammary gland ECM remodeling, stiffness, and mechanosignaling in normal development and tumor progression. *Cold Spring Harb Perspect Biol* 3 (1):a003228.

Schittny, J. C. and P. D. Yurchenco. 1989. Basement membranes: Molecular organization and function in development and disease. *Curr Opin Cell Biol* 1 (5):983–8.

Shayan, R., M. G. Achen, and S. A. Stacker. 2006. Lymphatic vessels in cancer metastasis: Bridging the gaps. *Carcinogenesis* 27 (9):1729–38.

Shekhar, M. P., J. Werdell, S. J. Santner, R. J. Pauley, and L. Tait. 2001. Breast stroma plays a dominant regulatory role in breast epithelial growth and differentiation: Implications for tumor development and progression. *Cancer Res* 61 (4):1320–6.

Simonsen, N., P. van't Veer, J. J. Strain, J. M. Martin-Moreno, J. K. Huttunen, J. F. Navajas, B. C. Martin et al. 1998. Adipose tissue omega-3 and omega-6 fatty acid content and breast cancer in the EURAMIC study. European Community Multicenter Study on Antioxidants, Myocardial Infarction, and Breast Cancer. *Am J Epidemiol* 147 (4):342–52.

Simonsen, N. R., J. Fernandez-CrehuetNavajas, J. M. Martin-Moreno, J. J. Strain, J. K. Huttunen, B. C. Martin, M. Thamm et al. 1998. Tissue stores of individual monounsaturated fatty acids and breast cancer: The EURAMIC study. European Community Multicenter Study on Antioxidants, Myocardial Infarction, and Breast Cancer. *Am J Clin Nutr* 68 (1):134–41.

Sims, A. H., A. Howell, S. J. Howell, and R. B. Clarke. 2007. Origins of breast cancer subtypes and therapeutic implications. *Nat Clin Pract Oncol* 4 (9):516–25.

Sinkus, R., J. Lorenzen, D. Schrader, M. Lorenzen, M. Dargatz, and D. Holz. 2000. High-resolution tensor MR elastography for breast tumour detection. *Phys Med Biol* 45 (6):1649–64.

Snell, R. S. 2004. *Clinical Anatomy: An Illustrated Review with Questions and Explanations.* Philadelphia, PA: Lippincott Williams & Wilkins.

Sodunke, T. R., K. K. Turner, S. A. Caldwell, K. W. McBride, M. J. Reginato, and H. M. Noh. 2007. Micropatterns of Matrigel for three-dimensional epithelial cultures. *Biomaterials* 28 (27):4006–16.

Song, H. H., K. M. Park, and S. Gerecht. 2014. Hydrogels to model 3D *in vitro* microenvironment of tumor vascularization. *Adv Drug Deliv Rev* 79–80:19–29.

Sorisky, A. 1999. From preadipocyte to adipocyte: Differentiation-directed signals of insulin from the cell surface to the nucleus. *Crit Rev Clin Lab Sci* 36 (1):1–34.

Speroni, L., G. S. Whitt, J. Xylas, K. P. Quinn, A. Jondeau-Cabaton, C. Barnes, I. Georgakoudi, C. Sonnenschein, and A. M. Soto. 2014. Hormonal regulation of epithelial organization in a three-dimensional breast tissue culture model. *Tissue Eng Part C Methods* 20 (1):42–51.

Sternlicht, M. D. 2006. Key stages in mammary gland development: The cues that regulate ductal branching morphogenesis. *Breast Cancer Res* 8 (1):201.

Sternlicht, M. D., H. Kouros-Mehr, P. Lu, and Z. Werb. 2006. Hormonal and local control of mammary branching morphogenesis. *Differentiation* 74 (7):365–81.

Stillaert, F. B., P. Blondeel, M. Hamdi, K. Abberton, E. Thompson, and W. A. Morrison. 2006. Adipose tissue induction *in vivo*. *Adv Exp Med Biol* 585:403–12.

Taubenberger, A. V. 2014. *In vitro* microenvironments to study breast cancer bone colonisation. *Adv Drug Deliv Rev* 79–80:135–44.

Tozeren, A., C. W. Coward, and S. P. Petushi. 2005. Origins and evolution of cell phenotypes in breast tumors. *J Theor Biol* 233 (1):43–54.

Trujillo, M. E. and P. E. Scherer. 2006. Adipose tissue-derived factors: Impact on health and disease. *Endocr Rev* 27 (7):762–78.

Van Houten, E. E., M. M. Doyley, F. E. Kennedy, J. B. Weaver, and K. D. Paulsen. 2003. Initial *in vivo* experience with steady-state subzone-based MR elastography of the human breast. *J Magn Reson Imaging* 17 (1):72–85.

Villadsen, R. 2005. In search of a stem cell hierarchy in the human breast and its relevance to breast cancer evolution. *Apmis* 113 (11–12):903–21.

Wang, F., S. Gao, F. Chen, Z. Fu, H. Yin, X. Lu, J. Yu, and C. Lu. 2014. Mammary fat of breast cancer: Gene expression profiling and functional characterization. *PLoS One* 9 (10):e109742.

Wang, X., M. R. Reagan, and D. L. Kaplan. 2010. Synthetic adipose tissue models for studying mammary gland development and breast tissue engineering. *J Mammary Gland Biol Neoplasia* 15 (3):365–76.

Wang, X., L. Sun, M. V. Maffini, A. Soto, C. Sonnenschein, and D. L. Kaplan. 2010. A complex 3D human tissue culture system based on mammary stromal cells and silk scaffolds for modeling breast morphogenesis and function. *Biomaterials* 31 (14):3920–9.

Wang, X., X. Zhang, L. Sun, B. Subramanian, M. V. Maffini, A. Soto, C.Sonnenschein, and D. L.Kaplan. 2009. Preadipocytes stimulate ductal morphogenesis and functional differentiation of human mammary epithelial cells on 3D silk scaffolds. *Tissue Eng Part A* 15 (10):3087–98.

Weaver, V. M., A. R. Howlett, B. Langton-Webster, O. W. Petersen, and M. J. Bissell. 1995. The development of a functionally relevant cell culture model of progressive human breast cancer. *Semin Cancer Biol* 6 (3):175–84.

Weigelt, B., C. M. Ghajar, and M. J. Bissell. 2014. The need for complex 3D culture models to unravel novel pathways and identify accurate biomarkers in breast cancer. *Adv Drug Deliv Rev* 69–70:42–51.

Wellman, P. S. and R. D. Howe. 1998. Breast tissue stiffness in compression is correlated to histological diagnosis. Harvard Bio-robotics Laboratory 1–15, https://biorobotics.harvard.edu/pubs/1999/mechprops.pdf

Welsch, C. W. 1992. Relationship between dietary fat and experimental mammary tumorigenesis: A review and critique. *Cancer Res* 52 (7 Suppl):2040s–8s.

Welsch, C. W. 1994. Interrelationship between dietary lipids and calories and experimental mammary gland tumorigenesis. *Cancer* 74 (3 Suppl):1055–62.

Wendel, M. and A. R. Heller. 2009. Anticancer actions of omega-3 fatty acids: Current state and future perspectives. *Anticancer Agents Med Chem* 9 (4):457–70.

Wiseman, B. S. and Z. Werb. 2002. Stromal effects on mammary gland development and breast cancer. *Science* 296 (5570):1046–9.

Xie, J. and S. Z. Haslam. 1997. Extracellular matrix regulates ovarian hormone-dependent proliferation of mouse mammary epithelial cells. *Endocrinology* 138 (6):2466–73.

Xu, W., J. Qian, Y. Zhang, A. Suo, N. Cui, J. Wang, Y. Yao, and H. Wang. 2016. A double-network poly(Nvarepsilon–acryloyl L-lysine)/hyaluronic acid hydrogel as a mimic of the breast tumor microenvironment. *Acta Biomater* 33:131–41.

Yalcin, B. 2013. Staging, risk assessment and screening of breast cancer. *Exp Oncol* 35 (4):238–45.

Yamada, K. M. and E. Cukierman. 2007. Modeling tissue morphogenesis and cancer in 3D. *Cell* 130 (4):601–10.

Zangani, D., K. M. Darcy, S. Shoemaker, and M. M. Ip. 1999. Adipocyte–epithelial interactions regulate the *in vitro* development of normal mammary epithelial cells. *Exp Cell Res* 247 (2):399–409.

Zhu, W., B. Holmes, R. I. Glazer, and L. G. Zhang. 2016. 3D printed nanocomposite matrix for the study of breast cancer bone metastasis. *Nanomedicine* 12 (1):69–79.

Zhu, W., M. Wang, Y. Fu, N. J. Castro, S. W. Fu, and L. G. Zhang. 2015. Engineering a biomimetic three-dimensional nanostructured bone model for breast cancer bone metastasis study. *Acta Biomater* 14:164–74.

Zhu, Z. R., J. Agren, S. Mannisto, P. Pietinen, M. Eskelinen, K. Syrjanen, and M. Uusitupa. 1995. Fatty acid composition of breast adipose tissue in breast cancer patients and in patients with benign breast disease. *Nutr Cancer* 24 (2):151–60.

10 Mineralized 3D Culture Systems for Studying Bone Metastatic Breast Cancer

Frank He, Siyoung Choi, Lara A. Estroff, and Claudia Fischbach

CONTENTS

10.1 Introduction 169
10.2 Relevance of Mineral to "Seed-and-Soil" Concept of Bone Metastasis 171
    10.2.1 Mammary Calcifications 171
    10.2.2 Bone Mineral 174
10.3 Experimental Models to Study Cell–Mineral Interactions 176
    10.3.1 Cell- and Tissue-Based Methods to Recapitulate Mineralized Microenvironments 176
    10.3.2 Incorporation of Synthetic HA into Scaffolds for Cell Culture 177
    10.3.3 Collagen as Substrates for Mineralization 181
10.4 Conclusion and Perspective 183
Acknowledgments 184
References 184

10.1 INTRODUCTION

Skeletal metastases occur in approximately 85% of breast cancer patients. Advancements in molecular biology and genetics have resulted in targeted therapeutics that can improve the clinical prognosis of patients with primary disease. However, once spread to the bone, metastatic breast cancer continues to be associated with short median survival times and high mortality rates. These grim statistics are due in part to an insufficient mechanistic understanding of the microenvironmental factors that regulate the progression from primary breast cancer to bone metastatic disease. In particular, hydroxyapatite (HA) mineral, present in mammary tissue as microcalcifications and an essential nanostructural constituent of bone tissue, is largely overlooked, but may play a critical role in driving breast cancer malignancy. While engineered tumor models are increasingly used to recapitulate the complex and heterogeneous tumor microenvironments at both the primary and secondary sites, very few of the current platforms incorporate mineral into their respective designs.

Breast cancer metastasis to bone is the leading cause of breast cancer-related deaths among women worldwide (Mundy 2002). Roughly 85% of patients with advanced breast cancer develop skeletal metastases, which are characterized by painful osteolytic lesions, pathological fractures, and poor clinical prognoses (Coleman and Rubens 1987). Despite the wide array of clinical treatments for breast cancer bone metastasis, including surgery, radio- and chemotherapy, analgesics, and adjuvant therapy with antiresorptive drugs, median survival time remains at a dismal two-year post-diagnosis (Kozlow and Guise 2005). This grim statistic is a reflection of an insufficient mechanistic understanding of this disease, and may be due to the use of model systems that do not accurately mimic appropriate pathological contexts.

Studies in standard two-dimensional (2D) cell culture have significantly increased our understanding of signaling mechanisms relevant to cancer (Hanahan and Weinberg 2000). However, 2D cultures typically fail to mimic the complex microenvironmental conditions that influence disease progression in patients. Indeed, increasing culture dimensionality from 2D to 3D has been shown to significantly alter cell protein expression (Fischbach et al. 2007; Kenny et al. 2007), proliferation (Wang et al. 1998), differentiation (Hosseinkhani et al. 2006), and metabolism (Rhodes et al. 2004). In addition, many other microenvironmental components such as the surrounding extracellular matrix (ECM), other neighboring cells, and cytokine gradients have been recapitulated with engineered model systems to reveal novel insights (Infanger et al. 2013). Despite these advances in modeling the dynamic and multifactorial interactions underlying tumorigenesis, it still remains poorly understood which specific properties need to be present at the primary and secondary sites in order to selectively enable bone metastasis.

The vast majority of the research efforts thus far have been focused on the biological mechanisms that govern the bone metastatic capability of breast cancer cells (Kozlow and Guise 2005; Mundy 2002; Weilbaecher et al. 2011). However, relatively little is known about the role of cell–ECM interactions in regulating these processes. In particular, the functional contribution of ECM-embedded hydroxyapatite—$(Ca_{10}(PO_4)_{6-x}(CO_3)_x(OH)_2)$ (HA)—to breast cancer bone metastasis remains almost completely unknown. Tumor cells are exposed to this mineral at both the primary and secondary sites as HA is a key component of breast microcalcifications (which are observed in 50% of breast cancer cases [Morgan et al. 2005]) and an essential nanostructural constituent of the bone metastatic site, respectively. In addition, *in vitro* studies have indicated that HA is a bioactive material that modulates key features of cancer cell aggressiveness, including migration (Cox et al. 2012a) and secretion of tumorigenic chemokines (Choi et al. 2015; Pathi et al. 2010, 2011). Hence, it is possible that HA may play a role in the progression from primary breast cancer to bone metastatic disease.

While engineered 3D tumor models including culture platforms based on polymeric scaffolds, hydrogel systems, and spheroid cultures (Hutmacher 2010; Nyga et al. 2011) can recapitulate the complex and heterogeneous tumor–microenvironment interactions that regulate breast cancer bone metastasis at both the primary and secondary sites, only a few of these systems consider mineral a vital design parameter. Here, we will summarize the current knowledge of tumor–mineral interactions relevant to bone metastasis, describe current efforts to develop mineralized culture systems, and provide a perspective on how such models may be expanded in the future to study the role of mineral in regulating breast cancer in general, and bone metastasis in particular.

10.2 RELEVANCE OF MINERAL TO "SEED-AND-SOIL" CONCEPT OF BONE METASTASIS

The clinically and experimentally supported "seed-and-soil" concept argues that site-specific metastasis occurs only if the target organ provides a fertile ground for tumor cells to seed (Paget 1889; Langley and Fidler 2011; Cox et al. 2012b). Also known as the premetastatic niche, this concept has formed the basis of investigations focused on the strong preference of metastatic breast cancer cells for bone. Indeed, breast cancer cells hijack molecular and cellular mechanisms used by hematopoietic stem cells in order to home to and grow within bone (Weilbaecher et al. 2011). For example, the chemokine receptor type 4 (CXCR4) expression of bone metastatic breast cancer cells renders them responsive to stromal cell-derived factor 1 (SDF-1) secreted by bone marrow-derived mesenchymal cells (Müller et al. 2001; Kang et al. 2003; Teicher and Fricker 2010). Furthermore, the specific physical properties (e.g., acidic pH, high extracellular calcium concentration, hypoxia) of the bone microenvironment promote tumor-cell growth (Kingsley et al. 2007). Once seeded in bone, tumor cells disrupt the homeostatic interplay between bone-forming osteoblasts and bone-degrading osteoclasts leading to the net effect of osteolysis. Bone degradation, in turn, further activates the vicious cycle of bone metastasis by releasing tumorigenic growth factors and cytokines, including transforming growth factor beta (TGF-beta) and insulin-like growth factor 1 (IGF-1) that foster secondary tumor development (Mundy 2002; Kozlow and Guise 2005; Weilbaecher et al. 2011).

Whether tumor–cell interactions with the inorganic mineral HA may impact the aforementioned processes by influencing both the seed and the soil remains unknown. For example, one may hypothesize that HA at the primary site may prime tumor cells for seeding to bone, for example, by upregulating genes typically associated with bone metastasis (Kang et al. 2003). Furthermore, it is also conceivable that tumor cells leverage specific HA nanostructural and physicochemical properties in bone in order to home and colonize effectively. When trying to answer some of these questions, it needs to be kept in mind that the material properties and formation mechanisms of HA in microcalcifications in the mammary tissue and in the bone matrix vary significantly. Hence, a basic understanding of the respective similarities and differences in both sites is necessary when designing *in vitro* model systems to study the functional influence of HA on bone metastasis.

10.2.1 MAMMARY CALCIFICATIONS

Breast microcalcifications are pathological mineral deposits that have been used for diagnosing early stage, nonpalpable breast cancer in routine mammographic screenings (Moon et al. 2000; Morgan et al. 2005; Bazin et al. 2012) (Figure 10.1a). Nearly 93% of ductal carcinomas *in situ* and 40% of mammary carcinomas (Castronovo and Bellahcene 1998) present radiologically detectable mineral deposits (Hofvind et al. 2011), the shape, size, distribution, and density of which can be further used to predict the level of breast cancer malignancy (Stomper et al. 2003; Tabar et al. 2004; Tse et al. 2008). While the vast majority of detected calcifications are benign, it has been established that certain clustering patterns

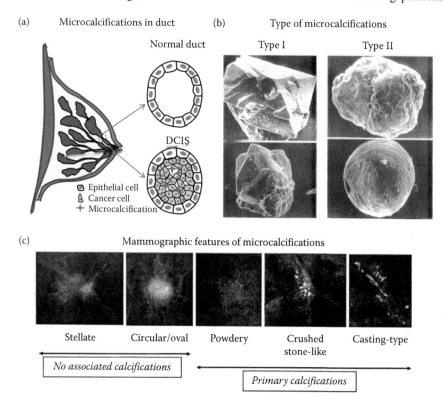

FIGURE 10.1 Mammary microcalcifications. (a) Microcalcifications are most frequently detected in ductal carcinoma *in situ* (DCIS) when cancerous cells fill the lumen of mammary ducts and mineral deposits develop due in part to cell death. (b) SEM micrograph revealing the morphology of a type I microcalcification of a sclerocystic mastopathy (top) and of an *in situ* lobular carcinoma (bottom). Morphology of a type II microcalcification in an infiltrating adenocarcinoma of the breast with irregular (top) and smooth surface (bottom). (Reproduced from *Hum Pathol*, 15 (9), Frappart, L. et al., Structure and composition of microcalcifications in benign and malignant lesions of the breast: Study by light microscopy, transmission and scanning electron microscopy, microprobe analysis, and X-ray diffraction, 880–9, Copyright 1984, W. B. Saunders Co., with permission from Elsevier, Inc.) (c) Mammographic features of breast carcinoma. (Tabar, L. et al.: Mammographic tumor features can predict long-term outcomes reliably in women with 1–14-mm invasive breast carcinoma. *Cancer*. 2004. 101. 1745–59. Copyright Wiley-VCH Verlag GmbH & Co. KGaA. Reproduced with permission.)

and morphologies implicate different subtypes or invasive grades of malignant disease. For instance, benign calcifications typically have a scattered distribution and are coarser with smooth margins, whereas malignant calcifications typically have a clustered, pleomorphic appearance and are finer with linear branching patterns (Muttarak et al. 2009) (Figure 10.1c). Moreover, breast cancer patients with microcalcifications exhibit decreased survival and increased lymph node involvement (Holme et al. 1993), suggesting their correlation with a more aggressive phenotype.

Mammary microcalcifications are classified into two distinct subgroups and can be distinguished by differences in structure and composition (Frappart et al. 1984, 1986). Type I microcalcifications exhibit pronounced crystalline structures and are predominantly composed of calcium oxalate dihydrate ($CaC_2O_4 \cdot 2H_2O$) (CO) (Kozlow and Guise 2005), while type II microcalcifications are composed of poorly defined, heterogeneous structures, and consist mainly of HA (Frappart et al. 1984) (Figure 10.1b). Interestingly, CO has been strictly found in benign growths (Barth et al. 1977; Büsing et al. 1981; Frappart et al. 1986; Going et al. 1990), but HA is commonly associated with more invasive disease (Hassler 1969; Frappart et al. 1986; Haka et al. 2002). Furthermore, variations of HA composition (e.g., carbonate substitution of HA) may be used to assess the malignant potential of breast cancer. More specifically, breast microcalcifications with decreased carbonate content may be linked with more aggressive disease relative to their more carbonated counterparts, implicating that compositional variations of microcalcifications may serve as prognostic indicators (Haka et al. 2002; Baker et al. 2010).

Although the exact mechanisms underlying the genesis of breast microcalcifications are unclear, experimental evidence implicates synergistic interactions between mammary tumor cells and their surrounding microenvironments. It has traditionally been thought that the more crystalline type I calcifications are formed through cell secretions, whereas the aggregated type II calcium deposits result from cellular degeneration and necrosis (Büsing et al. 1981; Haka et al. 2002; Muttarak et al. 2009). However, similar to deposition mechanisms of vascular and other pathological calcifications, the formation of HA in breast tissue could also be due to active cell-mediated processes (Cox and Morgan 2013). Indeed, Cox and coworkers have suggested that tumor cells themselves can deposit HA (Cox et al. 2012a), but other cell types may play a similarly important role. For example, not only bone marrow-derived mesenchymal stem cells are actively recruited by tumors, but they can also spontaneously calcify (Yoon et al. 2004; Breitbach et al. 2007). In particular, morphogens released by activated immune cells may play a role in this process (Abedin et al. 2004). In addition to the cells, mammary tumors contain appreciable levels of ECM components known to play a key role in mineral formation, such as bone sialoprotein (BSP), an arginine-glycine-aspartic acid (RGD)-containing phosphoprotein known to initiate HA deposition (Bellahcene et al. 2008), and osteopontin (OPN) (Bellahcene and Castronovo 1995; Bellahcene et al. 2008), an inhibitor of ectopic calcification depending on its phosphorylation state (Gericke et al. 2005; Addison et al. 2010).

10.2.2 BONE MINERAL

In bone, mineral occurs in the form of HA platelets that are embedded into collagen fibrils (Figure 10.2a). The composite of collagen fibrils and co-aligned HA mineral platelets composes the fundamental building block of bone (Traub et al. 1989; Landis et al. 1993), and, thus, influences bone hierarchical structure and mechanical performance (Weiner and Traub 1992; Fratzl and Weinkamer 2007; Pazzaglia et al. 2012; Reznikov et al. 2014). This collagen–mineral arrangement optimizes the toughness of the protein with the stiffness of the mineral to provide both rigidity and resistance against fracture. Should the geometric arrangement or integrity of each of these two components be altered in some way, the mechanical performance of bone tissue would be compromised (Fratzl et al. 2004). Relatively little is known currently about the modulating effect of breast cancer bone metastasis on bone mineral properties. However, a number of related findings indeed suggest that bone mineral changes in the presence of breast cancer cells and should, thus, be considered when studying bone metastasis.

Clinical studies causally associate high bone turnover with cancer metastasis (Zheng et al. 2013), and inhibiting bone resorption can prevent the growth of tumor cells in the bone (Zheng et al. 2013). After homing to bone, breast cancer cells release factors that cause visible degradation in the bone structure (Mundy 2002; Kingsley et al. 2007; Weilbaecher et al. 2011). In animal models of bone metastasis, these osteolytic lesions most frequently occur in the proximal tibiae and in the distal femurs (Kang et al. 2003; Zhang et al. 2009). The activity of bone degrading cells known as osteoclasts are enhanced by breast cancer cell-associated activation of the receptor activator of nuclear factor kappa-B ligand (RANKL) pathway (Mundy 2002). However, RANKL-independent osteolytic mechanisms via interleukin 8 (IL-8) signaling (Bendre et al. 2003, 2005) and lysyl oxidase (LOX) (Cox et al. 2015) can also contribute to bone degradation. While little is known about whether and how breast tumors change HA in the bone, it has been shown for prostate cancer that the metastasized tumor engenders significant changes in the collagen mineralization, carbonate substitution, mineral crystallinity, and carbonate:matrix ratio (Bi et al. 2013), significantly disrupting the nano- and microscale integrity of the bone structure (Figure 10.2c). Interestingly, recent experimental evidence suggests that breast tumors may be able to significantly modulate the bone structure even in the absence of skeletal metastasis (Thorpe et al. 2011; Cox et al. 2015). These data implicate that remotely located mammary cancer cells release factors into the circulation (e.g., growth factors, exosomes [Peinado et al. 2012]) that cause premetastatic remodeling of the bone niche, ultimately enhancing tumor-cell homing (Cox et al. 2015). How this increased bone homing relates to bone HA and the tumor-mediated changes in its properties remains to be demonstrated.

Indeed, other pathologies such as osteogenesis imperfecta (OI), osteoporosis, pycnodysostosis, and fluorosis have been shown to worsen bone quality by altering the mineral–collagen structural composite (Fratzl et al. 2010; Gamsjaeger et al. 2014). OI, a condition characterized by highly brittle bone (Rauch and Glorieux 2004), is a particularly well-studied example of how bone disease influences mineral nanostructure. Notably, the collagen fibrils in OI (oim/oim) mice exhibit only half the mechanical

Mineralized 3D Culture Systems

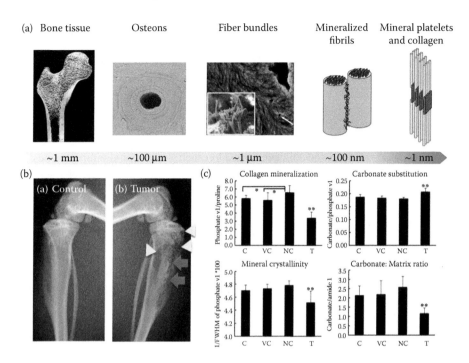

FIGURE 10.2 Bone structure is affected by cancer metastasis. (a) Hierarchical structure of mammalian bone. Important features are shown at the progressively decreasing length scales from left to right. (From Fratzl, P. et al. 2004. Structure and mechanical quality of the collagen-mineral nano-composite in bone. *J Mat Chem* no. 14 (14):2115–2123. Reproduced by permission of The Royal Society of Chemistry; Reproduced from *Prog Mat Sci*, 52 (8), Fratzl, P. and R. Weinkamer. 2007, Nature's hierarchical materials, 1263–1334, Copyright 2007, with permission from Elsevier; Pazzaglia, U. E. et al.: Morphometry and patterns of lamellar bone in human Haversian systems. *Anat Rec (Hoboken)*. 2012. 295. 1421–9. Copyright Wiley-VCH Verlag GmbH & Co. KGaA. Reproduced with permission.) (b) Prostate cancer metastasis engenders large lesions in the proximal tibiae. Yellow and red arrows indicate osteolytic and osteoblastic lesions, respectively. (Reproduced from *Bone*, 56 (2), Bi, X. et al., Prostate cancer metastases alter bone mineral and matrix composition independent of effects on bone architecture in mice—A quantitative study using microCT and Raman spectroscopy, 454–60, Copyright 2013, with permission from Elsevier.) (c) Raman spectroscopy reveals that the collagen mineralization, carbonate substitution, mineral crystallinity, and carbonate: matrix ratio is significantly affected by the bone metastasis shown in (b). C, VC, NC, and T indicate the contralateral control, vehicle injection control, noninjection control, and tumor conditions, respectively. (Reproduced from *Bone*, 56 (2), Bi, X. et al., Prostate cancer metastases alter bone mineral and matrix composition independent of effects on bone architecture in mice—A quantitative study using microCT and Raman spectroscopy, 454–60, Copyright 2013, with permission from Elsevier.)

strength as those from control mice (Misof et al. 1997), which could be explained by abnormal collagen mineralization patterns: some regions of bone do not exhibit any mineralization (Traub et al. 1994), whereas others are overmineralized and are comprised of abnormally thin and variably aligned particles (Traub et al. 1994; Fratzl et al. 1996; Grabner et al. 2001; Vanleene et al. 2012). OI bones also exhibit changes in mineral crystallinity (Vetter et al. 1993), collagen cross-links (Vetter et al. 1993; Carriero et al. 2014), and collagen fibril diameters (Cassella and Ali 1992). Thorough characterization studies like these have not yet been performed on breast cancer-associated bone mineral and collagen fibrils. Yet such studies could inform the design of experimental culture models incorporating relevant mineral particle characteristics to investigate their influence on tumor-cell behavior and signaling.

10.3 EXPERIMENTAL MODELS TO STUDY CELL–MINERAL INTERACTIONS

Adapting bioinspired tissue engineering strategies has enabled researchers to model tumors with context-appropriate cell types, ECM components, and proteins (Kretlow and Mikos 2007; Hutmacher et al. 2010; Infanger et al. 2013). In these settings, biomaterials derived from natural and synthetic sources typically serve as scaffolds that not only function to provide structural support and mimic the signaling function of organic ECM components, but can also be modified to integrate mineral. The following sections provide an overview on current approaches used for engineering mineralized matrices, each with their respective advantages and limitations for use in bone metastasis model systems.

10.3.1 Cell- and Tissue-Based Methods to Recapitulate Mineralized Microenvironments

Given their physiologic nature and intrinsic signaling capacities, cell- and tissue-based methods are attractive for use in model systems aimed at studying tumor-cell behavior within mineralized environments. Physiologically complex *in vitro* approaches including the long-term bioreactor culture of bone cells can result in the formation of mineralized, multiple cell-layer tissue (Dhurjati et al. 2006). Introduction of breast cancer cells into such systems permits modeling secondary tumor progression in bone-like environments of varying tissue maturity (Dhurjati et al. 2008) and pro-inflammatory cytokine profiles (Sosnoski et al. 2015). While attractive for examining the complex cell–microenvironment interactions that modulate tumor-cell behavior in bone, the investigation of isolated mineral-specific effects on tumor-cell behavior remains complicated with such technologies. This challenge may be addressed with cell-free approaches. Matrigel®, a mix of isolated basement membrane components of the Engelbreth-Holm-Swarm (EHS) mouse sarcoma, has been routinely applied to study the formation of polarized acini as a function of impaired cell ECM (Lee et al. 2007). Furthermore, Matrigel® can enhance the mineralization competence of mesenchymal stem cells (Kang et al. 2012) and fibroblast progenitor cells (Yamashiro et al. 2007). However, Matrigel's® inherent batch-to-batch variability, unsuitable mechanical performance, and lack of the main bone ECM components collagen type I and HA clearly limit its ability to recapitulate the multifactorial interplay influencing tumor-cell behavior in mineralized tissues.

To overcome these limitations, one could use decellularized matrices deposited by bone cells. Primary osteoblasts and stem cells cultured in osteogenic media produce mineralized ECM; once decellularized, these matrices can be used to study tumor-cell behavior in response to certain features of the bone ECM (Reichert et al. 2010; Taubenberger et al. 2013) (Figure 10.3a). Indeed, bone metastatic breast cancer cells in contact with these mineralized matrices exhibit increased alignment and invasiveness suggesting a functional role of these substrates in driving malignancy (Taubenberger et al. 2013). Recent technological advancements have made it possible to generate such ECM environments *in vitro* more robustly: by covalently anchoring human mesenchymal stem cell (hMSC)-derived ECM to a culture substrate, Prewitz and colleagues have showed that the molecular, structural, and mechanical properties of this tethered-ECM could mediate the expansion and differentiation of bone marrow stem cells (Prewitz et al. 2013) (Figure 10.3b). While such studies are important advancements that may also accelerate the study of breast cancer cells, cell-derived matrices are still lacking much of the complexity of the actual bone ECM *in vivo*. Furthermore, cells are cultured on top of these matrices, which may not fully mimic their engagement of adhesion receptors in the body. Decellularized native bone may help to circumvent some of these shortcomings. Indeed, decellularized bone can induce osteogenic differentiation of various progenitor cell types (Mauney et al. 2004; Marolt et al. 2012) and has also been used to construct tumor-cell bone niches (Villasante et al. 2014). However, it has to be kept in mind that bone samples harvested from different sites feature differences in matrix architecture and mineral content, which may independently influence cell behavior (Marcos-Campos et al. 2012) (Figure 10.3c). Furthermore, other parameters common to native bone should be kept in mind when interpreting findings. For example, changes in the curvature of native bone surfaces that could result from spatial variations in bone remodeling may affect tumor-cell growth independent of other parameters (Rumpler et al. 2008; Bidan et al. 2013) (Figure 10.4a).

Even though the aforementioned approaches have the tremendous advantage of mimicking physiological complexity, they typically do not allow sophisticated experimental control, are low-throughput, and exhibit batch-to-batch variations, limiting their use in investigations of how specific structural, chemical, or topological properties of mineral in the bone or microcalcifications could drive cancer cell behavior. Thus, in order to address these shortcomings, researchers have developed synthetic approaches that enable control over the physiochemical properties of mineralized matrices.

10.3.2 Incorporation of Synthetic HA into Scaffolds for Cell Culture

Various approaches using synthetic HA as a scaffolding material have been developed in the context of bone regeneration and may be adapted for application in bone metastasis studies. For example, scaffolds purely composed of HA have been used as *in vivo* models to study tumor progression in a bone-like environment. These HA scaffolds were preloaded with bone morphogenetic protein-2 (BMP-2) and have been

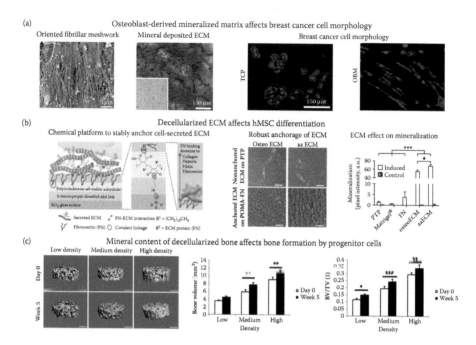

FIGURE 10.3 Cell- and tissue-derived mineralized matrices. (a) Mineralized matrix deposited by human primary osteoblasts consists of an oriented dense fibrillar meshwork (arrow indicates fibril direction) containing mineral as confirmed by Alizarin Red S staining. Inset: mineral staining under nonosteogenic conditions. When cultured on ECMs deposited by osteoblasts (OBM) breast cancer cells change their morphology relative to the same cells cultured on tissue culture polystyrene (TCP). (Taubenberger, A. V. et al.: Delineating breast cancer cell interactions with engineered bone microenvironments. *J Bone Miner Res*. 2013. no. 28. 1399–411. Copyright Wiley-VCH Verlag GmbH & Co. KGaA. Reproduced with permission.) (b) Decellularized matrices can be created more robustly when generated on substrates previously modified with poly(octadecene-alt-maleic anhydride) and fibronectin (POMA-FN). Micrographs show ECMs deposited by human mesenchymal stem cells (hMSCs) in media containing osteogenic supplements and ascorbic acid (aa) either on POMA-FN or plasma-treated culture plastic (PTP). Decellularized ECMs deposited by hMSCs on POMA-FN surfaces stimulate mineral deposition more relative to PTP, Matrigel® and FN. (Reprinted by permission from Springer Nature. *Nat Methods*, Prewitz, M. C. et al. Tightly anchored tissue-mimetic matrices as instructive stem cell microenvironments. no. 10 (8):788–94, Copyright 2013.) (c) Trabecular bone can be decellularized and used for subsequent studies of cell behavior. In the shown example, bone was harvested from bovine wrists, sorted by density and mesenchymal progenitors derived from human embryonic stem cells (hESCs) were cultured in these scaffolds in osteogenic media. Deposition of new mineral was analyzed by μCT; the analysis revealed that the initial mineral content of trabecular bone influences the amount of newly formed mineralized matrix. (Reproduced from *Biomaterials*, no. 33 (33), Marcos-Campos, I. et al., Bone scaffold architecture modulates the development of mineralized bone matrix by human embryonic stem cells, 8329–42, Copyright 2012, with permission from Elsevier.)

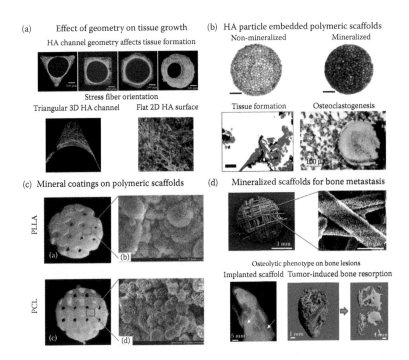

FIGURE 10.4 Synthetic approaches to incorporate HA into 3D scaffolds. (a) HA can be sintered to form substrates of various shapes, which has revealed that 3D curvature of scaffolds influences the local growth rate of tissue from murine osteoblasts. This may be attributed to changes in cell orientation as triangular HA channels exhibit stress fibers parallel to the tissue surface at the corner whereas randomly oriented stress fibers are observed when cells are cultured on flat HA surfaces. (Adapted from Rumpler, M. et al. 2008. The effect of geometry on three-dimensional tissue growth. *J R Soc Interface* no. 5 (27):1173–80. Reproduced with permission from The Royal Society.) (b) 3D mineral-containing PLG scaffolds can be fabricated by incorporating HA nanoparticles during the fabrication process. When seeded with breast cancer cells, HA-containing scaffolds enable coherent tissue formation (pink) around HA particles (black, von Kossa stained), and conditioned media collected from HA-containing tumor-cell cultures induce osteoclastogenesis relative to media from cultures without HA. (Adapted from Pathi, S. P. et al. 2010. A novel 3-D mineralized tumor model to study breast cancer bone metastasis. *PLoS One* no. 5 (1):e8849 under Creative Commons Attribution (CC BY) license.) (c) Porous scaffolds can be retrospectively mineralized using simulated body fluids (SBF). Using this approach, continuous mineral coatings can be formed on biodegradable poly(L-lactic acid) (PLLA) and poly(ε-caprolactone) (PCL) scaffolds. (Saito, E. et al.: Biomineral coating increases bone formation by ex vivo BMP-7 gene therapy in rapid prototyped poly(L-lactic acid) (PLLA) and poly(epsilon-caprolactone) (PCL) porous scaffolds. *Adv Healthc Mater.* 2015. no. 4. 621–32. Copyright Wiley-VCH Verlag GmbH & Co. KGaA. Reproduced with permission.) (d) SBF-mineralized electrospun polycaprolactone scaffolds allow generating humanized bone metastasis environments. The mineralized scaffolds were cultured with human osteoblastic cells and implanted into NOD/SCID mice. Following their intracardiac injection, metastatic breast cancer cells located to these scaffolds and formed mineral-degrading lesions. (Adapted from Thibaudeau, L. et al. 2014. A tissue-engineered humanized xenograft model of human breast cancer metastasis to bone. *Dis Model Mech* no. 7 (2):299–309 under Creative Commons Attribution (CC BY) license.)

employed as a murine bioreactor; the osteoid layer that formed on these scaffolds significantly enhanced the growth of a mammary tumor-cell line (Halpern et al. 2006). However, scaffolds composed solely of sintered HA are limited by porous structures that cannot be tightly controlled with regard to their architecture and exhibit poor mechanical properties.

Porous polymeric scaffolds consisting of biodegradable polymers (e.g., poly(lactide-*co*-glycolide) [PLG]) into which HA can be incorporated during the fabrication process may provide suitable alternatives. Such constructs permit better control over scaffold architecture and improved mechanical performance while enabling cellular organization into 3D tumor-like structures (Hutmacher et al. 2001; Fischbach et al. 2007). Being able to modulate scaffold microarchitecture is not only important for the essential transport of oxygen and nutrients, but also for the control of cell proliferation and migration, which are dependent on pore diameter and shape (Peyton et al. 2011; Bidan et al. 2013). Additionally, differences in scaffold microarchitecture may influence cell shape, which can regulate many different cellular features relevant to bone metastasis including hMSC differentiation (McBeath et al. 2004) and geometry-dependent cell growth and viability (Chen et al. 1997). The relevance of PLG-based systems to studies of bone metastasis can be further improved by incorporation of HA nanoparticles during their fabrication by a gas foaming/particulate leaching technique (Pathi et al. 2010, 2011) (Figure 10.4b). Using this approach, we previously showed that the behavior of breast cancer cells changes in the presence of HA and that introduction of mechanical stimulation further alters their gene expression (Lynch et al. 2013). Moreover, culturing breast cancer cells on PLG scaffolds containing HA nanoparticles of varying chemical and physical properties has shown that HA size and crystallinity regulates tumor-cell adhesion, proliferation, and osteolytic factor secretion (Pathi et al. 2011).

While the above described approach integrated previously synthesized HA particles into the scaffolds during the fabrication process, it is also possible to mineralize surfaces or scaffolds after their fabrication. Such biomimetic mineralization approaches have been developed originally for mechanistic studies of calcium phosphate mineral formation and for various tissue engineering applications. They are performed near physiological temperature and pH; that is, conditions which are optimal for the incorporation of temperature-sensitive biomaterials and biological molecules (Rodriguez et al. 2014; Marelli et al. 2015). This could be relevant to future studies testing the effect of morphogens on the mineral response of tumor cells during bone metastasis. A commonly used mineralizing solution is simulated body fluid (SBF), which is composed of solely inorganic constituents of human blood plasma (Kokubo 1996). When using SBF approaches, the mineralizing substrate should be designed to present active chemical groups for heterogeneous nucleation and growth of mineral (Taguchi et al. 2001; Murphy and Mooney 2002). SBF approaches are valued for their versatility to form HA on a wide variety of materials and thus there are many successful examples (Figure 10.4c and d), which include the mineralization of both natural and synthetic biocompatible materials in many forms (e.g., films, fibers, microspheres, scaffolds and hydrogels) (Chen et al. 2006; Kumar et al. 2008; Al-Munajjed et al. 2009; Zhong and Chu 2012; Davis et al. 2013; Ye et al. 2014; Saito et al. 2015). Hence, it may become possible to study either independent or combined effects of bone ECM topography and mineral presentation as they pertain to bone metastasis. Previous studies have shown that HA surfaces formed on polymeric scaffolds from SBF solutions promote cell adhesion and proliferation. Indeed, breast cancer cells adhere and proliferate better when seeded onto SBF-mineralized versus control scaffolds (Ye et al. 2014); additionally, the subcutaneous implantation of mineral-coated polymeric scaffolds seeded with primary human osteoblasts served as bone homing sites for breast cancer cells (Thibaudeau et al. 2014) (Figure 10.4d). When compared to approaches that require harsh conditions, these more physiologic methods offer more control over the composition of the mineral itself. For instance, the properties of pathological mammary microcalcifications may be mimicked by synthesizing HA surfaces with varying carbonate composition simply through varying the carbonate concentration in the used SBF. Indeed, this process not only changed the chemical and physical properties of the HA surfaces, but the resulting properties were also biologically relevant as they mediated differences in protein adsorption and breast cancer cell behavior (Choi et al. 2015).

Though completely synthetic approaches for controlling mineral properties allow for a degree of control that is not possible with tissue- or cell- derived approaches, their main disadvantage is their inability to recapitulate the physiological complexity of native ECM. In particular, the ECM in bone is not only composed of mineral, but mineral is deposited into pre-existing collagen type I fibrils. Collagen type I properties may vary in response to tumor-secreted factors (e.g., LOX or TGF-beta) (Leask and Abraham 2004; Yamauchi and Shiiba 2008; Cox et al. 2013), which may, in turn, affect mineral deposition. In order to address these possibilities and assess their possible functional impact on bone metastasis, researchers are now working toward synthesizing native-like bone ECM with which both collagen and mineral properties may be controlled. The next section will focus specifically on efforts to mineralize naturally derived collagen fibrils.

10.3.3 Collagen as Substrates for Mineralization

Collagen is the most abundant ECM component of the bone matrix and of many primary tumors. Through self-assembly mechanisms, it can form mesh networks of fibrils (Parry 1988; Mouw et al. 2014) within hydrogels that exhibit structural similarity to ECM of various tissues (Drury and Mooney 2003; DeForest and Anseth 2012). Nonmineralized collagen has been used to build tunable stromal environments for 3D cancer models and its physical properties have been explored for their ability to modulate cancer cell behavior. For example, breast cancer cell invasive behavior was observed to be dependent on collagen fibril diameter and pore size of 3D collagen networks (Sapudom et al. 2015). In addition, tuning collagen stiffness was found to have a dramatic effect on tumor-cell morphology (Paszek et al. 2005), growth patterns (Paszek et al. 2005), and invasion characteristics (Provenzano et al. 2009).

In efforts to mimic native bone, researchers are developing methods of incorporating HA into the collagen fibrillar microstructure. SBF-based mineralization methods form mineral on the surface of the collagen fibrils (Falini et al. 2008; Al-Munajjed et al. 2009) while co-precipitation of mineral during collagen fibrillogenesis generates co-aligned HA nanocrystals (Nudelman et al. 2010). Successful HA platelet infiltration of collagen fibrils has been achieved by the use of highly negatively charged polymers such as polyaspartic acid and OPN to stabilize the formation of the amorphous calcium phosphate precursor (Olszta et al. 2007; Deshpande and Beniash 2008; Jee et al. 2010; Nudelman et al. 2010; Rodriguez et al. 2014) (Figure 10.5a). This polymer-mediated process has also shown its ability to mineralize demineralized matrices from bone. (Rodriguez et al. 2014) (Figure 10.5b). Hence, it may be used to control mineral properties of decellularized native bone constructs that were already described in Section 10.3.1. While the mineralization of collagen fibrils can generate synthetic ultrastructures that resemble the native ECM in bone (Li and Aparicio 2013), one limitation is their general tunability. As explained previously, the collagen fibrils and mineral platelets of bone tissue may be modified during cancer premetastatic remodeling (Thorpe et al. 2011; Cox et al. 2015). Thus, the development of novel methods will be required to control for these changes in reconstituted, fibrillar collagen matrices.

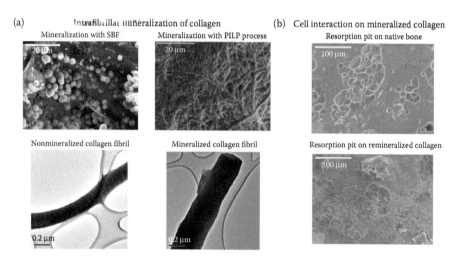

FIGURE 10.5 Mineralization of collagen fibrils. (a) SBF can also be used to mimic bone-like collagen-HA composites. Simply adding SBF to collagen fibers yields HA clusters on the collagen surface, but using a polymer-induced liquid-precursor (PILP) process enables physiologically relevant collagen intrafibrillar mineralization. TEM images show that the native periodic banding pattern of nonmineralized collagen disappears due to intrafibrillar mineralization of collagen. (Reproduced from *Acta Biomater*, no. 6 (9), Jee, S. S. et al., Development of bone-like composites via the polymer-induced liquid-precursor (PILP) process. Part 1: Influence of polymer molecular weight, 3676–86, Copyright 2010, with permission from Elsevier.) (b) Inclusion of noncollagenous proteins such as osteopontin during the PILP process similarly results in intrafibrillar collagen mineralization of bone that was previously demineralized, but additionally activates osteoclast activity ultimately resulting in resorption pit formation when these cells are seeded onto mineralized collagen. (Reproduced from *Acta Biomater*, 10 (1), Rodriguez, D. E. et al., Multifunctional role of osteopontin in directing intrafibrillar mineralization of collagen and activation of osteoclasts, 494–507, Copyright 2014, with permission from Elsevier.)

10.4 CONCLUSION AND PERSPECTIVE

There is currently a variety of *in vitro* approaches for modeling cell–mineral interactions, ranging from ECM derived from cells and tissues to synthetic bone-like ECM generated from the mineralization of collagen fibrils. There is a value to all of the described methods for their respective advantages, but collectively, there are still shortcomings that will need to be addressed in the future.

One limitation of the aforementioned approaches is their lack of throughput. Recently, there have been efforts to construct 2D and 3D matrices within multiwell plates to allow the systematic and reproducible analysis of cellular responses to environmental cues in a format that is compatible with screening assays and automated imaging systems. A number of cancer studies conducted with high-throughput assays have determined the drug efficacy profiles of a large number of cancer cell-targeting compounds across a variety of *in vitro* model systems (Markovitz-Bishitz et al. 2010; Evensen et al. 2013; Hongisto et al. 2013). However, despite the wide use of matrix materials in high-throughput systems, there are very few studies that have assayed cellular responses to mineralized matrices. One can even think about co-opting array-based hydrogel photopatterning techniques to assay various mineral properties in the context of altered ECM mechanics and biochemistry, which would allow assessing their combinatorial effect on cell behavior (Mosiewicz et al. 2013).

Another consideration is that many mineral responses could be regulated at the organ, or whole body level particularly, as cells responding to mineral at the primary site may alter mineral properties at the secondary site. Yet, most culture approaches focus at the cellular or tissue scale. Microfluidic "organ-on-a-chip" devices provide spatial and temporal control of biochemical, biophysical, and mechanical cues, and have been used to mimic the structure and function of various tissues and organs and their communication with one another (Esch et al. 2015). Examples of how such devices have been used in the context of bone include the modeling of hematopoietic niches, screening the would-healing potential of specific biomaterials, and assaying the invasive dynamics of breast cancer cells (Lee et al. 2012; Bersini et al. 2014; Torisawa et al. 2014). Collectively, these studies suggest that "bone-on-a-chip" models could effectively recreate 3D bone environments with multiple cellular and matrix components under conditions of dynamic flow; thereby, it is conceivable that methods to produce mineralized matrices can be co-opted for developing microfluidic systems. However, many current devices are limited to individual cells or organs. In order to recapitulate the complex metastatic cascade, the system-like integration of multiple organs will be required.

Advances in molecular biology and genetics have yielded an enormous amount of insight into the biology, diagnostics and therapeutics of breast cancer, which is now classified into subtypes based on gene expression profiles, cell-surface markers, and other methods. These efforts have improved treatment strategies with the development of drugs that are not only targeted against specific proteins or processes but are also appropriate for the unique subpopulations of breast cancer patients. However, mortality from breast cancer remains high, with bone metastasis and drug resistance being critical issues that have not been sufficiently addressed.

Fortunately, the push to generate pathologically relevant data is gaining more traction. Development of pathologically relevant *in vitro* assays and drug testing platforms will be paramount if we are to improve treatment and prognostic strategies for cancer patients. For patients suffering from bone metastatic breast cancer, the delivery of chemotherapeutics may be optimized by better understanding drug transport within bone. This is not only relevant as bone is a mechanically active tissue in which tumors may compromise convective transport by altering interstitial fluid flow (Lynch and Fischbach 2014), but also because certain drugs can interact with mineral. For instance, the family of osteoclast-inhibiting bisphosphonates has a unique affinity for HA, resulting in variations in uptake and release from bone cells (Nancollas et al. 2006). Hence, HA-containing cell culture substrates will not only advance basic understanding of tumor-cell–mineral interactions as they pertain to bone metastasis, but also inform more efficacious treatment of patients with already available drugs by considering their bioavailability and signaling capacity. Collectively, mineralized tumor models offer a tremendous potential to improve clinical strategies aimed at interfering with bone metastasis and, thus, may ultimately improve the prognosis of breast cancer patients afflicted with this condition.

ACKNOWLEDGMENTS

We acknowledge financial support through NCI (R01CA173083), NSF (Graduate Research Fellowship to FH), and the Alexander von Humboldt Foundation (Fellowship for Experienced Researchers to CF).

REFERENCES

Abedin, M., Y. Tintut, and L. L. Demer. 2004. Vascular calcification: Mechanisms and clinical ramifications. *Arterioscler Thromb Vasc Biol* no. 24 (7):1161–70.

Addison, W. N., D. L. Masica, J. J. Gray, and M. D. McKee. 2010. Phosphorylation-dependent inhibition of mineralization by osteopontin ASARM peptides is regulated by PHEX cleavage. *J Bone Miner Res* no. 25 (4):695–705.

Al-Munajjed, A. A., N. A. Plunkett, J. P. Gleeson, T. Weber, C. Jungreuthmayer, T. Levingstone, J. Hammer, and F. J. O'Brien. 2009. Development of a biomimetic collagen-hydroxyapatite scaffold for bone tissue engineering using a SBF immersion technique. *J Biomed Mater Res B Appl Biomater* no. 90 (2):584–91.

Baker, R., K. D. Rogers, N. Shepherd, and N. Stone. 2010. New relationships between breast microcalcifications and cancer. *Br J Cancer* no. 103 (7):1034–9.

Barth, V., E. D. Franz, and A. Scholl. 1977. Microcalcifications in mammary glands. *Naturwissenschaften* no. 64 (5):278–9.

Bazin, D., M. Daudon, C. Combes, and C. Rey. 2012. Characterization and some physicochemical aspects of pathological microcalcifications. *Chem Rev* no. 112 (10):5092–120.

Bellahcene, A. and V. Castronovo. 1995. Increased expression of osteonectin and osteopontin, two bone matrix proteins, in human breast cancer. *Am J Pathol* no. 146 (1):95–100.

Bellahcene, A., V. Castronovo, K. U. Ogbureke, L. W. Fisher, and N. S. Fedarko. 2008. Small integrin-binding ligand N-linked glycoproteins (SIBLINGs): Multifunctional proteins in cancer. *Nat Rev Cancer* no. 8 (3):212–26.

Bendre, M. S., A. G. Margulies, B. Walser, N. S. Akel, S. Bhattacharrya, R. A. Skinner, F. Swain et al. 2005. Tumor-derived interleukin-8 stimulates osteolysis independent of the receptor activator of nuclear factor-kappaB ligand pathway. *Cancer Res* no. 65 (23):11001–09.

Bendre, M. S., D. C. Montague, T. Peery, N. S. Akel, D. Gaddy, and L. J. Suva. 2003. Interleukin-8 stimulation of osteoclastogenesis and bone resorption is a mechanism for the increased osteolysis of metastatic bone disease. *Bone* no. 33 (1):28–37.

Bersini, S., J. S. Jeon, G. Dubini, C. Arrigoni, S. Chung, J. L. Charest, M. Moretti, and R. D. Kamm. 2014. A microfluidic 3D *in vitro* model for specificity of breast cancer metastasis to bone. *Biomaterials* no. 35 (8):2454–61.

Bi, X., J. A. Sterling, A. R. Merkel, D. S. Perrien, J. S. Nyman, and A. Mahadevan-Jansen. 2013. Prostate cancer metastases alter bone mineral and matrix composition independent of effects on bone architecture in mice—A quantitative study using microCT and Raman spectroscopy. *Bone* no. 56 (2):454–60.

Bidan, C. M., K. P. Kommareddy, M. Rumpler, P. Kollmannsberger, P. Fratzl, and J. W. Dunlop. 2013. Geometry as a factor for tissue growth: Towards shape optimization of tissue engineering scaffolds. *Adv Healthc Mater* no. 2 (1):186–94.

Breitbach, M., T. Bostani, W. Roell, Y. Xia, O. Dewald, J. M. Nygren, J. W. Fries et al. 2007. Potential risks of bone marrow cell transplantation into infarcted hearts. *Blood* no. 110 (4):1362–69.

Büsing, C. M., U. Keppler, and V. Menges. 1981. Differences in microcalcification in breast tumors. *Virchows Archiv A* no. 393 (3):307–13.

Carriero, A., E. A. Zimmermann, A. Paluszny, S. Y. Tang, H. Bale, B. Busse, T. Alliston, G. Kazakia, R. O. Ritchie, and S. J. Shefelbine. 2014. How tough is brittle bone? Investigating osteogenesis imperfecta in mouse bone. *J Bone Miner Res* no. 29 (6):1392–401.

Cassella, J. P. and S. Y. Ali. 1992. Abnormal collagen and mineral formation in osteogenesis imperfecta. *Bone Miner* no. 17 (2):123–8.

Castronovo, V. and A. Bellahcene. 1998. Evidence that breast cancer associated microcalcifications are mineralized malignant cells. *Int J Oncol* no. 12 (2):305–8.

Chen, C. S., M. Mrksich, S. Huang, G. M. Whitesides, and D. E. Ingber. 1997. Geometric control of cell life and death. *Science* no. 276 (5317):1425–8.

Chen, J., B. Chu, and B. S. Hsiao. 2006. Mineralization of hydroxyapatite in electrospun nanofibrous poly(L-lactic acid) scaffolds. *J Biomed Mater Res A* no. 79 (2):307–17.

Choi, S., S. Coonrod, L. Estroff, and C. Fischbach. 2015. Chemical and physical properties of carbonated hydroxyapatite affect breast cancer cell behavior. *Acta Biomater* no. 24:333–42.

Coleman, R. E. and R. D. Rubens. 1987. The clinical course of bone metastases from breast cancer. *Br J Cancer* no. 55 (1):61–66.

Cox, R. F., A. Hernandez-Santana, S. Ramdass, G. McMahon, J. H. Harmey, and M. P. Morgan. 2012a. Microcalcifications in breast cancer: Novel insights into the molecular mechanism and functional consequence of mammary mineralisation. *Br J Cancer* no. 106 (3):525–37.

Cox, R. F. and M. P. Morgan. 2013. Microcalcifications in breast cancer: Lessons from physiological mineralization. *Bone* no. 53 (2):437–50.

Cox, T. R., D. Bird, A. M. Baker, H. E. Barker, M. W. Ho, G. Lang, and J. T. Erler. 2013. LOX-mediated collagen crosslinking is responsible for fibrosis-enhanced metastasis. *Cancer Res* no. 73 (6):1721–32.

Cox, T. R., A. Gartland, and J. T. Erler. 2012b. The pre-metastatic niche: Is metastasis random? *Bonekey Rep* no. 1 (May 2):80.

Cox, T. R., R. M. Rumney, E. M. Schoof, L. Perryman, A. M. Hoye, A. Agrawal, D. Bird et al. 2015. The hypoxic cancer secretome induces pre-metastatic bone lesions through lysyl oxidase. *Nature* no. 522 (7554):106–10.

Davis, H. E., B. Y. Binder, P. Schaecher, D. D. Yakoobinsky, A. Bhat, and J. K. Leach. 2013. Enhancing osteoconductivity of fibrin gels with apatite-coated polymer microspheres. *Tissue Eng Part A* no. 19 (15–16):1773–82.

DeForest, C. A. and K. S. Anseth. 2012. Advances in bioactive hydrogels to probe and direct cell fate. *Annu Rev Chem Biomol Eng* no. 3:421–44.

Deshpande, A. S. and E. Beniash. 2008. Bio-inspired synthesis of mineralized collagen fibrils. *Cryst Growth Des* no. 8 (8):3084–90.

Dhurjati, R., V. Krishnan, L. A. Shuman, A. M. Mastro, and E. A. Vogler. 2008. Metastatic breast cancer cells colonize and degrade three-dimensional osteoblastic tissue in vitro. *Clin Exp Metastasis* no. 25 (7):741–52.

Dhurjati, R., X. Liu, C. V. Gay, A. M. Mastro, and E. A. Vogler. 2006. Extended-term culture of bone cells in a compartmentalized bioreactor. *Tissue Eng* no. 12 (11):3045–54.

Drury, J. L. and D. J. Mooney. 2003. Hydrogels for tissue engineering: Scaffold design variables and applications. *Biomaterials* no. 24 (24):4337–51.

Esch, E. W., A. Bahinski, and D. Huh. 2015. Organs-on-chips at the frontiers of drug discovery. *Nat Rev Drug Discov* no. 14 (4):248–60.

Evensen, N. A., J. Li, J. Yang, X. Yu, N. S. Sampson, S. Zucker, and J. Cao. 2013. Development of a high-throughput three-dimensional invasion assay for anti-cancer drug discovery. *PLoS One* no. 8 (12):e82811

Falini, G., S. Fermani, B. Palazzo, and N. Roveri. 2008. Helical domain collagen substrates mineralization in simulated body fluid. *J Biomed Mater Res A* no. 87 (2):470–6.

Fischbach, C., R. Chen, T. Matsumoto, T. Schmelzle, J. S. Brugge, P. J. Polverini, and D. J. Mooney. 2007. Engineering tumors with 3D scaffolds. *Nat Methods* no. 4 (10):855–60.

Frappart, L., M. Boudeulle, J. Boumendil, H. C. Lin, I. Martinon, C. Palayer, Y. Mallet-Guy et al. 1984. Structure and composition of microcalcifications in benign and malignant lesions of the breast: Study by light microscopy, transmission and scanning electron microscopy, microprobe analysis, and X-ray diffraction. *Hum Pathol* no. 15 (9):880–9.

Frappart, L., I. Remy, H. C. Lin, A. Bremond, D. Raudrant, B. Grousson, and J. L. Vauzelle. 1986. Different types of microcalcifications observed in breast pathology. Correlations with histopathological diagnosis and radiological examination of operative specimens. *Virchows Arch A Pathol Anat Histopathol* no. 410 (3):179–87.

Fratzl, P., H. S. Gupta, E. P. Paschalis, and P. Roschger. 2004. Structure and mechanical quality of the collagen-mineral nano-composite in bone. *J Mat Chem* no. 14 (14):2115–2123.

Fratzl, P., H. S. Gupta, P. Roschger, and K. Klaushofer. 2010. Bone nanostructure and its relevance for mechanical performance, disease and treatment. In *Nanotechnology*. Berlin: Wiley-VCH Verlag GmbH & Co. KGaA.

Fratzl, P., O. Paris, K. Klaushofer, and W. J. Landis. 1996. Bone mineralization in an osteogenesis imperfecta mouse model studied by small-angle x-ray scattering. *J Clin Invest* no. 97 (2):396–402.

Fratzl, P. and R. Weinkamer. 2007. Nature's hierarchical materials. *Prog Mat Sci* no. 52 (8):1263–334.

Gamsjaeger, S., R. Mendelsohn, A. L. Boskey, S. Gourion-Arsiquaud, K. Klaushofer, and E. P. Paschalis. 2014. Vibrational spectroscopic imaging for the evaluation of matrix and mineral chemistry. *Curr Osteoporos Rep* no. 12 (4):454–64.

Gericke, A., C. Qin, L. Spevak, Y. Fujimoto, W. T. Butler, E. S. Sorensen, and A. L. Boskey. 2005. Importance of phosphorylation for osteopontin regulation of biomineralization. *Calcif Tissue Int* no. 77 (1):45–54.

Going, J. J., T. J. Anderson, P. R. Crocker, and D. A. Levison. 1990. Weddellite calcification in the breast: Eighteen cases with implications for breast cancer screening. *Histopathology* no. 16 (2):119–24.

Grabner, B., W. J. Landis, P. Roschger, S. Rinnerthaler, H. Peterlik, K. Klaushofer, and P. Fratzl. 2001. Age- and genotype-dependence of bone material properties in the osteogenesis imperfecta murine model (oim). *Bone* no. 29 (5):453–57.
Haka, A. S., K. E. Shafer-Peltier, M. Fitzmaurice, J. Crowe, R. R. Dasari, and M. S. Feld. 2002. Identifying microcalcifications in benign and malignant breast lesions by probing differences in their chemical composition using Raman spectroscopy. *Cancer Res* no. 62 (18):5375–80.
Halpern, J., C. C. Lynch, J. Fleming, D. Hamming, M. D. Martin, H. S. Schwartz, L. M. Matrisian, and G. E. Holt. 2006. The application of a murine bone bioreactor as a model of tumor: Bone interaction. *Clin Exp Metastasis* no. 23 (7–8):345–56.
Hanahan, D. and R. A. Weinberg. 2000. The hallmarks of cancer. *Cell* no. 100 (1):57–70.
Hassler, O. 1969. Microradiographic investigations of calcifications of the female breast. *Cancer* no. 23 (5):1103–9.
Hofvind, S., B. F. Iversen, L. Eriksen, B. M. Styr, K. Kjellevold, and K. D. Kurz. 2011. Mammographic morphology and distribution of calcifications in ductal carcinoma *in situ* diagnosed in organized screening. *Acta Radiol* no. 52 (5):481–87.
Holme, T. C., M. M. Reis, A. Thompson, A. Robertson, D. Parham, P. Hickman, and P. E. Preece. 1993. Is mammographic microcalcification of biological significance? *Eur J Surg Oncol* no. 19 (3):250–53.
Hongisto, V., S. Jernstrom, V. Fey, J. P. Mpindi, K. Kleivi Sahlberg, O. Kallioniemi, and M. Perala. 2013. High-throughput 3D screening reveals differences in drug sensitivities between culture models of JIMT1 breast cancer cells. *PLoS One* no. 8 (10):e77232.
Hosseinkhani, H., M. Hosseinkhani, F. Tian, H. Kobayashi, and Y. Tabata. 2006. Osteogenic differentiation of mesenchymal stem cells in self-assembled peptide-amphiphile nanofibers. *Biomaterials* no. 27 (22):4079–86.
Hutmacher, D. W. 2010. Biomaterials offer cancer research the third dimension. *Nat Mater* no. 9 (2):90–93.
Hutmacher, D. W., D. Loessner, S. Rizzi, D. L. Kaplan, D. J. Mooney, and J. A. Clements. 2010. Can tissue engineering concepts advance tumor biology research? *Trends Biotechnol* no. 28 (3):125–33.
Hutmacher, D. W., T. Schantz, I. Zein, K. W. Ng, S. H. Teoh, and K. C. Tan. 2001. Mechanical properties and cell cultural response of polycaprolactone scaffolds designed and fabricated via fused deposition modeling. *J Biomed Mater Res* no. 55 (2):203–16.
Infanger, D. W., M. E. Lynch, and C. Fischbach. 2013. Engineered culture models for studies of tumor-microenvironment interactions. *Annu Rev Biomed Eng* no. 15:29–53.
Jee, S. S., T. T. Thula, and L. B. Gower. 2010. Development of bone-like composites via the polymer-induced liquid-precursor (PILP) process. Part 1: Influence of polymer molecular weight. *Acta Biomater* no. 6 (9):3676–86.
Kang, B. J., H. H. Ryu, S. S. Park, Y. Kim, H. M. Woo, W. H. Kim, and O. K. Kweon. 2012. Effect of matrigel on the osteogenic potential of canine adipose tissue-derived mesenchymal stem cells. *J Vet Med Sci* no. 74 (7):827–36.
Kang, Y., P. M. Siegel, W. Shu, M. Drobnjak, S. M. Kakonen, C. Cordon-Cardo, T. A. Guise, and J. Massague. 2003. A multigenic program mediating breast cancer metastasis to bone. *Cancer Cell* no. 3 (6):537–49.
Kenny, P. A., G. Y. Lee, C. A. Myers, R. M. Neve, J. R. Semeiks, P. T. Spellman, K. Lorenz et al. 2007. The morphologies of breast cancer cell lines in three-dimensional assays correlate with their profiles of gene expression. *Mol Oncol* no. 1 (1):84–96.
Kingsley, L. A., P. G. Fournier, J. M. Chirgwin, and T. A. Guise. 2007. Molecular biology of bone metastasis. *Mol Cancer Ther* no. 6 (10):2609–17.
Kokubo, T. 1996. Vitrification, Transformation and Crytallization of Glasses. Formation of biologically active bone-like apatite on metals and polymers by a biomimetic process. *Thermochimica Acta* no. 280:479–90.

Kozlow, W. and T. A. Guise. 2005. Breast cancer metastasis to bone: Mechanisms of osteolysis and implications for therapy. *J Mammary Gland Biol Neoplasia* no. 10 (2):169–80.

Kretlow, J. D. and A. G. Mikos. 2007. Review: Mineralization of synthetic polymer scaffolds for bone tissue engineering. *Tissue Eng* no. 13 (5):927–38.

Kumar, R., K. H. Prakash, P. Cheang, L. Gower, and K. A. Khor. 2008. Chitosan-mediated crystallization and assembly of hydroxyapatite nanoparticles into hybrid nanostructured films. *J R Soc Interface* no. 5 (21):427–39.

Landis, W. J., M. J. Song, A. Leith, L. McEwen, and B. F. McEwen. 1993. Mineral and organic matrix interaction in normally calcifying tendon visualized in three dimensions by high-voltage electron microscopic tomography and graphic image reconstruction. *J Struct Biol* no. 110 (1):39–54.

Langley, R. R. and I. J. Fidler. 2011. The seed and soil hypothesis revisited—the role of tumor–stroma interactions in metastasis to different organs. *Int J Cancer* no. 128 (11):2527–35.

Leask, A. and D. J. Abraham. 2004. TGF-beta signaling and the fibrotic response. *Faseb J* no. 18 (7):816–27.

Lee, G. Y., P. A. Kenny, E. H. Lee, and M. J. Bissell. 2007. Three-dimensional culture models of normal and malignant breast epithelial cells. *Nat Methods* no. 4 (4):359–65.

Lee, J. H., Y. Gu, H. Wang, and W. Y. Lee. 2012. Microfluidic 3D bone tissue model for high-throughput evaluation of wound-healing and infection-preventing biomaterials. *Biomaterials* no. 33 (4):999–1006.

Li, Y. and C. Aparicio. 2013. Discerning the subfibrillar structure of mineralized collagen fibrils: A model for the ultrastructure of bone. *PLoS One* no. 8 (9):e76782.

Lynch, M. E., D. Brooks, S. Mohanan, M. J. Lee, P. Polamraju, K. Dent, L. J. Bonassar, M. C. van der Meulen, and C. Fischbach. 2013. In vivo tibial compression decreases osteolysis and tumor formation in a human metastatic breast cancer model. *J Bone Miner Res* no. 28 (11):2357–67.

Lynch, M. E. and C. Fischbach. 2014. Biomechanical forces in the skeleton and their relevance to bone metastasis: Biology and engineering considerations. *Adv Drug Deliv Rev* no. 79–80:119–34.

Marcos-Campos, I., D. Marolt, P. Petridis, S. Bhumiratana, D. Schmidt, and G. Vunjak-Novakovic. 2012. Bone scaffold architecture modulates the development of mineralized bone matrix by human embryonic stem cells. *Biomaterials* no. 33 (33):8329–42.

Marelli, B., C. E. Ghezzi, Y. L. Zhang, I. Rouiller, J. E. Barralet, and S. N. Nazhat. 2015. Fibril formation pH controls intrafibrillar collagen biomineralization *in vitro* and *in vivo*. *Biomaterials* no. 37:252–59.

Markovitz-Bishitz, Y., Y. Tauber, E. Afrimzon, N. Zurgil, M. Sobolev, Y. Shafran, A. Deutsch, S. Howitz, and M. Deutsch. 2010. A polymer microstructure array for the formation, culturing, and high throughput drug screening of breast cancer spheroids. *Biomaterials* no. 31 (32):8436–44.

Marolt, D., I. M. Campos, S. Bhumiratana, A. Koren, P. Petridis, G. Zhang, P. F. Spitalnik, W. L. Grayson, and G. Vunjak-Novakovic. 2012. Engineering bone tissue from human embryonic stem cells. *Proc Natl Acad Sci USA* no. 109 (22):8705–09.

Mauney, J. R., S. Sjostorm, J. Blumberg, R. Horan, J. P. O'Leary, G. Vunjak-Novakovic, V. Volloch, and D. L. Kaplan. 2004. Mechanical stimulation promotes osteogenic differentiation of human bone marrow stromal cells on 3-D partially demineralized bone scaffolds *in vitro*. *Calcif Tissue Int* no. 74 (5):458–68.

McBeath, R., D. M. Pirone, C. M. Nelson, K. Bhadriraju, and C. S. Chen. 2004. Cell shape, cytoskeletal tension, and RhoA regulate stem cell lineage commitment. *Dev Cell* no. 6 (4):483–95.

Misof, K., W. J. Landis, K. Klaushofer, and P. Fratzl. 1997. Collagen from the osteogenesis imperfecta mouse model (OIM) shows reduced resistance against tensile stress. *J Clin Invest* no. 100 (1):40–5.

Moon, W. K., J. G. Im, Y. H. Koh, D. Y. Noh, and I. A. Park. 2000. US of mammographically detected clustered microcalcifications. *Radiology* no. 217 (3):849–54.

Morgan, M. P., M. M. Cooke, and G. M. McCarthy. 2005. Microcalcifications associated with breast cancer: An epiphenomenon or biologically significant feature of selected tumors? *J Mammary Gland Biol Neoplasia* no. 10 (2):181–87.

Mosiewicz, K. A., L. Kolb, A. J. van der Vlies, M. M. Martino, P. S. Lienemann, J. A. Hubbell, M. Ehrbar, and M. P. Lutolf. 2013. In situ cell manipulation through enzymatic hydrogel photopatterning. *Nat Mater* no. 12 (11):1072–78.

Mouw, J. K., G. Ou, and V. M. Weaver. 2014. Extracellular matrix assembly: A multiscale deconstruction. *Nat Rev Mol Cell Biol* no. 15 (12):771–85.

Müller, A., B. Homey, H. Soto, N. Ge, D. Catron, M. E. Buchanan, T. McClanahan et al. Involvement of chemokine receptors in breast cancer metastasis. *Nature* no. 410 (6824):50–56.

Mundy, G. R. 2002. Metastasis to bone: Causes, consequences and therapeutic opportunities. *Nat Rev Cancer* no. 2 (8):584–93.

Murphy, W. L. and D. J. Mooney. 2002. Bioinspired growth of crystalline carbonate apatite on biodegradable polymer substrata. *J Am Chem Soc* no. 124 (9):1910–17.

Muttarak, M., P. Kongmebhol, and N. Sukhamwang. 2009. Breast calcifications: Which are malignant? *Singapore Med J* no. 50 (9):907–13.

Nancollas, G. H., R. Tang, R. J. Phipps, Z. Henneman, S. Gulde, W. Wu, A. Mangood, R. G. Russell, and F. H. Ebetino. 2006. Novel insights into actions of bisphosphonates on bone: Differences in interactions with hydroxyapatite. *Bone* no. 38 (5):617–27.

Nudelman, F., K. Pieterse, A. George, P. H. Bomans, H. Friedrich, L. J. Brylka, P. A. Hilbers, G. de With, and N. A. Sommerdijk. 2010. The role of collagen in bone apatite formation in the presence of hydroxyapatite nucleation inhibitors. *Nat Mater* no. 9 (12):1004–09.

Nyga, A., U. Cheema, and M. Loizidou. 2011. 3D tumour models: Novel *in vitro* approaches to cancer studies. *J Cell Commun Signal* no. 5 (3):239–48.

Olszta, M. J., X. Cheng, S. S. Jee, R. Kumar, Y.-Y. Kim, M. J. Kaufman, E. P. Douglas, and L. B. Gower. 2007. Bone structure and formation: A new perspective. *Mater Sci Eng: R Rep* no. 58 (3–5):77–116.

Paget, S. 1889. The Distribution of secondary growths in cancer of the breast. *Lancet* no. 133 (3421):571–73.

Parry, D. A. 1988. The molecular and fibrillar structure of collagen and its relationship to the mechanical properties of connective tissue. *Biophys Chem* no. 29 (1–2):195–209.

Paszek, M. J., N. Zahir, K. R. Johnson, J. N. Lakins, G. I. Rozenberg, A. Gefen, C. A. Reinhart-King et al. 2005. Tensional homeostasis and the malignant phenotype. *Cancer Cell* no. 8 (3):241–54.

Pathi, S. P., C. Kowalczewski, R. Tadipatri, and C. Fischbach. 2010. A novel 3-D mineralized tumor model to study breast cancer bone metastasis. *PLoS One* no. 5 (1):e8849.

Pathi, S. P., D. D. Lin, J. R. Dorvee, L. A. Estroff, and C. Fischbach. 2011. Hydroxyapatite nanoparticle-containing scaffolds for the study of breast cancer bone metastasis. *Biomaterials* no. 32 (22):5112–22.

Pazzaglia, U. E., T. Congiu, M. Marchese, F. Spagnuolo, and D. Quacci. 2012. Morphometry and patterns of lamellar bone in human Haversian systems. *Anat Rec (Hoboken)* no. 295 (9):1421–29.

Peinado, H., M. Aleckovic, S. Lavotshkin, I. Matei, B. Costa-Silva, G. Moreno-Bueno, M. Hergueta-Redondo et al. 2012. Melanoma exosomes educate bone marrow progenitor cells toward a pro-metastatic phenotype through MET. *Nat Med* no. 18 (6):883–91.

Peyton, S. R., Z. I. Kalcioglu, J. C. Cohen, A. P. Runkle, K. J. Van Vliet, D. A. Lauffenburger, and L. G. Griffith. 2011. Marrow-derived stem cell motility in 3D synthetic scaffold is governed by geometry along with adhesivity and stiffness. *Biotechnol Bioeng* no. 108 (5):1181–93.

Prewitz, M. C., F. P. Seib, M. von Bonin, J. Friedrichs, A. Stissel, C. Niehage, K. Muller et al. 2013. Tightly anchored tissue-mimetic matrices as instructive stem cell microenvironments. *Nat Methods* no. 10 (8):788–94.

Provenzano, P. P., D. R. Inman, K. W. Eliceiri, and P. J. Keely. 2009. Matrix density-induced mechanoregulation of breast cell phenotype, signaling and gene expression through a FAK-ERK linkage. *Oncogene* no. 28 (49):4326–43.

Rauch, F. and F. H. Glorieux. 2004. Osteogenesis imperfecta. *Lancet* no. 363 (9418):1377–85.

Reichert, J. C., V. M. Quent, L. J. Burke, S. H. Stansfield, J. A. Clements, and D. W. Hutmacher. 2010. Mineralized human primary osteoblast matrices as a model system to analyse interactions of prostate cancer cells with the bone microenvironment. *Biomaterials* no. 31 (31):7928–36.

Reznikov, N., R. Shahar, and S. Weiner. 2014. Bone hierarchical structure in three dimensions. *Acta Biomater* no. 10 (9):3815–26.

Rhodes, N. P., J. K. Srivastava, R. F. Smith, and C. Longinotti. 2004. Metabolic and histological analysis of mesenchymal stem cells grown in 3-D hyaluronan-based scaffolds. *J Mater Sci Mater Med* no. 15 (4):391–95.

Rodriguez, D. E., T. Thula-Mata, E. J. Toro, Y. W. Yeh, C. Holt, L. S. Holliday, and L. B. Gower. 2014. Multifunctional role of osteopontin in directing intrafibrillar mineralization of collagen and activation of osteoclasts. *Acta Biomater* no. 10 (1):494–507.

Rumpler, M., A. Woesz, J. W. Dunlop, J. T. van Dongen, and P. Fratzl. 2008. The effect of geometry on three-dimensional tissue growth. *J R Soc Interface* no. 5 (27):1173–80.

Saito, E., D. Suarez-Gonzalez, W. L. Murphy, and S. J. Hollister. 2015. Biomineral coating increases bone formation by ex vivo BMP-7 gene therapy in rapid prototyped poly(L-lactic acid) (PLLA) and poly(epsilon-caprolactone) (PCL) porous scaffolds. *Adv Healthc Mater* no. 4 (4):621–32.

Sapudom, J., S. Rubner, S. Martin, T. Kurth, S. Riedel, C. T. Mierke, and T. Pompe. 2015. The phenotype of cancer cell invasion controlled by fibril diameter and pore size of 3D collagen networks. *Biomaterials* no. 52:367–75.

Sosnoski, D. M., R. J. Norgard, C. D. Grove, S. J. Foster, and A. M. Mastro. 2015. Dormancy and growth of metastatic breast cancer cells in a bone-like microenvironment. *Clin Exp Metastasis* no. 32 (4):335–44.

Stomper, P. C., J. Geradts, S. B. Edge, and E. G. Levine. 2003. Mammographic predictors of the presence and size of invasive carcinomas associated with malignant microcalcification lesions without a mass. *AJR Am J Roentgenol* no. 181 (6):1679–84.

Tabar, L., H. H. Tony Chen, M. F. Amy Yen, T. Tot, T. H. Tung, L. S. Chen, Y. H. Chiu, S. W. Duffy, and R. A. Smith. 2004. Mammographic tumor features can predict long-term outcomes reliably in women with 1–14-mm invasive breast carcinoma. *Cancer* no. 101 (8):1745–59.

Taguchi, T., Y. Muraoka, H. Matsuyama, A. Kishida, and M. Akashi. 2001. Apatite coating on hydrophilic polymer-grafted poly(ethylene) films using an alternate soaking process. *Biomaterials* no. 22 (1):53–58.

Taubenberger, A. V., V. M. Quent, L. Thibaudeau, J. A. Clements, and D. W. Hutmacher. 2013. Delineating breast cancer cell interactions with engineered bone microenvironments. *J Bone Miner Res* no. 28 (6):1399–411.

Teicher, B. A. and S. P. Fricker. 2010. CXCL12 (SDF-1)/CXCR4 pathway in cancer. *Clin Cancer Res* no. 16 (11):2927–31.

Thibaudeau, L., A. V. Taubenberger, B. M. Holzapfel, V. M. Quent, T. Fuehrmann, P. Hesami, T. D. Brown et al. 2014. A tissue-engineered humanized xenograft model of human breast cancer metastasis to bone. *Dis Model Mech* no. 7 (2):299–309.

Thorpe, M. P., R. J. Valentine, C. J. Moulton, A. J. Wagoner Johnson, E. M. Evans, and D. K. Layman. 2011. Breast tumors induced by N-methyl-N-nitrosourea are damaging to bone strength, structure, and mineralization in the absence of metastasis in rats. *J Bone Miner Res* no. 26 (4):769–76.

Torisawa, Y. S., C. S. Spina, T. Mammoto, A. Mammoto, J. C. Weaver, T. Tat, J. J. Collins, and D. E. Ingber. 2014. Bone marrow-on-a-chip replicates hematopoietic niche physiology in vitro. *Nat Methods* no. 11 (6):663–69.

Traub, W., T. Arad, U. Vetter, and S. Weiner. 1994. Ultrastructural studies of bones from patients with osteogenesis imperfecta. *Matrix Biol* no. 14 (4):337–45.

Traub, W., T. Arad, and S. Weiner. 1989. Three-dimensional ordered distribution of crystals in turkey tendon collagen fibers. *Proc Natl Acad Sci USA* no. 86 (24):9822–26.

Tse, G. M., P. H. Tan, A. L. Pang, A. P. Tang, and H. S. Cheung. 2008. Calcification in breast lesions: Pathologists' perspective. *J Clin Pathol* no. 61 (2):145–51.

Vanleene, M., A. Porter, P. V. Guillot, A. Boyde, M. Oyen, and S. Shefelbine. 2012. Ultrastructural defects cause low bone matrix stiffness despite high mineralization in osteogenesis imperfecta mice. *Bone* no. 50 (6):1317–23.

Vetter, U., M. A. Weis, M. Morike, E. D. Eanes, and D. R. Eyre. 1993. Collagen crosslinks and mineral crystallinity in bone of patients with osteogenesis imperfecta. *J Bone Miner Res* no. 8 (2):133–37.

Villasante, A., A. Marturano-Kruik, and G. Vunjak-Novakovic. 2014. Bioengineered human tumor within a bone niche. *Biomaterials* no. 35 (22):5785–94.

Wang, F., V. M. Weaver, O. W. Petersen, C. A. Larabell, S. Dedhar, P. Briand, R. Lupu, and M. J. Bissell. 1998. Reciprocal interactions between beta1-integrin and epidermal growth factor receptor in three-dimensional basement membrane breast cultures: A different perspective in epithelial biology. *Proc Natl Acad Sci U S A* no. 95 (25):14821–26.

Weilbaecher, K. N., T. A. Guise, and L. K. McCauley. 2011. Cancer to bone: A fatal attraction. *Nat Rev Cancer* no. 11 (6):411–25.

Weiner, S. and W. Traub. 1992. Bone structure: From angstroms to microns. *FASEB J* no. 6 (3):879–85.

Yamashiro, T., L. Zheng, Y. Shitaku, M. Saito, T. Tsubakimoto, K. Takada, T. Takano-Yamamoto, and I. Thesleff. 2007. Wnt10a regulates dentin sialophosphoprotein mRNA expression and possibly links odontoblast differentiation and tooth morphogenesis. *Differentiation* no. 75 (5):452–62.

Yamauchi, M. and M. Shiiba. 2008. Lysine hydroxylation and cross-linking of collagen. *Methods Mol Biol* no. 446:95–108.

Ye, M., P. Mohanty, and G. Ghosh. 2014. Biomimetic apatite-coated porous PVA scaffolds promote the growth of breast cancer cells. *Mater Sci Eng C: Mater Biol Appl* no. 44:310–16.

Yoon, Y. S., J. S. Park, T. Tkebuchava, C. Luedeman, and D. W. Losordo. 2004. Unexpected severe calcification after transplantation of bone marrow cells in acute myocardial infarction. *Circulation* no. 109 (25):3154–57.

Zhang, X. H., Q. Wang, W. Gerald, C. A. Hudis, L. Norton, M. Smid, J. A. Foekens, and J. Massague. 2009. Latent bone metastasis in breast cancer tied to Src-dependent survival signals. *Cancer Cell* no. 16 (1):67–78.

Zheng, Y., H. Zhou, C. R. Dunstan, R. L. Sutherland, and M. J. Seibel. 2013. The role of the bone microenvironment in skeletal metastasis. *J Bone Oncol* no. 2 (1):47–57.

Zhong, C. and C. C. Chu. 2012. Biomimetic mineralization of acid polysaccharide-based hydrogels: Towards porous 3-dimensional bone-like biocomposites. *J Mater Chem* no. 22 (13):6080–87.

11 Design Considerations for 3D Cardiovascular Tissue Scaffolds

Scott Cooper, Christopher Moraes, and Richard L. Leask

CONTENTS

11.1 Introduction 193
    11.1.1 3D Structure of the Cardiovascular System 195
        11.1.1.1 Myocardium 3D Environment 195
        11.1.1.2 Heart Valve 3D Environment..196
        11.1.1.3 Blood Vessel 3D Environment..198
    11.1.2 Current Challenges in Cardiovascular *In Vitro* Tissue Modeling.....199
11.2 Scaffold Considerations...201
    11.2.1 Common Scaffolds 201
        11.2.1.1 Polydimethylsiloxane 202
        11.2.1.2 Synthetic Hydrogel Matrices 202
        11.2.1.3 Electrospun Matrices 202
        11.2.1.4 Decellularized Matrices..203
    11.2.2 Scaffold Microenvironment..203
        11.2.2.1 Surface Properties and Cellular Adhesion.......................203
        11.2.2.2 Scaffold Pore Size 204
        11.2.2.3 Remodeling of Extracellular Matrix................................204
        11.2.2.4 Cell-to-Cell Communication 205
        11.2.2.5 Mechanical Properties 206
11.3 Conclusion and Perspective 207
Acknowledgment 207
References..207

11.1 INTRODUCTION

Cardiovascular disease remains a leading cause of death and disability in the developed world (Go et al. 2014). Our understanding of the mechanisms that lead to cardiovascular disease has been significantly advanced by *in vitro* modeling. These idealized models allow researchers to isolate important variables to answer research questions about cell/tissue response and mechanobiology. The significance of the three-dimensional (3D) tissue environment for proper cell structure and function *in vitro* has been well documented in cardiovascular research (Akins et al. 2010). Advances in 3D *in vitro* models have allowed for the design of scaffolds for cell and tissue transplantation (Mata et al. 2009; Hussain et al. 2013; Mei et al. 2014), drug screening (Truskey 2010; Moraes et al. 2013; Leung et al. 2015), and dynamic bioreactors (Barron et al. 2003; Mironov et al. 2006; Moraes et al. 2010). Paramount to these advances has been the recognition of realistic mechanical environments through tuning of material elasticity, dynamic force application, biochemically improved transport, and surface functionalization. This chapter highlights some of the advances made in 3D cardiovascular models as well as remaining challenges and potential applications.

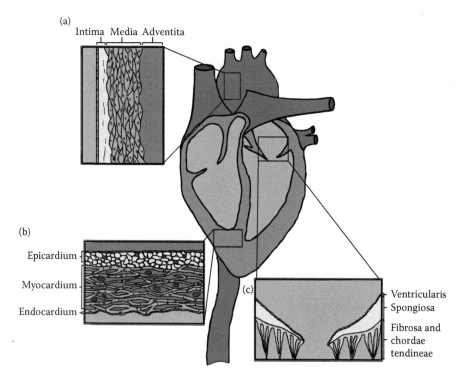

FIGURE 11.1 Cartoon of the arterial tree and the composition of its major components. (a) Ascending Aorta: The intima is in contact with the blood flow and is comprised of a layer of endothelial cells on an elastic membrane. The media supports this layer and contains alternating layers of smooth muscle cells and elastin fibers and is encased by the adventitia. (b) Myocardium: The epicardium consists of a layer of endothelial cells in contact with blood in the interior of the heart chambers. The myocardium itself consists of a network of vascularized cardiomyocytes, which is encased in the epicardium forming the outer surface of the heart. (c) Mitral valve: A valve consisting of two leaflets with the ventricularis, a layer of endothelial cells supported by a layer of elastic fibers, facing incoming blood flow. Under this layer is the spongiosa, which is predominantly proteoglycans and is supported by a dense layer of collagen called the fibrosa. Finally, the chordae tendineae helps maintain a closed valve during the ejection of the ventricle.

11.1.1 3D STRUCTURE OF THE CARDIOVASCULAR SYSTEM

The cardiovascular system is comprised of a series of organized structures including the myocardium, valves, aorta, and the supporting vasculature, Figure 11.1. The myocardium is the "workhorse" of the heart, which generates the pressure to pump blood through the body, valves prevent backflow and allow pressurization of the chambers of the heart, and the aorta delivers blood to the rest of the vasculature. When healthy, this coordinated system allows for the delivery and removal of nutrients and waste products, maintaining homeostasis in the human body. Details of the major structures of the cardiovascular system, their pathology, and *in vitro* model considerations will be further described in this section.

11.1.1.1 Myocardium 3D Environment

The heart wall is organized in three layers: a thin inner layer of epithelial cells called the endothelium, which is in contact with the blood, the middle layer of cardiac muscle called the myocardium and the epicardium, the outer layer of connective tissue. The pumping of the heart occurs through a coordinated contraction of the myocardium, Figure 11.2. Contraction decreases the heart chamber volumes, increasing the pressure, resulting in blood being pumped through one of four heart valves. This dynamic contraction happens in multiple planes of the tissue with radial, longitudinal, and circumferential forces

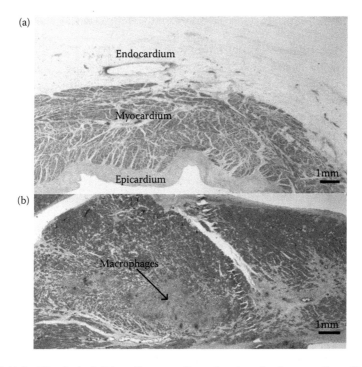

FIGURE 11.2 Histological slides of hematoxylin and eosin stained myocardium. (a) Healthy myocardium oriented with the epicardium on the bottom and endocardium on the top. (b) Constrictive myocardium thickened with fibrosis (smooth pink) and macrophages (blue dots).

generated. The myocardium causes the contractile forces, and is comprised predominantly of specialized striated smooth muscle cells called cardiomyocytes. In its healthy state, the coordinated contraction of the myocardium leads to efficient force production through a shortening and twisting of the left and right ventricles.

The benefits of 3D myocardial tissue models have been known since the 1950s (Landau and Marsland 1952; Moscona and Moscona 1952). When cultured in flat plates, cardiac myocytes will form a rhythmically pulsating monolayer that, over time, can detach forming cardiac sheets (Eschenhagen and Zimmermann 2005). Cardiomyocytes are autorhythmic and, without pacing by the conduction system of the heart, they can spontaneously beat when cultured in medium containing serum. Without a physiologically representative mechanical load, once detached, cultured sheets lose their ability to beat. This emphasizes the necessity for a dynamic 3D environment. The importance of extracellular matrix (ECM) proteins and their orientation as well as 3D mechanical stimulation for proper cell attachment, function, and differentiation was recognized over 40 years ago, prompting an increased interest in 3D scaffold design (Chambard et al. 1981; Hall et al. 1982; Terracio et al. 1988) More recent research has focused on improved material properties, nutrient transport and cell sources for engineering myocardial tissue in these matrices (Mata et al. 2009; Louch et al. 2011; Hussain et al. 2013; Mei et al. 2014). To further investigate pathologies such as hypertrophic remodeling, it is important to be able to mimic the dynamic contractile nature of the myocardium and the importance of fibrotic regions on its mechanics, which can only be fully examined in 3D environments.

11.1.1.2 Heart Valve 3D Environment

Within the heart, the different chambers are separated by valves, which ensure the unidirectional flow of blood through the vasculature. Valves are secured to a fibrous ring of tissue and are comprised of two or three leaflets, which open and close as the heart beats. Leaflets are formed from three distinct layers: the ventricularis, spongiosa, and fibrosa. The fibrosa is a dense extension of collagen from the fibrous ring and supports most of the load of the leaflet. On top of this layer is the spongiosa, which consists predominantly of proteoglycans found in a collagen network that is sometimes referred to as the "shock absorber" of the leaflet (Liu et al. 2007). Finally, the ventricularis is the layer in contact with incoming blood and is composed primarily of elastin fibers, coated with a layer of endothelial cells. These three layers interact to maintain valve integrity by communicating and supporting one another, providing a robust valve capable of withstanding the environmental pressures of the heart. Each layer is important and damage to one, such as ventricularis inflammation and stenosis, can affect stresses on and phenotypes of the other layers, suggesting that 3D models that recapitulate this complexity are critical for *in vitro* studies. Throughout the internal structure of the leaflet are valve interstitial cells (VICs), which help maintain the ECM and play a role in immune response (Taylor et al. 2003). Recent evidence suggests that the VIC population is heterogeneous with distinct functions in separate layers of the valve leaflet, contributing to the complexity of this 3D structure (Moraes et al. 2013). The endothelial cells lining the ventricularis tend to align circumferentially with the valve that differs from the rest of the vasculature and this is hypothesized to be due to the pressure effects across the valve

Design Considerations for 3D Cardiovascular Tissue Scaffolds   197

dominating the mechanotransductive regulation of morphology (Deck 1986). These pressure gradients are dependent on the shape and morphology of the entire valve structure. The interplay between the layers helps to provide heart valves the ability to retain the unidirectional flow of blood while avoiding potentially harmful hemodynamics and damaging mechanical stress to its components.

Valve disease is commonly associated with the formation of calcific lesions, which limit the effectiveness of leaflets leading to regurgitation or incompetence, Figure 11.3 (Schoen 2005). The calcification of valves obstructs the outflow leading to a gradual increase in pressure gradient across the valve, which leads to a decline in cardiac function. VICs play a crucial role in the calcification process as their various phenotypes have been shown to modulate leaflet inflammation and repair (Liu et al. 2007). Several VIC phenotypes have been observed. The most relevant to disease are myofibroblast-differentiated VICs as these cells respond to valve injury due to pathological conditions, altered matrix composition, and disturbed hemodynamics.

Two-dimensional (2D) static culture of VICs has shown to initiate disease states, making it challenging to study healthy samples in a simple Petri dish. Hence, several researchers have set up dynamic experimental conditions such as cyclic stretch or ECM stiffness in 3D structures (Butcher and Nerem 2004; Yip et al. 2009; Moraes et al. 2010). Furthermore, combinations of these factors and the presence of ECM proteins and soluble factors can synergistically affect VIC phenotype from each of the layers (Moraes et al. 2013), and inversely the expressed phenotype of VICs can

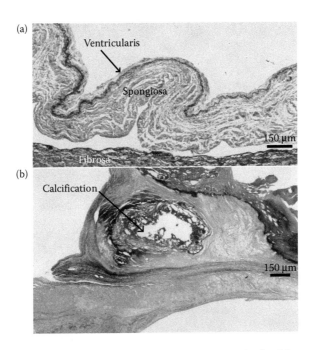

FIGURE 11.3 Histological slides of heart valves stained with elastic trichrome. (a) Healthy pulmonary valve oriented with the ventricularis (top), spongiosa (middle), and fibrosa (bottom). (b) Senile stenotic aortic valve with calcific lesion and mature collagen (blue).

remodel the ECM (Liu et al. 2007). This remodeling can lead to clinically significant pathologies. VICs also interact with the endothelial cells, which line the leaflets, and *in vitro* their coculture results in a more physiologically relevant quiescent VIC phenotype (Butcher and Nerem 2004).

11.1.1.3 Blood Vessel 3D Environment

The cardiovascular system branches from the heart into a vast network of arteries and veins, which bring blood and nutrients to bodily tissues and return it to the heart. Arteries have three layers: the tunica intima, the tunica media, and the tunica adventitia, Figure 11.4. The intima is the innermost layer acting as a barrier between the vessel and blood flow and is a monolayer of endothelial cells (ECs), which is supported by an internal elastic membrane. The medial layer is largely responsible for the vascular tone and mechanical function of the artery. It contains mainly smooth muscle cells and elastic tissue. The organization and content of elastin and smooth muscle cells in the media vary along the arterial tree. The aorta is dominated by elastic fibers but the quantity of these decreases along the length of the vessel (Harkness et al. 1957). The elastic components help aid in energy redistribution, whereas smooth

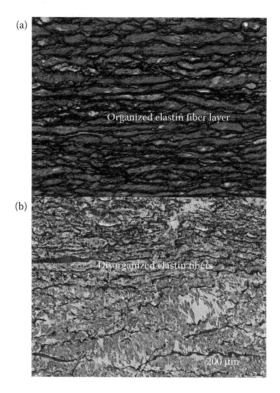

FIGURE 11.4 Histological slides of the ascending aorta. (a) Healthy tissue comprised of alternating layers of smooth muscle cells (red) and elastin fibers (black) with small amounts of collagen (yellow) and mucopolysaccharides (blue). (b) Diseased tissue in a dilated aorta with loss of smooth muscle cells, increased collagen and fragmented elastin.

muscles help to regulate the vascular tone of the artery. Encasing the media is the tunica adventitia, a fibrous layer comprised mostly of collagen. Arteries bifurcate and reduce in size along the vasculature, allowing for efficient nutrient transport through capillaries and venules. Veins have a similar structure to arteries, comprised of the same three layers. However, veins have significantly less muscular tone than arteries and some contain valves to prevent backflow in the venous network.

Atherosclerosis is the most ubiquitous of arterial diseases and can progress to the formation of plaques, which can occlude vessels or dislodge, leading to myocardial infarction or stroke (Sakakura et al. 2013). Atherosclerosis is an inflammatory disease involving the endothelium and a cascade of biochemical events, which results in the accumulation of macromolecules, macrophages, and T lymphocytes, thickening the intima/medial layer that changes the 3D environment. Arterial stiffness also increases with age as characterized by increased collagen content, fragmentation of elastic fibers in the media, and intimal hyperplasia (Cecelja and Chowienczyk 2012). This increased stiffness decreases the compliance of the arterial tree and causes hypertension.

The importance of mechanical stimulation for proper vascular cell function has been known for decades (Fry 1968; Dewey et al. 1981). In the late 1970s, Ross and Glomset hypothesized that mechanical forces can lead to the development and progression of atherosclerosis (Ross and Glomset 1976). Since then, the sensitivity of endothelial cells and smooth muscle cells to mechanical forces has been well documented (Dewey et al. 1981; Dartsch and Betz 1989; Tzima et al. 2001). Furthermore, the interaction between these cells and the ECM is vital in cell function and response (Tzima et al. 2001). To help model this 3D environment, tubular scaffolds for research and replacement grafts have shown promise (Vaz et al. 2005; Soffer et al. 2008; Shalumon et al. 2011).

11.1.2 CURRENT CHALLENGES IN CARDIOVASCULAR *IN VITRO* TISSUE MODELING

The majority of early *in vitro* cardiovascular models was 2D in nature and allowed for some significant insights into the fundamentals of cardiovascular cellular and physical properties. Many of these consisted of culturing of a monolayer (or very few layers) of cells onto a glass or polymer substrate. As only a thin layer of cells was cultured, there were no mass transport limitations through cell layers so it was very easy to stimulate the cells in a uniform manner and support their nutritional needs. Furthermore, analysis was simplified as imaging, staining, and blotting techniques could easily be performed on cells grown on glass cover slips to determine cell phenotype. These 2D models lacked a realistic tissue environment and cellular interactions rendering them unable to properly mimic the complex structures described in the previous section.

In vitro cardiovascular tissue modeling has progressed to a 3D dynamic environment with multiple cell types; however, the dynamic 3D environment produces additional challenges. There are several factors, which can affect cell function, including environmental variables like oxygen concentration, carbon dioxide concentration, temperature, pH, and sterility. In 2D monolayer culture, mass transfer limitations are minimal so supplying a steady amount of nutrients in an incubator simply involves a frequent replenishing of media (Sato and Kan 2001). However,

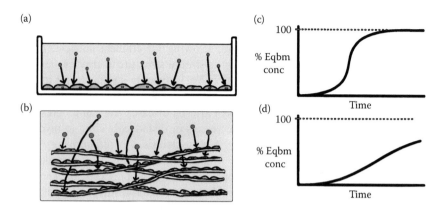

FIGURE 11.5 Demonstration of the mass transfer limitations in 2D versus 3D culture. Reference equilibrium concentration is a point far away from the cells. (a) a 2D culture where molecules can easily diffuse to whole cell population and (b) a woven 3D scaffold where the fibers lead to a tortuous path for molecules leading to decreased diffusion and subsequently decreased concentration deeper in the structure. Time course of the concentration of an added molecule to the media of (c) a 2D culture where the cell surface very quickly reaches equilibrium with the bulk concentration and (d) a 3D culture where deeper in the structure the concentration reaches equilibrium at a much slower rate.

in 3D models such as scaffolds, passive diffusion will not always be able to supply nutrients to the cells deeper in the structure due to mass transfer limitations, Figure 11.5 (Leung et al. 2015). In cases where diffusion limits cell penetration and nutrient transport, a necrotic core may form. The inclusion of channels into scaffolds during production (Durham et al. 2013), modular construction of scaffolds (Corstorphine and Sefton 2011) and casting sacrificial templates (Miller et al. 2012) have all been shown as useful tools in ensuring cell and nutrient migration through scaffolds. Agitation and perfusion can be used to address mass transport limitations (Martin et al. 2004), and studies of cardiomyocytes have found that higher cell viabilities can also be achieved in rotating vessels (laminar flow) versus simple stirred flasks (turbulent flow) (Carrier et al. 1999). "Hanging drop" cultures have also been developed that allow for the formation of 3D aggregation of cardiomyocytes, which naturally determine their limiting size (Beauchamp et al. 2015).

Changing cell phenotype is a factor, which must also be considered in model design. The goal is usually to measure a phenotypical change brought on by a factor of the experiment; however, sometimes other changes might occur, which may confound the results. These changes can be as profound as cell dedifferentiation (Xu et al. 2004; Zhang et al. 2010; Kikuchi 2015) or as subtle as slight changes in protein or cytokine expression (LaFramboise et al. 2007; Davies et al. 2013). Nonuniform or changing phenotype can be caused by solubility and transport limitations and temporal bioavailability of nutrients (Tchao et al. 2014). Proper binding of adherent cells such as endothelial cells and smooth muscle cells is another factor that is necessary for cell survival and maintaining phenotype (Hynes 1999). On a mechanical level, the stiffness of substrates (McDaniel et al. 2007) and applied stresses (Sugden 2001) and their directionality (Malek and Izumo 1996) can affect phenotype. Devices have been developed to test the impact that unidirectional or bidirectional stresses have on cell differentiation with great success. Three-dimensional scaffolds have been increasingly utilized to better define the effects of mechanical loads on cells and to better explain cellular differentiation mechanics (Moraes et al. 2010).

The need for a dynamic environment brings additional challenges when striving to mimic physiological conditions. In cardiovascular research, cell media is used as a blood substitute but lacks blood's non-Newtonian properties. Cell culture media lacks the complexity of the protein and cellular makeup of whole blood. The aggregation and break up of red blood cells within blood gives shear-thinning properties to it, meaning the viscosity of the fluid decreases with increasing shear. This discrepancy has an effect on the shear rate and stress imposed on vessel walls (Gijsen et al. 1999). This can lead to inaccurate shear stress profiles in complex flows where secondary flow patterns may be attenuated because of cell media's Newtonian properties. Engineers turn to dimensionless analysis using parameters, such as the Reynolds number and Womersley and Dean's numbers, for pulsatile and curved flow, respectively, to better replicate physiological conditions (Frame et al. 1998; Comerford et al. 2008). This results in the fine tuning of model geometry or the addition of viscous agents such as dextran to media to match these dimensionless numbers as closely as possible (Farcas et al. 2009; Lu et al. 2009). Similarly, ambient pressures differ between *in vivo* tissues and *in vitro* models as tissues are part of a system with many surrounding structures, whereas models are typically exposed directly to an open-air or liquid environment. This can have effects on the external pressure applied to a scaffold structure as well as the diffusivity of biomolecules and nutrients through a model (Gutierrez and Crumpler 2008).

11.2 SCAFFOLD CONSIDERATIONS

The importance of recreating the 3D mechanical and biochemical environment in basic cardiovascular research and tissue engineering is well documented (Akins et al. 2010). The complexity and unique structure of cardiovascular tissue make recreating this environment *in vitro* challenging. Organ culture and transplantation allow for the preservation of native structure; however, a lack of human tissue has necessitated the development of synthetic engineered scaffolds and *ex vivo* expansion of cells.

11.2.1 COMMON SCAFFOLDS

Practical concerns in cost and repeatability limit scaffold development for various applications (Hutmacher et al. 2004). Many scaffolds are fabricated under carefully controlled environmental conditions but homogeneity can become an issue leading to inconsistent results. The development of new materials such as chitosan–alginate (Kievit et al. 2010) and techniques like solid freeform fabrication (Leong et al. 2003) and 3D printing (Ventola 2014) has ushered a new era of cheaper, better-defined scaffolds.

11.2.1.1 Polydimethylsiloxane

Synthetic polydimethylsiloxane (PDMS) scaffolds are commonly used for *in vitro* studies due to resistance to degradation but are not suitable for *in vivo* deployment (Mata et al. 2009). Commercially available polymers such as Sylgard® have the benefits of having a tunable modulus, can be cast in any shape, and they are not biodegradable. Monomer techniques generally print layers of PDMS, which are then stacked to form the final scaffold structure. The printing techniques used allow careful control of factors, such as pore size, surface texture and geometry, which increases the usefulness in specific applications.

These PDMS scaffolds have the benefits of flexibility, optical transparency, and high gas diffusivity, which along with their ease of use make them very attractive for research purposes (Regehr et al. 2009). However, confounding issues exist such as their ability to absorb small hydrophobic molecules (such as estrogen), leeching of uncured polymer into media, and polymer chain diffusivity that can lead to variable surface properties especially after surface treatment (Toepke and Beebe 2006; Regehr et al. 2009; Berthier et al. 2012).

11.2.1.2 Synthetic Hydrogel Matrices

Hydrogels offer distinct advantages owing to their extremely high retention of fluid, which allows for effective mass transport while maintaining a structure that has similar flexibility and viscoelastic properties to native tissue (Dahliwal 2012). These scaffolds can be formed with natural (fibrinogen, hyaluronic acid, collagen, and chitosan) or synthetic polymers (polyethylene glycol [PEG], polylactide, and polyvinyl alcohol) with various techniques and advantages.

The chemical and material properties of synthetic hydrogels can be easily tuned, making them useful in a variety of applications, and their biodegradability allows them to be used for transplantation of engineered tissue (Dhandayuthapani et al. 2010; Li et al. 2014). However, synthetic polymers tend to exhibit cytotoxicity, are also difficult to remodel, and only a limited number of them have been approved for human use (Li et al. 2014). Cellular remodeling is a technical challenge, which has been overcome with new approaches such as peptide synthesis (Levesque and Shoichet 2007) and PEG incorporation (Sridhar et al. 2015), but both impeded remodeling and cytotoxicity have created a major impetus to develop matrices with natural polymers.

11.2.1.3 Electrospun Matrices

Electrospinning is a technique that involves the synthesis of natural polymer fibers on the scale of nanometers to microns into nonwoven structures (Ortega et al. 2013). The process generally consists of forcing a polymer through an electrostatic field forming a jet, which breaks up into fibers of definable diameter. Control of the process parameters can allow for multilayered scaffolds to be produced with varying pore and fiber sizes, creating unique structures for research applications (Shalumon et al. 2011).

Scaffolds produced with this technique have the advantages of resembling native ECM, high surface area to volume ratio to promote cell attachment, interconnected pores to increase efficiency of diffusive processes, and they can be formed with numerous (to date >50) polymers that can help tune mechanical and adhesive properties of the scaffolds (Khorshidi et al. 2016). They can have limitations on their macroscale strength, and although they have a high external surface area, it can be difficult for cells to migrate into the interior of their structures. When working with synthetic polymers, these too can exhibit high cytotoxicity.

11.2.1.4 Decellularized Matrices

In the field of tissue regeneration of the myocardium and valves, researchers have turned to the decellularization of the ECM, which leaves it as a viable scaffold for cell culture. The mostly intact ECM is isolated by removing the supported cells and soluble material in the tissue through methods, such as freeze/thaw cycling and treatment with enzymatic (trypsin) and/or chemical (sodium dodecyl sulfate) solutions (Song and Ott 2011).

Using native tissue scaffolds helps decrease the xenogenic contents, which could cause tissue rejection if used in transplantation. The scaffold will also leave a sort of "cellular footprint" with the proper functionalization and locations already present for new tissue growth to occur and ECM to be laid down (Song and Ott 2011). For example, the CryoValve® SG Pulmonary Valve is a commercially available decellularized human cardiac pulmonary valve used in various cardiac valve replacement surgeries (Brown et al. 2010). Though promising, decellularized tissues pose some serious challenges for research and clinical purposes. The inability to control various aspects of decellularized matrices prevents hypothesis-driven testing. The treatment technique used in the decellularization protocol has been found to affect the cytotoxicity of the matrix (Crapo et al. 2011). Finally, availability of native tissue and the time required to grow sufficient cells for recolonization are likely unable to meet the demands for engineering replacement tissues using this technique.

11.2.2 SCAFFOLD MICROENVIRONMENT

11.2.2.1 Surface Properties and Cellular Adhesion

The adhesion-dependent nature of many cell lines used in cardiovascular research has led to the development of novel approaches to overcome cell adhesion inefficiencies in 3D models. In 2D models, cells are cultured on to glass or plastic slides, which can have poor adhesive properties. Surface treatments are used to increase their adhesiveness such as plasma treatment of polystyrene and PDMS to decrease hydrophobicity (Owen and Smith 1994), and receptor-mediated adhesion can be achieved through protein attachment through surface or electrochemistry. In 3D models where cell adhesion is desired throughout the matrix, as is the case with mimicking myocardial tissue, it can be difficult to treat the inner structure of scaffolds with traditional methods. Printing scaffolds in layers and absorbing functional protein fragments into the scaffold can get much higher penetration of functionalization, increasing cell adhesion throughout the structure (Mata et al. 2009; Seras-Franzoso et al. 2013).

Adhesive cells such as ECs bind to ECM proteins through integrin binding, which is an important consideration in vascular studies. These heterodimeric transmembrane proteins bind to fibronectin, laminin, and collagen among other proteins (Miranti 2002). *In vivo,* these extracellular proteins are readily available for cells to adhere to in neighboring tissues. *In vitro,* however, many surfaces used for developing 3D models are synthetic and lack an ECM. This further highlights the importance of functionalization and the necessity to overcome the added difficulties of 3D environments.

Novel materials and methods for 3D scaffold development have been addressing cellular adhesion concerns. Researchers have tuned electrospun compounds, particularly polysaccharides such as chitosan (Hussain et al. 2013), cellulose (Kumbar et al. 2011), or polycaprolactone (Hutmacher et al. 2001) to increase cell adhesion. These hydrophilic compounds allow for better interactions with adhesive proteins and growth factors, which make them ideal for promoting cell adhesion. They can also be effectively treated with fibronectin and laminin (Stamati et al. 2014), further increasing their adhesive properties.

11.2.2.2 Scaffold Pore Size

The size and shape of pores and scaffold thickness can affect the properties of the scaffold. Generally speaking, as the pore size becomes smaller, diffusion limitations can decrease nutrient dispersion and cell migration due to size exclusion. Conversely, as the pore size is increased, the specific surface area will decrease, lowering the final cell density. Cardiomyocytes have been effectively cultured in scaffolds of different materials with the most efficient pore sizes between 50 and 200 µm (Gonnerman et al. 2012; Chiu et al. 2014). Pore sizes on this scale have been shown to not pose a significant resistance to nutrient transport and can therefore sustain cell cultures. These pore sizes also allowed for adequate proliferation and motility of the cells to create dense and uniformly dispersed cultures.

Small pore sizes can also affect the ability of cells to migrate through a scaffold resulting in stagnant zones within its interior. Innovative production methods of scaffolds have started to alleviate these difficulties. Disc electrospinning and air impedance techniques can create a diverse range of micropores and macropores, which have the benefit of maintaining the high surface area to promote dense cultures while providing larger voids to allow the migration of the cells through this structure (Li et al. 2014; Yin et al. 2014).

11.2.2.3 Remodeling of Extracellular Matrix

As cells proliferate and mature in the 3D environment, natural processes will begin to occur in remodeling the ECM. Typically, higher levels of remodeling occur in disease states and during early cellular development so it is an important consideration in the 3D scaffold design (Daley et al. 2008). This process occurs from signals through integrins, laminin, or syndecans, which interact with the matrix. The remodeling is important for cellular homeostasis, cell migration, and to accommodate cellular function. Matrix metalloproteinases (MMPs) are enzymes produced by cells throughout the entire cardiovascular system, which can degrade structural components of the ECM, leading to scaffold biodegradation. For example, scaffolds produced with collagen, laminin, or fibrin included in their structure will be sensitive to biodegradation by MMPs as these ECM proteins have specific cleavage sites for the enzymes (Zhu and Marchant 2011). Because of this potential remodeling, consideration of whether it will negatively or positively affect the efficacy of a scaffold should be considered. For scaffolds to be deployed *in vivo*, this degradation can be quite useful but for *in vitro* experimentation it may confound results as changes in the mechanical properties of the scaffold may occur.

11.2.2.4 Cell-to-Cell Communication

Cell phenotype can be dependent on the type and density of surrounding cells. Research questions are often best answered in pure cultures free of exogenous signaling from other cell types. Researchers often use primary cultures extracted from tissue for experimentation, but need to verify cell purity to properly interpret the results. For example, a carefully dissected piece of myocardium may be predominantly cardiomyocytes but there will also be other cell types, which are found *in vivo* such as fibroblasts. To account for this, commercially available kits can be used to eliminate unwanted cells and allow for isolation of cardiomyocytes and other cell lines (Louch et al. 2011).

Coculture studies, however, are better at replicating the *in vivo* environment by incorporating the natural interactions of multiple cell types within all areas of the cardiovascular system. The interaction between endothelial and other vascular cells (smooth muscle cells, cardiac myocytes, fibroblasts, leukocytes, or valvular interstitial cells) is important for paracrine cell signaling, which more closely resembles the *in vivo* environment (Truskey 2010). Coculturing can be accomplished by growing endothelial cells and other vascular cells on opposite sides of a membrane (Chiu et al. 2003), culturing endothelial cells on scaffolds containing other vascular cells (Hussain et al. 2013), or directly culturing endothelial cells on other cells (Niwa et al. 2004).

Porous membranes have been used to investigate the interaction with smooth muscle and endothelial cells in expression of cellular adhesion molecules (CAMs) in vascular studies (Chiu et al. 2003; Srigunapalan et al. 2011). Both cell types were cultured on to either side of a porous membrane and allowed to proliferate. When endothelial cells are exposed to wall shear stress, smooth muscle cell coculture attenuates the increased gene expression of ICAM-1 in endothelial cells when compared to controls, demonstrating the effect of intracellular signaling from a typical monoculture. Porous membrane experiments such as these help simplify the number of variables by limiting the complexity of the cell–cell interactions. Furthermore, nutrient delivery to both cell types is simplified as both cultures can be exposed directly to growth media.

Biocompatible 3D scaffolds have been implemented for the coculture of cardiomyocytes with either endothelial cells or fibroblasts (Hussain et al. 2013). Researchers found that they could achieve a high long-term cell viability in this scaffold (over 3 weeks) when cultured with fibroblasts but not with endothelial cells. The cardiomyocyte/fibroblast coculture expressed high levels of important functional proteins and was therefore deemed suitable for such applications as *ex vivo* tissue engineering of muscle mass to implant in patients post cardiac infarction. This study exemplified the advantages of allowing cell signaling to better mimic the complex structures found in myocardial tissue without any barrier between cell–cell interactions like in membrane separated cultures. However, there is a loss in uniformity from the cell seeding methods, which could result in inconsistent findings.

To closely mimic the actual *in vitro* environment of the vascular endothelium, culturing of endothelial cells directly on to smooth muscle cells has been performed. Using this technique, the absorption of low density lipoproteins found that the uptake of this molecule implicated in atherosclerosis was greater in coculture than endothelial cell monoculture (Niwa et al. 2004). Although this method of coculture best mimics the *in vivo* environment, it can be difficult to maintain the health and phenotype of the underlying smooth muscle cells as nutrients must diffuse through the endothelial cell layer.

Coculturing has allowed researchers to begin moving past some of the fundamental issues of *in vitro* models, helping elucidate the interactions that the cells have with their neighboring tissues and promoting cell viability. Studies have shown that increased long-term viability of engineered tissue can be seen in coculture in 3D matrices and other models, giving credence to the importance of coculture consideration (Hussain et al. 2013).

11.2.2.5 Mechanical Properties

The mechanical properties of substrates can affect cell phenotype and potentially confound experimental results. In the simplest example, components found in the ECM (including proteins especially integrins) directly communicate with the cellular cytoskeleton and can provide different cell responses based on substrate stiffness (Discher et al. 2005). *In vivo*, biological tissues which act as the cell substrate have elastic moduli on the order of 0.1–100 kPa, whereas *in vitro* substrates such as glass are on the order of GPa (Levental et al. 2007). This is particularly important in scaffold design when engineering tissue. Development of the 3D myocardium models relies on maintaining viable, beating cardiomyocytes, and this viability has been directly linked to scaffold stiffness (Shapira-Schweitzer and Seliktar 2007; Mei et al. 2014).

It has been demonstrated that cells sense their environment and can therefore control motility and morphology based on substrate stiffness, a process termed "durotaxis." Researchers studying mouse fibroblasts observed that they preferentially moved in the direction of stiffer polyacrylamide gel gradients and that these cells could produce more traction on stiffer substrates (Lo et al. 2000).

The need to control substrate elasticity has contributed toward the increased use of polymeric substrates in the 3D models. Polymers allow for greater control over the mechanical properties of the substrate and therefore researchers can mimic the native environments for their cells. Numerous studies have used a silicone elastomer (Sylgard 184) to develop vascular models (Doyle et al. 2009; Farcas et al. 2009) and testing has shown that this material has an elastic moduli of 1–300 kPa (Gutierrez and Groisman 2011) falling in a similar range of arterial stiffness of 1–4 kPa (Stroka and Aranda-Espinoza 2011). Novel processing techniques have also been developed to allow fabrication of intrinsically soft microstructures (<20 μm) in PDMS elastomers as soft as 1.5 kPa (Moraes et al. 2015). Gelatin–collagen blends (elastic moduli of 60–200 kPa) have also been used to closely mimic the stiffness of native myocardium (elastic moduli of approximately 10 kPa) in scaffolds (Mei et al. 2014). Advancements in materials engineering have allowed researches to better tune the stiffness of scaffolds and membranes used in cell culture studies, helping create conditions closely replicating the native environment of cells. This tuning lays the groundwork of choosing the appropriate substrate needed for a specific 3D model.

11.3 CONCLUSION AND PERSPECTIVE

Advancements in the field of *in vitro* modeling have allowed researchers to develop structures to closely mimic the cardiovascular environment. These models began as simple 2D constructs and have developed into intricate 3D domains, which can be used for both fundamental research and clinical treatments. By taking into account the important biological interactions, which occur *in vitro*, innovative new materials and methods have been produced to help address some of the current challenges faced in the research of cardiovascular disease.

ACKNOWLEDGMENT

The authors would like to acknowledge the contribution of Alexander Emmott for providing histological slide images for the chapter.

REFERENCES

Akins, R. E. Jr., D. Rockwood, K. G. Robinson, D. Sandusky, J. Rabolt, and C. Pizarro. 2010. Three-dimensional culture alters primary cardiac cell phenotype. *Tissue Eng Part A* no. 16 (2):629–41.

Barron, V., E. Lyons, C. Stenson-Cox, P. E. McHugh, and A. Pandit. 2003. Bioreactors for cardiovascular cell and tissue growth: A review. *Ann Biomed Eng* no. 31 (9):1017–30.

Beauchamp, P., W. Moritz, J. M. Kelm, N. D. Ullrich, I. Agarkova, B. D. Anson, T. M. Suter, and C. Zuppinger. 2015. Development and characterization of a scaffold-free 3D spheroid model of induced pluripotent stem cell-derived human cardiomyocytes. *Tissue Eng Part C: Methods* no. 21 (8):852–61.

Berthier, E., E. W. Young, and D. Beebe. 2012. Engineers are from PDMS-land, biologists are from polystyrenia. *Lab Chip* no. 12 (7):1224–37.

Brown, J. W., R. C. Elkins, D. R. Clarke, J. S. Tweddell, C. B. Huddleston, J. R. Doty, J. W. Fehrenbacher, and J. J. Takkenberg. 2010. Performance of the CryoValve SG human decellularized pulmonary valve in 342 patients relative to the conventional CryoValve at a mean follow-up of four years. *J Thorac Cardiovasc Surg* no. 139 (2):339–48.

Butcher, J. T. and R. M. Nerem. 2004. Porcine aortic valve interstitial cells in three-dimensional culture: Comparison of phenotype with aortic smooth muscle cells. *J Heart Valve Dis* no. 13 (3):478–85; discussion 485-6.

Carrier, R. L., M. Papadaki, M. Rupnick, F. J. Schoen, N. Bursac, R. Langer, L. E. Freed, and G. Vunjak-Novakovic. 1999. Cardiac tissue engineering: Cell seeding, cultivation parameters, and tissue construct characterization. *Biotechnol Bioeng* no. 64 (5):580–9.

Cecelja, M. and P. Chowienczyk. 2012. Role of arterial stiffness in cardiovascular disease. *JRSM Cardiovasc Dis* no. 1 (4): 1–11; doi: 10.1258/cvd.2012.012016.

Chambard, M., J. Gabrion, and J. Mauchamp. 1981. Influence of collagen gel on the orientation of epithelial cell polarity: Follicle formation from isolated thyroid cells and from preformed monolayers. *J Cell Biol* no. 91 (1):157–66.

Chiu, J. J., L. J. Chen, P. L. Lee, C. I. Lee, L. W. Lo, S. Usami, and S. Chien. 2003. Shear stress inhibits adhesion molecule expression in vascular endothelial cells induced by coculture with smooth muscle cells. *Blood* no. 101 (7):2667–74.

Chiu, Y. W., W. P. Chen, C. C. Su, Y. C. Lee, P. H. Hsieh, and Y. L. Ho. 2014. The arrhythmogenic effect of self-assembling nanopeptide hydrogel scaffolds on neonatal mouse cardiomyocytes. *Nanomedicine* no. 10 (5):1065–73.

Comerford, A., M. J. Plank, and T. David. 2008. Endothelial nitric oxide synthase and calcium production in arterial geometries: An integrated fluid mechanics/cell model. *J Biomech Eng* no. 130 (1):011010.

Corstorphine, L. and M. V. Sefton. 2011. Effectiveness factor and diffusion limitations in collagen gel modules containing HepG2 cells. *J Tissue Eng Regen Med* no. 5 (2):119–29.

Crapo, P. M., T. W. Gilbert, and S. F. Badylak. 2011. An overview of tissue and whole organ decellularization processes. *Biomaterials* no. 32 (12):3233–43.

Dahliwal, A. 2012. 3D cell culture: A review. *Mater Methods* no. 2: 162; doi: 10.13070/mm.en.2.162.

Daley, W. P., S. B. Peters, and M. Larsen. 2008. Extracellular matrix dynamics in development and regenerative medicine. *J Cell Sci* no. 121 (Pt 3):255–64.

Dartsch, P. C. and E. Betz. 1989. Response of cultured endothelial cells to mechanical stimulation. *Basic Res Cardiol* no. 84 (3):268–81.

Davies, P. F., M. Civelek, Y. Fang, and I. Fleming. 2013. The atherosusceptible endothelium: Endothelial phenotypes in complex haemodynamic shear stress regions *in vivo*. *Cardiovasc Res* no. 99 (2):315–27.

Deck, J. D. 1986. Endothelial cell orientation on aortic valve leaflets. *Cardiovasc Res* no. 20 (10):760–7.

Dewey, C. F. Jr., S. R. Bussolari, M. A. Gimbrone Jr., and P. F. Davies. 1981. The dynamic response of vascular endothelial cells to fluid shear stress. *J Biomech Eng* no. 103 (3):177–85.

Dhandayuthapani, B., U. M. Krishnan, and S. Sethuraman. 2010. Fabrication and characterization of chitosan-gelatin blend nanofibers for skin tissue engineering. *J Biomed Mater Res B: Appl Biomater* no. 94 (1):264–72.

Discher, D. E., P. Janmey, and Y. L. Wang. 2005. Tissue cells feel and respond to the stiffness of their substrate. *Science* no. 310 (5751):1139–43.

Doyle, B. J., T. J. Corbett, A. J. Cloonan, M. R. O'Donnell, M. T. Walsh, D. A. Vorp, and T. M. McGloughlin. 2009. Experimental modelling of aortic aneurysms: Novel applications of silicone rubbers. *Med Eng Phys* no. 31 (8):1002–12.

Durham, E. R., E. Ingham, and S. J. Russell. 2013. Technique for internal channelling of hydroentangled nonwoven scaffolds to enhance cell penetration. *J Biomater Appl* no. 28 (2):241–9.

Eschenhagen, T. and W. H. Zimmermann. 2005. Engineering myocardial tissue. *Circ Res* no. 97 (12):1220–31.

Farcas, M. A., L. Rouleau, R. Fraser, and R. L. Leask. 2009. The development of 3-D, *in vitro*, endothelial culture models for the study of coronary artery disease. *Biomed Eng Online* no. 8:30.

Frame, M. D., G. B. Chapman, Y. Makino, and I. H. Sarelius. 1998. Shear stress gradient over endothelial cells in a curved microchannel system. *Biorheology* no. 35 (4–5):245–61.

Fry, D. L. 1968. Acute vascular endothelial changes associated with increased blood velocity gradients. *Circ Res* no. 22 (2):165–97.

Gijsen, F. J., F. N. van de Vosse, and J. D. Janssen. 1999. The influence of the non-Newtonian properties of blood on the flow in large arteries: Steady flow in a carotid bifurcation model. *J Biomech* no. 32 (6):601–8.

Go, A. S., D. Mozaffarian, V. L. Roger, E. J. Benjamin, J. D. Berry, M. J. Blaha, S. Dai et al. 2014. Executive summary: Heart disease and stroke statistics—2014 update: A report from the American Heart Association. *Circulation* no. 129 (3):399–410.

Gonnerman, E. A., D. O. Kelkhoff, L. M. McGregor, and B. A. Harley. 2012. The promotion of HL-1 cardiomyocyte beating using anisotropic collagen-GAG scaffolds. *Biomaterials* no. 33 (34):8812–21.

Gutierrez, E. and A. Groisman. 2011. Measurements of elastic moduli of silicone gel substrates with a microfluidic device. *PLoS One* no. 6 (9):e25534.

Gutierrez, R. A. and E. T. Crumpler. 2008. Potential effect of geometry on wall shear stress distribution across scaffold surfaces. *Ann Biomed Eng* no. 36 (1):77–85.

Hall, H. G., D. A. Farson, and M. J. Bissell. 1982. Lumen formation by epithelial cell lines in response to collagen overlay: A morphogenetic model in culture. *Proc Natl Acad Sci USA* no. 79 (15):4672–6.

Harkness, M. L., R. D. Harkness, and D. A. McDonald. 1957. The collagen and elastin content of the arterial wall in the dog. *Proc R Soc Lond B: Biol Sci* no. 146 (925):541–51.

Hussain, A., G. Collins, D. Yip, and C. H. Cho. 2013. Functional 3-D cardiac co-culture model using bioactive chitosan nanofiber scaffolds. *Biotechnol Bioeng* no. 110 (2):637–47.

Hutmacher, D. W., T. Schantz, I. Zein, K. W. Ng, S. H. Teoh, and K. C. Tan. 2001. Mechanical properties and cell cultural response of polycaprolactone scaffolds designed and fabricated via fused deposition modeling. *J Biomed Mater Res* no. 55 (2):203–16.

Hutmacher, D. W., M. Sittinger, and M. V. Risbud. 2004. Scaffold-based tissue engineering: Rationale for computer-aided design and solid free-form fabrication systems. *Trends Biotechnol* no. 22 (7):354–62.

Hynes, R. O. 1999. Cell adhesion: Old and new questions. *Trends Cell Biol* no. 9 (12):M33–7.

Khorshidi, S., A. Solouk, H. Mirzadeh, S. Mazinani, J. M. Lagaron, S. Sharifi, and S. Ramakrishna. 2016. A review of key challenges of electrospun scaffolds for tissue-engineering applications. *J Tissue Eng Regen Med.* 10 (9): 715–38; doi: 10.1002/term.1978

Kievit, F. M., S. J. Florczyk, M. C. Leung, O. Veiseh, J. O. Park, M. L. Disis, and M. Zhang. 2010. Chitosan-alginate 3D scaffolds as a mimic of the glioma tumor microenvironment. *Biomaterials* no. 31 (22):5903–10.

Kikuchi, K. 2015. Dedifferentiation, transdifferentiation, and proliferation: Mechanisms underlying cardiac muscle regeneration in zebrafish. *Curr Pathobiol Rep* no. 3 (1):81–8.

Kumbar, S. G., U. S. Toti, M. Deng, R. James, C. T. Laurencin, A. Aravamudhan, M. Harmon, and D. M. Ramos. 2011. Novel mechanically competent polysaccharide scaffolds for bone tissue engineering. *Biomed Mater* no. 6 (6):065005. doi: 10.1088/1748-6041/6/6/065005

LaFramboise, W. A., D. Scalise, P. Stoodley, S. R. Graner, R. D. Guthrie, J. A. Magovern, and M. J. Becich. 2007. Cardiac fibroblasts influence cardiomyocyte phenotype *in vitro*. *Am J Physiol Cell Physiol* no. 292 (5):C1799–808. doi: 10.1152/ajpcell.00166.2006

Landau, J. and D. Marsland. 1952. Temperature-pressure studies on the cardiac rate in tissue culture explants from the heart of the tadpole (*Rana pipiens*). *J Cell Physiol* no. 40 (3):367–81.

Leong, K. F., C. M. Cheah, and C. K. Chua. 2003. Solid freeform fabrication of three-dimensional scaffolds for engineering replacement tissues and organs. *Biomaterials* no. 24 (13):2363–78.

Leung, B. M., C. Moraes, S. P. Cavnar, K. E. Luker, G. D. Luker, and S. Takayama. 2015. Microscale 3D collagen cell culture assays in conventional flat-bottom 384-well plates. *J Lab Autom* no. 20 (2):138–45.

Levental, I., P. C. Georges, and P. A. Janmey. 2007. Soft biological materials and their impact on cell function. *Soft Matter* no. 3 (3):299–306.

Levesque, S. G. and M. S. Shoichet. 2007. Synthesis of enzyme-degradable, peptide-cross-linked dextran hydrogels. *Bioconjug Chem* no. 18 (3):874–85.

Li, D., T. Wu, N. He, J. Wang, W. Chen, L. He, C. Huang, H. A. Ei-Hamshary, S. S. Al-Deyab, Q. Ke, and X. Mo. 2014. Three-dimensional polycaprolactone scaffold via needle-less electrospinning promotes cell proliferation and infiltration. *Colloids Surf B: Biointerfaces* no. 121:432–43.

Liu, A. C., V. R. Joag, and A. I. Gotlieb. 2007. The emerging role of valve interstitial cell phenotypes in regulating heart valve pathobiology. *Am J Pathol* no. 171 (5):1407–18.

Lo, C. M., H. B. Wang, M. Dembo, and Y. L. Wang. 2000. Cell movement is guided by the rigidity of the substrate. *Biophys J* no. 79 (1):144–52.

Louch, W. E., K. A. Sheehan, and B. M. Wolska. 2011. Methods in cardiomyocyte isolation, culture, and gene transfer. *J Mol Cell Cardiol* no. 51 (3):288–98.

Lu, K. W., J. Perez-Gil, and H. Taeusch. 2009. Kinematic viscosity of therapeutic pulmonary surfactants with added polymers. *Biochim Biophys Acta* no. 1788 (3):632–7.

Malek, A. M. and S. Izumo. 1996. Mechanism of endothelial cell shape change and cytoskeletal remodeling in response to fluid shear stress. *J Cell Sci* no. 109 (Pt 4):713–26.

Martin, I., D. Wendt, and M. Heberer. 2004. The role of bioreactors in tissue engineering. *Trends Biotechnol* no. 22 (2):80–6.

Mata, A., E. J. Kim, C. A. Boehm, A. J. Fleischman, G. F. Muschler, and S. Roy. 2009. A three-dimensional scaffold with precise micro-architecture and surface micro-textures. *Biomaterials* no. 30 (27):4610–7.

McDaniel, D. P., G. A. Shaw, J. T. Elliott, K. Bhadriraju, C. Meuse, K. H. Chung, and A. L. Plant. 2007. The stiffness of collagen fibrils influences vascular smooth muscle cell phenotype. *Biophys J* no. 92 (5):1759–69.

Mei, J. C., A. Y. Wu, P. C. Wu, N. C. Cheng, W. B. Tsai, and J. Yu. 2014. Three-dimensional extracellular matrix scaffolds by microfluidic fabrication for long-term spontaneously contracted cardiomyocyte culture. *Tissue Eng Part A* no. 20 (21–22):2931–41.

Miller, J. S., K. R. Stevens, M. T. Yang, B. M. Baker, D. H. Nguyen, D. M. Cohen, E. Toro, A. A. Chen, P. A. Galie, X. Yu, R. Chaturvedi, S. N. Bhatia, and C. S. Chen. 2012. Rapid casting of patterned vascular networks for perfusable engineered three-dimensional tissues. *Nat Mater* no. 11 (9):768–74.

Miranti, C. K. 2002. Application of cell adhesion to study signaling networks. *Methods Cell Biol* no. 69:359–83.

Mironov, V., V. A. Kasyanov, M. J. Yost, R. Visconti, W. Twal, T. Trusk, X. Wen, I. Ozolanta, A. Kadishs, G. D. Prestwich, L. Terracio, and R. R. Markwald. 2006. Cardiovascular tissue engineering I. Perfusion bioreactors: A review. *J Long Term Eff Med Implants* no. 16 (2):111–30.

Moraes, C., J. M. Labuz, Y. Shao, J. Fu, and S. Takayama. 2015. Supersoft lithography: Candy-based fabrication of soft silicone microstructures. *Lab Chip* no. 15 (18):3760–5.

Moraes, C., M. Likhitpanichkul, C. J. Lam, B. M. Beca, Y. Sun, and C. A. Simmons. 2013. Microdevice array-based identification of distinct mechanobiological response profiles in layer-specific valve interstitial cells. *Integr Biol (Camb)* no. 5 (4):673–80.

Moraes, C., G. Wang, Y. Sun, and C. A. Simmons. 2010. A microfabricated platform for high-throughput unconfined compression of micropatterned biomaterial arrays. *Biomaterials* no. 31 (3):577–84.

Moscona, A. and H. Moscona. 1952. The dissociation and aggregation of cells from organ rudiments of the early chick embryo. *J Anat* no. 86 (3):287–301.

Niwa, K., T. Kado, J. Sakai, and T. Karino. 2004. The effects of a shear flow on the uptake of LDL and acetylated LDL by an EC monoculture and an EC-SMC coculture. *Ann Biomed Eng* no. 32 (4):537–43.

Ortega, I., A. J. Ryan, P. Deshpande, S. MacNeil, and F. Claeyssens. 2013. Combined microfabrication and electrospinning to produce 3-D architectures for corneal repair. *Acta Biomater* no. 9 (3):5511–20.

Owen, M. J. and P. J. Smith. 1994. Plasma treatment of polydimethylsiloxane. *J. Adhesion Sci Technol* no. 8 (10):1063–75.

Regehr, K. J., M. Domenech, J. T. Koepsel, K. C. Carver, S. J. Ellison-Zelski, W. L. Murphy, L. A. Schuler, E. T. Alarid, and D. J. Beebe. 2009. Biological implications of polydimethylsiloxane-based microfluidic cell culture. *Lab Chip* no. 9 (15):2132–9.

Ross, R. and J. A. Glomset. 1976. The pathogenesis of atherosclerosis (second of two parts). *N Engl J Med* no. 295 (8):420–5.

Sakakura, K., M. Nakano, F. Otsuka, E. Ladich, F. D. Kolodgie, and R. Virmani. 2013. Pathophysiology of atherosclerosis plaque progression. *Heart Lung Circ* no. 22 (6):399–411.

Sato, J. D. and M. Kan. 2001. Media for culture of mammalian cells. *Curr Protoc Cell Biol* no. Chapter 1:Unit 1.2.

Schoen, F. J. 2005. Cardiac valves and valvular pathology: Update on function, disease, repair, and replacement. *Cardiovasc Pathol* no. 14 (4):189–94.

Seras-Franzoso, J., C. Steurer, M. Roldan, M. Vendrell, C. Vidaurre-Agut, A. Tarruella, L. Saldana, N. Vilaboa, M. Parera, E. Elizondo, I. Ratera, N. Ventosa, J. Veciana, A. J. Campillo-Fernandez, E. Garcia-Fruitos, E. Vazquez, and A. Villaverde. 2013. Functionalization of 3D scaffolds with protein-releasing biomaterials for intracellular delivery. *J Control Release* no. 171 (1):63–72.

Shalumon, K. T., P. R. Sreerekha, D. Sathish, H. Tamura, S. V. Nair, K. P. Chennazhi, and R. Jayakumar. 2011. Hierarchically designed electrospun tubular scaffolds for cardiovascular applications. *J Biomed Nanotechnol* no. 7 (5):609–20.

Shapira-Schweitzer, K. and D. Seliktar. 2007. Matrix stiffness affects spontaneous contraction of cardiomyocytes cultured within a PEGylated fibrinogen biomaterial. *Acta Biomater* no. 3 (1):33–41.

Soffer, L., X. Wang, X. Zhang, J. Kluge, L. Dorfmann, D. L. Kaplan, and G. Leisk. 2008. Silk-based electrospun tubular scaffolds for tissue-engineered vascular grafts. *J Biomater Sci Polym Ed* no. 19 (5):653–64.

Song, J. J. and H. C. Ott. 2011. Organ engineering based on decellularized matrix scaffolds. *Trends Mol Med* no. 17 (8):424–32.

Sridhar, B. V., J. L. Brock, J. S. Silver, J. L. Leight, M. A. Randolph, and K. S. Anseth. 2015. Development of a cellularly degradable PEG hydrogel to promote articular cartilage extracellular matrix deposition. *Adv Healthc Mater* no. 4 (5):702–13.

Srigunapalan, S., C. Lam, A. R. Wheeler, and C. A. Simmons. 2011. A microfluidic membrane device to mimic critical components of the vascular microenvironment. *Biomicrofluidics* no. 5 (1):13409.

Stamati, K., J. V. Priestley, V. Mudera, and U. Cheema. 2014. Laminin promotes vascular network formation in 3D *in vitro* collagen scaffolds by regulating VEGF uptake. *Exp Cell Res* no. 327 (1):68–77.

Stroka, K. M. and H. Aranda-Espinoza. 2011. Endothelial cell substrate stiffness influences neutrophil transmigration via myosin light chain kinase-dependent cell contraction. *Blood* no. 118 (6):1632–40.

Sugden, P. H. 2001. Mechanotransduction in cardiomyocyte hypertrophy. *Circulation* no. 103 (10):1375–7.

Taylor, P. M., P. Batten, N. J. Brand, P. S. Thomas, and M. H. Yacoub. 2003. The cardiac valve interstitial cell. *Int J Biochem Cell Biol* no. 35 (2):113–8.

Tchao, J., L. Han, B. Lin, L. Yang, and K. Tobita. 2014. Combined biophysical and soluble factor modulation induces cardiomyocyte differentiation from human muscle derived stem cells. *Sci Rep* no. 4:6614.

Terracio, L., B. Miller, and T. K. Borg. 1988. Effects of cyclic mechanical stimulation of the cellular components of the heart: In vitro. *In Vitro Cell Dev Biol* no. 24 (1):53–8.

Toepke, M. W. and D. J. Beebe. 2006. PDMS absorption of small molecules and consequences in microfluidic applications. *Lab Chip* no. 6 (12):1484–6.

Truskey, G. A. 2010. Endothelial cell vascular smooth muscle cell co-culture assay for high throughput screening assays for discovery of anti-angiogenesis agents and other therapeutic molecules. *Int J High Throughput Screen* no. 2010 (1):171–81.

Tzima, E., M. A. del Pozo, S. J. Shattil, S. Chien, and M. A. Schwartz. 2001. Activation of integrins in endothelial cells by fluid shear stress mediates Rho-dependent cytoskeletal alignment. *EMBO J* no. 20 (17):4639–47.

Vaz, C. M., S. van Tuijl, C. V. Bouten, and F. P. Baaijens. 2005. Design of scaffolds for blood vessel tissue engineering using a multi-layering electrospinning technique. *Acta Biomater* no. 1 (5):575–82.

Ventola, C. L. 2014. Medical applications for 3D printing: Current and projected uses. *P T* no. 39 (10):704–11.

Xu, W., X. Zhang, H. Qian, W. Zhu, X. Sun, J. Hu, H. Zhou, and Y. Chen. 2004. Mesenchymal stem cells from adult human bone marrow differentiate into a cardiomyocyte phenotype *in vitro*. *Exp Biol Med (Maywood)* no. 229 (7):623–31.

Yin, A., J. Li, G. L. Bowlin, D. Li, I. A. Rodriguez, J. Wang, T. Wu, H. A. Ei-Hamshary, S. S. Al-Deyab, and X. Mo. 2014. Fabrication of cell penetration enhanced poly (l-lactic acid-co-varepsilon-caprolactone)/silk vascular scaffolds utilizing air-impedance electrospinning. *Colloids Surf B: Biointerfaces* no. 120:47–54.

Yip, C. Y., J. H. Chen, R. Zhao, and C. A. Simmons. 2009. Calcification by valve interstitial cells is regulated by the stiffness of the extracellular matrix. *Arterioscler Thromb Vasc Biol* no. 29 (6):936–42.

Zhang, Y., T. S. Li, S. T. Lee, K. A. Wawrowsky, K. Cheng, G. Galang, K. Malliaras, M. R. Abraham, C. Wang, and E. Marban. 2010. Dedifferentiation and proliferation of mammalian cardiomyocytes. *PLoS One* no. 5 (9):e12559.

Zhu, J. and R. E. Marchant. 2011. Design properties of hydrogel tissue-engineering scaffolds. *Expert Rev Med Devices* no. 8 (5):607–26.

Section III

Biological Considerations

12 Pro- and Anti-Inflammatory Cytokine Signaling within 3D Tissue Models

Stephen L. Rego, Tian McCann, and Didier Dréau

CONTENTS

12.1 Introduction 215
12.2 Pro- and Anti-Inflammatory Cytokines 216
    12.2.1 Cytokines Eliciting Inflammatory Immune Responses 217
    12.2.2 Cytokines Eliciting Anti-Inflammatory Immune Responses 219
    12.2.3 Cytokine Signaling Pathways 220
    12.2.4 Spatial and Dynamic Involvement in Tissue Maintenance/
           Remodeling and Immune Responses..221
12.3 3D models of Cell Behaviors and Cytokines..222
    12.3.1 Pro-Inflammatory Cytokines in an *In Vitro* 3D Culture
           Model of Osteoarthritis 222
    12.3.2 Endogenous and Exogenous Inflammatory Signals in
           Neutrophil Chemotaxis...223
    12.3.3 Bone Marrow, Biomaterials, Bone Remodeling, and
           Mesenchymal Stromal Cell Derived Cytokines 223
    12.3.4 Cytokines and Identification of Neural Progenitor Cells
           Using 3D Models 224
    12.3.5 Inflammasomes and 3D *In Vitro* Models...225
12.4 Conclusion and Perspective 225
References..226

12.1 INTRODUCTION

Tissue engineering and three-dimensional (3D) biological modeling raise exciting possibilities for generating functional organ replacements as well as studying complex physiologic processes *in vitro*. A number of techniques including some using extracellular matrix (ECM) proteins have been developed to generate functional 3D tissue models. Those 3D models allow studies of the development and pathophysiology of most tissue in the body (Streuli et al. 1991; Petersen et al. 1992; Rego et al. 2015, 2016; Lance et al. 2016). Furthermore, utilizing 3D models to anticipate appropriate pharmacologic responses has proven useful in many drug screening applications (Lan and Starly 2011; Leonard et al. 2012; Malpass 2013; Fong et al. 2014). Indeed, as conventional two-dimensional (2D) models lack the appropriate spatial arrangement of cells observed *in vivo*, investigations of cellular behaviors in response to signaling molecules using 3D models have been shown to be more predictive of *in vivo* activities than 2D models (Griffith and Swartz 2006).

Cytokines are fundamental soluble protein signaling molecules that have key roles in mediating immune responses as well as contributing to numerous other critical physiologic processes (Dreau et al. 2000; Medzhitov et al. 2011; Li et al. 2015). Cytokines are secreted by most cells in the body and act via binding to their cognate receptors in autocrine or paracrine manners to activate downstream signaling cascades that lead to changes in cellular function or phenotype (Leonard and Lin 2000; Bezbradica and Medzhitov 2009; Huang and August 2015). Cytokines are instrumental in mediating inflammation and a number of cytokines are clinical targets for various inflammatory diseases including rheumatoid arthritis (Genovese et al. 2014; von Pawel et al. 2014; Fischer et al. 2015; Iwata 2015). In addition to their critical roles in immune responses, cytokines (pro and anti inflammatory) are expressed by nearly every cell type in the body and have essential roles mediating cellular behavior (Brusnahan et al. 2010; Ballotta et al. 2014; Asada et al. 2015; Cornejo et al. 2015; Lee et al. 2015).

2D *in vitro* models have assisted in studying the effects of cytokines on cellular behaviors; however, 2D models do not always translate to *in vivo* activities, due to inappropriate cellular architecture and organization (Zdzisinska et al. 2009). Animal models are also useful to investigate the activities of cytokines but are costly, time consuming, and may not possess homologous functions to their human counterparts. 3D models provide improved approaches for investigating the effects of human cytokines on cellular behaviors in a setting that mimics the organization of cells in their native environment (Kenny et al. 2007; Inman and Bissell 2010; Rouaud-Tinguely et al. 2015). 3D models have been utilized to investigate the role of pro- and anti-inflammatory cytokines in modulating the behaviors of both immune cell (such as macrophages and neutrophils) and nonimmune cell (such as epithelial, stromal, and endothelial cells) populations (Lehman et al. 2013; Hopkins et al. 2015; Lombardo Bedran et al. 2015). Importantly, the role of cytokines in tissue repair by altering the behaviors of diverse cell populations (immune and nonimmune) is an area of research that benefits from relevant 3D models (Xu et al. 2014).

Here, the role of pro- and anti-inflammatory cytokines in regulating inflammatory or wound healing processes as well as the use and potential of 3D models in identifying and studying cytokine signaling is detailed.

12.2 PRO- AND ANTI-INFLAMMATORY CYTOKINES

Cytokines are soluble signaling peptides that elicit responses by binding to their cognate receptors (Leonard and Lin 2000). Although there are many different classification systems used for cytokines, most recently they have been grouped into superfamilies based on their structural and sequence similarities. The tumor necrosis factor (TNF)/TNF receptor superfamily includes TNFα, lymphotoxins, CD40L,

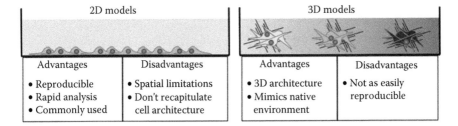

FIGURE 12.1 Comparison of 2D and 3D models. Schematic representation of 2D and 3D models highlighting the advantages and disadvantages of each approach. Difference in shade intensity indicates cytokine gradients.

and CD95. The TNF superfamily modulates immune cell phenotype, migration, or survival (stimulate apoptosis) (Locksley et al. 2001). The interleukin 1 (IL1)/IL1 receptor superfamily contains IL1α, IL1β, IL-receptor antagonist, IL-18, IL-33, and Toll-like receptors (TLRs). Those cytokines mediate host-defense function and microbial recognition (Pantschenko et al. 2003; Rifkin et al. 2005; Marshak-Rothstein 2006). In this chapter, cytokines are grouped functionally based on their ability to elicit (1) inflammatory immune responses or (2) anti-inflammatory (wound healing) immune responses.

The type of response elicited by a specific cytokine varies depending on its temporal and spatial availability as well as the receptor expression profile on the target cell(s). 3D models coupled with *in vivo* studies have been instrumental in determining the importance of cytokine gradients in mediating cellular responses. A comparison of 2D and 3D modeling is outlined in Figure 12.1 and illustrates the limitations of 2D systems in studying cytokine activities.

12.2.1 Cytokines Eliciting Inflammatory Immune Responses

Cytokines mediate inflammation through activation of a number of different cell types including macrophages, neutrophils, natural killer (NK) cells, mast cells, and eosinophils (Dreau et al. 2000; Leonard and Lin 2000). Most cytokines elicit pleiotropic effects on cells. Those include activating/deactivating immune cells, upregulating reactive oxygen species (ROS) and adhesion molecules, stimulating cell migration (chemotaxis), and inducing cell death (apoptosis) (Watkins et al. 1995; Zhang and An 2007). The most studied (nonexhaustive list) pro-inflammatory cytokines and their actions are presented in Table 12.1.

TNFα (also referred to as TNF as TNFβ is now commonly denoted as lymphotoxin) resides at the apex of inflammatory signaling (Locksley et al. 2001). TNF is secreted primarily by monocytes; however, it is also expressed by a number of other immune and nonimmune cell types (Dreau et al. 2000). Responses elicited by TNF include apoptosis, cachexia, inflammation, and inhibition of tumorigenesis (Aggarwal et al. 2012). TNF acts by binding to one of its two cognate receptors; TNF receptor 1 (TNFR1) and TNFR2, where both lead to activation of downstream signaling cascades (outlined in Section 2.3) (Henkler et al. 2003; Wajant et al. 2003).

TABLE 12.1
Pro-Inflammatory Cytokines

Cytokine	Receptor(s)	Primary Cell Source(s)	Major Function(s)
TNF	TNFR1/2	Monocytes	Monocyte activation/differentiation
		T cells	Tumor cell apoptosis
		B cells	Cachexia
IFNγ	IFNγR1/2	Macrophages	Inhibit viral replication
		T cells	Activate macrophages
		B cells	Stimulate antigen presentation
IL1	IL1RI	Macrophages	Adhesion molecule expression
		Fibroblasts	ROS production
		Dendritic cells	Matrix degradation
IL6[a]	IL6R/gp130	Monocytes	B cell proliferation
		Fibroblasts	Antibody production
		T cells	T cell proliferation
IL8	CXCR1/CXCR2	Macrophages	Induce chemotaxis
		Epithelial cells	Stimulate phagocytosis
		Smooth muscle cells	Angiogenesis
GCSF	GCSFR (CD114)	Endothelial cells	Granulocyte differentiation/proliferation
		Macrophages	Chemotaxis
GMCSF	GMCSFR (CD116)	Macrophages	Granulocyte differentiation/proliferation
		T cells	Monocyte differentiation/proliferation
		Mast cells	ROS production

[a] Has anti-inflammatory properties also.

Interferon gamma (IFNγ) is an inflammatory cytokine that was originally discovered through its ability to hinder viral replication (Komatsu et al. 1996; Zhang et al. 1997). IFNγ is primarily expressed by leukocytes and functions to inhibit viral replication, activate macrophages and cellular immune responses, stimulate antigen presentation, and induce tumor cell death (Schroder et al. 2004). The binding of IFNγ to its heterodimeric receptors consisting of IFNγ receptor 1 (IFNγR1) and IFNγR2 leads to the activation of the Janus kinase/signal transducers and activators of transcription (JAK/STAT) intracellular signaling cascades (Schroder et al. 2004).

IL1 family members are expressed by macrophages, fibroblasts, dendritic cells, lymphocytes, and epithelial cells, and play important roles in promoting inflammatory cell recruitment and act as a potent pyrogen (Barsky et al. 2007). IL1 signaling occurs through binding of type I IL1 receptor (IL1RI), which then recruits a coreceptor necessary for signal transduction (Martin and Wesche 2002). IL1 family members play major roles in inflammatory disorders including rheumatoid arthritis and periodontitis (Barsky et al. 2007). IL1 receptor antagonist (IL1Ra, see below) is another key cytokine within the IL1 family that functions to inhibit downstream signaling through the IL1R (Fearon and Fearon 2008).

Interleukin-6 (IL6) is an inflammatory cytokine, which belongs to a superfamily that includes oncostatin M and leukemia inhibitory factor. IL-6 is secreted by monocytes, fibroblasts, B cells, and T cells (Akira et al. 1990). IL6 is critical in inducing fever in response to pathogens. Cellular signaling of IL6 requires binding of IL6 to its receptor (IL6R), which in turn activates the coreceptor glycoprotein 130 (gp130), thus, leading to signaling through the JAK/STAT pathway (Schneiders et al. 2015). Interestingly, the IL6R can be shed from cells by the enzyme tumor necrosis factor converting enzyme (TACE) and modulate the inflammatory response through trans-signaling (Rego et al. 2014). Along with its inflammatory properties, IL6 also acts as an anti-inflammatory factor in muscle (Scheller et al. 2011).

IL8 is an inflammatory cytokine that falls under the subcategory of chemokines (Baggiolini and Clark-Lewis 1992). Macrophages are the primary producers of IL8; however, other cells including epithelial cells, smooth muscle cells, and endothelial cells have also been shown to release IL8 (Gahler et al. 2000; Carneiro-Lobo et al. 2014; Sakai et al. 2014; Ibusuki et al. 2015). The major functions of IL8 include cell recruitment, stimulating phagocytosis, and angiogenesis. IL8 can activate a number of different cell surface receptors including the chemokine receptors CXCR1 and CXCR2, which often leads to activation of the nuclear factor kappa-light-chain-enhancer of activated B cells (NFκB) transcription factor (Min et al. 2008). Regulation of IL6 and IL8 expression is highly dependent on the 3D microenvironment, as evidenced by the increased expression of these cytokines in 3D cocultures of breast cancer cells and fibroblasts compared to 2D cultures (Estrada et al. 2016).

12.2.2 Cytokines Eliciting Anti-Inflammatory Immune Responses

Anti-inflammatory cytokines are immuno-regulatory factors that function to curb the inflammatory immune response (see mainly studied Table 12.2 (nonexhaustive list)). Examples include soluble proteins that bind to cell surface receptors leading

TABLE 12.2
Anti-Inflammatory Cytokines

Cytokine	Receptor(s)	Primary Cell Source(s)	Major Function(s)
IL10	IL10R1/2	Monocytes	Decrease Th1 cytokines
		T cells	Decrease ROS
		B cells	Induce anergy
IL4	IL4Rα	T cells	Th2 differentiation/survival
		NK cells	B cell differentiation
			Increase adhesion molecules
IL13	IL4Rα	T cells	Increase ECM degradation
			Mucus secretion
IL1Ra	IL1RI	Monocytes	Inhibits IL1 signaling
IL11	IL11Rα/gp130	Stromal cells	Megakaryocyte maturation
IL6[a]	IL6R/gp130	Myocytes	Increase IL1Ra and IL10 activation
			Decrease TNF and IL1 activities

[a] Has pro-inflammatory properties also.

to the activation of anti-inflammatory signaling pathways or the inhibition of pro-inflammatory signaling pathways.

IL10 is a soluble protein primarily expressed by monocytes but can also be expressed by dendritic cells, T cells, B cells, epithelial cells, and keratinocytes (Trifunovic et al. 2015; von Haehling et al. 2015). IL10 dampens the inflammatory response by downregulating the expression of Th1 cytokines and inhibiting pro-inflammatory macrophage functions such as decreasing levels of reactive oxygen species and costimulatory molecule expression (Trifunovic et al. 2015). IL10 also stimulates the regulatory immune response by activating T regulatory cells and inducing anergy (Maris et al. 2007). In response to IL10, fibroblasts reduce two activities essential for appropriate wound healing: matrix metalloprotease expression and collagen release (Balaji et al. 2015). IL10 signaling involves two IL10 receptors IL10R1 and IL10R2, which form heteromers once bound to IL10. This binding and heteromerization lead to activation of STAT3 signaling and inhibition of the NFκB signaling pathway (Riley et al. 1999; Tanaka et al. 2005).

IL4 is an anti-inflammatory cytokine expressed by NK cells, basophils, and specific subsets of T cells (Chatterjee et al. 2014). IL4 stimulates T and B cell proliferation and differentiation and can induce macrophages to express an alternative phenotype that promotes wound healing functions (Chatterjee et al. 2014). The receptor for IL4, IL4Rα, exists in three distinct forms throughout the body and can be activated by both IL4 and IL13, all having similar biologic functions (Ito et al. 2009; Andrews et al. 2013).

IL1Ra is an anti-inflammatory cytokine that belongs to the IL1 superfamily. IL1Ra is produced by monocytes and acts by binding to the IL1R and inhibiting activation of this receptor by the inflammatory cytokine IL1 (Fearon and Fearon 2008).

Some cytokines exhibit both pro- and anti-inflammatory effects, such as IL6. Along with its pro-inflammatory effects, IL6 possesses anti-inflammatory properties in skeletal muscle tissues (Munoz-Canoves et al. 2013). By activating distinct signaling pathways in muscle cells (myocytes) compared to macrophages, IL6 stimulates inflammation in some areas of the body while blunting the inflammatory response in muscles.

12.2.3 Cytokine Signaling Pathways

Cytokines elicit their effects by binding to their cognate receptors on target cells and activating an array of signaling cascades, including but not limited to those summarized in Figure 12.2. The signaling cascades activated by cytokines are context and cell specific and it is not uncommon for a single cytokine to activate multiple signaling pathways. For example, the canonical inflammatory cytokine, TNF, upon binding to its receptor activates both caspase dependent and independent signaling events (Rath and Aggarwal 1999; Koul et al. 2006). The activated TNFR recruits a number of effector proteins including TNFR-Associated Death Domain protein (TRADD) which in turn recruits Fas-Associated Death Domain (FADD), TNF Receptor-Associated Factor-2 (TRAF2), and Receptor-Interacting Protein (RIP). TRADD and FADD recruitment to the TNFR leads to activation of the caspase cascade and ultimately apoptosis. TRAF2 and RIP lead to activation of the Activation

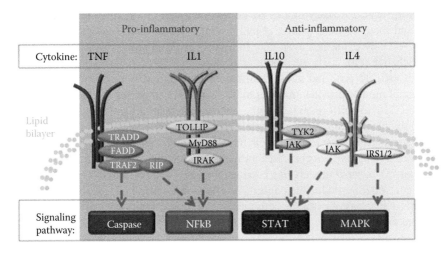

FIGURE 12.2 Basic schematic of pro- and anti-inflammatory signaling pathways. Major proteins involved in the pro-inflammatory signaling cascades triggered by the cytokines TNF and IL1 leading to the activation of the caspase and NFκB pathways, respectively, are presented on the left (highlighted in pink). On the right, key proteins associated with the anti-inflammatory signaling cascades, JAK/STAT and MAPK, which are activated by the IL10 and IL4 cytokines, are presented. Abbreviations: Toll-Interacting Protein (TOLLIP), Myeloid Differentiation primary response gene-88 (MyD88), IL-1 Receptor-Associated Kinase 1/2 (IRS1/2), and Insulin Receptor Substrate (IRAK).

Protein-1 (AP-1) and NFκB pathways that have pleiotropic effects on cellular behaviors (Henkler et al. 2003; Wajant et al. 2003).

The anti-inflammatory cytokine also activates numerous signaling cascades. For example, upon activation, the IL10 receptors (IL10R1 and IL10R2) form heteromers, leading to phosphorylation of their associated proteins JAK and Tyrosine Kinase-2 (TYK2) (Shouval et al. 2014; Shouval et al. 2014). Subsequently, STAT3 is recruited to the receptor complexes and phosphorylated. Following phosphorylation, STAT3 dimerizes and activates the expression of antiapoptotic and cell cycle genes, leading to cell survival. IL10 also activates other anti-inflammatory signaling pathways and inhibits the pro-inflammatory NFκB pathway (Riley et al. 1999).

12.2.4 SPATIAL AND DYNAMIC INVOLVEMENT IN TISSUE MAINTENANCE/REMODELING AND IMMUNE RESPONSES

The pleiotropic nature of cytokines makes classification extremely difficult as evidenced by the number of distinct classification systems (Akira et al. 1990; Baggiolini and Clark-Lewis 1992; Zlotnik and Yoshie 2000; Barsky et al. 2007; Bezbradica and Medzhitov 2009; Aggarwal et al. 2012). Furthermore, inflammatory lesions are dynamic environments where different cells under cytokine control contribute to a number of different processes, such as the resolution of an infection and ultimately scarring or tissue healing (Ballotta et al. 2014; Barrientos et al. 2014; Balaji et al.

2015; Koob et al. 2015). Cytokines are key at every stage of inflammation and wound repair and their dynamic temporal and spatial organization is essential; therefore, models to study cytokines must take into account these properties (Zhang and An 2007; Scheller et al. 2011; Barrientos et al. 2014).

To investigate pro- and anti-inflammatory cytokine activities, immuno-competent animal models provide an intact niche, which encompasses the 3D architecture of the ECM and cell organization and appropriate spatial and temporal organization of soluble proteins including cytokines. Nevertheless, given cross-species differences are often observed and their inherent complexity, reproducibility using *in vivo* models remains a concern. In contrast, the reductionist approach using the conventional 2D *in vitro* models has been extensively used to study of cytokines in a highly controlled reproducible context. As shown in Figure 12.1, 3D *in vitro* models allow investigations of cytokine activities in a 3D context with controlled spatial and temporal organization.

12.3 3D MODELS OF CELL BEHAVIORS AND CYTOKINES

The importance of 3D architecture and the ECM in mediating cellular behaviors was highlighted by Mina Bissell's group who demonstrated that although normal breast epithelial cells cultured in Matrigel® formed well-organized acinus-like structures, tumor cells formed easily distinguished disorganized structures (Streuli et al. 1991; Streuli and Bissell 1991; Schmidhauser et al. 1992). The role of the ECM in mediating cell behaviors was well established by the Bissell group who identified a number of ECM proteins important in modulating normal and cancer cell behaviors. 3D models also recapitulated the paracrine effects of various cell types observed *in vivo*. For example, the growth promoting effects of fibroblasts on metastatic tumor cells were observed in 3D models and led to the identification of multiple key growth factors (Karagiannis et al. 2012). A large number of studies have used diverse 3D *in vitro* culture systems to further our understanding of pro- and anti-inflammatory cytokine activities. Below are highlighted examples of pro- and anti-inflammatory cytokine activities investigated in *in vitro* 3D culture models.

12.3.1 Pro-Inflammatory Cytokines in an *In Vitro* 3D Culture Model of Osteoarthritis

The role of inflammatory cytokines in osteoarthritis has been investigated in a human *in vitro* 3D cartilage system (Sun et al. 2011). 3D cultures were generated through seeding of primary chondrocytes in silk protein scaffolds and cultured for up to 21 days. The effects of the administration of pro-inflammatory cytokines IL-1β and TNFα or the addition of macrophage conditioned medium (CM) were assessed by RNA and protein expressions. Both pro-inflammatory cytokines and the macrophage CM regulated matrix-related gene expression of chondrocytes were different. Whereas cytokines suppressed aggrecan formation and left collagen type II expression unchanged, macrophage CM suppressed collagen type II and upregulated aggrecan. Conversely, cytokines and macrophage CM both enhanced expression of matrix metalloproteinases (MMPs). Furthermore, pro-inflammatory cytokines and macrophage CM differentially affected functional hypertrophy and apoptosis of chondrocytes. Using a 3D chondrocyte human tissue system, this study highlights key effects of pro-inflammatory cytokines in the origin and outcome of osteoarthritis (Sun et al. 2011).

12.3.2 Endogenous and Exogenous Inflammatory Signals in Neutrophil Chemotaxis

How neutrophils distinguish between multiple and competing endogenous and exogenous chemoattractants to reach their target site remained unclear until studies conducted using agarose assays (Heit et al. 2002). Agarose assays utilize the gel-forming ability of the polysaccharide agarose, which has easily tunable properties (Heit et al. 2002; Kajiwara et al. 2009). In this particular assay, researchers utilized a 1.2% agarose gel embedded with cytokines to investigate the migration of cells through 3D gels toward varying concentrations of pro- and anti-inflammatory cytokines (Heit et al. 2002). Under those 3D conditions, migration of neutrophils toward stronger exogenous chemoattractants was mediated through the p38 mitogen activated protein kinase (MAPK) pathway, whereas endogenous chemoattractants activated the phospho-inositide 3-kinase (PI3K)/protein kinase B (Akt) signaling pathway. Those observations highlighted a signaling hierarchy with preferential migration of neutrophils toward exogenous stimuli compared to endogenous stimuli. Furthermore, the adhesion molecules involved in these chemotactic responses to exogenous and endogenous signals were identified as macrophage antigen 1 (Mac1) and lymphocyte function-associated antigen 1 (LFA1), respectively. This study demonstrated that cells migrating away from a local chemoattractant toward distant agonists do so in part by "remembering" signals they encounter in their local environment (Foxman et al. 1999). These findings provide another theory as to how neutrophils are guided to their specific destination within target tissues by specific temporally mediated combinations of chemoattractants (Foxman et al. 1999). Using cytokine gradients and 3D models highlighted the presence of hierarchical signaling pathways in neutrophils that likely contribute to neutrophils migration toward the vasculature then to the location of the primary source of inflammation (Foxman et al. 1999).

12.3.3 Bone Marrow, Biomaterials, Bone Remodeling, and Mesenchymal Stromal Cell Derived Cytokines

The cytokine production of bone marrow stromal cells from multiple myeloma patients after exposure to a myeloma cell line in 2D and 3D cultures has been compared (Zdzisinska et al. 2009). Gelatin sponge scaffolds were used in *in vitro* 3D culture systems. As mentioned above, the expression of various cytokines was different in 2D culture conditions compared to 3D culture conditions. Indeed, in 3D culture conditions bone marrow stromal cells produced more IL-11 and hepatocyte growth factor (HGF) and less IL-10 than in 2D culture conditions. Upon addition of multiple myeloma cells, bone marrow stromal cells in 3D culture conditions secreted more soluble IL-6R than in 2D culture conditions. This difference in both basal expression of cytokines and cytokine production in response to other cells underlines that *in vitro* 3D culture conditions may be more appropriate platforms investigate cancers including multiple myeloma (Zdzisinska et al. 2009).

Mesenchymal stromal cells (MSCs) rely on interactions with leukocytes to promote their wound healing properties. 3D models allow the study of MSC–leukocyte interactions in controlled environments that can incorporate fluid flow, which these cells experience in circulation. Indeed, in 3D models, leukocytes seeded on 3D scaffolds consistently secreted numerous immuno-modulatory proteins, whereas MSCs under the same circumstances secreted trophic factors (Ballotta et al. 2014). Seeded together and under pulsatile flow, leukocytes and MSCs synergistically upregulated CXCL12 and fibroblast growth factor production (Ballotta et al. 2014).

Furthermore, as MSCs immuno-modulatory properties are associated with the generation of anti-inflammatory microenvironment, their presence at the interface with biomaterials may prevent or limit negative immune host responses. Indeed, in 3D culture conditions, cocultures of embedded MSCs within hydrogels and macrophages led to altered stromal protein expression by MSCs and cytokine profiles by macrophages. Specifically, MSCs upregulated the expression of collagen-I, collagen-III, pro-collagen, and matrix metalloproteinase-9 genes in embedded hydrogels compared to controls (King et al. 2014). Macrophages overexpressed immuno-regulatory cytokines including pro-inflammatory (i.e., IL-1β, TNFα, IFNγ, and IL-12) and anti-inflammatory (e.g., IL-10) cytokines along with other factors (i.e., macrophage inflammatory protein-1α, vascular endothelial growth factor, and hepatocyte growth factor) when exposed to MSC embedded hydrogels. These observations suggest that MSCs regulate immune cells toward an immune response, facilitating the use bioengineered implants (King et al. 2014).

The beneficial effects of cytokines released by MSCs in bone remodeling and the migratory patterns of MSCs within bone have also been demonstrated through novel 3D modeling techniques. The essential role of stromal cell-derived factor 1 (SDF1/CXCL12) in mediating MSC chemotaxis within bone was revealed utilizing 3D biomimetic scaffolds (King et al. 2014). In those 3D models, SDF1 led to complete colonization of scaffolds, supporting the use of SDF1 to promote the healing of local bone defects (King et al. 2014).

12.3.4 Cytokines and Identification of Neural Progenitor Cells Using 3D Models

Transcriptomic expression in neural progenitor cells cultured on a 2D substrate, onto 3D porous polystyrene scaffold, or onto 3D neurospheres implanted *in vivo* was determined (Lai et al. 2011). Neural progenitor cells expressed markedly different cytokine levels in 2D versus 3D culture conditions. Also, cytokine transcriptomic expressions differentiated the 2D from the 3D culture conditions with the expression of 16 cytokines that distinguished 2D models from 3D scaffolds and neurospheres. Transcripts upregulated in 3D cultures included bone morphogenic protein 8 (BMP8), CCL13, fibroblast growth factor 5 (FGF5), IL-11, IL-1, and vascular endothelial growth factor (VEGF). These results highlight that cytokine gene expression differs between cells that are cultured using 2D versus 3D culture conditions and that 3D models may provide a more accurate approach to study cytokine expression (Lai et al. 2011).

12.3.5 INFLAMMASOMES AND 3D IN VITRO MODELS

3D models have been instrumental in demonstrating the central role of inflammasomes in regulating the inflammatory process and in a number of disease states (Christenson et al. 2013; Peeters et al. 2014). Inflammasomes are intracellular protein complexes, which include key inflammatory signaling molecules; they regulate the production of active IL-1β (Meraz et al. 2012). Although highly present in immune cells, especially playing a key role in regulating the innate immune system (De Nardo et al. 2014), inflammasomes are also active in multiple cells including epithelial cells (Lombardo Bedran et al. 2015). *In vitro* studies have demonstrated the ability of metals, such as silica and gold, to induce an inflammatory response through activation of inflammasomes in myeloid and epithelial cells (Niikura et al. 2013; Peeters et al. 2014). In 3D cultures of neutrophils, the role of inflammasomes in apoptosis was investigated. In those 3D conditions, neutrophils isolated from healthy individuals promoted inflammasome activation and their death, whereas neutrophils isolated from patients with rheumatoid arthritis expressing lower levels of IL-1β failed to promote the inflammasome (Christenson et al. 2013). These observations highlight the link between IL-1β activation by the inflammasome and the sensitivity of neutrophils to apoptotic signals, and may explain the sustained inflammation in patients with rheumatoid arthritis (Christenson et al. 2013). Along with macrophages and neutrophils, dendritic cells have also been shown to rely heavily on inflammasome-mediated signaling (Meraz et al. 2012).

12.4 CONCLUSION AND PERSPECTIVE

The importance of cytokines in normal immune cell and nonimmune cell functioning is well established. Furthermore, the clinical use of anticytokine therapies such as anti-TNF and IL6 for the treatment of multiple inflammatory disorders highlights their importance in diseases. Although these therapies have transformed the treatment of patients with severe inflammatory arthritis, there remain significant limiting factors regarding treatment failure in some patients along with safety concerns and off-target effects.

3D models are valuable in studying the effects of cytokines in various microenvironments involving immune and nonimmune cell populations and will assist in the development of strategies to target and modulate cytokine activities. 3D models will likely have a significant impact is the understanding and derivation of clinical protocols for tissue repairs, which are especially reliant on cytokine signaling. As 3D models are generated to provide a controlled environment to study the responses of multiple cell types (immune and nonimmune) to cytokines, identification the respective roles of each cytokines involved in normal and diseased states may become possible.

Beyond current specific 3D systems (e.g., 3D model of osteoarthritis or breast tissues), new imaging approach should allow in the future real-time analysis of less reductionist 3D systems encompassing a variety of cells and cytokines. Such approaches will enhance our understanding of cell–cell, cell–ECM interactions and communications as well as improve our protocol to treat inflammatory disorders.

REFERENCES

Aggarwal, B. B., S. C. Gupta, and J. H. Kim. 2012. Historical perspectives on tumor necrosis factor and its superfamily: 25 years later, a golden journey. *Blood* no. 119 (3):651–65.

Akira, S., T. Hirano, T. Taga, and T. Kishimoto. 1990. Biology of multifunctional cytokines: IL 6 and related molecules (IL 1 and TNF). *FASEB J* no. 4 (11):2860–7.

Andrews, A. L., I. K. Nordgren, G. Campbell-Harding, J. W. Holloway, S. T. Holgate, and D. E. Davies. 2013. The association of the cytoplasmic domains of interleukin 4 receptor alpha and interleukin 13 receptor alpha 2 regulates interleukin 4 signaling. *Mol Biosyst.* no. 9 (12):3009–14.

Asada, Y., S. Nakae, W. Ishida, K. Hori, J. Sugita, K. Sudo, K. Fukuda et al. 2015. Roles of epithelial cell-derived type 2-initiating cytokines in experimental allergic conjunctivitis. *Invest Ophthalmol Vis Sci* no. 56 (9):5194–202.

Baggiolini, M. and I. Clark-Lewis. 1992. Interleukin-8, a chemotactic and inflammatory cytokine. *FEBS Lett* no. 307 (1):97–101.

Balaji, S., A. King, E. Marsh, M. LeSaint, S. S. Bhattacharya, N. Han, Y. Dhamija et al. 2015. The role of interleukin-10 and hyaluronan in murine fetal fibroblast function *in vitro*: Implications for recapitulating fetal regenerative wound healing. *PLoS One* no. 10 (5):e0124302.

Ballotta, V., A. I. Smits, A. Driessen-Mol, C. V. Bouten, and F. P. Baaijens. 2014. Synergistic protein secretion by mesenchymal stromal cells seeded in 3D scaffolds and circulating leukocytes in physiological flow. *Biomaterials* no. 35 (33):9100–13.

Barrientos, S., H. Brem, O. Stojadinovic, and M. Tomic-Canic. 2014. Clinical application of growth factors and cytokines in wound healing. *Wound Repair Regen* no. 22 (5):569–78.

Barsky, L. E., J. E. Trainor, M. R. Torres, and B. E. Aguirre. 2007. Managing volunteers: FEMA's Urban Search and Rescue programme and interactions with unaffiliated responders in disaster response. *Disasters* no. 31 (4):495–507.

Bezbradica, J. S. and R. Medzhitov. 2009. Integration of cytokine and heterologous receptor signaling pathways. *Nat Immunol* no. 10 (4):333–9.

Brusnahan, S. K., T. R. McGuire, J. D. Jackson, J. T. Lane, K. L. Garvin, B. J. O'Kane, A. M. Berger, S. R. Tuljapurkar, M. A. Kessinger, and J. G. Sharp. 2010. Human blood and marrow side population stem cell and Stro-1 positive bone marrow stromal cell numbers decline with age, with an increase in quality of surviving stem cells: Correlation with cytokines. *Mech Ageing Dev* no. 131 (11–12):718–22.

Carneiro-Lobo, T. C., M. T. Lima, A. Mariano-Oliveira, A. Dutra-Oliveira, S. M. Oba-Shinjo, S. K. Marie, M. C. Sogayar, and R. Q. Monteiro. 2014. Expression of tissue factor signaling pathway elements correlates with the production of vascular endothelial growth factor and interleukin-8 in human astrocytoma patients. *Oncol Rep* no. 31 (2):679–86.

Chatterjee, P., V. L. Chiasson, K. R. Bounds, and B. M. Mitchell. 2014. Regulation of the anti-inflammatory cytokines interleukin-4 and interleukin-10 during pregnancy. *Front Immunol* no. 5:253.

Christenson, K., L. Bjorkman, A. Karlsson, and J. Bylund. 2013. Regulation of neutrophil apoptosis differs after *in vivo* transmigration to skin chambers and synovial fluid: A role for inflammasome-dependent interleukin-1beta release. *J Innate Immun* no. 5 (4):377–88.

Cornejo, M. C., S. K. Cho, C. Giannarelli, J. C. Iatridis, and D. Purmessur. 2015. Soluble factors from the notochordal-rich intervertebral disc inhibit endothelial cell invasion and vessel formation in the presence and absence of pro-inflammatory cytokines. *Osteoarthritis Cartilage* no. 23 (3):487–96.

De Nardo, D., C. M. De Nardo, and E. Latz. 2014. New insights into mechanisms controlling the NLRP3 inflammasome and its role in lung disease. *Am J Pathol* no. 184 (1):42–54.

Dreau, D., D. S. Morton, M. Foster, N. Fowler, and G. Sonnenfeld. 2000. Effects of 2-deoxy-D-glucose administration on cytokine production in BDF1 mice. *J Interferon Cytokine Res* no. 20 (2):247–55.

Estrada, M. F., S. P. Rebelo, E. J. Davies, M. T. Pinto, H. Pereira, V. E. Santo, M. J. Smalley et al. 2016. Modelling the tumour microenvironment in long-term microencapsulated 3D co-cultures recapitulates phenotypic features of disease progression. *Biomaterials* no. 78:50–61.

Fearon, W. F. and D. T. Fearon. 2008. Inflammation and cardiovascular disease: Role of the interleukin-1 receptor antagonist. *Circulation* no. 117 (20):2577–9.

Fischer, J. A., A. J. Hueber, S. Wilson, M. Galm, W. Baum, C. Kitson, J. Auer et al. 2015. Combined inhibition of tumor necrosis factor alpha and interleukin-17 as a therapeutic opportunity in rheumatoid arthritis: Development and characterization of a novel bispecific antibody. *Arthritis Rheumatol* no. 67 (1):51–62.

Fong, E. L., M. Martinez, J. Yang, A. G. Mikos, N. M. Navone, D. A. Harrington, and M. C. Farach-Carson. 2014. Hydrogel-based 3D model of patient-derived prostate xenograft tumors suitable for drug screening. *Mol Pharm* no. 11 (7):2040–50.

Foxman, E. F., E. J. Kunkel, and E. C. Butcher. 1999. Integrating conflicting chemotactic signals. The role of memory in leukocyte navigation. *J Cell Biol* no. 147 (3):577–88.

Gahler, A., T. Stallmach, J. Schwaller, M. F. Fey, and A. Tobler. 2000. Interleukin-8 expression by fetal and neonatal pulmonary cells in hyaline membrane disease and amniotic infection. *Pediatr Res* no. 48 (3):299–303.

Genovese, M. C., M. Greenwald, C. S. Cho, A. Berman, L. Jin, G. S. Cameron, O. Benichou et al. 2014. A phase II randomized study of subcutaneous ixekizumab, an anti-interleukin-17 monoclonal antibody, in rheumatoid arthritis patients who were naive to biologic agents or had an inadequate response to tumor necrosis factor inhibitors. *Arthritis Rheumatol* no. 66 (7):1693–704.

Griffith, L. G. and M. A. Swartz. 2006. Capturing complex 3D tissue physiology *in vitro*. *Nat Rev Mol Cell Biol* no. 7 (3):211–24.

Heit, B., S. Tavener, E. Raharjo, and P. Kubes. 2002. An intracellular signaling hierarchy determines direction of migration in opposing chemotactic gradients. *J Cell Biol* no. 159 (1):91–102.

Henkler, F., B. Baumann, M. Fotin-Mleczek, M. Weingartner, R. Schwenzer, N. Peters, A. Graness et al. 2003. Caspase-mediated cleavage converts the tumor necrosis factor (TNF) receptor-associated factor (TRAF)-1 from a selective modulator of TNF receptor signaling to a general inhibitor of NF-kappaB activation. *J Biol Chem* no. 278 (31):29216–30.

Hopkins, A. M., E. DeSimone, K. Chwalek, and D. L. Kaplan. 2015. 3D *in vitro* modeling of the central nervous system. *Prog Neurobiol* no. 125:1–25.

Huang, W. and A. August. 2015. The signaling symphony: T cell receptor tunes cytokine-mediated T cell differentiation. *J Leukoc Biol* no. 97 (3):477–85, doi: 10.1189/jlb.1RI0614-293R.

Ibusuki, K., T. Sakiyama, S. Kanmura, T. Maeda, Y. Iwashita, Y. Nasu, F. Sasaki et al. 2015. Human neutrophil peptides induce interleukin-8 in intestinal epithelial cells through the P2 receptor and ERK1/2 signaling pathways. *Int J Mol Med* no. 35 (6):1603–9, doi: 10.3892/ijmm.2015.2156.

Inman, J. L. and M. J. Bissell. 2010. Apical polarity in three-dimensional culture systems: Where to now? *J Biol* no. 9 (1):2.

Ito, T., S. Suzuki, S. Kanaji, H. Shiraishi, S. Ohta, K. Arima, G. Tanaka et al. 2009. Distinct structural requirements for interleukin-4 (IL-4) and IL-13 binding to the shared IL-13 receptor facilitate cellular tuning of cytokine responsiveness. *J Biol Chem* no. 284 (36):24289–96.

Iwata, Y. 2015. Three cases of previous smokers with rheumatoid arthritis who did not respond to tumor necrosis factor inhibitors were treated successfully with an anti-interleukin-6 receptor antibody. *Case Rep Rheumatol* no. 2015:806725.

Kajiwara, Y., S. Panchabhai, D. D. Liu, M. Kong, J. J. Lee, and V. A. Levin. 2009. Melding a new 3-dimensional agarose colony assay with the E(max) model to determine the effects of drug combinations on cancer cells. *Technol Cancer Res Treat* no. 8 (2):163–76.

Karagiannis, G. S., T. Poutahidis, S. E. Erdman, R. Kirsch, R. H. Riddell, and E. P. Diamandis. 2012. Cancer-associated fibroblasts drive the progression of metastasis through both paracrine and mechanical pressure on cancer tissue. *Mol Cancer Res* no. 10 (11):1403–18.

Kenny, P. A., G. Y. Lee, C. A. Myers, R. M. Neve, J. R. Semeiks, P. T. Spellman, K. Lorenz et al. 2007. The morphologies of breast cancer cell lines in three-dimensional assays correlate with their profiles of gene expression. *Mol Oncol* no. 1 (1):84–96.

King, S. N., S. E. Hanson, X. Chen, J. Kim, P. Hematti, and S. L. Thibeault. 2014. *In vitro* characterization of macrophage interaction with mesenchymal stromal cell-hyaluronan hydrogel constructs. *J Biomed Mater Res A* no. 102 (3):890–902.

Komatsu, T., Z. Bi, and C. S. Reiss. 1996. Interferon-gamma induced type I nitric oxide synthase activity inhibits viral replication in neurons. *J Neuroimmunol* no. 68 (1–2):101–8.

Koob, T. J., J. J. Lim, N. Zabek, and M. Massee. 2015. Cytokines in single layer amnion allografts compared to multilayer amnion/chorion allografts for wound healing. *J Biomed Mater Res B: Appl Biomater* no. 103 (5):1133–40.

Koul, D., Y. Takada, R. Shen, B. B. Aggarwal, and W. K. Yung. 2006. PTEN enhances TNF-induced apoptosis through modulation of nuclear factor-kappaB signaling pathway in human glioma cells. *Biochem Biophys Res Commun* no. 350 (2):463–71.

Lai, Y., A. Asthana, K. Cheng, and W. S. Kisaalita. 2011. Neural cell 3D microtissue formation is marked by cytokines' up-regulation. *PLoS One* no. 6 (10):e26821.

Lan, S. F. and B. Starly. 2011. Alginate based 3D hydrogels as an *in vitro* co-culture model platform for the toxicity screening of new chemical entities. *Toxicol Appl Pharmacol* no. 256 (1):62–72.

Lance, A., C. C. Yang, M. Swamydas, D. Dean, S. Deitch, K. J. Burg, and D. Dreau. 2016. Increased extracellular matrix density decreases MCF10A breast cell acinus formation in 3D culture conditions. *J Tissue Eng Regen Med* no. 10 (1):71–80.

Lee, Y. H., O. Shynlova, and S. J. Lye. 2015. Stretch-induced human myometrial cytokines enhance immune cell recruitment via endothelial activation. *Cell Mol Immunol* no. 12 (2):231–42.

Lehman, H. L., E. J. Dashner, M. Lucey, P. Vermeulen, L. Dirix, S. Van Laere, and K. L. van Golen. 2013. Modeling and characterization of inflammatory breast cancer emboli grown *in vitro*. *Int J Cancer* no. 132 (10):2283–94.

Leonard, F., H. Ali, E. M. Collnot, B. J. Crielaard, T. Lammers, G. Storm, and C. M. Lehr. 2012. Screening of budesonide nanoformulations for treatment of inflammatory bowel disease in an inflamed 3D cell-culture model. *Altex* no. 29 (3):275–85.

Leonard, W. J. and J. X. Lin. 2000. Cytokine receptor signaling pathways. *J Allergy Clin Immunol* no. 105 (5):877–88.

Li, G. X., S. S. Zhao, X. G. Zhang, W. H. Wang, J. Liu, K. W. Xue, X. Y. Li, Y. X. Guo, and L. H. Wang. 2015. Comparison of the proliferation, cytotoxic activity and cytokine secretion function of cascade primed immune cells and cytokine-induced killer cells *in vitro*. *Mol Med Rep* no. 12 (2):2629–35.

Locksley, R. M., N. Killeen, and M. J. Lenardo. 2001. The TNF and TNF receptor superfamilies: Integrating mammalian biology. *Cell* no. 104 (4):487–501.

Lombardo Bedran, T. B., D. Palomari Spolidorio, and D. Grenier. 2015. Green tea polyphenol epigallocatechin-3-gallate and cranberry proanthocyanidins act in synergy with cathelicidin (LL-37) to reduce the LPS-induced inflammatory response in a three-dimensional co-culture model of gingival epithelial cells and fibroblasts. *Arch Oral Biol* no. 60 (6):845–53.

Malpass, K. 2013. Neurodegenerative disease: A novel 3D culture model of tauopathy shows promise as a screening tool for Alzheimer disease therapies. *Nat Rev Neurol* no. 9 (1):2.

Maris, C. H., C. P. Chappell, and J. Jacob. 2007. Interleukin-10 plays an early role in generating virus-specific T cell anergy. *BMC Immunol* no. 8:8.

Marshak-Rothstein, A. 2006. Toll-like receptors in systemic autoimmune disease. *Nat Rev Immunol* no. 6 (11):823–35.

Martin, M. U. and H. Wesche. 2002. Summary and comparison of the signaling mechanisms of the Toll/interleukin-1 receptor family. *Biochim Biophys Acta* no. 1592 (3):265–80.

Medzhitov, R., E. M. Shevach, G. Trinchieri, A. L. Mellor, D. H. Munn, S. Gordon, P. Libby et al. 2011. Highlights of 10 years of immunology in Nature Reviews Immunology. *Nat Rev Immunol* no. 11 (10):693–702.

Meraz, I. M., B. Melendez, J. Gu, S. T. Wong, X. Liu, H. A. Andersson, and R. E. Serda. 2012. Activation of the inflammasome and enhanced migration of microparticle-stimulated dendritic cells to the draining lymph node. *Mol Pharm* no. 9 (7):2049–62.

Min, K. S., H. I. Kim, H. S. Chang, H. R. Kim, H. O. Pae, H. T. Chung, S. H. Hong et al. 2008. Involvement of mitogen-activated protein kinases and nuclear factor-kappa B activation in nitric oxide-induced interleukin-8 expression in human pulp cells. *Oral Surg Oral Med Oral Pathol Oral Radiol Endod* no. 105 (5):654–60.

Munoz-Canoves, P., C. Scheele, B. K. Pedersen, and A. L. Serrano. 2013. Interleukin-6 myokine signaling in skeletal muscle: A double-edged sword? *FEBS J* no. 280 (17):4131–48.

Niikura, K., T. Matsunaga, T. Suzuki, S. Kobayashi, H. Yamaguchi, Y. Orba, A. Kawaguchi et al. 2013. Gold nanoparticles as a vaccine platform: Influence of size and shape on immunological responses *in vitro* and *in vivo*. *ACS Nano* no. 7 (5):3926–38.

Pantschenko, A. G., I. Pushkar, K. H. Anderson, Y. Wang, L. J. Miller, S. H. Kurtzman, G. Barrows, and D. L. Kreutzer. 2003. The interleukin-1 family of cytokines and receptors in human breast cancer: Implications for tumor progression. *Int J Oncol* no. 23 (2):269–84.

Peeters, P. M., I. M. Eurlings, T. N. Perkins, E. F. Wouters, R. P. Schins, P. J. Borm, W. Drommer, N. L. Reynaert, and C. Albrecht. 2014. Silica-induced NLRP3 inflammasome activation *in vitro* and in rat lungs. *Part Fibre Toxicol* no. 11:58.

Petersen, O. W., L. Ronnov-Jessen, A. R. Howlett, and M. J. Bissell. 1992. Interaction with basement membrane serves to rapidly distinguish growth and differentiation pattern of normal and malignant human breast epithelial cells. *Proc Natl Acad Sci USA* no. 89 (19):9064–8.

Rath, P. C. and B. B. Aggarwal. 1999. TNF-induced signaling in apoptosis. *J Clin Immunol* no. 19 (6):350–64.

Rego, S. L., R. S. Helms, and D. Dreau. 2014. Tumor necrosis factor-alpha-converting enzyme activities and tumor-associated macrophages in breast cancer. *Immunol Res* no. 58 (1):87–100.

Rego, S. L., S. Raghavan, E. Zakhem, and K. N. Bitar. 2015. Enteric neural differentiation in innervated, physiologically functional, smooth muscle constructs is modulated by bone morphogenic protein 2 secreted by sphincteric smooth muscle cells. *J Tissue Eng Regen Med*, doi: 10.1002/term.2027.

Rego, S. L., E. Zakhem, G. Orlando, and K. N. Bitar. 2016. Bioengineering functional human sphincteric and non-sphincteric gastrointestinal smooth muscle constructs. *Methods* no. 99:128–34.

Rifkin, I. R., E. A. Leadbetter, L. Busconi, G. Viglianti, and A. Marshak-Rothstein. 2005. Toll-like receptors, endogenous ligands, and systemic autoimmune disease. *Immunol Rev* no. 204:27–42.

Riley, J. K., K. Takeda, S. Akira, and R. D. Schreiber. 1999. Interleukin-10 receptor signaling through the JAK-STAT pathway. Requirement for two distinct receptor-derived signals for anti-inflammatory action. *J Biol Chem* no. 274 (23):16513–21.

Rouaud-Tinguely, P., D. Boudier, L. Marchand, V. Barruche, S. Bordes, H. Coppin, M. P. Roth, and B. Closs. 2015. From the morphological to the transcriptomic characterization of a compromised three-dimensional *in vitro* model mimicking atopic dermatitis. *Br J Dermatol* no. 173 (4):1006–14.

Sakai, Y., E. Nemoto, S. Kanaya, M. Shimonishi, and H. Shimauchi. 2014. Calcium phosphate particles induce interleukin-8 expression in a human gingival epithelial cell line via the nuclear factor-kappaB signaling pathway. *J Periodontol* no. 85 (10):1464–73.

Scheller, J., A. Chalaris, D. Schmidt-Arras, and S. Rose-John. 2011. The pro- and anti-inflammatory properties of the cytokine interleukin-6. *Biochim Biophys Acta* no. 1813 (5):878–88.

Schmidhauser, C., G. F. Casperson, C. A. Myers, K. T. Sanzo, S. Bolten, and M. J. Bissell. 1992. A novel transcriptional enhancer is involved in the prolactin- and extracellular matrix-dependent regulation of beta-casein gene expression. *Mol Biol Cell* no. 3 (6):699–709.

Schneiders, J., F. Fuchs, J. Damm, C. Herden, R. Gerstberger, D. M. Soares, J. Roth, and C. Rummel. 2015. The transcription factor nuclear factor interleukin 6 mediates pro- and anti-inflammatory responses during LPS-induced systemic inflammation in mice. *Brain Behav Immun* no. 48:147–64.

Schroder, K., P. J. Hertzog, T. Ravasi, and D. A. Hume. 2004. Interferon-gamma: An overview of signals, mechanisms and functions. *J Leukoc Biol* no. 75 (2):163–89.

Shouval, D. S., A. Biswas, J. A. Goettel, K. McCann, E. Conaway, N. S. Redhu, I. D. Mascanfroni et al. 2014. Interleukin-10 receptor signaling in innate immune cells regulates mucosal immune tolerance and anti-inflammatory macrophage function. *Immunity* no. 40 (5):706–19.

Shouval, D. S., J. Ouahed, A. Biswas, J. A. Goettel, B. H. Horwitz, C. Klein, A. M. Muise, and S. B. Snapper. 2014. Interleukin 10 receptor signaling: Master regulator of intestinal mucosal homeostasis in mice and humans. *Adv Immunol* no. 122:177–210.

Streuli, C. H., N. Bailey, and M. J. Bissell. 1991. Control of mammary epithelial differentiation: Basement membrane induces tissue-specific gene expression in the absence of cell–cell interaction and morphological polarity. *J Cell Biol* no. 115 (5):1383–95.

Streuli, C. H. and M. J. Bissell. 1991. Mammary epithelial cells, extracellular matrix, and gene expression. *Cancer Treat Res* no. 53:365–81.

Sun, L., X. Wang, and D. L. Kaplan. 2011. A 3D cartilage–inflammatory cell culture system for the modeling of human osteoarthritis. *Biomaterials* no. 32 (24):5581–9.

Tanaka, N., Y. Hoshino, J. Gold, S. Hoshino, F. Martiniuk, T. Kurata, R. Pine, D. Levy, W. N. Rom, and M. Weiden. 2005. Interleukin-10 induces inhibitory C/EBPbeta through STAT-3 and represses HIV-1 transcription in macrophages. *Am J Respir Cell Mol Biol* no. 33 (4):406–11.

Trifunovic, J., L. Miller, Z. Debeljak, and V. Horvat. 2015. Pathologic patterns of interleukin 10 expression—a review. *Biochem Med (Zagreb)* no. 25 (1):36–48.

von Haehling, S., K. Wolk, C. Hoflich, S. Kunz, B. H. Grunberg, W. D. Docke, U. Reineke et al. 2015. Interleukin-10 receptor-1 expression in monocyte-derived antigen-presenting cell populations: Dendritic cells partially escape from IL-10's inhibitory mechanisms. *Genes Immun* no. 16 (1):8–14.

von Pawel, J., J. H. Harvey, D. R. Spigel, M. Dediu, M. Reck, C. L. Cebotaru, R. C. Humphreys, M. J. Gribbin, N. L. Fox, and D. R. Camidge. 2014. Phase II trial of mapatumumab, a fully human agonist monoclonal antibody to tumor necrosis factor-related apoptosis-inducing ligand receptor 1 (TRAIL-R1), in combination with paclitaxel and carboplatin in patients with advanced non-small-cell lung cancer. *Clin Lung Cancer* no. 15 (3):188–96.e2.

Wajant, H., K. Pfizenmaier, and P. Scheurich. 2003. Tumor necrosis factor signaling. *Cell Death Differ* no. 10 (1):45–65.

Watkins, L. R., S. F. Maier, and L. E. Goehler. 1995. Immune activation: The role of pro-inflammatory cytokines in inflammation, illness responses and pathological pain states. *Pain* no. 63 (3):289–302.

Xu, N., X. Ye, D. Wei, J. Zhong, Y. Chen, G. Xu, and D. He. 2014. 3D artificial bones for bone repair prepared by computed tomography-guided fused deposition modeling for bone repair. *ACS Appl Mater Interfaces* no. 6 (17):14952–63.

Zdzisinska, B., J. Rolinski, T. Piersiak, and M. Kandefer-Szerszen. 2009. A comparison of cytokine production in 2-dimensional and 3-dimensional cultures of bone marrow stromal cells of multiple myeloma patients in response to RPMI8226 myeloma cells. *Folia Histochem Cytobiol* no. 47 (1):69–74.

Zhang, J. M. and J. An. 2007. Cytokines, inflammation, and pain. *Int Anesthesiol Clin* no. 45 (2):27–37.

Zhang, X., D. R. Hinton, D. J. Cua, S. A. Stohlman, and M. M. Lai. 1997. Expression of interferon-gamma by a coronavirus defective-interfering RNA vector and its effect on viral replication, spread, and pathogenicity. *Virology* no. 233 (2):327–38.

Zlotnik, A. and O. Yoshie. 2000. Chemokines: A new classification system and their role in immunity. *Immunity* no. 12 (2):121–7.

13 Cell–Cell Communications through Gap Junctions and Cancer in 3D Systems

Stephanie Nicole Shishido and
Thu Annelise Nguyen

CONTENTS

13.1 Introduction 233
13.2 Intercellular Communication..234
13.3 Gap Junctional Intercellular Communication..234
13.4 Gap Junctions/Connexins in Cancer Initiation and Promotion 237
13.5 Gap Junctions/Connexins in Cancer Progression..240
13.6 Gap Junctions/Connexins in 3D Systems 240
13.7 Conclusion and Perspective 242
References..242

13.1 INTRODUCTION

Two-dimensional (2D) substrates, such as tissue culture polystyrene and the surface of tissue analogs, make an enormous contribution to modern *in vitro* cell studies; however, traditional 2D platforms cannot accurately mimic the complex 3D architecture of the extracellular matrix (ECM) where native cells reside. In 2D culture, cell monolayers experience media and growth factors in bulk with homogenous concentration of nutrients and growth factors that induce artificial cell environments and cell–cell interactions, yielding a flat and stretched morphology. Recent studies have shown that the morphological differences of cells cultured in 2D and 3D can also exhibit several striking differences in subtle cellular processes, such as proliferation, apoptosis, differentiation, gene expression, migration, and drug sensitivies (Chitcholtan et al. 2012; He et al. 2014; Imamura et al. 2015). The *in vitro* 3D model system provides an alternative to poorly representative 2D systems and animal models that are expensive, time-consuming, and ethically challenging. Indeed, the 3D model systems can account for both the ECM complexity and the relevant physiology of different *in vivo* organs. In this chapter, the role of gap junctions in cell-to-cell communication, especially in cancer initiation and progression, is reviewed with a focus on 3D systems.

13.2 INTERCELLULAR COMMUNICATION

Multicellular organisms are composed of complex networks of cells that form tissues and organs to perform specific functions in maintaining homeostasis. Optimal cell, tissue, and organ functions depend on maintaining the limits of the internal environment, which involves a variety of regulatory mechanisms and the co-ordination of a vast number of physiological activities, such as intermediary metabolism, cellular communication, cell growth, and cell differentiation. Cells are able to communicate with one another by releasing soluble factors that affect other cells either locally or distantly. There are several modes of transmitting information between cells: direct communication between adjacent cells, autocrine and paracrine signaling, and neurotransmitters and hormones produced by neurons and endocrine cells, respectively (Brucher and Jamall 2014; Howard and Baudino 2014).

Adjacent cells may be connected to each other through tight junction, desmosomes, gap junctions, and adherens to facilitate passage of signaling molecules from cell to cell (Dréau 2010). Tight junctions, or zonula occludens, form a virtually impermeable barrier to fluid between closely associated cells by joining the membranes together. These are typically more apically located. Desmosomes, or macula adherens, support cell–cell adhesion by attaching to intermediate filaments of keratin in the cytosol. Adherens, or zonula adherens, form strong mechanical attachments by forming a bridge connecting the actin cytoskeleton of neighboring cells. These protein complexes are composed of cadherins and catenins, and are usually more basally located. Gap junctions form direct intracellular connections between adjacent cells allowing for intercellular communication via the transfer of low molecular weight molecules.

The integrity of epithelial cell layers is maintained by tight junctions, adherens, and desmosomes, whereas gap junctions provide a route for intercellular communication, allowing a single cell to directly influence the behavior of neighboring cells in a specific manner. Intercellular communication between groups of specialized cells within organs/tissues regulates proliferation, apoptosis, and differentiation to maintain tissue homeostasis.

13.3 GAP JUNCTIONAL INTERCELLULAR COMMUNICATION

Gap junctions consist of aggregated transmembrane proteins that form channels between adjacent cells directly connecting their cytoplasms. Unlike other modes of intercellular communication, gap junctions are present in all animals and provide direct exchange of molecular signals between cells. Gap junctions are present in all vertebrate cell types, with a few exceptions: red blood cell, platelets, some neurons, mature skeletal muscle fibers, and spermatozoids (Willecke et al. 2002). The diffusion of molecules between adjacent cells through gap junctions is termed gap junctional intercellular communication (GJIC). This process is vital in maintaining homeostasis, synchronizing cellular activities, and regulating proliferation and apoptosis (Ruch 1994). GJIC is critical for normal embryogenesis and development, neural activity, gamete production, endocrine function, immune function, smooth muscle function, and cardiovascular function. For example, smooth muscle cells express connexin that mediates Ca^{2+} movement between cells, leading to smooth muscle cell contraction (Halidi et al. 2012; Lagaud et al. 2002). Defects in GJIC can lead to teratogenesis, neuropathy, infertility, diabetes, autoimmunity, atherosclerosis, and cancer (Trosko et al. 1998; Saez et al. 2003).

Gap junctions are protein channels made of the protein connexin (Cx). Connexins have four hydrophobic membrane spanning domains: two conserved, extracellular domains involved in paired hemichannel docking and three cytoplasmic domains (Figure 13.1) (Saez et al. 2003). Intercellular channels are formed through oligomerization of six connexins into a hexameric hemichannel called a connexon, which is trafficked to the plasma membrane. Hemichannels allow communication between cytoplasm and extracellular space. On the membrane, the connexon floats laterally until it docks with a second connexon on the adjacent cell to form an intact gap junction channel. Groups of these channels form gap junctional plaques, allowing the flow of small molecules between the cytosol of neighboring cells.

The cytoplasmic regions of the connexin have variable amino acid sequences, leading to different connexin types (Bennett et al. 1991). Vertebrates have approximately 20 different connexins (Willecke et al. 2002; Goodenough and Paul 2003; Saez et al. 2003), commonly designated with numerical suffixes identifying the molecular weight of the sequence in kilodaltons (kDa) (Saez et al. 2003). Vertebrate gap junctions have a permeability size of 1.2 kDa, allowing amino acids, sugars, nucleotides, most secondary messengers, water, and other small molecules to diffuse between cells (Simon et al. 1997; Willecke et al. 2002; Saez et al. 2003). This allows adjacent cells to share a common intracellular environment through the formation

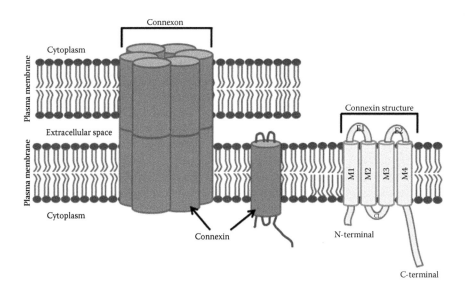

FIGURE 13.1 Structure of the gap junction. Connexins have four transmembrane domains (M1–M4) with the C and N cytoplasmic termini, a cytoplasmic loop (CL) and two extracellular loops (E1 and E2). The connexon is formed from the assembly of six connexins. Two connexons come together to form the gap junction.

of gap junctions. GJIC provides cells a route to share information to function as a single metabolic unit, creating a local environment that leads to regional functionality (Kam et al. 1986).

Gap junction channels are not typically formed exclusively of one connexin subtype (homotypic), but rather consist of multiple distinct connexin isoforms forming a heteromeric channel (Wang and Peracchia 1998). The formation of heteromeric connexons increases the complexity of regulation. GJIC is regulated by activation of protein kinases (Shi et al. 2001; Duncan and Fletcher 2002; Cottrell et al. 2003) and protein phosphatases (John et al. 2003). Phosphorylation induces channel gating: The molecular transition leads to gap junction channel opening or closing (Kanno et al. 1984; Azarnia et al. 1988). Channels are regulated by various stimuli, including changes in pH, voltage, and phosphorylation stage of the C-terminal tail (Simon et al. 1997; Lampe and Lau 2000; Willecke et al. 2002; Saez et al. 2003). Biological studies in the 3D model system require a specific condition in order to be able to preserve the structure and function of gap junction channels. Mammalian cells need the basic nutrients for growth, including amino acids, monosaccharides, vitamins, hormones, osmotic pressure, and suitable pH. Thus, the changes in these nutrients play a significant role in the regulation of gap junction channels.

Furthermore, the connexin proteins are regulated by protein kinases that phosphorylate serine and threonine residues of the connexin carboxyl terminal region (Lampe and Lau 2004; Warn-Cramer and Lau 2004). Studies have shown that the mitogen-activated protein kinase (MAPK) and protein kinase C (PKC) mediate phosphorylation of the C-terminal end to close Cx43 hemichannels (Goodenough and Paul 2003). Phosphorylation of gap junctions occurs after membrane insertion and deposition into gap junction plaques (Musil and Goodenough 1991).

There are three kinetic routes of gap junctional control: fast, intermediate, and long-term. The fast control involves gating responses that result in an effect within milliseconds of the initial response. These immediate effects may be the result of rapid changes in ion concentration, pH, protein kinases, phosphatases, or lipid composition of the membrane (Crow et al. 1990; Hyrc and Rose 1990; Malewicz et al. 1990). The intermediate control is conducted by vesicular withdrawal or insertion of connexins in the membrane, which takes minutes. This is possible due to a perimembrane pool of connexins that is present within cytoplasmic vesicles, determined by the observation that connexins can be inserted into the plasma membrane despite the presence of inhibitors of protein synthesis (Epstein and Gilula 1977). Last, the long-term control is regulated at a transcriptional level, where connexin mRNA is altered, adjusting the connexin protein pools within the cell. This takes hours from the initial stimuli. Gap junctions are dynamic plasma membrane structures with rapid turnover rates (Jordan et al. 1999; Gaietta et al. 2002; Lauf et al. 2002). The half-life of the connexin protein is between 2 and 5 h in cultured cells and tissues (Crow et al. 1990; Musil et al. 1990; Laird et al. 1991; Lampe 1994; Beardslee et al. 1998). There is controversy as to whether all the connexin proteins are conventionally synthesized in the endoplasmic reticulum, transported through the Golgi, and exported to the plasma membrane.

Gap junctions provide regional functions. First, they buffer the harmful effects of xenobiotic metabolites by dispersing them outward from the exposure point into the tissue. Pinto and colleagues (2010) demonstrated that normal human skin fibroblast cells preassembled with functional gap junctions and structural/functional extracellular matrix in 3D cultures produced bystander signaling and the consequent signal transduction. The reverse effect is often seen in the 3D system of cancerous cells in which the effect of anticancer drug is significantly lower under 3D culture conditions compared to that under 2D culture conditions (Bohovic et al. 2015). Second, healthy cells can provide nourishment for deprived or sick cells through shared metabolites. This gives the tissue plasticity as long as there is functional GJIC. However, the loss of GJIC in cancer cells (Loewenstein 1979; Yamasaki and Naus 1996) is one of the reasons why the positive anticancer effect observed in 2D cultures often failed during *in vivo* testing. Third, they function in the rapid exchange of electrical signals and regulators. Fourth, they distribute metabolites vital for cellular proliferation/health (i.e., cAMP). This is important in that not all cells within a tissue have the same metabolic capacity, requiring that essential metabolites are shared between cells (Peterson 1983). Last, gap junctions function to eliminate waste or unwanted byproducts.

13.4 GAP JUNCTIONS/CONNEXINS IN CANCER INITIATION AND PROMOTION

Defects in critical signaling pathways that regulate cellular properties, such as proliferation, differentiation, and apoptosis, result in the formation of cancer. Tumorigenesis may be affected by secondary mechanisms not related to direct gene damage (Lijinsky 1989, 1990; Trosko 1989). This is a category of carcinogens classified as nongenotoxic, which indirectly stimulate hyperplastic growth, without altering DNA sequence or structure. Nongenotoxic carcinogens elicit a mechanism of cancer induction that includes receptor- and nonreceptor-mediated endocrine modulation, tumor promoters, toxicity responses, inflammatory responses, or deficiencies in GJIC. Many nongenotoxic carcinogens inhibit or reduce GJIC, including chlordane (Rivedal and Witz 2005), 2,3,7,8-tetrachlorodibenzodioxin (TCDD) (Gakhar et al. 2009), dichlorodiphenyltrichloroethane (DDT) (IARC 1991), phenobarbital (IARC 1991), and acetamide (IARC 1999). The absence of genotoxicity and the tendency of being tissue specific make nongenotoxic mechanisms challenging to identify and characterize.

A deficiency in GJIC affects tumorigenesis in two main ways: (1) the loss of GJIC leads to a lack of homeostasis resulting in cellular damage and (2) excessive proliferation may occur due to hormones, metabolites, or secondary messengers not being effectively distributed to adjacent cells. Tumor formation is a multistage process in which epithelial cells go through series of changes forming multiple premalignant phenotypes, ultimately developing into an invasive cancer (Figure 13.2). Loewenstein and Kanno (1966) first reported a lack of electrical coupling in rat hepatomas. This was observed in chemically induced and transplanted hepatomas (Loewenstein and Kanno 1966; Loewenstein and Kanno 1967), which differed significantly from the normally well-coupled liver cells. Similar results were obtained in transplanted thyroid tumors (Jamakosmanovic and Loewenstein 1968) and carcinomas of the stomach (Kanno and Matsui 1968). The lack of electrical coupling

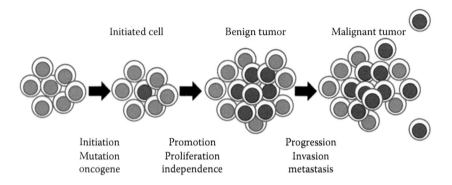

FIGURE 13.2 The stages of tumorigenesis. A tumor is generated by a three-step process: initiation, promotion, and progression. Blue represents the normal healthy cell. Red indicates a cell that has been transformed through either genomic instability or oncogenic activation.

soon became a common characteristic found in solid tumors, whether chemically induced, transplanted, or spontaneously formed. This was true for various species across an array of tissue types.

Multiple studies confirmed that a deficiency in gap junctions, and thus GJIC, is associated with the cancer phenotype (Loewenstein 1979; Yamasaki and Naus 1996; Mesnil 2002). There is a clear correlation between reduced GJIC and the promotion and progression stages of cancer formation (Trosko and Chang 1985; Nicolson 1987; Ruch et al. 1987; Trosko 1988, 1989; Trosko and Chang 1989; Yamasaki 1990; Krutovskikh et al. 1991). Inhibition of GJIC in initiated tissue, that is, which have initiated cells, leads to tumor promotion of a chemically induced carcinogenesis (Murray and Fitzgerald 1979; Yotti et al. 1979; Mesnil et al. 1988; Yamasaki 1990). Many tumor-promoting agents have been found to be inhibitors of GJIC (Murray and Fitzgerald 1979; Yotti et al. 1979; Budunova and Williams 1994), reinforcing the hypothesis that a deficiency of GJIC leads to tumorigenesis. Most known oncogenes (i.e., *ras, raf, neu, src*) downregulate GJIC, whereas tumor suppressor genes upregulate GJIC (Ruch 1994; Zhang et al. 1994; Na et al. 2000). In primary cells isolated from human breast cancer (Lee et al. 1992), rat mammary carcinomas (Laird et al. 1999), and transformed breast cancer cell lines (Laird et al. 1999; Singal et al. 2000), a deficiency in Cx26 and Cx43 has been observed. In fact, cell lines are known to have less gap junctions than their corresponding normal tissue cells (Enomoto and Yamasaki 1985; Yamasaki and Katoh 1988). There is a distinct inverse relationship between cell growth and GJIC in transformed cell lines, where the induction of GJIC leads to the inhibition of growth, whereas the inhibition of GJIC promotes cellular proliferation (Mehta et al. 1986).

Loss of connexin is an early event in cancer development, though researchers have been unable to clearly identify at which stage of tumorigenesis the decreased expression of connexins occurs. There are two routes to explain this early development: (1) clonal expansion of adult stem cells that do not express connexins, therefore, resulting in a lack of GJIC at very early stages; or (2) differential expression of connexins after initiation, in that the expression level and/or function is reduced by the onset of oncogenic activities as malignancy progresses (Mesnil et al. 2005). This second explanation covers why only some cancers express connexins at early stages. In many cancer cases, loss of connexin expression is observed during dysplasia of the precancerous lesion, such as a reduction in Cx43 in cervical dysplasia (King et al. 2000). In addition in lobular or ductal mammary carcinomas, Cx43 is not detectable, indicating that Cx43 is a marker for early oncogenesis (Laird et al. 1999). Reduced connexin expression may also be observed in the later stages of tumorigenesis. As an example, there is a decrease in Cx43 expression during the late stages of prostate cancer, but not in the benign stages (Tsai et al. 1996). This observation indicates that loss of connexin expression in not required for initiation of prostate cancer (Tsai et al. 1996). In support of the hypothesis that loss of GJIC is important in carcinogenesis, there are studies showing that re-expression of connexins in cancer cells causes normalization of cell growth control and reduced tumor growth. In normal mammary tissue, Cx26 is not detected, but it is upregulated in invasive breast carcinoma lesions (Jamieson et al. 1998).

The observable lack of GJIC in neoplastic cells is not only due to a lack of connexin expression, but also due to aberrant localization of connexin proteins. Many studies demonstrate expression of connexins in neoplastic cells, but abnormally located in the cytoplasm *in vitro* and *in vivo*. In more than 50% of invasive breast carcinomas, Cx26 is located in the cytoplasm (Jamieson et al. 1998), whereas about 90% of advanced grade tumors have cytoplasmic expression of Cx43 (Kanczuga-Koda et al. 2005). Cx32 has been shown to be cytoplasmic in liver cancer cell lines and tumors (Yano et al. 2001). This is also true for chemically induced tumors, in which Cx32 and Cx26 have been identified to be cytoplasmically located in 7,12-dimethylbenz(a) anthracene (DMBA)-induced rat hepatomas (Neveu et al. 1994). Aberrant connexin localization may be due to impaired trafficking of connexins to the membrane. This is seen with human colon cancer cells, which express Cx43 cytoplasmically, and the overexpression of Cx43 via transfection of cDNA does not improve localization at the membrane or restore GJIC (McMasters et al. 1998). Other reports have suggested that it may be due to a lack of cell–cell recognition. Neoplasms often show a decrease in E-cadherin, a cell–cell recognition transmembrane protein, which is lost with a transition in phenotype. Overexpression of E-cadherin produces a more epithelial phenotype with restoration of GJIC (Mege et al. 1988). In addition, nuclear localization of connexins has been reported, but no reasonable explanation has been provided. Specifically, Cx43 is localized in the nucleus in rat liver cells that have been transformed by the oncogenes *src* or *neu* (de Feijter et al. 1996). In addition, in HeLa human cervical cancer cells, the Cx43 carboxyl terminus is anchored in the nucleus, inhibiting cellular proliferation (Dang et al. 2003).

The alterations in the expression levels of connexin proteins may be due to genetic mutations in the neoplastic cells, such as a series of mutations in a tumor suppressor gene, or a specific gene mutation that affects connexin production (Mesnil 2002). Mutations in tumor suppressor genes may lead to a lack of connexin expression directly by altering the gene sequence, or indirectly via changes in regulatory factors. An example of the indirect route is in liver tumors where altered expression of the transcription factor hepatocyte nuclear factor 1α (HNF-1α) downregulated Cx32 (Flodby et al. 1995; Kalkuhl et al. 1996; Wang et al. 1998). Alterations in the expression of connexins may also be due to mutations in the noncoding sequence of the genes, thus, modulating the regulation of expression.

13.5 GAP JUNCTIONS/CONNEXINS IN CANCER PROGRESSION

Metastasis is a complex process involving cellular dissociation, tissue invasion, transport of metastatic cells via blood or lymph, extravasation to a distant site, and formation of a secondary tumor. Loss of GJIC has been observed in metastatic disease (Nicolson et al. 1988; Behrens et al. 1989; Klaunig et al. 1990; Ren et al. 1990; Yamasaki 1990; Birchmeier et al. 1991). There are two steps in which gap junctions play a role in metastasis: (1) cellular dissociation and invasion and (2) extravasation at the secondary site. Evidence indicates that a loss of GJIC correlates with metastatic potential of the primary tumor. In a metastatic breast cancer cell line, transfection with the breast metastasis suppressor 1 (BRMS1) complementary DNA (cDNA) restores GJIC by increasing Cx43 expression and reducing Cx32, resulting in a more normal phenotype (Saunders et al. 2001). E-cadherin expression also correlates positively with GJIC (Mege et al. 1988; Jongen et al. 1991). A reduction in E-cadherin indicates a loss of co-operation between neighboring cells and reduced GJIC, leading to cellular dissociation in invasive tumors.

Interestingly, low metastatic potential cells do not establish functional GJIC with the surrounding cells, but highly malignant mammary carcinoma or melanoma rat cells have been shown to readily transfer dye to endothelial cells at a secondary site (el-Sabban and Pauli 1991). Extravasation of malignant cells involves diapedesis across the endothelial barrier into the tissue prior to secondary tumor formation. This has been observed in breast cancer cells, which require GJIC between tumor cells and endothelial cells at the secondary site (Kanczuga-Koda et al. 2005; Pollmann et al. 2005). El-Sabban and Pauli showed an increase in cellular adhesion and communication by highly metastatic lung carcinoma cells, presumably to facilitate extravasation during the metastatic process (el-Sabban and Pauli 1994). These studies exemplify the importance of GJIC in the establishment of metastatic foci, though more research is needed into the role of gap junctions in extravasation. During the process of metastasis, data suggests a change in connexin profile from a loss of GJIC during tissue invasion to functional GJIC during extravasation.

13.6 GAP JUNCTIONS/CONNEXINS IN 3D SYSTEMS

The importance of 3D systems is becoming evident as more and more studies benefit from the biomaterials that gives us more control over the microenvironment of a tissue. Current approaches for the development of *in vitro* tumor models aim to recapitulate the native microenvironment of gap junctions *in vivo* using 3D scaffolds in order to create better preclinical cancer models. Studies of human glioma U118 spheroid demonstrated that pharmacological inhibitor of gap junctions or silencing connexin 43 expression increases cell migration from the spheroid (Aftab, Sin, and Naus 2015). Furthermore, overexpression of Cx43 in human mammary adenocarcinoma,

MDA-MB-231, cells decreased cell growth in 3D cultures and associated with β-catenin, α-catenin, and ZO-2 (Talhouk et al. 2013). In addition, Cx43 silencing induced a change in 3D growth morphology of MCF10A, non-neoplastic human breast cell, colonies where there is an evident shift from the spheroid colonies to tubular connected growth morphology (Talhouk et al. 2013). Interestingly, the levels of c-myc and cyclin-D1 were slightly downregulated in 3D cultures of MDA-MB-231 cells compared to a significant decrease in p21 levels (Syed-Picard et al. 2013). This finding demonstrated that cyclin-D1 protein expression levels were decreased on in 3D cultures of MDA-MB-231 cells in line with the previous studies as an alteration in cyclin-D1 is caused by G_0/G_1 arrest (Weng et al. 2002).

Layered cardiomyocyte sheets directly onto the heart surface promote mesothelial cell trans-differentiation and cardiomyocyte, bridging the intact areas and subsequently leading to functional gap junction formation (Sekine et al. 2006). Earlier work also showed that engineered 3D heart tissues by gelling a mixture of cardiomyocytes and liquid collagen promote formation of gap junctions/connexins between grafts and the host myocardium (Zimmermann et al. 2002). Sekine and coworkers demonstrated that the migration of bridging cardiomyocytes mainly occurred from the tissue graft into the heart. This may due to the immaturity of the bioengineered myocardial tissue grafts, which were composed of neonatal cardiomyocytes. Furthermore, random migration and extension of graft cardiomyocytes may occasionally contact cardiomyocytes of the hearts and form functional gap junctions (Sekine et al. 2006). Bioengineered 3D tissue graft model contributes to the improvement of the damaged heart function via gap junction communication between graft and host.

A scaffoldless 3D model has been used to provide a proper spatial organization during tissue development in part cell–cell interactions in human dental pulp cells (Syed-Picard et al. 2013). Scaffoldless self-assembled 3D constructs are formed by first culturing cells to confluence on a 2D substrate and monolayers of cell sheet self-assemble into a solid cylindrical tissue anchored to the plate by the pins (Hairfield-Stein et al. 2007). During development, gap junction channels provide a conduit for molecules to form expression gradients in a community of cells (Loewenstein 1979). Syed-Picard and colleagues (2013) showed that Cx43 is necessary for proper bone and dentin differentiation from bone marrow stromal cell and dental pulp cells in scaffoldless 3D culture. Thus, scaffolding material can affect cellular functions and should be taken in consideration when selecting material for tissue engineering component.

Research in the field of pancreatic β-cells showed that the 3D culture system produced more insulin-secreting cells than the traditional 2D monolayer system and promoted differentiated cells form islet-like tissue structures with greater similarities to adult pancreatic islets (Bhandari et al. 2011; Guo-Parke et al. 2012). Communication between β cells suppressed basal insulin secretion but enhanced glucose-stimulated insulin secretion (GSIS) (Ravier et al. 2005; Luther et al. 2006). Mouse insulioma 6 (NIN6) cells in the 3D culture system had an increase in Cx36 gene expression and more gap junction formation by Cx36 (Liu et al. 2014). Furthermore, Liu and coworkers demonstrated that Cx36 protein was involved in aggregate formation and insulin secretion under the 3D culture system.

13.7 CONCLUSION AND PERSPECTIVE

Recent studies of soft sarcoma cell lines in the 3D systems provided insight into the changes of GJ genes. Analysis of gap junction molecules showed significant changes in the gene and protein expression profiles under 3D conditions. These changes affected cell-to-cell communication and were mainly associated with biological processes such as cell proliferation and apoptosis. Human osteosarcoma, HOSS1, cells in 3D cultures showed an abundant expression of Cx26, Cx43, and Cx45 compared to the absent in 2D cultures (Bai et al. 2015). As previously indicated, gap junction molecules such as Cx43 contribute to cell–cell interactions and their expression differs in various cell types. Currently, it is unknown why re-expression of connexins occurs in 3D culture of HOSS1 cell spheroid. Thus, the 3D systems are being increasingly employed in cancer research, as well as in tissue engineering and developmental and cell biology. Cell responsiveness is an important issue and there are major differences in 3D gap junction communication compared to the 2D culture systems.

REFERENCES

Aftab, Q., W. C. Sin, and C. C. Naus. 2015. Reduction in gap junction intercellular communication promotes glioma migration. *Oncotarget* no. 6 (13):11447–64.

Azarnia, R., S. Reddy, T. E. Kmiecik, D. Shalloway, and W. R. Loewenstein. 1988. The cellular src gene product regulates junctional cell-to-cell communication. *Science* no. 239 (4838):398–401.

Bai, C., M. Yang, Z. Fan, S. Li, T. Gao, and Z. Fang. 2015. Associations of chemo- and radio-resistant phenotypes with the gap junction, adhesion and extracellular matrix in a three-dimensional culture model of soft sarcoma. *J Exp Clin Cancer Res* no. 34:58.

Beardslee, M. A., J. G. Laing, E. C. Beyer, and J. E. Saffitz. 1998. Rapid turnover of connexin43 in the adult rat heart. *Circ Res* no. 83 (6):629–35.

Behrens, J., M. M. Mareel, F. M. Van Roy, and W. Birchmeier. 1989. Dissecting tumor cell invasion: Epithelial cells acquire invasive properties after the loss of uvomorulin-mediated cell-cell adhesion. *J Cell Biol* no. 108 (6):2435–47.

Bennett, M. V., L. C. Barrio, T. A. Bargiello, D. C. Spray, E. Hertzberg, and J. C. Saez. 1991. Gap junctions: New tools, new answers, new questions. *Neuron* no. 6 (3):305–20.

Bhandari, D. R., K. W. Seo, B. Sun, M. S. Seo, H. S. Kim, Y. J. Seo, J. Marcin, N. Forraz, H. L. Roy, D. Larry, M. Colin, and K. S. Kang. 2011. The simplest method for *in vitro* beta-cell production from human adult stem cells. *Differentiation* no. 82 (3):144–52.

Birchmeier, W., J. Behrens, K. M. Weidner, U. H. Frixen, and J. Schipper. 1991. Dominant and recessive genes involved in tumor cell invasion. *Curr Opin Cell Biol* no. 3 (5):832–40.

Bohovic, R., L. Demkova, M. Cihova, S. Skolekova, E. Durinikova, L. Toro, S. Tyciakova, Z. Kozovska, M. Matuskova, and L. Kucerova. 2015. 3D multicellular models reflect the efficiency of MSC-directed enzyme/prodrug treatment. *Neoplasma* no. 62 (4):521–30.

Brucher, B. L. and I. S. Jamall. 2014. Cell-cell communication in the tumor microenvironment, carcinogenesis, and anticancer treatment. *Cell Physiol Biochem* no. 34 (2):213–43.

Budunova, I. V. and G. M. Williams. 1994. Cell culture assays for chemicals with tumor-promoting or tumor-inhibiting activity based on the modulation of intercellular communication. *Cell Biol Toxicol* no. 10 (2):71–116.

Chitcholtan, K., P. H. Sykes, and J. J. Evans. 2012. The resistance of intracellular mediators to doxorubicin and cisplatin are distinct in 3D and 2D endometrial cancer. *J Transl Med* no. 10:38.

Cottrell, G. T., R. Lin, B. J. Warn-Cramer, A. F. Lau, and J. M. Burt. 2003. Mechanism of v-Src- and mitogen-activated protein kinase-induced reduction of gap junction communication. *Am J Physiol Cell Physiol* no. 284 (2):C511–20.

Crow, D. S., E. C. Beyer, D. L. Paul, S. S. Kobe, and A. F. Lau. 1990. Phosphorylation of connexin43 gap junction protein in uninfected and Rous sarcoma virus-transformed mammalian fibroblasts. *Mol Cell Biol* no. 10 (4):1754–63.

Dang, X., B. W. Doble, and E. Kardami. 2003. The carboxy-tail of connexin-43 localizes to the nucleus and inhibits cell growth. *Mol Cell Biochem* no. 242 (1–2):35–8.

de Feijter, A. W., D. F. Matesic, R. J. Ruch, X. Guan, C. C. Chang, and J. E. Trosko. 1996. Localization and function of the connexin 43 gap-junction protein in normal and various oncogene-expressing rat liver epithelial cells. *Mol Carcinog* no. 16 (4):203–12.

Dréau, D. 2010. Cell biology and biophysics of the the cell membrane. In R. Splinter (Ed.) *Handbook of Physics in Medicine and Biology*, 3–8. Boca Raton, FL: CRC Press.

Duncan, J. C. and W. H. Fletcher. 2002. alpha 1 Connexin (connexin43) gap junctions and activities of cAMP-dependent protein kinase and protein kinase C in developing mouse heart. *Dev Dyn* no. 223 (1):96–107.

el-Sabban, M. E. and B. U. Pauli. 1991. Cytoplasmic dye transfer between metastatic tumor cells and vascular endothelium. *J Cell Biol* no. 115 (5):1375–82.

el-Sabban, M. E. and B. U. Pauli. 1994. Adhesion-mediated gap junctional communication between lung-metastatatic cancer cells and endothelium. *Invasion Metastasis* no. 14 (1–6):164–76.

Enomoto, T. and H. Yamasaki. 1985. Phorbol ester-mediated inhibition of intercellular communication in BALB/c 3T3 cells: relationship to enhancement of cell transformation. *Cancer Res* no. 45 (6):2681–8.

Epstein, M. L. and N. B. Gilula. 1977. A study of communication specificity between cells in culture. *J Cell Biol* no. 75 (3):769–87.

Flodby, P., D. Z. Liao, A. Blanck, K. G. Xanthopoulos, and I. P. Hallstrom. 1995. Expression of the liver-enriched transcription factors C/EBP alpha, C/EBP beta, HNF-1, and HNF-4 in preneoplastic nodules and hepatocellular carcinoma in rat liver. *Mol Carcinog* no. 12 (2):103–9.

Gaietta, G., T. J. Deerinck, S. R. Adams, J. Bouwer, O. Tour, D. W. Laird, G. E. Sosinsky, R. Y. Tsien, and M. H. Ellisman. 2002. Multicolor and electron microscopic imaging of connexin trafficking. *Science* no. 296 (5567):503–7.

Gakhar, G., D. Schrempp, and T. A. Nguyen. 2009. Regulation of gap junctional intercellular communication by TCDD in HMEC and MCF-7 breast cancer cells. *Toxicol Appl Pharmacol* no. 235 (2):171–81.

Goodenough, D. A. and D. L. Paul. 2003. Beyond the gap: functions of unpaired connexon channels. *Nat Rev Mol Cell Biol* no. 4 (4):285–94, doi: 10.1038/nrm1072.

Guo-Parke, H., J. T. McCluskey, C. Kelly, M. Hamid, N. H. McClenaghan, and P. R. Flatt. 2012. Configuration of electrofusion-derived human insulin-secreting cell line as pseudoislets enhances functionality and therapeutic utility. *J Endocrinol* no. 214 (3):257–65, doi: 10.1530/joe-12-0188.

Hairfield-Stein, M., C. England, H. J. Paek, K. B. Gilbraith, R. Dennis, E. Boland, and P. Kosnik. 2007. Development of self-assembled, tissue-engineered ligament from bone marrow stromal cells. *Tissue Eng* no. 13 (4):703–10.

Halidi, N., F. Alonso, J. M. Burt, J. L. Beny, J. A. Haefliger, and J. J. Meister. 2012. Intercellular calcium waves in primary cultured rat mesenteric smooth muscle cells are mediated by connexin43. *Cell Commun Adhes* no. 19 (2):25–37.

He, W., Y. Kuang, X. Xing, R. J. Simpson, H. Huang, T. Yang, J. Chen, L. Yang, E. Liu, W. He, and J. Gu. 2014. Proteomic comparison of 3D and 2D glioma models reveals increased HLA-E expression in 3D models is associated with resistance to NK cell-mediated cytotoxicity. *J Proteome Res* no. 13 (5):2272–81.

Howard, C. M. and T. A. Baudino. 2014. Dynamic cell-cell and cell-ECM interactions in the heart. *J Mol Cell Cardiol* no. 70:19–26.

Hyrc, K. and B. Rose. 1990. The action of v-src on gap junctional permeability is modulated by pH. *J Cell Biol* no. 110 (4):1217–26.

IARC. 1991. Occupational exposures in insecticide application, and some pesticides. In Proceedings of the IARC Working Group on the Evaluation of Carcinogenic Risks to Humans, *Lyon, France,* 16–23 October 1990. *IARC Monogr Eval Carcinog Risks Hum* no. 53:5–586.

IARC. 1999. Re-evaluation of some organic chemicals, hydrazine and hydrogen peroxide. In Proceedings of the IARC Working Group on the Evaluation of Carcinogenic Risks to Humans, Lyon, France, 17–24 February 1998. *IARC Monogr Eval Carcinog Risks Hum* no. 71 (Pt 1):1–315.

Imamura, Y., T. Mukohara, Y. Shimono, Y. Funakoshi, N. Chayahara, M. Toyoda, N. Kiyota, S. Takao, S. Kono, T. Nakatsura, and H. Minami. 2015. Comparison of 2D- and 3D-culture models as drug-testing platforms in breast cancer. *Oncol Rep* no. 33 (4):1837–43.

Jamakosmanovic, A. and W. R. Loewenstein. 1968. Intercellular communication and tissue growth. 3. Thyroid cancer. *J Cell Biol* no. 38 (3):556–61.

Jamieson, S., J. J. Going, R. D'Arcy, and W. D. George. 1998. Expression of gap junction proteins connexin 26 and connexin 43 in normal human breast and in breast tumours. *J Pathol* no. 184 (1):37–43.

John, S., D. Cesario, and J. N. Weiss. 2003. Gap junctional hemichannels in the heart. *Acta Physiol Scand* no. 179 (1):23–31.

Jongen, W. M., D. J. Fitzgerald, M. Asamoto, C. Piccoli, T. J. Slaga, D. Gros, M. Takeichi, and H. Yamasaki. 1991. Regulation of connexin 43-mediated gap junctional intercellular communication by Ca2+ in mouse epidermal cells is controlled by E-cadherin. *J Cell Biol* no. 114 (3):545–55.

Jordan, K., J. L. Solan, M. Dominguez, M. Sia, A. Hand, P. D. Lampe, and D. W. Laird. 1999. Trafficking, assembly, and function of a connexin43-green fluorescent protein chimera in live mammalian cells. *Mol Biol Cell* no. 10 (6):2033–50.

Kalkuhl, A., K. Kaestner, A. Buchmann, and M. Schwarz. 1996. Expression of hepatocyte-enriched nuclear transcription factors in mouse liver tumours. *Carcinogenesis* no. 17 (3):609–12.

Kam, E., L. Melville, and J. D. Pitts. 1986. Patterns of junctional communication in skin. *J Invest Dermatol* no. 87 (6):748–53.

Kanczuga-Koda, L., S. Sulkowski, J. Tomaszewski, M. Koda, M. Sulkowska, W. Przystupa, J. Golaszewska, and M. Baltaziak. 2005. Connexins 26 and 43 correlate with Bak, but not with Bcl-2 protein in breast cancer. *Oncol Rep* no. 14 (2):325–9.

Kanno, Y., T. Enomoto, Y. Shiba, and H. Yamasaki. 1984. Protective effect of cAMP on tumor promoter-mediated inhibition of cell-cell communication. *Exp Cell Res* no. 152 (1):31–7.

Kanno, Y. and Y. Matsui. 1968. Cellular uncoupling in cancerous stomach epithelium. *Nature* no. 218 (5143):775–6.

King, T. J., L. H. Fukushima, A. D. Hieber, K. A. Shimabukuro, W. A. Sakr, and J. S. Bertram. 2000. Reduced levels of connexin43 in cervical dysplasia: Inducible expression in a cervical carcinoma cell line decreases neoplastic potential with implications for tumor progression. *Carcinogenesis* no. 21 (6):1097–109.

Klaunig, J. E., R. J. Ruch, J. A. Hampton, C. M. Weghorst, and J. A. Hartnett. 1990. Gap-junctional intercellular communication and murine hepatic carcinogenesis. *Prog Clin Biol Res* no. 331:277–91.

Krutovskikh, V. A., M. Oyamada, and H. Yamasaki. 1991. Sequential changes of gap-junctional intercellular communications during multistage rat liver carcinogenesis: direct measurement of communication *in vivo. Carcinogenesis* no. 12 (9):1701–6.

Lagaud, G., K. P. Davies, K. Venkateswarlu, and G. J. Christ. 2002. The physiology, pathophysiology and therapeutic potential of gap junctions in smooth muscle. *Curr Drug Targets* no. 3 (6):427–40.

Laird, D. W., P. Fistouris, G. Batist, L. Alpert, H. T. Huynh, G. D. Carystinos, and M. A. Alaoui-Jamali. 1999. Deficiency of connexin43 gap junctions is an independent marker for breast tumors. *Cancer Res* no. 59 (16):4104–10.

Laird, D. W., K. L. Puranam, and J. P. Revel. 1991. Turnover and phosphorylation dynamics of connexin43 gap junction protein in cultured cardiac myocytes. *Biochem J* no. 273 (Pt 1):67–72.

Lampe, P. D. 1994. Analyzing phorbol ester effects on gap junctional communication: a dramatic inhibition of assembly. *J Cell Biol* no. 127 (6 Pt 2):1895–905.

Lampe, P. D. and A. F. Lau. 2000. Regulation of gap junctions by phosphorylation of connexins. *Arch Biochem Biophys* no. 384 (2):205–15.

Lampe, P. D. and A. F. Lau. 2004. The effects of connexin phosphorylation on gap junctional communication. *Int J Biochem Cell Biol* no. 36 (7):1171–86.

Lauf, U., B. N. Giepmans, P. Lopez, S. Braconnot, S. C. Chen, and M. M. Falk. 2002. Dynamic trafficking and delivery of connexons to the plasma membrane and accretion to gap junctions in living cells. *Proc Natl Acad Sci USA* no. 99 (16):10446–51.

Lee, S. W., C. Tomasetto, D. Paul, K. Keyomarsi, and R. Sager. 1992. Transcriptional downregulation of gap-junction proteins blocks junctional communication in human mammary tumor cell lines. *J Cell Biol* no. 118 (5):1213–21.

Lijinsky, W. 1989. A view of the relation between carcinogenesis and mutagenesis. *Environ Mol Mutagen* no. 14 (Suppl 16):S78–S84.

Lijinsky, W. 1990. Non-genotoxic environmental carcinogens. *Environ Carcinogenesis Rev* no. 8 (1):45–87.

Liu, X., F. Yan, H. Yao, M. Chang, J. Qin, Y. Li, Y. Wang, and X. Pei. 2014. Involvement of RhoA/ROCK in insulin secretion of pancreatic beta-cells in 3D culture. *Cell Tissue Res* no. 358 (2):359–69.

Loewenstein, W. R. 1979. Junctional intercellular communication and the control of growth. *Biochim Biophys Acta* no. 560 (1):1–65.

Loewenstein, W. R. and Y. Kanno. 1966. Intercellular communication and the control of tissue growth: lack of communication between cancer cells. *Nature* no. 209 (5029):1248–9.

Loewenstein, W. R. and Y. Kanno. 1967. Intercellular communication and tissue growth. I. Cancerous growth. *J Cell Biol* no. 33 (2):225–34.

Luther, M. J., A. Hauge-Evans, K. L. Souza, A. Jorns, S. Lenzen, S. J. Persaud, and P. M. Jones. 2006. MIN6 beta-cell-beta-cell interactions influence insulin secretory responses to nutrients and non-nutrients. *Biochem Biophys Res Commun* no. 343 (1):99–104.

Malewicz, B., V. V. Kumar, R. G. Johnson, and W. J. Baumann. 1990. Lipids in gap junction assembly and function. *Lipids* no. 25 (8):419–27.

McMasters, R. A., R. L. Saylors, K. E. Jones, M. E. Hendrix, M. P. Moyer, and R. R. Drake. 1998. Lack of bystander killing in herpes simplex virus thymidine kinase-transduced colon cell lines due to deficient connexin43 gap junction formation. *Hum Gene Ther* no. 9 (15):2253–61.

Mege, R. M., F. Matsuzaki, W. J. Gallin, J. I. Goldberg, B. A. Cunningham, and G. M. Edelman. 1988. Construction of epithelioid sheets by transfection of mouse sarcoma cells with cDNAs for chicken cell adhesion molecules. *Proc Natl Acad Sci USA* no. 85 (19):7274–8.

Mehta, P. P., J. S. Bertram, and W. R. Loewenstein. 1986. Growth inhibition of transformed cells correlates with their junctional communication with normal cells. *Cell* no. 44 (1):187–96.

Mesnil, M. 2002. Connexins and cancer. *Biol Cell* no. 94 (7–8):493–500.

Mesnil, M., S. Crespin, J. L. Avanzo, and M. L. Zaidan-Dagli. 2005. Defective gap junctional intercellular communication in the carcinogenic process. *Biochim Biophys Acta* no. 1719 (1–2):125–45.

Mesnil, M., D. J. Fitzgerald, and H. Yamasaki. 1988. Phenobarbital specifically reduces gap junction protein mRNA level in rat liver. *Mol Carcinog* no. 1 (2):79–81.

Murray, A. W. and D. J. Fitzgerald. 1979. Tumor promoters inhibit metabolic cooperation in cocultures of epidermal and 3T3 cells. *Biochem Biophys Res Commun* no. 91 (2):395–401.

Musil, L. S., E. C. Beyer, and D. A. Goodenough. 1990. Expression of the gap junction protein connexin43 in embryonic chick lens: molecular cloning, ultrastructural localization, and post-translational phosphorylation. *J Membr Biol* no. 116 (2):163–75.

Musil, L. S. and D. A. Goodenough. 1991. Biochemical analysis of connexin43 intracellular transport, phosphorylation, and assembly into gap junctional plaques. *J Cell Biol* no. 115 (5):1357–74.

Na, H. K., M. R. Wilson, K. S. Kang, C. C. Chang, D. Grunberger, and J. E. Trosko. 2000. Restoration of gap junctional intercellular communication by caffeic acid phenethyl ester (CAPE) in a ras-transformed rat liver epithelial cell line. *Cancer Lett* no. 157 (1):31–8.

Neveu, M. J., J. R. Hully, K. L. Babcock, E. L. Hertzberg, B. J. Nicholson, D. L. Paul, and H. C. Pitot. 1994. Multiple mechanisms are responsible for altered expression of gap junction genes during oncogenesis in rat liver. *J Cell Sci* no. 107 (Pt 1):83–95.

Nicolson, G. L. 1987. Tumor cell instability, diversification, and progression to the metastatic phenotype: from oncogene to oncofetal expression. *Cancer Res* no. 47 (6):1473–87.

Nicolson, G. L., K. M. Dulski, and J. E. Trosko. 1988. Loss of intercellular junctional communication correlates with metastatic potential in mammary adenocarcinoma cells. *Proc Natl Acad Sci USA* no. 85 (2):473–6.

Peterson, J. A. 1983. The widespread nature of phenotypic variability in hepatomas and cell lines, in the form of a geometric series. *J Theor Biol* no. 102 (1):41–53.

Pinto, M., E. I. Azzam, and R. W. Howell. 2010. Investigation of adaptive responses in bystander cells in 3D cultures containing tritium-labeled and unlabeled normal human fibroblasts. *Radiat Res* no. 174 (2):216–27.

Pollmann, M. A., Q. Shao, D. W. Laird, and M. Sandig. 2005. Connexin 43 mediated gap junctional communication enhances breast tumor cell diapedesis in culture. *Breast Cancer Res* no. 7 (4):R522–34.

Ravier, M. A., M. Guldenagel, A. Charollais, A. Gjinovci, D. Caille, G. Sohl, C. B. Wollheim, K. Willecke, J. C. Henquin, and P. Meda. 2005. Loss of connexin36 channels alters beta-cell coupling, islet synchronization of glucose-induced Ca^{2+} and insulin oscillations, and basal insulin release. *Diabetes* no. 54 (6):1798–807.

Ren, J., J. Hamada, N. Takeichi, S. Fujikawa, and H. Kobayashi. 1990. Ultrastructural differences in junctional intercellular communication between highly and weakly metastatic clones derived from rat mammary carcinoma. *Cancer Res* no. 50 (2):358–62.

Rivedal, E. and G. Witz. 2005. Metabolites of benzene are potent inhibitors of gap-junction intercellular communication. *Arch Toxicol* no. 79 (6):303–11.

Ruch, R. J. 1994. The role of gap junctional intercellular communication in neoplasia. *Ann Clin Lab Sci* no. 24 (3):216–31.

Ruch, R. J., J. E. Klaunig, and M. A. Pereira. 1987. Inhibition of intercellular communication between mouse hepatocytes by tumor promoters. *Toxicol Appl Pharmacol* no. 87 (1):111–20.

Saez, J. C., V. M. Berthoud, M. C. Branes, A. D. Martinez, and E. C. Beyer. 2003. Plasma membrane channels formed by connexins: their regulation and functions. *Physiol Rev* no. 83 (4):1359–400.

Saunders, M. M., M. J. Seraj, Z. Li, Z. Zhou, C. R. Winter, D. R. Welch, and H. J. Donahue. 2001. Breast cancer metastatic potential correlates with a breakdown in homospecific and heterospecific gap junctional intercellular communication. *Cancer Res* no. 61 (5):1765–7.

Sekine, H., T. Shimizu, S. Kosaka, E. Kobayashi, and T. Okano. 2006. Cardiomyocyte bridging between hearts and bioengineered myocardial tissues with mesenchymal transition of mesothelial cells. *J Heart Lung Transplant* no. 25 (3):324–32.

Shi, X., B. Potvin, T. Huang, P. Hilgard, D. C. Spray, S. O. Suadicani, A. W. Wolkoff, P. Stanley, and R. J. Stockert. 2001. A novel casein kinase 2 alpha-subunit regulates membrane protein traffic in the human hepatoma cell line HuH-7. *J Biol Chem* no. 276 (3):2075–82.

Simon, A. M., D. A. Goodenough, E. Li, and D. L. Paul. 1997. Female infertility in mice lacking connexin 37. *Nature* no. 385 (6616):525–9.

Singal, R., Z. J. Tu, J. M. Vanwert, G. D. Ginder, and D. T. Kiang. 2000. Modulation of the connexin26 tumor suppressor gene expression through methylation in human mammary epithelial cell lines. *Anticancer Res* no. 20 (1a):59–64.

Syed-Picard, F. N., T. Jayaraman, R. S. Lam, E. Beniash, and C. Sfeir. 2013. Osteoinductivity of calcium phosphate mediated by connexin 43. *Biomaterials* no. 34 (15):3763–74.

Talhouk, R. S., M. B. Fares, G. J. Rahme, H. H. Hariri, T. Rayess, H. A. Dbouk, D. Bazzoun, D. Al-Labban, and M. E. El-Sabban. 2013. Context dependent reversion of tumor phenotype by connexin-43 expression in MDA-MB231 cells and MCF-7 cells: role of beta-catenin/connexin43 association. *Exp Cell Res* no. 319 (20):3065–80.

Trosko, J. E. 1988. A failed paradigm: Carcinogenesis is more than mutagenesis. *Mutagenesis* no. 3 (4):363–6.

Trosko, J. E. 1989. Towards understanding carcinogenic hazards: A crisis in paradigms. *Int J Toxicol* no. 8 (6):1121–32.

Trosko, J. E. and C. C. Chang. 1985. Role of tumor promotion in affecting the multi-hit nature of carcinogenesis. *Basic Life Sci* no. 33:261–84.

Trosko, J. E. and C. C. Chang. 1989. Stem cell theory of carcinogenesis. *Toxicol Lett* no. 49 (2–3):283–95.

Trosko, J. E., C. C. Chang, B. Upham, and M. Wilson. 1998. Epigenetic toxicology as toxicant-induced changes in intracellular signalling leading to altered gap junctional intercellular communication. *Toxicol Lett* no. 102–103:71–8.

Tsai, H., J. Werber, M. O. Davia, M. Edelman, K. E. Tanaka, A. Melman, G. J. Christ, and J. Geliebter. 1996. Reduced connexin 43 expression in high grade, human prostatic adenocarcinoma cells. *Biochem Biophys Res Commun* no. 227 (1):64–9.

Wang, X. G. and C. Peracchia. 1998. Chemical gating of heteromeric and heterotypic gap junction channels. *J Membr Biol* no. 162 (2):169–76.

Wang, W., Y. Hayashi, T. Ninomiya, K. Ohta, H. Nakabayashi, T. Tamaoki, and H. Itoh. 1998. Expression of HNF-1 alpha and HNF-1 beta in various histological differentiations of hepatocellular carcinoma. *J Pathol* no. 184 (3):272–8.

Warn-Cramer, B. J. and A. F. Lau. 2004. Regulation of gap junctions by tyrosine protein kinases. *Biochim Biophys Acta* no. 1662 (1–2):81–95.

Weng, S., M. Lauven, T. Schaefer, L. Polontchouk, R. Grover, and S. Dhein. 2002. Pharmacological modification of gap junction coupling by an antiarrhythmic peptide via protein kinase C activation. *FASEB J* no. 6 (9):1114–6.

Willecke, K., J. Eiberger, J. Degen, D. Eckardt, A. Romualdi, M. Guldenagel, U. Deutsch, and G. Sohl. 2002. Structural and functional diversity of connexin genes in the mouse and human genome. *Biol Chem* no. 383 (5):725–37.

Yamasaki, H. 1990. Gap junctional intercellular communication and carcinogenesis. *Carcinogenesis* no. 11 (7):1051–8.

Yamasaki, H. and F. Katoh. 1988. Further evidence for the involvement of gap-junctional intercellular communication in induction and maintenance of transformed foci in BALB/c 3T3 cells. *Cancer Res* no. 48 (12):3490–5.

Yamasaki, H. and C. C. Naus. 1996. Role of connexin genes in growth control. *Carcinogenesis* no. 17 (6):1199–213.

Yano, T., F. J. Hernandez-Blazquez, Y. Omori, and H. Yamasaki. 2001. Reduction of malignant phenotype of HEPG2 cell is associated with the expression of connexin 26 but not connexin 32. *Carcinogenesis* no. 22 (10):1593–600.

Yotti, L. P., C. C. Chang, and J. E. Trosko. 1979. Elimination of metabolic cooperation in Chinese hamster cells by a tumor promoter. *Science* no. 206 (4422):1089–91.

Zhang, Z. Q., Z. X. Lin, and Y. Y. Lu. 1994. Studies on the reduction of malignant phenotypes in a highly metastatic human lung carcinoma-correlated changes of intercellular communication, cytoskeletons, oncogenes and antioncogene. *Zhonghua Zhong liu za zhi [Chin J Oncol]* no. 16 (2):88–92.

Zimmermann, W. H., M. Didie, G. H. Wasmeier, U. Nixdorff, A. Hess, I. Melnychenko, O. Boy, W. L. Neuhuber, M. Weyand, and T. Eschenhagen. 2002. Cardiac grafting of engineered heart tissue in syngenic rats. *Circulation* no. 106 (12 Suppl 1):I151–7.

14 Advances in Breast Stem Cell Knowledge through 3D Systems

Kerri W. Kwist and Brian W. Booth

CONTENTS

14.1 Introduction 249
14.2 Advances Made Using Gel-Based Matrices 251
14.3 Free-Floating Mammosphere 3D System..253
14.4 Cancer Stem Cell Discoveries 256
14.5 Heterotypic 3D *In Vitro* Systems...256
14.6 Conclusion and Perspective 258
Acknowledgment 258
References..258

14.1 INTRODUCTION

Multicellular three-dimensional (3D) *in vitro* models have been used to generate tremendous advances in the fields of normal and cancer mammary somatic stem and progenitor cells. The 3D *in vitro* models are highly varied and can be composed of many different matrices and cell types. The ease of modification of the 3D models allows investigators to use different models to address specific scientific questions that the traditional two-dimensional (2D) *in vitro* models or *in vivo* models cannot readily answer.

In the recent past, considerable gain in our scientific knowledge of stem cells has been made. This has been especially true for somatic stem cells of the human breast and resident stem cells of the mouse mammary gland. The mammary gland provides an excellent model for the study of resident stem cells as the majority of growth and development occurs postnatal during puberty and any subsequent pregnancies and involutions. For years, the only definitive experiments to prove the existence and functionality of these stem cells were transplantation experiments. Although these *in vivo* models proved highly informative and successful, they are expensive and time consuming compared to *in vitro* assays.

The existence of stem cells in the adult mouse mammary gland and the adult human breast has been demonstrated using many different approaches. Mouse mammary stem cells were first demonstrated when portions of a minced gland were transplanted into juvenile mammary fat pads of syngeneic mice cleared of endogenous epithelium (Deome et al. 1959; Faulkin and Deome 1960). In order to fill the empty mammary fat pad, the transplanted cellular population must self-renew and expand. The resulting mammary regeneration and subsequent serial transplantations using both mammary fragments and dissociated mammary epithelial cells prove the existence of mammary stem cells in the adult female mouse (Deome et al. 1959; Daniel 1975).

Stem cells in the adult human breast were demonstrated using different approaches. The basic structure of the human breast is the terminal ductal lobular unit (TDLU) that consists of alveoli situated around a duct and side branches (Stirling and Chandler 1976). Within a TDLU, the X chromosome-linked gene inactivation is the same for all cells, suggesting that the population arose from a single progenitor (Diallo et al. 2001). A study of human breast epithelium demonstrated the presence of mammary epithelial cells possessing the ability to regenerate elaborate branching structures resembling TDLUs both by morphology and marker expression, *in vivo* using xenotransplantation models and *in vitro* (Gudjonsson et al. 2002).

Cancer stem cells (CSCs) are considered the subset of cells of a given tumor from which that tumor arose. CSCs are resistant to most chemo- and radio-therapies and are able to expand and regenerate tumors (Sinha et al. 2013; Faswaran et al. 2014). Most tumors are believed to contain a population of malignant cells with stem cell characteristics defined by their ability to initiate tumors when xenografted into immunocompromised mice. The initiating cell of a tumor can be a transformed stem cell or the result of a mutation in a more lineage-committed progenitor cell. Examples in human breast cancer could include undifferentiated triple negative breast cancers that arise from basal stem cells where tumors that express estrogen receptor (ER) or human epidermal growth factor (EGF) receptor 2 (HER2) arise from more differentiated luminal cells. Breast cancer is a highly heterogeneous disease on histological, molecular, and epidemiologic levels. There are six molecular subtypes based on gene expression: normal breast-like, luminal A, luminal B, basal-like, claudin-low, and HER2 over-expressing (Perou et al. 2000; Sorlie et al. 2001).

The growth and study of mammary and breast stem cells *in vitro* has been limited prior to the introduction of 3D models. When grown in the standard 2D culture systems, primary cells generally have limited expansion potential. The 2D cultures become senescent after fewer than 10 passages. This is a result of differentiation of the stem cells when placed in 2D cultures. Once the stem cells are extinguished through differentiation, the primary cultures can no longer be expanded resulting in the termination of experimental use (Bissell 1981). In addition, the traditional 2D *in vitro* systems do not accurately mimic *in vivo* conditions since cells *in vivo* exist and interact in three dimensions. The introduction and refinement of the 3D *in vitro* systems have allowed for increased cellular manipulations to occur, thus, generating an expanded knowledge base.

The innate flexibility of 3D culture systems, the capacity to interchange components including different cell types, allows for the recapitulation of crucial intercellular signaling required for certain morphological development. Figure 14.1 demonstrates different growth patterns when cells are grown on various matrices. Signaling originating from extracellular matrix (ECM) proteins is another component that is often overlooked in the 2D systems that can be readily modified into 3D models.

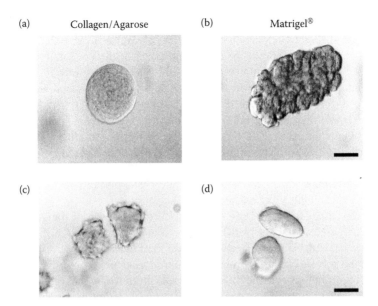

FIGURE 14.1 Morphological differences exhibited by cells grown in different 3D *in vitro* matrices. The cancer cell line 4T1 grown in (a) collagen/agarose or (b) Matrigel® and the normal mammary epithelial cell line NMuMG grown in (c) collagen/agarose or (d) Matrigel®. Scale bars are 40 μm. (Modified from previous publication Booth et al. 2013; http://www.tandfonline.com.)

In this chapter, we will highlight and discuss advancements in the field of normal and cancer breast/mammary stem cells that have been made using the 3D *in vitro* systems. We will focus on gel-based solid culture systems and the free-floating mammosphere culture system as well as heterotypic 3D systems.

14.2 ADVANCES MADE USING GEL-BASED MATRICES

The epithelial structures of the normal mouse mammary gland are comprised of polarized luminal epithelial cells encompassed by a layer of myoepithelial cells. This epithelial bilayer is separated from the surrounding stroma by the basement membrane (BM) (Ronnov-Jessen et al. 1996). The stroma is a mix of ECM, adipocytes, nerves, blood vessels, and other components. The surrounding stroma regulates many aspects of cellular development and differentiation through structural support and providing soluble factors (Lelievre et al. 1996; Weaver and Bissell 1999). Cellular behavior can be altered by modification of the surrounding environment such as changing stiffness, tissue density, fat and lipid content, and vascularity. Type I collagen and Matrigel® are the most frequently used matrices for 3D *in vitro* culture of mammary epithelial cells.

In the 1970s, floating collagen gels were shown to maintain epithelial structure and function of mammary and liver tissue fragments (Elsdale and Bard 1972; Emerman and Pitelka 1977). The maintained epithelial structures retained some of their differentiated capacity as the mammary structures produced the milk protein β-casein *de novo* and the liver cells produced albumin (Michalopoulos and Pitot 1975; Lee et al. 1985; Gudjonsson et al. 2002). It was later determined that it is not the collagen itself that allows for the maintenance of the epithelial structure and function but instead the ability to establish a BM layer. When grown in 2D, epithelial cells lose the ability to lay down BM and therefore lose the signaling interactions with the BM (Streuli and Bissell 1990; Boudreau et al. 1995).

The discovery that Engelbreth–Holm–Swarm mouse sarcoma cells produce and secrete copious amounts of BM components led to the introduction of Matrigel® (Kleinman et al. 1986). This substance has been called laminin-rich ECM, EHS extract, basement membrane-like gel, Cultrex® BME, and Matrigel®. This matrix is rich in laminins, collagens, heparin sulfate proteoglycans, and growth factors (Kleinman et al. 1982; Vukicevic et al. 1992).

Cells can either be grown embedded inside of or on top of the gel (Lee et al. 2007). Compared to cells grown in 2D on tissue culture flasks and dishes, cells grown using a gel-based matrix retain more of their *in vivo* properties. The BM proteins and the soft surface create more of an appropriate microenvironment for these cells. Cell morphology is different in gel-based cultures than the traditional 2D systems. Cells grown in the traditional 2D cultures look and grow the same no matter if they are cancerous or not. These same cells if grown cultured using a gel-based matrix will have very different characteristics depending on cell type. Malignant cells lose cellular organization; they proliferate rapidly, migrate, and grow large structures in Matrigel®-based systems (Lee et al. 2007). The specific 3D cellular structure will depend on what type of gene and protein expression that particular cell type will display. Cells with similar gene and protein expression will have a similar morphology (Kenny et al. 2007). In the case of a normal mammary epithelial cell line, HC-11, when expression of the signaling molecule Notch1 is reduced using shRNA, colony size is reduced when grown on Matrigel® (Figure 14.2) (Park et al. 2013).

Although malignant cells proliferate rapidly in Matrigel® systems, nonmalignant cells do not and instead are pushed down a differentiation pathway. The differentiated phenotype includes cell structure and gene expression, and is dependent on the cells of origin. This result is true either with primary cells or established cell lines. Primary cells have been shown to recapture many of their original tissue properties (Petersen et al. 1992). The cause of this is not readily known, but it most likely to do with the microenvironment of the Matrigel® matrix. Not only does the Matrigel® provide a change in extracellular stiffness compared to tissue culture plastic, but also because Matrigel® was isolated from basement membrane secreted by tumor cells, the cultured cells are being exposed to multiple factors, including hormones and proteins, that most likely cause this differentiation.

The most straightforward way to use Matrigel® is as a tissue test system to mimic breast tissue. By culturing cells in this environment, it can be determined, which signaling pathways are being activated or inhibited. As these pathways are regulated in this environment, this system becomes even more similar to the original tissue. By growing "normal" and "cancerous" cells in this 3D matrix, comparisons can be made about how the different cell types communicate and which pathways play important roles *in vivo* (Weaver et al. 1997). Another way to use this tissue test

Advances in Breast Stem Cell Knowledge through 3D Systems

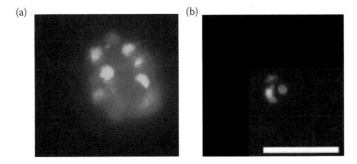

FIGURE 14.2 Role of Notch1 in colony formation. The normal mammary epithelial cell line HC-11 was grown on growth factor reduced Matrigel® (a) or cultured after receiving Notch1 specific shRNA (b). Scale bar is 50 μm. (Modified from previous publication Park, J. P. et al. 2013. *Stem Cells Dev* no. 22 (8):1297–306.)

system is the identification of biomarkers. Certain biomarkers have been associated with certain cancer types using cells grown in 2D conditions. In many cases, these biomarkers were found not to actually be relevant when studied *in vivo*. Researchers re-evaluating biomarkers discovered using 2D models and testing them using 3D cultures found that this system is more an accurate predictor of cancerous biomarkers. As potential chemotherapeutic drugs are developed, they can be tested on a smaller scale using these types of tissue test systems to validate how effective a possible treatment would be (Correia and Bissell 2012).

Many important discoveries have been made using gel-based matrices (Kleinman and Martin 2005; Weigelt et al. 2014). However, the *in vitro* environment created using gel-based matrices does not entirely mimic numerous *in vivo* conditions and results obtained from experiments that rely solely on cells grown in or on gel-based matrices may lead to misleading or limited conclusions. Matrigel® is a highly variable material, the contents of which are reasonably ill-defined. All *in vitro* culture models have inherent advantages and disadvantages, and if one understands how a given cell type will behave in a certain *in vitro* system one can more accurately predict how a similar cell type will behave in such an environment (Swamydas et al. 2010). Based on cell behaviors, the *in vitro* systems can be designed to study specific research questions and produce results that may more readily decipher the *in vivo* condition.

14.3 FREE-FLOATING MAMMOSPHERE 3D SYSTEM

In the past decade, growing nonadherent cell clusters, or mammospheres, has become a common technique in many research laboratories. The mammosphere system is based on the neurosphere system in which neural stem cells were isolated and expanded using a nonattachment 3D *in vitro* system. The theory behind the free-floating system is that only stem and early progenitor cells are capable of surviving anoikis, whereas differentiating cells require physical contact with either other cells or a BM to survive. The resulting cell death of the differentiating cells leaves a culture of stem cells and early progenitor cells that are then able to form clonal spheres comprised of their daughter cells. Glioblastoma stem cells (GSCs) were expanded using a clonogenic sphere technique. The GSCs are enriched for the neural stem cell markers CD133 and nestin, self-renew, proliferate, and differentiate *in vitro* into phenotypes identical to the original tumor *in situ* (Singh et al. 2003, 2004). Mammospheres were developed first using primary breast epithelial cells from reduction mammoplasties (Dontu et al. 2003). The mammospheres were enriched for breast stem/progenitor cells as determined by differentiation along all breast epithelial lines and the development of clonal 3D complexes. These mammospheres have many of the same characteristics as breast cancer stem cells (BCSCs). The mammospheres express similar proteins; they have the ability to differentiate into multiple cell types, can proliferate extensively, and have a high engraftment capacity regardless if they originated from normal or cancer cells. Because mammospheres can be grown *in vitro*, they provide a convenient platform to study CSCs. Signaling pathways studied in breast and mammary cells using mammosphere systems include Notch and the EGF family (Dontu et al. 2004; Booth et al. 2010). The EGF family member amphiregulin was found to influence the growth and self-renewal of duct-limited mammary progenitor cells in mammospheres (Booth et al. 2010).

Floating clusters of cells have been grown from many different types of cells. In focusing on only mammary cells, this has been done with breast tissue as well as cell lines (Ponti et al. 2005; Wang et al. 2014). Initially, the cells are grown using low attachment plates in serum free media. The cells that will eventually form mammospheres remain floating in the media and can be grown out for several days to several weeks resulting in spheres. If these cell clusters are allowed to grow for longer time periods, the differentiated cells will die off. From this point, the viable mammospheres can be used in their current state or dissociated back down to individual cells and passaged (Liu et al. 2005). This process can be repeated several times producing many generations of mammospheres. The resulting product can be collected for further experiments or screened for specific cell markers.

Applications being developed through the use of mammospheres include improved methods of cancer diagnosis, studies of CSC biomarkers, and signaling pathways, and new drugs for the treatment of cancer can be identified (Saadin and White 2013). This selecting for and growth of mammospheres in itself can serve as a cancer-screening tool. Simply put, the more mammospheres that can be isolated, the more likely that these cells could form tumors. The capacity to form mammosphere directly correlates to tumor aggressiveness (Kok et al. 2009). Samples can be taken either from a biopsy or a blood sample, and cells recovered from these samples can be grown in mammosphere-promoting conditions (Saadin and White 2013). Spheres that form in these conditions most likely originate from CSCs and can be screened for more specific cancer markers indicating certain disease characteristics. This allows for a personalized approach to treatment.

The most common use of mammospheres is to use them as an *in vitro* method to study BCSCs characteristics such as biomarkers expression by cancer cells. Mammospheres can be used to validate possible CSC markers. These markers are used to isolate and identify CSCs and may serve as future anticancer targets. The most common and most used of these markers are CD44 and CD24, but the presence of other markers such as ALDH1 and D4 can also be used to identify stem cells. Chen and coworkers used mammospheres to determine that not only was ANTXR1 a stem cell marker, but also determined its functionality by showing that it played a role in the Wnt signaling pathway (Chen et al. 2013). Ganglioside CD2 is another marker found in many CSCs and therefore found in mammospheres. By studying this marker on mammospheres, it was determined that it affected the enzyme GD3S, which is essential for BCSC function (Battula et al. 2012). By having a better understanding of which markers are and are not present on cancer cells, a cancer diagnosis can be more specific and with a better understanding of the individual disease. In addition, better and more effective treatment can be determined based on which markers are present.

A more recent development involving mammospheres is to determine which signaling pathways the CSCs use during sphere development and differentiation. Once identified, these pathways can be used as another way for cancer diagnosis and also for possible drug targets. Some pathways have been found to increase mammosphere formation and by knocking out these pathways, mammosphere formation is greatly reduced. One such pathway is the Hedgehog signaling pathway. Liu and coworkers showed that this pathway was active in BCSCs. An increase in this type of signaling increased not only the number of mammospheres formed, but also the size of them (Liu et al. 2006). In another example of using mammospheres to study signaling pathways, the Wnt signaling pathway was shown to be more active in cancerous tissue compared to noncancerous tissue. Much of this study was done using mammospheres for their stem-like activity (Lamb et al. 2013).

Once we know more about these BCSCs, how they operate and how they communicate with their environment, we can more effectively eliminate these cancerous cells from patients, leaving healthy cells intact. Again, in this respect, mammospheres can be used as a stand in for the BCSCs to test new drugs and treatment methods. Many times a drug will fail because although many chemotherapeutic agents will kill most cancers cells, it will not destroy the stem cells. Paclitaxel is one such drug. When this drug was tested on cancer cells and mammospheres, although the amount of cancer cells did decrease, when tested on mammospheres, their numbers did not change and in fact the size of the mammospheres increased. However, another compound, salinomycin, was able to significantly decrease the number of viable mammospheres as well as preventing their formation (Gupta et al. 2009). Similarly, the combination of prolactin and cisplatin inhibited mammosphere formation in erbB2 overexpressing cancer cells (Lee et al. 2015). By using mammospheres to study the Notch pathway, Lagadec and coworkers found that radiation-induced Notch signaling in mammospheres compared to cells grown in a monolayer. Using this information, studies to inhibit the Notch pathway are now in process and notch inhibitors are used along with radiation therapy (Lagadec et al. 2013).

The biggest hurdle of using mammospheres as a replacement for CSCs is the inefficient way they are produced. The current method of singling out individual cells and growing them in isolation is labor intensive and takes several days. Developments in microsystems in order to grow mammospheres are currently being explored, but it will take time to overcome some of the major hurdles with adjusting this system (Saadin and White 2013). From growth to analysis, on-chip systems for PCR and protein expression are more of a reality, but will take time to be adapted to this new type of cell culture.

14.4 CANCER STEM CELL DISCOVERIES

Normal mammary stem cells have a finite number of cell divisions or self-renewals. Following serial transplantations, generally 5–8 transplantations, the normal stem cells undergo senescence (Daniel 1975). However, unlike normal stem cells, mouse mammary CSCs or cells isolated from preneoplastic lesions do not possess a limited proliferative capacity. Tumor fragments and cells isolated from tumors or preneoplastic lesions will continue to initiate tumors and precancerous lesions indefinitely, that is, these cells are immortal (Daniel et al. 1975; Smith et al. 1978, 1980; Callahan and Smith 2000; Medina 2000, 2002; Maglione et al. 2001; Medina et al. 2002). These populations can be nontumorigenic, weakly tumorigenic, or highly tumorigenic (Medina and Kittrell 1993; Medina et al. 1993; Medina 2002).

CSCs were first isolated from human breast cancers by Al-Hajj and colleagues who demonstrated that uncultured cells isolated from pleural effusions of breast cancer patients formed tumors in immunodeficient mice (Al-Hajj et al. 2003). The cells were separated based on the CD24 and CD44 cell surface markers. When the researchers injected 200 $CD24^-/CD44^+$ cells, tumors were formed, whereas the injections of thousands of unsorted tumor cells failed to initiate tumors. Additional markers have since been used to isolate putative breast CSCs including CD133, ALDH1, and Hoechst-dye exclusion (Smalley and Clarke 2005; Ginestier et al. 2007; Wright et al. 2008).

Certain human breast cell lines have the capacity to form spheres. In the case of tumor cells, the spheres are termed tumorspheres. Immortal normal human breast cells (MCF10A), ER^+ breast cancer cells (MCF7), $HER2^+$ breast cancer cells (SUM149), and triple negative breast cancer cells (MDA-MB-231) were sorted for the CSC markers CD24 and CD44 as well as epithelial specific antigen (ESA) and cultured in sphere-forming conditions (Fillmore and Kuperwasser 2008). Populations derived from the parental cell lines sorted for $CD44^+/CD24^-/ESA^+$ were tumorigenic, formed tumorspheres, cycled slower, and were chemoresistant, all properties of stem cells thus confirming that breast cancer cell lines contain subpopulations of CSCs.

Long-term tumorsphere culture does not maintain a high number of CSCs. When MCF7 cells were sorted for $CD44^+/CD24^-$ and placed in tumorsphere-forming conditions, the number of $CD44^+/CD24^-$ CSCs decreased over time (Peng et al. 2011). This result indicates that there are still needed discoveries that will maintain a pure pool of breast CSCs for *in vitro* research.

14.5 HETEROTYPIC 3D *IN VITRO* SYSTEMS

The 3D systems discussed previously are monoculture systems. The intact human breast and mouse mammary gland are not comprised of only one cell type. To fully recapitulate the complexity of an *in vivo* environment, not only are BM components required as in the case of Matrigel®-based systems, but also additional cell types such as stromal cells need to be incorporated into 3D systems. The additional cell types will interact with the epithelial cells both physically and biochemically through the production of intercellular signaling molecules such as growth factors (Cunha and Hom 1996; Radisky et al. 2001).

Many heterotypic 3D systems have been developed. These systems incorporate epithelial cells in coculture with adipocytes, stromal fibroblasts, or immune cells such as macrophages and T cells (Noel et al. 1992; Ronnov-Jessen et al. 1995; Seidl et al. 2002; Olsen et al. 2010; Hou et al. 2011; Lanitis et al. 2014). The majority of the heterotypic systems use Matrigel® or collagen-based matrices and two cell types. These systems allow for researchers to alter the concentrations of matrix, modify the ratios of cell types, and use different culture media. Tunable heterotypic 3D systems have been used to study not only normal breast and mammary development but also tumor cell behavior in response to different environmental stimuli (Yang and Burg 2015).

CSCs relay mainly on mitochondrial metabolism compared to more differentiated tumor cells and this correlates with increased radio-resistance (Vlashi et al. 2014). Mitochondrial biogenesis is required for mammosphere formation and propagation by CSCs *in vitro* (De Luca et al. 2015). Mitochondrial metabolism is promoted by oxidative stress and autophagy in the tumor microenvironment. Metabolic synergy between the cancer cells and normal stromal cells occurs when glycolytic stromal cells and oxidative cancer cells interact. The glycolytic stromal cells are part of the Warburg effect and produce reactive oxygen species (ROS). High ROS levels in turn favor cancer cell mitochondrial metabolism and enhance tumor cell growth and tumor progression (Martinez-Outschoorn et al. 2014). The incorporation of cancer-related stromal cells and breast cancer cells in a 3D matrix will help address this phenomenon and provide new insights on how to combat this synergy in patients.

An important regulator of cellular function is ECM stiffness. The tumor microenvironment is stiffer than the normal microenvironment. The elastic modulus of Matrigel® is similar to that of the normal mouse mammary microenvironment, whereas the stiffness of tumor microenvironments is up to 20× higher (Paszek et al. 2005). The addition of additional components to the matrix such as collagen or agarose allows for researchers to adjust the elastic modulus of a given 3D system to more closely mimic the conditions found in normal and tumor situations *in vivo*.

Uncrosslinked collagen is readily remodeled by cells and therefore does not retain its initial 3D structure over time in culture. The addition of agarose to collagen matrices provides a stiffer substrate and therefore a more stable lattice for cell growth. Unlike collagen, cells do not remodel agarose; hence, a mix of the two allows a stable environment through which cells may traffic. Through the purposeful creation of a rigid, confining environment, we can drive metastatic cancer cells to differentiate rather than migrate (Booth et al. 2013). Conversely, by creating a permissive environment, we can induce normal cells to proliferate and migrate, mimicking a metastatic phenotype. By altering the surrounding environment, that is, changing the chemistry and/or matrix stiffness, one can fine-tune an *in vitro* system to answer specific biological questions.

Another variety of heterotypic 3D system has been developed in order to study disseminated breast cancer dormancy and metastasis initiation. Organotypic models of bone marrow and lung niches using different cell types and materials have been created. These models include microvascularization, microfluidics, and intravasation measurements (Ghajar et al. 2007, 2013; Hsu et al. 2013; Ehsan et al. 2014).

In summary, the heterotypic 3D systems allow scientists to manipulate multiple variables in order to answer questions that the traditional 2D culture systems simply cannot. The addition of multiple cell types, multiple chambers, and other factors means that heterotypic culture systems will be of great use in the future.

14.6 CONCLUSION AND PERSPECTIVE

Although the gold standard for stem cell functionality will always be *in vivo* experimentation, 3D *in vitro* platforms have served, and will continue to serve, as useful tools in the scientific exploration and understanding of normal and CSCs.

ACKNOWLEDGMENT

The authors acknowledge the Institute for Biological Interfaces of Engineering of Clemson University.

REFERENCES

Al-Hajj, M., M. S. Wicha, A. Benito-Hernandez, S. J. Morrison, and M. F. Clarke. 2003. Prospective identification of tumorigenic breast cancer cells. *Proc Natl Acad Sci USA* no. 100 (7):3983–8.

Battula, V. L., Y. Shi, K. W. Evans, R. Y. Wang, E. L. Spaeth, R. O. Jacamo et al. 2012. Ganglioside GD2 identifies breast cancer stem cells and promotes tumorigenesis. *J Clin Invest* no. 122 (6):2066–78.

Bissell, M. J. 1981. The differentiated state of normal and malignant cells or how to define a "normal" cell in culture. *Int Rev Cytol* no. 70:27–100.

Booth, B. W., C. A. Boulanger, L. H. Anderson, L. Jimenez-Rojo, C. Brisken, and G. H. Smith. 2010. Amphiregulin mediates self-renewal in an immortal mammary epithelial cell line with stem cell characteristics. *Exp Cell Res* no. 316 (3):422–32.

Booth, B. W., J. P. Park, and K. J. Burg. 2013. Evaluation of normal and metastatic mammary cells grown in different biomaterial matrices: Establishing potential tissue test systems. *J Biomater Sci Polym Ed* no. 24 (6):758–68.

Boudreau, N., C. Myers, and M. J. Bissell. 1995. From laminin to lamin: Regulation of tissue-specific gene expression by the ECM. *Trends Cell Biol* no. 5 (1):1–4.

Callahan, R. and G. H. Smith. 2000. MMTV-induced mammary tumorigenesis: Gene discovery, progression to malignancy and cellular pathways. *Oncogene* no. 19 (8): 992–1001.

Chen, D., P. Bhat-Nakshatri, C. Goswami, S. Badve, and H. Nakshatri. 2013. ANTXR1, a stem cell-enriched functional biomarker, connects collagen signaling to cancer stem-like cells and metastasis in breast cancer. *Cancer Res* no. 73 (18):5821–33.

Correia, A. L. and M. J. Bissell. 2012. The tumor microenvironment is a dominant force in multidrug resistance. *Drug Resist Updat* no. 15 (1–2):39–49.

Cunha, G. R. and Y. K. Hom. 1996. Role of mesenchymal-epithelial interactions in mammary gland development. *J Mammary Gland Biol Neoplasia* no. 1 (1):21–35.

Daniel, C. W. 1975. Regulation of cell division in aging mouse mammary epithelium. *Adv Exp Med Biol* no. 61:1–19.

Daniel, C. W., B. D. Aidells, D. Medina, and L. J. Faulkin, Jr. 1975. Unlimited division potential of precancerous mouse mammary cells after spontaneous or carcinogen-induced transformation. *Fed Proc* no. 34 (1):64–7.

De Luca, A., M. Fiorillo, M. Peiris-Pages, B. Ozsvari, D. L. Smith, R. Sanchez-Alvarez et al. 2015. Mitochondrial biogenesis is required for the anchorage-independent survival and propagation of stem-like cancer cells. *Oncotarget* no. 6 (17):14777–95.

Deome, K. B., L. J. Faulkin, Jr., H. A. Bern, and P. B. Blair. 1959. Development of mammary tumors from hyperplastic alveolar nodules transplanted into gland-free mammary fat pads of female C3H mice. *Cancer Res* no. 19 (5):515–20.

Diallo, R., K. L. Schaefer, C. Poremba, N. Shivazi, V. Willmann, H. Buerger, B. Dockhorn-Dworniczak, and W. Boecker. 2001. Monoclonality in normal epithelium and in hyperplastic and neoplastic lesions of the breast. *J Pathol* no. 193 (1):27–32.

Dontu, G., W. M. Abdallah, J. M. Foley, K. W. Jackson, M. F. Clarke, M. J. Kawamura, and M. S. Wicha. 2003. In vitro propagation and transcriptional profiling of human mammary stem/progenitor cells. *Genes Dev* no. 17 (10):1253–70.

Dontu, G., K. W. Jackson, E. McNicholas, M. J. Kawamura, W. M. Abdallah, and M. S. Wicha. 2004. Role of Notch signaling in cell-fate determination of human mammary stem/progenitor cells. *Breast Cancer Res* no. 6 (6):R605–15.

Easwaran, H., H. C. Tsai, and S. B. Baylin. 2014. Cancer epigenetics: Tumor heterogeneity, plasticity of stem-like states, and drug resistance. *Mol Cell* no. 54 (5):716–27.

Ehsan, S. M., K. M. Welch-Reardon, M. L. Waterman, C. C. Hughes, and S. C. George. 2014. A three-dimensional in vitro model of tumor cell intravasation. *Integr Biol (Camb)* no. 6 (6):603–10.

Elsdale, T. and J. Bard. 1972. Collagen substrata for studies on cell behavior. *J Cell Biol* no. 54 (3):626–37.

Emerman, J. T. and D. R. Pitelka. 1977. Maintenance and induction of morphological differentiation in dissociated mammary epithelium on floating collagen membranes. *In Vitro* no. 13 (5):316–28.

Faulkin, L. J., Jr. and K. B. Deome. 1960. Regulation of growth and spacing of gland elements in the mammary fat pad of the C3H mouse. *J Natl Cancer Inst* no. 24:953–69.

Fillmore, C. M. and C. Kuperwasser. 2008. Human breast cancer cell lines contain stem-like cells that self-renew, give rise to phenotypically diverse progeny and survive chemotherapy. *Breast Cancer Res* no. 10 (2):R25.

Ghajar, C. M., H. Peinado, H. Mori, I. R. Matei, K. J. Evason, H. Brazier et al. 2013. The perivascular niche regulates breast tumour dormancy. *Nat Cell Biol* no. 15 (7):807–17.

Ghajar, C. M., V. Suresh, S. R. Peyton, C. B. Raub, F. L. Meyskens, Jr., S. C. George, and A. J. Putnam. 2007. A novel three-dimensional model to quantify metastatic melanoma invasion. *Mol Cancer Ther* no. 6 (2):552–61.

Ginestier, C., M. H. Hur, E. Charafe-Jauffret, F. Monville, J. Dutcher, M. Brown et al. 2007. ALDH1 is a marker of normal and malignant human mammary stem cells and a predictor of poor clinical outcome. *Cell Stem Cell* no. 1 (5):555–67.

Gudjonsson, T., R. Villadsen, H. L. Nielsen, L. Ronnov-Jessen, M. J. Bissell, and O. W. Petersen. 2002. Isolation, immortalization, and characterization of a human breast epithelial cell line with stem cell properties. *Genes Dev* no. 16 (6):693–706.

Gupta, P. B., T. T. Onder, G. Jiang, K. Tao, C. Kuperwasser, R. A. Weinberg, and E. S. Lander. 2009. Identification of selective inhibitors of cancer stem cells by high-throughput screening. *Cell* no. 138 (4):645–59.

Hou, Z., D. J. Falcone, K. Subbaramaiah, and A. J. Dannenberg. 2011. Macrophages induce COX-2 expression in breast cancer cells: Role of IL-1beta autoamplification. *Carcinogenesis* no. 32 (5):695–702.

Hsu, Y. H., M. L. Moya, C. C. Hughes, S. C. George, and A. P. Lee. 2013. A microfluidic platform for generating large-scale nearly identical human microphysiological vascularized tissue arrays. *Lab Chip* no. 13 (15):2990–8.

Kenny, P. A., G. Y. Lee, C. A. Myers, R. M. Neve, J. R. Semeiks, P. T. Spellman et al. 2007. The morphologies of breast cancer cell lines in three-dimensional assays correlate with their profiles of gene expression. *Mol Oncol* no. 1 (1):84–96.

Kleinman, H. K. and G. R. Martin. 2005. Matrigel: Basement membrane matrix with biological activity. *Semin Cancer Biol* no. 15 (5):378–86.

Kleinman, H. K., M. L. McGarvey, J. R. Hassell, V. L. Star, F. B. Cannon, G. W. Laurie, and G. R. Martin. 1986. Basement membrane complexes with biological activity. *Biochemistry* no. 25 (2):312–8.

Kleinman, H. K., M. L. McGarvey, L. A. Liotta, P. G. Robey, K. Tryggvason, and G. R. Martin. 1982. Isolation and characterization of type IV procollagen, laminin, and heparan sulfate proteoglycan from the EHS sarcoma. *Biochemistry* no. 21 (24):6188–93.

Kok, M., R. H. Koornstra, T. C. Margarido, R. Fles, N. J. Armstrong, S. C. Linn, L. J. Van't Veer, and B. Weigelt. 2009. Mammosphere-derived gene set predicts outcome in patients with ER-positive breast cancer. *J Pathol* no. 218 (3):316–26.

Lagadec, C., E. Vlashi, Y. Alhiyari, T. M. Phillips, M. Bochkur Dratver, and F. Pajonk. 2013. Radiation-induced Notch signaling in breast cancer stem cells. *Int J Radiat Oncol Biol Phys* no. 87 (3):609–18.

Lamb, R., M. P. Ablett, K. Spence, G. Landberg, A. H. Sims, and R. B. Clarke. 2013. Wnt pathway activity in breast cancer sub-types and stem-like cells. *PLoS One* no. 8 (7):e67811.

Lanitis, E., J. B. Smith, D. Dangaj, S. Flingai, M. Poussin, S. Xu, B. J. Czerniecki, Y. F. Li, P. F. Robbins, and D. J. Powell, Jr. 2014. A human ErbB2-specific T-cell receptor confers potent antitumor effector functions in genetically engineered primary cytotoxic lymphocytes. *Hum Gene Ther* no. 25 (8):730–9.

Lee, E. H., A. S. Mount, D. W. Booth, and W. Y. Chen. 2015. Prolactin and cisplatin combination treatment inhibits tumorsphere formation and delays breast tumor growth in mice. *Int J Oncol* no. 2 (2):1–7.

Lee, E. Y., W. H. Lee, C. S. Kaetzel, G. Parry, and M. J. Bissell. 1985. Interaction of mouse mammary epithelial cells with collagen substrata: Regulation of casein gene expression and secretion. *Proc Natl Acad Sci USA* no. 82 (5):1419–23.

Lee, G. Y., P. A. Kenny, E. H. Lee, and M. J. Bissell. 2007. Three-dimensional culture models of normal and malignant breast epithelial cells. *Nat Methods* no. 4 (4):359–65.

Lelievre, S., V. M. Weaver, and M. J. Bissell. 1996. Extracellular matrix signaling from the cellular membrane skeleton to the nuclear skeleton: A model of gene regulation. *Recent Prog Horm Res* no. 51:417–32.

Liu, S., G. Dontu, I. D. Mantle, S. Patel, N. S. Ahn, K. W. Jackson, P. Suri, and M. S. Wicha. 2006. Hedgehog signaling and Bmi-1 regulate self-renewal of normal and malignant human mammary stem cells. *Cancer Res* no. 66 (12):6063–71.

Liu, S., G. Dontu, and M. S. Wicha. 2005. Mammary stem cells, self-renewal pathways, and carcinogenesis. *Breast Cancer Res* no. 7 (3):86–95.

Maglione, J. E., D. Moghanaki, L. J. Young, C. K. Manner, L. G. Ellies, S. O. Joseph, B. Nicholson, R. D. Cardiff, and C. L. MacLeod. 2001. Transgenic polyoma middle-T mice model premalignant mammary disease. *Cancer Res* no. 61 (22):8298–305.

Martinez-Outschoorn, U., F. Sotgia, and M. P. Lisanti. 2014. Tumor microenvironment and metabolic synergy in breast cancers: Critical importance of mitochondrial fuels and function. *Semin Oncol* no. 41 (2):195–216.

Medina, D. 2000. The preneoplastic phenotype in murine mammary tumorigenesis. *J Mammary Gland Biol Neoplasia* no. 5 (4):393–407.

Medina, D. 2002. Biological and molecular characteristics of the premalignant mouse mammary gland. *Biochim Biophys Acta* no. 1603 (1):1–9.

Medina, D. and F. S. Kittrell. 1993. Immortalization phenotype dissociated from the preneoplastic phenotype in mouse mammary epithelial outgrowths *in vivo*. *Carcinogenesis* no. 14 (1):25–8.

Medina, D., F. S. Kittrell, Y. J. Liu, and M. Schwartz. 1993. Morphological and functional properties of TM preneoplastic mammary outgrowths. *Cancer Res* no. 53 (3):663–7.

Medina, D., F. S. Kittrell, A. Shepard, L. C. Stephens, C. Jiang, J. Lu, D. C. Allred, M. McCarthy, and R. L. Ullrich. 2002. Biological and genetic properties of the p53 null preneoplastic mammary epithelium. *FASEB J* no. 16 (8):881–3.

Michalopoulos, G. and H. C. Pitot. 1975. Primary culture of parenchymal liver cells on collagen membranes. Morphological and biochemical observations. *Exp Cell Res* no. 94 (1):70–8.

Noel, A., C. Munaut, A. Boulvain, C. M. Calberg-Bacq, C. A. Lambert, B. Nusgens, C. M. Lapiere, and J. M. Foidart. 1992. Modulation of collagen and fibronectin synthesis in fibroblasts by normal and malignant cells. *J Cell Biochem* no. 48 (2):150–61.

Olsen, C. J., J. Moreira, E. M. Lukanidin, and N. S. Ambartsumian. 2010. Human mammary fibroblasts stimulate invasion of breast cancer cells in a three-dimensional culture and increase stroma development in mouse xenografts. *BMC Cancer* no. 10:444.

Park, J. P., A. Raafat, J. A. Feltracco, W. M. Blanding, and B. W. Booth. 2013. Differential gene expression in nuclear label-retaining cells in the developing mouse mammary gland. *Stem Cells Dev* no. 22 (8):1297–306.

Paszek, M. J., N. Zahir, K. R. Johnson, J. N. Lakins, G. I. Rozenberg, A. Gefen et al. 2005. Tensional homeostasis and the malignant phenotype. *Cancer Cell* no. 8 (3):241–54.

Peng, T., M. Qinghua, T. Zhenning, W. Kaifa, and J. Jun. 2011. Long-term sphere culture cannot maintain a high ratio of cancer stem cells: A mathematical model and experiment. *PLoS One* no. 6 (11):e25518.

Perou, C. M., T. Sorlie, M. B. Eisen, M. van de Rijn, S. S. Jeffrey, C. A. Rees et al. 2000. Molecular portraits of human breast tumours. *Nature* no. 406 (6797):747–52.

Petersen, O. W., L. Ronnov-Jessen, A. R. Howlett, and M. J. Bissell. 1992. Interaction with basement membrane serves to rapidly distinguish growth and differentiation pattern of normal and malignant human breast epithelial cells. *Proc Natl Acad Sci USA* no. 89 (19):9064–8.

Ponti, D., A. Costa, N. Zaffaroni, G. Pratesi, G. Petrangolini, D. Coradini, S. Pilotti, M. A. Pierotti, and M. G. Daidone. 2005. Isolation and *in vitro* propagation of tumorigenic breast cancer cells with stem/progenitor cell properties. *Cancer Res* no. 65 (13):5506–11.

Radisky, D., C. Hagios, and M. J. Bissell. 2001. Tumors are unique organs defined by abnormal signaling and context. *Semin Cancer Biol* no. 11 (2):87–95.

Ronnov-Jessen, L., O. W. Petersen, and M. J. Bissell. 1996. Cellular changes involved in conversion of normal to malignant breast: Importance of the stromal reaction. *Physiol Rev* no. 76 (1):69–125.

Ronnov-Jessen, L., O. W. Petersen, V. E. Koteliansky, and M. J. Bissell. 1995. The origin of the myofibroblasts in breast cancer. Recapitulation of tumor environment in culture unravels diversity and implicates converted fibroblasts and recruited smooth muscle cells. *J Clin Invest* no. 95 (2):859–73.

Saadin, K. and I. M. White. 2013. Breast cancer stem cell enrichment and isolation by mammosphere culture and its potential diagnostic applications. *Expert Rev Mol Diagn* no. 13 (1):49–60.

Seidl, P., R. Huettinger, R. Knuechel, and L. A. Kunz-Schughart. 2002. Three-dimensional fibroblast-tumor cell interaction causes downregulation of RACK1 mRNA expression in breast cancer cells *in vitro*. *Int J Cancer* no. 102 (2):129–36.

Singh, S. K., I. D. Clarke, M. Terasaki, V. E. Bonn, C. Hawkins, J. Squire, and P. B. Dirks. 2003. Identification of a cancer stem cell in human brain tumors. *Cancer Res* no. 63 (18):5821–8.

Singh, S. K., C. Hawkins, I. D. Clarke, J. A. Squire, J. Bayani, T. Hide, R. M. Henkelman, M. D. Cusimano, and P. B. Dirks. 2004. Identification of human brain tumour initiating cells. *Nature* no. 432 (7015):396–401.

Sinha, N., S. Mukhopadhyay, D. N. Das, P. K. Panda, and S. K. Bhutia. 2013. Relevance of cancer initiating/stem cells in carcinogenesis and therapy resistance in oral cancer. *Oral Oncol* no. 49 (9):854–62.

Smalley, M. J. and R. B. Clarke. 2005. The mammary gland "side population": A putative stem/progenitor cell marker? *J Mammary Gland Biol Neoplasia* no. 10 (1):37–47.

Smith, G. H., L. A. Arthur, and D. Medina. 1980. Evidence of separate pathways for viral and chemical carcinogenesis in C3H/StWi mouse mammary glands. *Int J Cancer* no. 26 (3):373–9.

Smith, G. H., R. J. Pauley, S. H. Socher, and D. Medina. 1978. Chemical carcinogenesis in C3H/StWi mice, a worthwhile experimental model for breast cancer. *Cancer Res* no. 38 (12):4504–9.

Sorlie, T., C. M. Perou, R. Tibshirani, T. Aas, S. Geisler, H. Johnsen et al. 2001. Gene expression patterns of breast carcinomas distinguish tumor subclasses with clinical implications. *Proc Natl Acad Sci USA* no. 98 (19):10869–74.

Stirling, J. W. and J. A. Chandler. 1976. The fine structure of the normal, resting terminal ductal-lobular unit of the female breast. *Virchows Arch A: Pathol Anat Histol* no. 372 (3):205–26.

Streuli, C. H. and M. J. Bissell. 1990. Expression of extracellular matrix components is regulated by substratum. *J Cell Biol* no. 110 (4):1405–15.

Swamydas, M., J. M. Eddy, K. J. Burg, and D. Dreau. 2010. Matrix compositions and the development of breast acini and ducts in 3D cultures. *In Vitro Cell Dev Biol Anim* no. 46 (8):673–84.

Vlashi, E., C. Lagadec, L. Vergnes, K. Reue, P. Frohnen, M. Chan, Y. Alhiyari, M. B. Dratver, and F. Pajonk. 2014. Metabolic differences in breast cancer stem cells and differentiated progeny. *Breast Cancer Res Treat* no. 146 (3):525–34.

Vukicevic, S., H. K. Kleinman, F. P. Luyten, A. B. Roberts, N. S. Roche, and A. H. Reddi. 1992. Identification of multiple active growth factors in basement membrane Matrigel suggests caution in interpretation of cellular activity related to extracellular matrix components. *Exp Cell Res* no. 202 (1):1–8.

Wang, R., Q. Lv, W. Meng, Q. Tan, S. Zhang, X. Mo, and X. Yang. 2014. Comparison of mammosphere formation from breast cancer cell lines and primary breast tumors. *J Thorac Dis* no. 6 (6):829–37.

Weaver, V. M. and M. J. Bissell. 1999. Functional culture models to study mechanisms governing apoptosis in normal and malignant mammary epithelial cells. *J Mammary Gland Biol Neoplasia* no. 4 (2):193–201.

Weaver, V. M., O. W. Petersen, F. Wang, C. A. Larabell, P. Briand, C. Damsky, and M. J. Bissell. 1997. Reversion of the malignant phenotype of human breast cells in three-dimensional culture and *in vivo* by integrin blocking antibodies. *J Cell Biol* no. 137 (1):231–45.

Weigelt, B., C. M. Ghajar, and M. J. Bissell. 2014. The need for complex 3D culture models to unravel novel pathways and identify accurate biomarkers in breast cancer. *Adv Drug Deliv Rev* no. 69–70:42–51.

Wright, M. H., A. M. Calcagno, C. D. Salcido, M. D. Carlson, S. V. Ambudkar, and L. Varticovski. 2008. Brca1 breast tumors contain distinct CD44+/CD24- and CD133+ cells with cancer stem cell characteristics. *Breast Cancer Res* no. 10 (1):R10.

Yang, C. C. and K. J. Burg. 2015. Designing a tunable 3D heterocellular breast cancer tissue test system. *J Tissue Eng Regen Med* no. 9 (3):310–4.

15 Shape Matters
Understanding the Breast through 3D Tissue Culture Models

Lucia Speroni, Ana M. Soto, and Carlos Sonnenschein

CONTENTS

15.1 Introduction 263
15.2 Characteristics of the Mammary Gland 264
15.3 Mammary Gland Development 264
15.4 Cancer in the Breast 266
15.5 *In Vitro* Models for the Study of Breast Tissue 266
15.6 3D Culture Models: Mammary Gland Biology and Carcinogenesis
      Studied from a Tissue-Level Perspective 267
15.7 Design of a 3D Culture Model of the Human Breast 268
      15.7.1 Mammary Epithelial Cell Types 268
      15.7.2 Stromal Cell Types 271
      15.7.3 Morphological Criteria to Distinguish between Normal and
             Abnormal Breast Epithelial Structures in 3D Culture 272
15.8 Biomechanical Factors Involved in Mammary Gland Morphogenesis 273
15.9 Interplay between Biomechanical Forces and Hormones 273
15.10 Data Acquisition and Analysis 276
15.11 Conclusion and Perspective 278
Acknowledgments 278
References 278

15.1 INTRODUCTION

During the last three decades, developmental biologists working at the cell and organ levels of biological complexity have contributed greatly to describing the structure and functions of the mammary gland. The data collected have enriched our understanding of events happening during the successive stages of mammary gland development under normal and pathological conditions, including cancer. We have proposed that cancer is, in fact, development gone awry, and thus much can be learned about mammary gland development by studying events that, from fetal life up to senescence, become part of the subject of mammary gland carcinogenesis (Sonnenschein et al. 2014; Soto and Sonnenschein 2014, 2011). For their part, molecular biologists also contributed significantly to describing structural phenomena and molecular interactions occurring during the development of the mammary gland while adopting the premise that species or strain-specific subcellular events will explain the phenotypic traits observed under *in vivo* conditions. To accomplish this aim, a variety of *in animal* and *in culture* models have been explored. During the second half of the last century and the current one, the tools generated by molecular biologists aimed at linking events taking place inside cells, such as those occurring during the cell cycle and/or during hormone-triggered induction of gene products, to the diverse phenotypes acquired by the gland during the lifetime of mammals.

Notwithstanding the staggering amount of data collected so far, there are aspects of normal mammary gland development and of cancer that still remain unknown. To cover these uncharted grounds, novel technological approaches have been added to the more traditional ones. In this chapter, we will discuss the three-dimensional (3D) culture models available to study the dynamics of normal and pathological breast development.

15.2 CHARACTERISTICS OF THE MAMMARY GLAND

The mammary gland is made up of two main tissue types, namely, (1) the parenchyma, represented by the epithelial cells, whose function is to generate milk to nourish the growing newborn and (2) the stroma which surrounds the glandular epithelium. The bilayered epithelium is comprised of luminal cuboidal epithelial cells and basally located myoepithelial cells. The stroma or connective tissue surrounding the epithelium is composed of various cell types (fibroblasts, adipocytes, and immune cells), blood vessels, nerves, and an extracellular fibrous matrix of which the main component is collagen (Howard and Gusterson 2000; Masso-Welch et al. 2000; Richert et al. 2000). In cycling adults, at the distal end of the small ductal tree, there are lobules composed of sacs or alveoli where milk is produced in response to hormonal cues. In human and primates, these structures are called terminal ductal lobular units and are the sites were breast tumors commonly develop starting as intraductal hyperplasia (Wellings et al. 1975). Throughout development, reciprocal interactions between the epithelium and the stroma are responsible for the phenotype of mammary glands. Perturbations of epithelial–stromal interactions can cause normal mammary gland development to go awry, leading to the eventual formation of tumors (Maffini et al. 2004).

15.3 MAMMARY GLAND DEVELOPMENT

The mammary gland undergoes morphological changes at each stage of development. Those stages of development have been extensively described in rodents and can be divided into fetal, prepubertal, puberty to adulthood, pregnancy, lactation, and involution. During mouse fetal development, the mammary placodes become visible between embryonic Day (E) 11 and 12 and they then develop into mammary buds by E13. At this time, several layers of mesenchyme condense surrounding the buds in a concentric fashion and they acquire a "light bulb" shape. In male embryos, the presence of testosterone instructs the mesenchyme to condense around the bud, which then separates from the epidermis impeding further epithelial development (Kratochwil 1971, 1977). In female mouse embryos, after a 24 h resting phase, the mammary bud sprouts as it pushes through the mesenchyme penetrating the presumptive fat pad made up of a cluster of adipocytes. At E18, the mammary epithelium consists of a rudimentary ductal tree (Balinsky 1950; Robinson et al. 1999). Apart from the action of testosterone described above, fetal mammary gland development in mice does not require the action of other hormones. However, fetal mammary morphogenesis can be altered by *in utero* exposure to hormonally active chemicals such as the xeno-estrogen Bisphenol-A (Vandenberg et al. 2007; Speroni et al. 2017). In rodents, the growth of the mammary gland is isometric until puberty. From puberty onward, the development of the mammary gland is subject to hormonal regulation resulting from complex feedback loops of the hypothalamic–pituitary–ovarian axis (HPOA). At the onset of puberty, estrogens secreted by the ovaries induce the formation of club-shaped structures at the end of the ducts, called terminal end buds (TEBs). Thereafter, the epithelium begins to fill the fat pad, and it increases its complexity due to the repetitive cycles of ovarian sex steroids. Progesterone facilitates side-branching through progesterone receptors (PRs) expressed in the epithelial cells. If pregnancy occurs, prolactin secreted by the pituitary, in combination with estrogen and progesterone, initiates a characteristic lobulo-alveolar development to enable milk production and eventual lactation (reviewed in Brisken and O'Malley 2010). When lactation ceases, involution of the alveolar structures occurs and the mammary gland returns to its resting state (i.e., non-lactating). Although certain hormones can be identified as the main drivers of rodent mammary gland development, at each stage there is basal activity of other hormones involved as suggested by evidence collected from knockout mice for hormone receptors. For example, prolactin receptor knockout mice show reduced ductal branching and failure of the TEBs to differentiate into alveolar buds at puberty (Brisken et al. 1999). Adult knockout mice for ERα (ERαKO) show a rudimentary epithelial tree lacking TEBs, pointing to the role of estrogen action in alveolar morphogenesis. This rudimentary tree is similar to that of a normal female mouse before puberty, suggesting that prenatal mammary gland development in the ERαKO could be influenced by maternal growth hormone (Bocchinfuso and Korach 1997).

The function and developmental stages of the mammary gland as well as the hormones involved are conserved between mice and humans. However, there are histological differences between the two species regarding the structure of the stroma. Namely, the human breast epithelium is in intimate contact with fibrous connective tissue and distant from the adipose tissue, whereas the mouse mammary ducts are dispersed in a stroma composed of fibroblasts and adipocytes (Parmar and Cunha 2004). Therefore, the 3D culture models that reproduce the human breast tissue architecture aim to provide insights into the role of stromal–epithelial interactions in human mammary gland development and neoplasia. In addition, given the complexity of the hormonal feedback loops that occur *in vivo*, hormone-sensitive 3D culture models are unique, desirable tools to help us understand hormone-induced mammary morphogenesis (Speroni et al. 2014).

15.4 CANCER IN THE BREAST

Breast carcinogenesis has received the dedicated attention of clinical and experimental researchers for over a century. In the nineteenth century, the availability of the light microscope and of new chemical stains dictated the agenda of those researchers. Since the second half of last century, with the advent of the molecular biology revolution, researchers have focused on the study of genes involved in breast cancer, a development that consolidated the hegemony of the somatic mutation theory (SMT). This reductionist approach favored exploring events happening within the confines of the cell's plasma membrane with special emphasis on a genetic perspective of cancer. As a result, hundreds of macromolecules present in the nucleus and cytoplasm of those cells and gene expression profiles as well as alleged molecular markers were thoroughly characterized. Notwithstanding, cancer at large and breast cancer in particular are still reliably diagnosed by pathologists who search and identify altered tissue organization in histological slides (Sonnenschein and Soto 1999; Soto and Sonnenschein 2011).

It is widely acknowledged that little progress has been made in the treatment of breast cancer and that a comprehensive explanation of breast carcinogenesis is far from having been reached (Hanahan 2014). This limited therapeutic progress in breast cancer has been attributed to two main factors: (1) the attempt to explain carcinogenesis by linear causality in a bottom-up approach from gene to cancer (Hanahan and Weinberg 2000, 2011) and (2) the use of two-dimensional (2D) cultures and models that generally involve only one cell type, the epithelium, which falls short in mimicking the features of the mammary gland architecture. Meanwhile, increasing evidence supports the alternative idea that carcinogenesis is due to alterations at the tissue level of biological organization as stated under the premises of the tissue organization field theory (TOFT). Briefly, those premises posit that (a) cancer is a tissue-based disease and that (b) proliferation with variation and motility are the default states of all cells (Sonnenschein and Soto 1999).

Mammary gland biology has benefited from the contribution of two main experimental approaches, namely (i) a biophysical one that centers on mechanical forces, which are the main determinants of shape and regulates the interaction between the epithelium and the stroma (Paszek et al. 2005; Barnes et al. 2014; Elosegui-Artola et al. 2014) and (ii) an endocrine one by which natural and synthetic hormones influence the different stages of stromal/epithelial morphogenesis. Based on these considerations, we will discuss the use of physiologically relevant culture systems for the study of the breast from a tissue-level perspective.

15.5 *IN VITRO* MODELS FOR THE STUDY OF BREAST TISSUE

Normal mammary gland morphogenesis and breast cancer, respectively, depend on normal and pathological reciprocal interactions between the stroma and the epithelium and their respective extracellular matrices. The complexity of the organ makes it difficult to study the interaction between compartments *in vivo*. To overcome this limitation, a variety of culture models have been developed. Conventional 2D cultures of epithelial cells remain as relevant models to study hormonal regulation of cell proliferation (Soto and Sonnenschein 1984; Soto et al. 1986) and of gene expression (Chalbos et al. 1982; Vignon et al. 1983; Soto et al. 1986). However, morphogenic processes such as the formation of ducts and acini, which are 3D structures, require appropriate substrates that allow cells to proliferate, move, and organize in a 3D space. In addition, remodeling of the extracellular matrix accompanies the morphogenic process. Thus, 3D culture models serve as effective tools to reproduce breast morphogenesis *in vitro*. Unlike 2D cultures, the 3D culture systems allow for the dynamic study of epithelial morphogenesis and the organization of the stroma. Morphological parameters are indicators of normal and diseased states for the study of normal breast development and breast cancer since both processes involve those dynamic changes in tissue architecture.

The aim of developing a 3D culture model is to mimic the *in vivo* conditions prevailing in a living organism. Thus, the design of a 3D culture model requires adopting several basic conditions, namely (1) define the main characteristics of the target tissue that the 3D culture model aims to reproduce, (2) identify whether the 3D culture model will mimic either the normal or the diseased state of the *in vivo* tissue, and (3) in the case of breast tissue, define which stage of mammary gland development the investigator is interested in reproducing *in vitro*.

15.6 3D CULTURE MODELS: MAMMARY GLAND BIOLOGY AND CARCINOGENESIS STUDIED FROM A TISSUE-LEVEL PERSPECTIVE

Increasingly complex 3D models aimed to provide a more accurate example of breast tissue than the 2D culture models. This requires choosing the appropriate cell types (epithelial and stromal), the varied matrices in which those cells will be placed and the type of culture vessels the 3D model will use. Epithelial–stromal interactions can be studied using 3D co-cultures of epithelial and stromal cells by analyzing matrix remodeling and epithelial morphogenesis. With regard to matrices, there are a number of different materials being used but the most biologically relevant ones should provide the structure and rigidity of the model tissue that allows the cellular components to attain characteristics seen in the breast. There are a variety of matrices and scaffolds that can be used to grow mammary epithelial cells in 3D culture; they can be made out of natural materials such as silk (Wang et al. 2010) or collagen (Krause et al. 2008, 2010; Dhimolea et al. 2010, 2012, 2014; Krause et al. 2012; Barnes et al. 2014; Speroni et al. 2014) or synthetic materials (Pavlovich et al. 2010; Miroshnikova et al. 2011). Silk scaffolds support the growth of monocultures of breast epithelial cells or co-cultures with stromal cells (Wang et al. 2010). The use of synthetic matrices has provided valuable information on the role of mechanical cues in epithelial morphogenesis. For example, self-assembly peptide gels (Miroshnikova et al. 2011) and polydimethylsiloxane (PDMS) substrates (Cassereau et al. 2015) can be used to study the role of matrix stiffness in collagen gels without significantly altering the architecture of the fibrillar matrix with respect to pore size and fiber diameter. Scaffolds and synthetic substrates often need to be supplemented with collagen type I, Matrigel®, or other basement membrane proteins such as laminin in order for the cells to grow or to organize into polarized epithelial structures. In this chapter, we focus on collagen-based matrices since collagen is a main component of the mammary stroma and allows for human mammary epithelial cells to self-organize into structures that closely resemble those observed *in vivo* (Krause et al. 2008, 2012; Dhimolea et al. 2010; Barnes et al. 2014; Speroni et al. 2014). In addition, collagen-based matrices are transparent and allow for live imaging throughout the culture period (Barnes et al. 2014). Another requirement of the "ideal" 3D culture model is that it should be technically feasible to measure the desired endpoints with physiologically relevant metrics. In a typical experiment using 3D cultures, the number of epithelial structures formed should allow for a large enough sampling to be used for quantitative analysis. This is more desirable than, for instance, to have a single acinus (or a hand-picked few) on which to base assumptions and conclusions.

15.7 DESIGN OF A 3D CULTURE MODEL OF THE HUMAN BREAST

In the normal mammary gland, ducts are predominant in the resting state (non-lactating), whereas acinar structures are abundantly present during pregnancy and lactation. Most 3D cultures of the mammary gland reproduce acini (Debnath et al. 2003; Lee et al. 2007). However, ducts are the main structures found in the resting mammary gland, structures where carcinomas most frequently arise. Although normal epithelial structures *in vivo* are characterized by the presence of lumen and cell polarization, abnormal or (neoplastic) structures are characterized by luminal filling, loss of polarization, and during the invasive stages, a disruption of the basement membrane.

The mammary stroma also exhibits differential characteristics between normalcy and neoplasia. High mammographic density, a risk factor for developing breast cancer (Boyd et al. 2007), is associated with changes in the stromal compartment, such as higher collagen content (Alowami et al. 2003). Different arrangements of collagen fiber alignment have also been associated with different stages of tumor growth in mice. Higher stromal density was also observed as tumors grew in size and collagen fibers aligned radially with respect to the tumor boundary, suggesting that this could favor invasion and metastasis (Provenzano et al. 2006, 2008). Matrix stiffness has also been linked to neoplasia, as shown by the increased stiffness of mouse mammary tumors in comparison with the normal mammary gland (Paszek et al. 2005).

15.7.1 MAMMARY EPITHELIAL CELL TYPES

3D cultures of the breast have used several established cell lines and primary cells. MCF10A has been the most widely studied "normal" breast epithelial cell line (Soule et al. 1990). In 3D culture, MCF10A cells are excellent tools for studying branching and acinar morphogenesis (Krause et al. 2008; Dhimolea et al. 2010) (Figure 15.1) and the mechanics involved in these processes such as cell movement (Tanner et al. 2012), tissue stiffness (Paszek et al. 2005; Barnes et al. 2014; Venugopalan et al. 2014), and transmission of forces through organization of collagen fibers (Guo et al. 2012; Barnes et al. 2014). The phenotype of the epithelial structures is highly dependent on the culture conditions. MCF10A cells form acini when cultured in

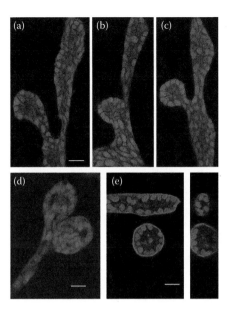

FIGURE 15.1 MCF10A cells grown in 3D culture conditions mimic the normal breast epithelium. (a) Branching duct, (b, c) budding ducts, and (d) ductal tip resembling a terminal end. Images of carmine stained-whole mounts obtained using confocal microscopy. (e) Duct (top) and an acinus (bottom) in a staining for F-actin (red). Nuclei were stained with DAPI (blue). Slice of a confocal 3D stack and its corresponding orthogonal view shows polarized nuclei. Scale bars: 20 μm.

matrices containing high concentrations of reconstituted basement membrane, that is, Matrigel® (Krause et al. 2008), or in an "on top assay" using laminin-1 as a matrix (Benton et al. 2009). Meanwhile, MCF10A cells form ducts when embedded in a collagen type 1 matrix, or when grown as monolayers when using the same matrix in an "on top assay" (Benton et al. 2009). Although MCF10A cells are excellent tools to study acinar and branching morphogenesis, they are unsuitable for the study of hormone action on the breast epithelium since these cells lack receptors for estrogen, progesterone, and prolactin. In the normal mammary gland, 10%–15% of the epithelial cells express ER and 96% of them coexpress PR. Of note, in the normal mammary gland, a cell population expresses Ki67 but not ER, suggesting that the effects of estrogen on cell proliferation are regulated through paracrine cues (Clarke et al. 1997; Clarke 2004; Brisken 2013).

Exposure to prolonged high levels of estrogen is a main risk for developing breast cancer (Key et al. 2002; Baglietto et al. 2010) and 70%–80% of breast tumors are ER+, of which approximately half are also PR+ (Keen and Davidson 2003). Currently, there are a few human hormone receptor-positive cell lines available, all of them derived from metastatic tumors, such as MCF7 and T47D. They express ER, PR, and prolactin receptors and exhibit a typical cell-proliferation pattern in response to estrogen (Figure 15.2) In contrast, MCF12A cells, derived from normal tissue, have been reported to be estrogen-sensitive as the expression of a subset of genes was estrogen-sensitive (Marchese and Silva 2012). Thus, hormone-responsive 3D culture

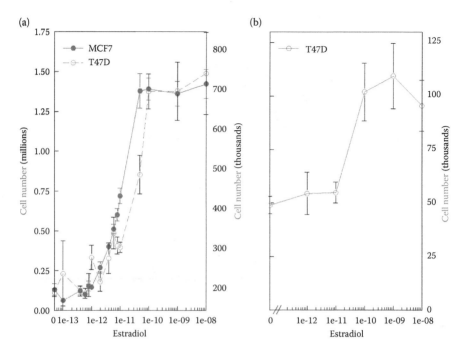

FIGURE 15.2 Dose–response curves of breast epithelial cells in the presence of 17β-estradiol for 7 days. (a) MCF7 and T47D cells in 2D culture conditions and (b) T47D cells in 3D culture conditions.

breast models are also relevant for the study of carcinogenesis and the testing of cancer therapies of cells that are genuinely sensitive to hormone action. In this regard, the influence of the microenvironment in the reversion of the malignant phenotype was studied in MCF7 cells grown in 3D culture (Krause et al. 2010; D'Anselmi et al. 2013). T47D cells grown in 3D culture were proven useful for the study of hormone-regulated epithelial organization and stromal remodeling and biomechanical factors associated with this process (Barcus et al. 2013; Speroni et al. 2014).

In principle, primary breast cells are a preferred choice for 3D culture models since they most closely resemble fresh tissue. However, when freshly harvested human tissue microstructures were exposed for 24 h to 17β-estradiol (E2) and promegestone (R5020), an analogue of progesterone, only the latter, but not E2, induced changes in the proliferative index and increased RANKL mRNA levels (Tanos et al. 2013). The standardization of models that use primary breast cells (Graham et al. 2009; Tanos et al. 2013) is somewhat challenging due to the heterogeneity of individual breast tissue samples given that the cell type composition and density vary between different tissue areas, and the lack of correlation between parameters like menstrual cycle status and parity and the proliferative response to E2 and R5020. Lack of stability regarding hormone receptor expression in primary cultures is another disadvantage when using primary cultures. To the contrary, the available established cell lines retain their hormone receptor status and show comparable dose–response proliferation curves through a large number of passages. Information on cell maintenance practices and passage number used is fundamental to guarantee reproducibility. Charcoal-stripped serum, which renders it steroid-free, is recommended to supplement the media when serum is required (Soto et al. 1995). To assure an estrogen-free in culture environment, culture media, plastic materials, and membrane filters should be evaluated for the presence of hormonally active synthetic compounds (Soto et al. 1991).

15.7.2 STROMAL CELL TYPES

The stroma is composed of several cell types, fibroblasts and adipocytes being the most abundant, as well as endothelial cells and inflammatory cells such as mast cells and macrophages. Although the stroma is a main contributor to mammary epithelial morphogenesis and neoplasia, our knowledge of the contribution of each stromal cell type is limited. Nonetheless, tissue recombination experiments have shown that mammary epithelium can develop into salivary-gland structures when recombined with salivary mesenchyme, suggesting that the surrounding stroma plays a main role (Kratochwil 1969; Sakakura et al. 1976). Moreover, when the stroma is affected by a carcinogenic insult, the result is neoplastic development (Barcellos-Hoff and Ravani 2000; Maffini et al. 2004). Recombination of stroma exposed to the mammary carcinogen N-nitrosomethylurea with vehicle-exposed epithelial cells resulted in neoplasms, whereas the reverse combination did not (Maffini et al. 2004). In addition, the mammary stroma is able to instruct tumor cells to develop into normal ducts (Maffini et al. 2005).

Fibroblasts and adipocytes have been co-cultured with epithelial cells in order to achieve a more complex 3D culture system of the breast. Fibroblasts from diverse anatomical sites are morphologically similar and typically stain positive for vimentin expression but negative for markers of epithelial, smooth muscle, endothelial, perineural, and histiocytic cells. However, fibroblasts exhibit topographical differences at the gene-expression level (Chang et al. 2002). Because these differences are maintained *in vitro* (Chang et al. 2002), we use fibroblasts isolated from reduction mammoplasties (RMF) in our 3D co-cultures with human breast epithelial cells (Krause et al. 2008; Dhimolea et al. 2010; Krause et al. 2012). RMF are commercially available and can be used for up to six passages. Fibroblasts can also be isolated from normal or neoplastic fresh tissue (Castello-Cros and Cukierman 2009).

Ductal elongation was accelerated in co-cultures of MCF10A and RMFs in collagen gels (Dhimolea et al. 2010). RMFs were able to induce tubulogenesis in a collagen matrix containing high levels of Matrigel®, a condition under which epithelial cells alone will only form acini (Krause et al. 2008). RMFs in close proximity to MCF10A epithelial cells promoted tubulogenesis in a "sandwich" gel system whereby epithelial cells were present inside a 50% Matrigel® matrix and fibroblasts were placed into a collagen type I gel separated by a membrane. Neither fibroblast-conditioned medium nor HGF was sufficient to promote tubulogenesis after 2 weeks in culture in 50% Matrigel® (Krause et al. 2012). These results suggest that ductal formation in the presence of fibroblasts is most likely due to physical factors such as remodeling of the collagen network rather than due to secreted molecules.

Adipocytes are abundant in the mammary stroma and have a key role in the development of the mammary epithelium. In the mouse, the mammary fat pad is visible at E14 and gradually grows in size. At E16, the mammary epithelium sprouts and penetrates the fat pad. On E18, the main duct has grown and branched into the fat pad. The development of the characteristic mammary epithelium architecture seems to be determined by the mammary fat pad as shown in tissue recombination experiments (Sakakura et al. 1982). Using a mouse model, it was shown that ablation of adipocytes at different development stages affects mammary epithelial morphogenesis. Ductal growth was inhibited and the number of TEBs and branching points was reduced in mammary glands that had been adipocyte-depleted during puberty. This effect was reversed upon adipocyte restoration. Ablation of adipocytes during adulthood resulted in an increase of tertiary branching and premature lobuloaveolar development reminiscent of the lactating mammary gland (Landskroner-Eiger et al. 2010). Human preadipocytes can be differentiated in a 3D culture system and co-cultured with mammary epithelial cells. Similar to co-cultures with RMFs, in collagen gels containing 50% Matrigel® adipocytes promote tubulogenesis (Krause et al. 2012). Mouse 3T3-L1 differentiated preadipocytes facilitated branching in microfabricated cultures of mammary epithelial tubules embedded within collagen gels (Pavlovich et al. 2010).

In the non-lactating mammary gland during each ovarian cycle (Chua et al. 2010), during puberty (Gouon-Evans et al. 2000; Van Nguyen and Pollard 2002), pregnancy, lactation (Pollard and Hennighausen 1994), and involution (O'Brien et al. 2012), macrophages are involved in mammary gland development. The 3D culture systems of the breast that include macrophages could provide insights on the role of these cells in remodeling the stroma. For instance, a 3D co-culture of mouse mammary epithelial cells and preadipocytes in porous 3D collagen-based scaffolds was infiltrated with macrophages. Similar to what is observed *in vivo,* macrophages became closely associated with epithelial structures and the epithelial cells switch their phenotype to express markers characteristic of the involution state (Campbell et al. 2014).

15.7.3 Morphological Criteria to Distinguish between Normal and Abnormal Breast Epithelial Structures in 3D Culture

Normal epithelial structures show a clear lumen surrounded by polarized cells, which express apico-basal markers such as integrins and sialomucin. In addition, these cells secrete basement membrane proteins such as laminin and collagen IV (Petersen et al. 1992; Weaver et al. 1997; Krause et al. 2008, 2012). After stimulation with lactogenic hormones, the epithelial structures also secrete the milk protein β-casein (Streuli et al. 1995; Lance et al. 2016). In contrast, abnormal epithelial structures are disorganized, that is, they lack proper polarization and do not have a patent lumen (Petersen et al. 1992; Weaver et al. 1997; Krause et al. 2010); these characteristics are found in intraductal hyperplasias and breast carcinoma *in situ.* Normalization of the malignant phenotype has been shown *in vivo* (Maffini et al. 2004, 2005) and reproduced *in vitro* (Krause et al. 2010; D'Anselmi et al. 2013). MCF7 cells growing alone in a 3D collagen type 1 matrix form round and solid clusters. To the contrary, these cells organize into quasinormal epithelial structures when they are co-cultured with mammary fibroblasts in the same matrix (Krause et al. 2010). Also, this normalization can be achieved by selecting the appropriate matrix; for instance, MCF7 cells growing alone in a mixed matrix containing Matrigel® and collagen type 1 organized into epithelial structures and display cell death in the center suggesting the formation of a lumen (Krause et al. 2010). MCF7 cells form duct-like structures, which produce β-casein when grown in the presence of egg white proteins (D'Anselmi et al. 2013).

15.8 BIOMECHANICAL FACTORS INVOLVED IN MAMMARY GLAND MORPHOGENESIS

Molecular pathways are insufficient to fully explain organ shape. For example, the development of the lung in chickens and humans has been shown to share molecular pathways, yet the resulting organ architecture is different (Kim et al. 2013). Most likely, mechanical forces are needed to shape organs. For example, in the developing lung, apical constriction drives monopodial budding (Kim et al. 2013). In the developing heart, mechanical forces, due to actin polymerization, drive cardiac bending during c-looping (Latacha et al. 2005; Gjorevski and Nelson 2010). Biomechanical cues play a role in mammary gland morphogenesis. For example, single breast epithelial cells rotate multiple times in the process of acinar formation (Tanner et al. 2012). MCF10A rotational movement is associated with the assembling of laminin, a basement membrane protein related to polarity. By virtue of their agentivity, that is, their ability to generate action, mammary epithelial cells organize collagen fibers (Figure 15.3) (Dhimolea et al. 2010; Barnes et al. 2014). Collagen type I fibers, a major component of the breast stroma, are aligned near epithelial structures as early as 7 h after seeding, even prior to changes in cell morphology are detected. When ducts are formed, localized collagen fiber alignment facilitates ductal elongation and branching (Barnes et al. 2014). By using bundles of collagen fibers, epithelial cells are able to transmit forces at a long distance range (Guo et al. 2012). These findings support the idea of a feedback loop between tissue organization and matrix remodeling. Indeed, the mechanical properties of the ECM are manipulated by the cells to influence epithelial morphogenesis, and in turn, matrix rigidity and fiber alignment exert shaping forces on the epithelium. Epithelial cells form normal acini in a matrix that matches the stiffness of a normal mammary gland, whereas increasing the matrix stiffness drives cellular organization toward abnormal phenotypes (Paszek et al. 2005; Miroshnikova et al. 2011). In our 3D culture model using MCF10A cells, the distribution of acini and ducts can vary by affecting the initial collagen fiber network. MCF10A cells form mostly ducts in a fibrillar network (collagen only), whereas the proportion of acini increases as the matrix becomes more globular (collagen plus increasing concentrations of Matrigel®) (Krause et al. 2012; Barnes et al. 2014).

15.9 INTERPLAY BETWEEN BIOMECHANICAL FORCES AND HORMONES

Most of what we know about the influence of hormones in mammary gland development and in neoplasia comes from studies on animal models. The complex feedback

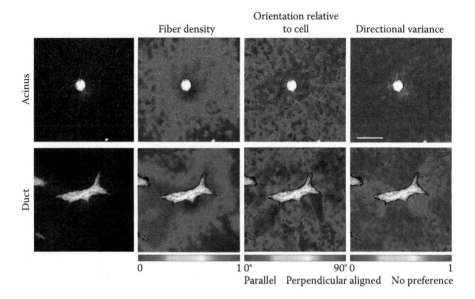

FIGURE 15.3 Representative fiber maps of MCF10A epithelial structures, an acinus (top) and a branching duct (bottom) at Day 5. Although both acini and ducts demonstrate greater fiber density closer to the epithelium, the local orientation of the fibers is substantially different. The mean fiber direction surrounding acini was perpendicular to the nearest cell surface; however, the high directional variance indicates that the strength of alignment in this mean direction is relatively weak. Conversely, elongated and branching ducts exhibit regions of fiber orientation that alternate from being parallel to perpendicular to the cell surface. Substantial changes in directional variance are found surrounding these structures with particularly low values in dense regions of fibers oriented perpendicular to the cell surface. Scale bar, 50 μm. (Reproduced with permission Barnes, C. et al. 2014. *PLoS One* no. 9 (4):e93325.)

between sex steroid hormones and the HPOA makes it difficult to assess direct versus indirect effects of the hormones on the mammary tissue. A few studies have explored the link between hormones and mechanical forces under 2D culture conditions of human cells and tissues of nonclassical estrogen targets. Though some have used hormone concentrations that fall outside of a physiological range, overall these studies seem to indicate that mechanical changes occur during the culture's response to hormonal cues and that biomechanical forces influence the culture's response to hormones. Evidence suggests that estrogen affects the biomechanical properties of cells, and that a mechanical stimulus, such as substrate stiffness, mechanical load, or tension, affects the culture's response to estrogen. In this regard, female athletes are more likely to suffer from ligament injuries than male athletes, suggesting a role of sex hormones in these types of injuries. Fibroblasts isolated from the anterior cruciate ligament (ACL) were cultured as a monolayer in the presence of a range of 10^{-11}–10^{-7} M 17β-estradiol and subjected to equibiaxial cyclic tensile stress to mimic physiological mechanical loading of the fibroblasts in the ACL. The results showed a dose-dependent decreased synthesis of collagen types I and III after mechanical load (Lee et al. 2004). In addition, treatment with estradiol decreased the stiffness of

Shape Matters

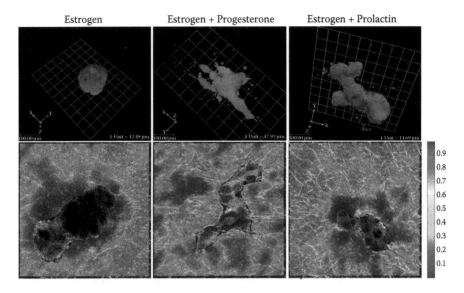

FIGURE 15.4 Hormone-induced epithelial morphogenesis in a 3D culture model. Top: treatment with hormones induces the formation of epithelial structures, side-branching, and budding. Bottom: maps of collagen fibers generated to quantify collagen organization surrounding the epithelial structures. (Adapted from publication Speroni, L. et al. 2014. *Tissue Eng Part C: Methods* no. 20 (1):42–51.)

the cornea (Spoerl et al. 2007), and in another study using human endothelial cells, it decreased cell stiffness and induced smoothing of surfaces (Hillebrand et al. 2008).

We have developed a hormone-sensitive 3D culture model of the breast where hormones influence epithelial morphology similar to what is observed *in vivo* by altering the pattern of collagen fiber organization (Speroni et al. 2014). In this 3D culture system, different patterns of epithelial organization are observed after 2 weeks of exposure to estradiol alone or when combined with prolactin or promegestone (Figure 15.4) Estradiol influenced T47D epithelial cells to organize into round, elongated, and irregular structures, which showed basolateral expression of E-cadherin and F-actin. In contrast, only clusters of 2–3 cells were observed when these cells were cultured in the hormone-depleted CD-FBS medium. Addition of promegestone to the culture medium containing estradiol induced flattening of epithelial structures. These structures displayed cytoplasmic projections reminiscent of side-branching. Finally, in the presence of estradiol, prolactin modified the pattern of epithelial cell organization, resulting in the formation of budding structures, and shifted the distribution of phenotypes toward more elongated structures. In addition, quantitative analysis of collagen fiber organization revealed that the pattern varied with the different hormone-induced epithelial morphologies. The mean fiber density was lower in structures resulting from the treatment with estradiol alone compared with that in the structures resulting from the combined treatments. However, combined hormone treatment of estrogen with promegestone or prolactin resulted in higher collagen density variability in close proximity to the epithelial structures.

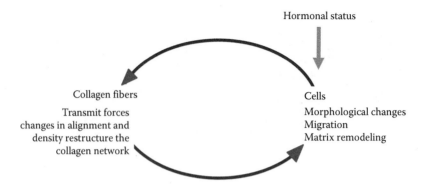

FIGURE 15.5 Schematic showing how hormonal status may alter the biomechanical properties of the breast tissue by affecting the loop between collagen fiber organization and transmission of forces, which contribute to epithelial morphogenesis.

This result is consistent with the finding that the structures in the combined treatments are more irregular in shape and branched when compared to those observed in estradiol alone (Speroni et al. 2014). Others have also investigated the link between another biomechanical parameter, matrix stiffness, and hormone action in breast epithelial morphogenesis. Variations in matrix stiffness change the organization of T47D epithelial structures in response to prolactin (Barcus et al. 2013). Therefore, a hypothesis emerges where hormonal status may alter the biomechanical properties of the breast tissue by affecting the loop between collagen fiber organization and transmission of forces, which contribute to epithelial morphogenesis (Figure 15.5) Finally, 3D hormone-sensitive models enable researchers to explore the link between exposure to hormones and high mammographic density, which are the main risks factors for developing breast cancer.

15.10 DATA ACQUISITION AND ANALYSIS

3D cultures enable data acquisition at the tissue level since there are several parameters that can be assessed in the epithelial structures and in the stroma. The dynamics of epithelial morphogenesis can be followed by live imaging of 3D cultures (Tanner et al. 2012; Ewald 2013; Barnes et al. 2014). After harvesting, in addition to conventional processing for histological analysis and immunohistochemistry, additional parameters can be assessed directly in whole mounts. Relevant parameters in morphological analysis include size, shape, and lumen of the epithelial structures. Quantitative data can be obtained either by analysis of the intact epithelial structures in images of whole mounts acquired using a stereoscope (Speroni et al. 2014) or in images of the live tissue acquired by confocal microscopy (Barnes et al. 2014). Relevant parameters on lumen development and acinar, that is, sphericity and ductal morphology, that is, complexity, branching, and alveolar development, can be obtained by using the Software for Automated Morphological Analysis (SAMA) (Figure 15.6) (Paulose et al. 2016). SAMA is a user-friendly set of customized macros operated via FIJI (http://fiji.sc/Fiji), an open-source image analysis platform in

Shape Matters

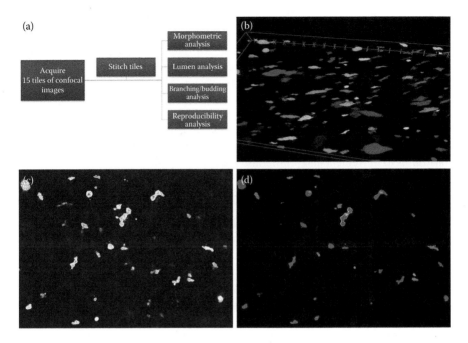

FIGURE 15.6 SAMA analysis of epithelial structure morphology under 3D culture conditions. (a) Steps of SAMA analysis. Whole-mounted gels stained with carmine alum are imaged using confocal microscopy. Samples are excited with the HeNe 633 nm laser given that the Carmine dye fluoresces at this wavelength. Images are acquired at 20× magnification using a MultiTime macro, which enables automated imaging of multiple frames of z-stacks, which are then stitched using 20% overlap of images to obtain 5 × 3 image tiles. Users have a choice to carry out basic morphometrics (such as elongation and sphericity), complexity (branching/budding analysis), and lumen analysis either simultaneously or independently. Basic morphometric analysis includes the counting of (b) all the structures in the 3D image. (b) 3D projection of structures identified in the stitched image and (c) optical slice of the 3D stack. (d) Morphological parameters for each individual structure can be obtained by selecting the structure of interest (outlined in yellow) in the image object map.

combination with a set of functions in R (http://www.r-project.org/), an open-source program for statistical analysis. SAMA enables a rapid, exhaustive, and quantitative 3D analysis of the shape of a population of structures in a 3D image. SAMA is licensed under the GPLv3 and available at http://montevil.theobio.org/content/sama. The epithelial structures are imaged, reconstructed in 3D, and analyzed with minimum human intervention and, therefore, bias. Matrix remodeling can be assessed by analyzing collagen fiber organization and by measuring matrix compliance (Peng et al. 2013; Cassereau et al. 2015; Lance et al. 2016) or deformation (Piotrowski et al. 2015) surrounding the epithelial structures. Images of the collagen fiber network can be acquired using Second Harmonic Generation (SHG) imaging (Speroni et al. 2014) or confocal reflection microscopy (Barnes et al. 2014). The laser power required for SHG may result in photodamage during time-lapse imaging over the course of lengthy periods of observation; to preclude this outcome, confocal reflection microscopy can be used instead. Analytical tools are available to obtain quantitative information of collagen fiber density and orientation in pixel (2D) (Barnes et al. 2014) and voxel (3D) (Liu et al. 2015) units. Finally, the data gathered in 3D cultures can serve as a basis for mathematical modeling of the process of breast epithelial morphogenesis; based on these two premises, namely (i) the default state of cells is proliferation with variation and motility and (ii) organismal constraints normally prevent the expression of the default state (Longo et al. 2015). We propose a mathematical model for the formation of ducts and acini where cells generate forces that are transmitted to neighboring cells and collagen fibers, which in turn create constraints to movement and proliferation (Montevil et al. 2016).

15.11 CONCLUSION AND PERSPECTIVE

The incorporation of 3D culture models has contributed to a better understanding of the process of normal and pathological breast/mammary organogenesis. These culture systems allow for the evaluation of cell–cell interactions and cell–matrix interactions happening under hormonal influences in 3D similar to how it occurs *in vivo*. Finally, the development of 3D cultures has also motivated improvements of analytical tools such as software that helps to obtain quantitative 2D and 3D data on epithelial morphology, such as size, complexity, and presence of lumen, and on matrix characteristics, such as collagen fiber orientation and density. Altogether, the knowledge already accumulated and referred to in this chapter plus input from novel technologies now under development will increase our understanding of normal and neoplastic development in the breast.

ACKNOWLEDGMENTS

We greatly appreciate the editorial contributions by Cheryl Schaeberle. This research was supported by the NIEHS/NIH ES 08314 and U01 ES20888 and the Avon Foundation Grant #02-2011-095. The content is solely the responsibility of the authors and does not necessarily represent the official views of the National Institute of Environmental Health Sciences or the National Institutes of Health or the Avon Foundation.

REFERENCES

Alowami, S., S. Troup, S. Al-Haddad, I. Kirkpatrick, and P. H. Watson. 2003. Mammographic density is related to stroma and stromal proteoglycan expression. *Breast Cancer Res* no. 5 (5):R129–35.

Baglietto, L., G. Severi, D. R. English, K. Krishnan, J. L. Hopper, C. McLean, H. A. Morris, W. D. Tilley, and G. G. Giles. 2010. Circulating steroid hormone levels and risk of breast cancer for postmenopausal women. *Cancer Epidemiol Biomarkers Prev* no. 19 (2):492–502.

Balinsky, B. I. 1950. On the prenatal growth of the mammary gland rudiment in the mouse. *J Anat* no. 84 (3):227–35.

Barcellos-Hoff, M. H. and S. A. Ravani. 2000. Irradiated mammary gland stroma promotes the expression of tumorigenic potential by unirradiated epithelial cells. *Cancer Res* no. 60 (5):1254–60.

Barcus, C. E., P. J. Keely, K. W. Eliceiri, and L. A. Schuler. 2013. Stiff collagen matrices increase tumorigenic prolactin signaling in breast cancer cells. *J Biol Chem* no. 288 (18):12722–32.

Barnes, C., L. Speroni, K. P. Quinn, M. Montevil, K. Saetzler, G. Bode-Animashaun et al. 2014. From single cells to tissues: Interactions between the matrix and human breast cells in real time. *PLoS One* no. 9 (4):e93325.

Benton, G., E. Crooke, and J. George. 2009. Laminin-1 induces E-cadherin expression in 3-dimensional cultured breast cancer cells by inhibiting DNA methyltransferase 1 and reversing promoter methylation status. *FASEB J* no. 23 (11):3884–95.

Bocchinfuso, W. P. and K. S. Korach. 1997. Mammary gland development and tumorigenesis in estrogen receptor knockout mice. *J Mammary Gland Biol Neoplasia* no. 2 (4):323–34.

Boyd, N. F., H. Guo, L. J. Martin, L. Sun, J. Stone, E. Fishell et al. 2007. Mammographic density and the risk and detection of breast cancer. *N Engl J Med* no. 356 (3):227–36.

Brisken, C. 2013. Progesterone signalling in breast cancer: A neglected hormone coming into the limelight. *Nat Rev Cancer* no. 13 (6):385–96.

Brisken, C., S. Kaur, T. E. Chavarria, N. Binart, R. L. Sutherland, R. A. Weinberg, P. A. Kelly, and C. J. Ormandy. 1999. Prolactin controls mammary gland development via direct and indirect mechanisms. *Dev Biol* no. 210 (1):96–106.

Brisken, C. and B. O'Malley. 2010. Hormone action in the mammary gland. *Cold Spring Harb Perspect Biol* no. 2 (12):a003178.

Campbell, J. J., L. A. Botos, T. J. Sargeant, N. Davidenko, R. E. Cameron, and C. J. Watson. 2014. A 3-D *in vitro* co-culture model of mammary gland involution. *Integr Biol (Camb)* no. 6 (6):618–26.

Cassereau, L., Y. A. Miroshnikova, G. Ou, J. Lakins, and V. M. Weaver. 2015. A 3D tension bioreactor platform to study the interplay between ECM stiffness and tumor phenotype. *J Biotechnol* no. 193:66–9.

Castello-Cros, R. and E. Cukierman. 2009. Stromagenesis during tumorigenesis: Characterization of tumor-associated fibroblasts and stroma-derived 3D matrices. *Methods Mol Biol* no. 522:275–305.

Chalbos, D., F. Vignon, I. Keydar, and H. Rochefort. 1982. Estrogens stimulate cell proliferation and induce secretory proteins in a human breast cancer cell line (T47D). *J Clin Endocrinol Metab* no. 55 (2):276–83.

Chang, H. Y., J. T. Chi, S. Dudoit, C. Bondre, M. van de Rijn, D. Botstein, and P. O. Brown. 2002. Diversity, topographic differentiation, and positional memory in human fibroblasts. *Proc Natl Acad Sci USA* no. 99 (20):12877–82.

Chua, A. C., L. J. Hodson, L. M. Moldenhauer, S. A. Robertson, and W. V. Ingman. 2010. Dual roles for macrophages in ovarian cycle-associated development and remodelling of the mammary gland epithelium. *Development* no. 137 (24):4229–38.

Clarke, R. B. 2004. Complementary yet distinct roles for oestrogen receptor-alpha and oestrogen receptor-beta in mouse mammary epithelial proliferation. *Breast Cancer Res* no. 6 (3):135–6.

Clarke, R. B., A. Howell, C. S. Potten, and E. Anderson. 1997. Dissociation between steroid receptor expression and cell proliferation in the human breast. *Cancer Res* no. 57 (22):4987–91.

D'Anselmi, F., M. G. Masiello, A. Cucina, S. Proietti, S. Dinicola, A. Pasqualato et al. 2013. Microenvironment promotes tumor cell reprogramming in human breast cancer cell lines. *PLoS One* no. 8 (12):e83770.

Debnath, J., S. K. Muthuswamy, and J. S. Brugge. 2003. Morphogenesis and oncogenesis of MCF-10A mammary epithelial acini grown in three-dimensional basement membrane cultures. *Methods* no. 30 (3):256–68.

Dhimolea, E., M. V. Maffini, A. M. Soto, and C. Sonnenschein. 2010. The role of collagen reorganization on mammary epithelial morphogenesis in a 3D culture model. *Biomaterials* no. 31 (13):3622–30.

Dhimolea, E., A. M. Soto, and C. Sonnenschein. 2012. Breast epithelial tissue morphology is affected in 3D cultures by species-specific collagen-based extracellular matrix. *J Biomed Mater Res A* no. 100 (11):2905–12.

Dhimolea, E., P. R. Wadia, T. J. Murray, M. L. Settles, J. D. Treitman, C. Sonnenschein, T. Shioda, and A. M. Soto. 2014. Prenatal exposure to BPA alters the epigenome of the rat mammary gland and increases the propensity to neoplastic development. *PLoS One* no. 9 (7):e99800.

Elosegui-Artola, A., E. Bazellieres, M. D. Allen, I. Andreu, R. Oria, R. Sunyer et al. 2014. Rigidity sensing and adaptation through regulation of integrin types. *Nat Mater* no. 13 (6):631–7.

Ewald, A. J. 2013. Practical considerations for long-term time-lapse imaging of epithelial morphogenesis in three-dimensional organotypic cultures. *Cold Spring Harb Protoc* no. 2013 (2):100–17.

Gjorevski, N. and C. M. Nelson. 2010. Branch formation during organ development. *Wiley Interdiscip Rev Syst Biol Med* no. 2 (6):734–41.

Gouon-Evans, V., M. E. Rothenberg, and J. W. Pollard. 2000. Postnatal mammary gland development requires macrophages and eosinophils. *Development* no. 127 (11):2269–82.

Graham, J. D., P. A. Mote, U. Salagame, J. H. van Dijk, R. L. Balleine, L. I. Huschtscha, R. R. Reddel, and C. L. Clarke. 2009. DNA replication licensing and progenitor numbers are increased by progesterone in normal human breast. *Endocrinology* no. 150 (7):3318–26.

Guo, C. L., M. Ouyang, J. Y. Yu, J. Maslov, A. Price, and C. Y. Shen. 2012. Long-range mechanical force enables self-assembly of epithelial tubular patterns. *Proc Natl Acad Sci USA* no. 109 (15):5576–82.

Hanahan, D. 2014. Rethinking the war on cancer. *Lancet* no. 383 (9916):558–63.

Hanahan, D. and R. A. Weinberg. 2000. The hallmarks of cancer. *Cell* no. 100 (1):57–70.

Hanahan, D. and R. A. Weinberg. 2011. Hallmarks of cancer: The next generation. *Cell* no. 144 (5):646–74.

Hillebrand, U., M. Hausberg, D. Lang, C. Stock, C. Riethmuller, C. Callies, and E. Bussemaker. 2008. How steroid hormones act on the endothelium—insights by atomic force microscopy. *Pflugers Arch* no. 456 (1):51–60.

Howard, B. A. and B. A. Gusterson. 2000. Human breast development. *J Mammary Gland Biol Neoplasia* no. 5 (2):119–37.

Keen, J. C. and N. E. Davidson. 2003. The biology of breast carcinoma. *Cancer* no. 97 (3 Suppl):S825–33.

Key, T., P. Appleby, I. Barnes, and G. Reeves. 2002. Endogenous sex hormones and breast cancer in postmenopausal women: Reanalysis of nine prospective studies. *J Natl Cancer Inst* no. 94 (8):606–16.

Kim, H. Y., V. D. Varner, and C. M. Nelson. 2013. Apical constriction initiates new bud formation during monopodial branching of the embryonic chicken lung. *Development* no. 140 (15):3146–55.

Kratochwil, K. 1969. Organ specificity in mesenchymal induction demonstrated in the embryonic development of the mammary gland of the mouse. *Dev Biol* no. 20 (1):46–71.

Kratochwil, K. 1971. In vitro analysis of the hormonal basis for the sexual dimorphism in the embryonic development of the mouse mammary gland. *J Embryol Exp Morphol* no. 25 (1):141–53.

Kratochwil, K. 1977. Development and loss of androgen responsiveness in the embryonic rudiment of the mouse mammary gland. *Dev Biol* no. 61 (2):358–65.

Krause, S., A. Jondeau-Cabaton, E. Dhimolea, A. M. Soto, C. Sonnenschein, and M. V. Maffini. 2012. Dual regulation of breast tubulogenesis using extracellular matrix composition and stromal cells. *Tissue Eng Part A* no. 18 (5–6):520–32.

Krause, S., M. V. Maffini, A. M. Soto, and C. Sonnenschein. 2008. A novel 3D *in vitro* culture model to study stromal–epithelial interactions in the mammary gland. *Tissue Eng Part C: Methods* no. 14 (3):261–71.

Krause, S., M. V. Maffini, A. M. Soto, and C. Sonnenschein. 2010. The microenvironment determines the breast cancer cells' phenotype: Organization of MCF7 cells in 3D cultures. *BMC Cancer* no. 10:263.

Lance, A., C. C. Yang, M. Swamydas, D. Dean, S. Deitch, K. J. Burg, and D. Dreau. 2016. Increased extracellular matrix density decreases MCF10A breast cell acinus formation in 3D culture conditions. *J Tissue Eng Regen Med* no. 10 (1):71–80.

Landskroner-Eiger, S., J. Park, D. Israel, J. W. Pollard, and P. E. Scherer. 2010. Morphogenesis of the developing mammary gland: Stage-dependent impact of adipocytes. *Dev Biol* no. 344 (2):968–78.

Latacha, K. S., M. C. Remond, A. Ramasubramanian, A. Y. Chen, E. L. Elson, and L. A. Taber. 2005. Role of actin polymerization in bending of the early heart tube. *Dev Dyn* no. 233 (4):1272–86.

Lee, C. Y., X. Liu, C. L. Smith, X. Zhang, H. C. Hsu, D. Y. Wang, and Z. P. Luo. 2004. The combined regulation of estrogen and cyclic tension on fibroblast biosynthesis derived from anterior cruciate ligament. *Matrix Biol* no. 23 (5):323–9.

Lee, G. Y., P. A. Kenny, E. H. Lee, and M. J. Bissell. 2007. Three-dimensional culture models of normal and malignant breast epithelial cells. *Nat Methods* no. 4 (4):359–65.

Liu, Z., K. P. Quinn, L. Speroni, L. Arendt, C. Kuperwasser, C. Sonnenschein, A.M. Soto, and I. Georgakoudi. 2015. Rapid three-dimensional quantification of voxel-wise collagen fiber orientation. *Biomed Opt Express* no. 6 (7):2294–310.

Longo, G., M. Montevil, C. Sonnenschein, and A. M. Soto. 2015. In search of principles for a Theory of Organisms. *J Biosci* no. 40 (5):955–68.

Maffini, M. V., J. M. Calabro, A. M. Soto, and C. Sonnenschein. 2005. Stromal regulation of neoplastic development: Age-dependent normalization of neoplastic mammary cells by mammary stroma. *Am J Pathol* no. 167 (5):1405–10.

Maffini, M. V., A. M. Soto, J. M. Calabro, A. A. Ucci, and C. Sonnenschein. 2004. The stroma as a crucial target in rat mammary gland carcinogenesis. *J Cell Sci* no. 117 (Pt 8):1495–502.

Marchese, S. and E. Silva. 2012. Disruption of 3D MCF-12A breast cell cultures by estrogens--an *in vitro* model for ER-mediated changes indicative of hormonal carcinogenesis. *PLoS One* no. 7 (10):e45767.

Masso-Welch, P. A., K. M. Darcy, N. C. Stangle-Castor, and M. M. Ip. 2000. A developmental atlas of rat mammary gland histology. *J Mammary Gland Biol Neoplasia* no. 5 (2):165–85.

Miroshnikova, Y. A., D. M. Jorgens, L. Spirio, M. Auer, A. L. Sarang-Sieminski, and V. M. Weaver. 2011. Engineering strategies to recapitulate epithelial morphogenesis within synthetic three-dimensional extracellular matrix with tunable mechanical properties. *Phys Biol* no. 8 (2):026013.

Montevil, M., L. Speroni, C. Sonnenschein, and A. M. Soto. 2016. Modeling mammary organogenesis from biological first principles: Cells and their physical constraints. *Prog Biophys Mol Biol* no. 122 (1):58–69.

O'Brien, J., H. Martinson, C. Durand-Rougely, and P. Schedin. 2012. Macrophages are crucial for epithelial cell death and adipocyte repopulation during mammary gland involution. *Development* no. 139 (2):269–75.

Parmar, H. and G. R. Cunha. 2004. Epithelial–stromal interactions in the mouse and human mammary gland *in vivo*. *Endocr Relat Cancer* no. 11 (3):437–58.

Paszek, M. J., N. Zahir, K. R. Johnson, J. N. Lakins, G. I. Rozenberg, A. Gefen et al. 2005. Tensional homeostasis and the malignant phenotype. *Cancer Cell* no. 8 (3):241–54.

Paulose, T., M. Montevil, L. Speroni, F. Cerruti, C. Sonnenschein, and A. M. Soto. 2016. SAMA: A method for 3D morphological analysis. *PLoS One* no. 11 (4):e0153022.

Pavlovich, A. L., S. Manivannan, and C. M. Nelson. 2010. Adipose stroma induces branching morphogenesis of engineered epithelial tubules. *Tissue Eng Part A* no. 16 (12):3719–26.

Peng, B., C. A. C. Alonzo, L. Xia, L. Speroni, I. Georgakoudi, A. M. Soto, C. Sonnenschein, and M. Cronin-Colomb. 2013. Evaluating cell matrix mechanics using an integrated nonlinear optical tweezer-confocal imaging system. In *Paper read at Proc. SPIE 8810, Optical Trapping and Optical Micromanipulation X, 88101O.*

Petersen, O. W., L. Ronnov-Jessen, A. R. Howlett, and M. J. Bissell. 1992. Interaction with basement membrane serves to rapidly distinguish growth and differentiation pattern of normal and malignant human breast epithelial cells. *Proc Natl Acad Sci USA* no. 89 (19):9064–8.

Piotrowski, A. S., V. D. Varner, N. Gjorevski, and C. M. Nelson. 2015. Three-dimensional traction force microscopy of engineered epithelial tissues. *Methods Mol Biol* no. 1189:191–206.

Pollard, J. W. and L. Hennighausen. 1994. Colony stimulating factor 1 is required for mammary gland development during pregnancy. *Proc Natl Acad Sci USA* no. 91 (20):9312–6.

Provenzano, P. P., K. W. Eliceiri, J. M. Campbell, D. R. Inman, J. G. White, and P. J. Keely. 2006. Collagen reorganization at the tumor–stromal interface facilitates local invasion. *BMC Med* no. 4 (1):38.

Provenzano, P. P., D. R. Inman, K. W. Eliceiri, J. G. Knittel, L. Yan, C. T. Rueden, J. G. White, and P. J. Keely. 2008. Collagen density promotes mammary tumor initiation and progression. *BMC Med* no. 6:11.

Richert, M. M., K. L. Schwertfeger, J. W. Ryder, and S. M. Anderson. 2000. An atlas of mouse mammary gland development. *J Mammary Gland Biol Neoplasia* no. 5 (2):227–41.

Robinson, G. W., A. B. Karpf, and K. Kratochwil. 1999. Regulation of mammary gland development by tissue interaction. *J Mammary Gland Biol Neoplasia* no. 4 (1):9–19.

Sakakura, T., Y. Nishizuka, and C. J. Dawe. 1976. Mesenchyme-dependent morphogenesis and epithelium-specific cytodifferentiation in mouse mammary gland. *Science* no. 194 (4272):1439–41.

Sakakura, T., Y. Sakagami, and Y. Nishizuka. 1982. Dual origin of mesenchymal tissues participating in mouse mammary gland embryogenesis. *Dev Biol* no. 91 (1):202–7.

Sonnenschein, C. and A. M. Soto. 1999. *The Society of Cells: Cancer and Control of Cell Proliferation*. New York: Springer-Verlag, 154 p.

Sonnenschein, C., A. M. Soto, A. Rangarajan, and P. Kulkarni. 2014. Competing views on cancer. *J Biosci* no. 39 (2):281–302.

Soto, A. M., H. Justicia, J. W. Wray, and C. Sonnenschein. 1991. p-Nonyl-phenol: An estrogenic xenobiotic released from "modified" polystyrene. *Environ Health Perspect* no. 92:167–73.

Soto, A. M., J. T. Murai, P. K. Siiteri, and C. Sonnenschein. 1986. Control of cell proliferation: Evidence for negative control on estrogen-sensitive T47D human breast cancer cells. *Cancer Res* no. 46 (5):2271–5.

Soto, A. M. and C. Sonnenschein. 1984. Mechanism of estrogen action on cellular proliferation: Evidence for indirect and negative control on cloned breast tumor cells. *Biochem Biophys Res Commun* no. 122 (3):1097–103.

Soto, A. M. and C. Sonnenschein. 2011. The tissue organization field theory of cancer: A testable replacement for the somatic mutation theory. *Bioessays* no. 33 (5):332–40.

Soto, A. M. and C. Sonnenschein. 2014. One hundred years of somatic mutation theory of carcinogenesis: Is it time to switch? *Bioessays* no. 36 (1):118–20.

Soto, A. M., C. Sonnenschein, K. L. Chung, M. F. Fernandez, N. Olea, and F. O. Serrano. 1995. The E-SCREEN assay as a tool to identify estrogens: An update on estrogenic environmental pollutants. *Environ Health Perspect* no. 103 (Suppl 7):S113–22.

Soule, H. D., T. M. Maloney, S. R. Wolman, W. D. Peterson, Jr., R. Brenz, C. M. McGrath, J. Russo, R. J. Pauley, R. F. Jones, and S. C. Brooks. 1990. Isolation and characterization of a spontaneously immortalized human breast epithelial cell line, MCF-10. *Cancer Res* no. 50 (18):6075–86.

Speroni, L., G. S. Whitt, J. Xylas, K. P. Quinn, A. Jondeau-Cabaton, C. Barnes, I. Georgakoudi, C. Sonnenschein, and A. M. Soto. 2014. Hormonal regulation of epithelial organization in a three-dimensional breast tissue culture model. *Tissue Eng Part C Methods* no. 20 (1):42–51.

Speroni, L., M. Voutilainen, M. L. Mikkola, S. A. Klager, C. M. Schaeberle, C. Sonnenschein, and A. M. Soto. 2017. New insights into fetal mammary gland morphogenesis: Differential effects of natural and environmental estrogens. *Sci Rep* 7: 40806.

Spoerl, E., V. Zubaty, F. Raiskup-Wolf, and L. E. Pillunat. 2007. Oestrogen-induced changes in biomechanics in the cornea as a possible reason for keratectasia. *Br J Ophthalmol* no. 91 (11):1547–50.

Streuli, C. H., C. Schmidhauser, N. Bailey, P. Yurchenco, A. P. Skubitz, C. Roskelley, and M. J. Bissell. 1995. Laminin mediates tissue-specific gene expression in mammary epithelia. *J Cell Biol* no. 129 (3):591–603.

Tanner, K., H. Mori, R. Mroue, A. Bruni-Cardoso, and M. J. Bissell. 2012. Coherent angular motion in the establishment of multicellular architecture of glandular tissues. *Proc Natl Acad Sci USA* no. 109 (6):1973–8.

Tanos, T., G. Sflomos, P. C. Echeverria, A. Ayyanan, M. Gutierrez, J. F. Delaloye et al. 2013. Progesterone/RANKL is a major regulatory axis in the human breast. *Sci Transl Med* no. 5 (182):182ra55.

Van Nguyen, A. and J. W. Pollard. 2002. Colony stimulating factor-1 is required to recruit macrophages into the mammary gland to facilitate mammary ductal outgrowth. *Dev Biol* no. 247 (1):11–25.

Vandenberg, L. N., M. V. Maffini, P. R. Wadia, C. Sonnenschein, B. S. Rubin, and A. M. Soto. 2007. Exposure to environmentally relevant doses of the xenoestrogen bisphenol-A alters development of the fetal mouse mammary gland. *Endocrinology* no. 148 (1):116–27.

Venugopalan, G., D. B. Camarillo, K. D. Webster, C. D. Reber, J. A. Sethian, V. M. Weaver, D. A. Fletcher, H. El-Samad, and C. H. Rycroft. 2014. Multicellular architecture of malignant breast epithelia influences mechanics. *PLoS One* no. 9 (8):e101955.

Vignon, F., S. Bardon, D. Chalbos, and H. Rochefort. 1983. Antiestrogenic effect of R5020, a synthetic progestin in human breast cancer cells in culture. *J Clin Endocrinol Metab* no. 56 (6):1124–30.

Wang, X., L. Sun, M. V. Maffini, A. Soto, C. Sonnenschein, and D. L. Kaplan. 2010. A complex 3D human tissue culture system based on mammary stromal cells and silk scaffolds for modeling breast morphogenesis and function. *Biomaterials* no. 31 (14):3920–9.

Weaver, V. M., O. W. Petersen, F. Wang, C. A. Larabell, P. Briand, C. Damsky, and M. J. Bissell. 1997. Reversion of the malignant phenotype of human breast cells in three-dimensional culture and *in vivo* by integrin blocking antibodies. *J Cell Biol* no. 137 (1):231–45.

Wellings, S. R., H. M. Jensen, and R. G. Marcum. 1975. An atlas of subgross pathology of the human breast with special reference to possible precancerous lesions. *J Natl Cancer Inst* no. 55 (2):231–73.

16 Cells and Tissue Structures in Cardiovascular 3D Tissue Systems

Justin McMahan, Rachel Hybart, and C. LaShan Simpson

CONTENTS

16.1 Introduction 285
16.2 Limitations of 3D Tissue Systems 286
16.3 Considerations for Cardiovascular 3D Tissue Systems 287
    16.3.1 Arterial Structure and Composition 287
    16.3.2 Cardiac Tissue Structure and Composition 288
    16.3.3 Scaffolds for Cardiovascular Tissue Models 289
        16.3.3.1 Scaffolds for Cardiac Tissue Development 290
        16.3.3.2 Scaffolds for Blood Vessel Development 291
        16.3.3.3 Culture Conditions for 3D Vascular Tissue Models 291
16.4 Approaches to Cardiovascular 3D Tissue Systems 291
    16.4.1 Decellularized Scaffolds... 291
        16.4.1.1 Tubular Scaffolds for Vessel Modeling............................. 292
        16.4.1.2 Myocardial Tissue Patches for Cardiac Tissue Engineering... 292
    16.4.2 Cell Sheet Engineering 292
16.5 Conclusion and Perspective 295
References... 295

16.1 INTRODUCTION

As the mechanisms behind cellular functions become better known, researchers are realizing that two-dimensional (2D) cell cultures are not the most effective manner of studying human, cellular responses. For instance, studying how cardiac cells react to environmental stimuli found in the human body varies greatly depending upon the dimensionality of the culture environment. In the human body, the cardiac tissues contract in response to electrical stimuli from the body due to the extracellular electric field (Tung and Borderies 1992). Also, when cells are placed under 2D culture conditions, their morphology gets altered (Pontes Soares et al. 2012b).

This is in part because the 2D environment, although it provides nutrients for growth, is significantly different from the three-dimensional (3D) natural microenvironment. Factors that affect this include specific cell-to-cell interactions, nutrient supply via growth medium, and gravity.

For these reasons, 3D tissue systems are models to study cells and how cells are altered in different diseases. The 3D cardiac systems have been developed to investigate genetic heart defects, such as irregular contractile function (de Lange et al. 2011b). The 3D tissue systems improve the study of these conditions because they allow the formation into shape and the functions that closely mimic those observed in their natural environment. Such 3D models permit investigations of novel ways to overcome genetic defects and the generation of artery and valve replacements (Nugent and Edelman 2003). Furthermore, cardiac tissue can also be grown into 3D multilayered sheets (Sakaguchi et al. 2015). Multilayered sheets are more akin to *in vivo* contractile cardiac tissue.

When cells are placed under 2D culture conditions, both the morphology and gene expression are drastically altered compared to 3D environment, highlighting the difference in stimuli under these two conditions (Fan et al. 2009). 3D culture conditions allow the study of cells from multiple angles, especially their interactions with one another at cell–cell junctions as well as other locations within the 3D structure (Donoghue et al. 2014). The latter is a key to address the role of gravity and the likely different responses between cells located in the center and at the edge of the 3D structure, respectively.

16.2 LIMITATIONS OF 3D TISSUE SYSTEMS

The current 3D cardiovascular tissue systems still face several limitations that need to be addressed before they can be used routinely. Among those are cell survival, model reproducibility, proper scaffold choice, growth, and scaffold permeability.

One of the first steps of generating a 3D structure is deciding on what type of scaffold to use. The scaffold must allow cellular permeation/infiltration and create cell-to-cell junctions to permit survival. If the scaffold does not allow cells access to the appropriate amount of nutrients, cell growth will be inhibited much like that observed with cells grown under 2D conditions (Akins et al. 2010). Deciding what type of scaffold is the best for cells to proliferate in a 3D structure is more difficult than deciding what media contain the proper nutrients for a 2D cell culture. Consider cardiac tissue models, for example, the 3D scaffold must be able to mimic the properties of the cardiac muscle, that is, the scaffold must be porous and contain channels and elastomers similar to the cardiac muscle. In an approach where cells are seeded in a specialized, preformed matrix, the matrix must contain these properties since the cells will not be creating their own. Further, when cells are cultured onto a scaffold that allows their proliferation, differentiation into specialized cells will require the application of additional stimuli. Such an approach permits cell guidance toward a 3D system that most closely fits the biological tissue mimicked (Vunjak-Novakovic et al. 2010).

Once these cells begin to proliferate, the next challenge is to ensure that the cells will grow and behave like the tissue which they are intended to replace. This is difficult because it often requires external stimuli to mimic the physiological environment. These stimuli can be chemical, electrical, or physical and applied in bioreactors. For example, electrical stimuli have been used in 3D cardiac tissues whose main functions rely on electrical impulses (Jin et al. 2015), whereas osteons in bones would require a more mechanical test.

Additionally, 3D model reproducibility remains a challenge (Chen et al. 2015). Since components of scaffolds used in the 3D models originate from animal tissues, the matrices of these scaffolds are likely to differ, thus, decreasing the reproducibility of those models. Nevertheless, the ability to investigate new methods to treat, analyze and/or alter cells within the 3D models mimicking *in vivo* conditions remains attractive.

16.3 CONSIDERATIONS FOR CARDIOVASCULAR 3D TISSUE SYSTEMS

To closely mimic the *in vivo* behavior and characteristics of functional tissues and organs, it is imperative to understand how a large number of cell and tissue types that constitute organs, varying in 3D structures, interact and behave with one another. When considering the reconstruction of tissues and organs of the cardiovascular system for modeling or regenerative purposes, specific cells are required. The tissues of the cardiovascular system, besides blood, are vessels (i.e., arteries, veins, lymphatic system, and capillaries) and the heart (i.e., cardiac muscle).

16.3.1 ARTERIAL STRUCTURE AND COMPOSITION

As illustrated in Figure 16.1, arterial walls can be divided into three regions: the tunica intima, the tunica media, and the tunica adventitia.

The innermost layer of the arteries, the tunica intima, is comprised primarily of a layer of flattened, condensed endothelial cells and is supported by a subendothelium that includes dispersed smooth muscle cells within an extracellular matrix (ECM) mostly composed of a network of collagen types I and III (Gasser et al. 2006).

The middle layer of the artery, the tunica media, consists primarily of a 3D network of smooth muscle cells, elastin, and predominantly types I and III collagen fibril bundles (Clark and Glagov 1979). The presence of smooth muscle cells in the medial portion of the artery permits vasodilation and vasoconstriction in response to numerous regulations including blood flow, whereas the elastin accommodates changes in cross-sectional area by providing a large degree of flexibility and extensibility to the artery (Zou and Zhang 2012). Circumferential alignments of collagen along with the smooth muscle cells allow resistance to loads applied in the circumferential direction.

The last and outermost layer of the artery is the tunica adventitia. The adventitia is comprised mainly of fibroblasts and fibrocytes, histological ground substance, and thick bundles of collagen fibers. The collagens of the adventitia provide stability and strength at its crimped state to permit expansion. However, once collagens reach their straightened lengths with significant strain levels, the artery's mechanical response may change to that of a stiff tube to prevent overstretching and rupture (Gasser et al. 2006).

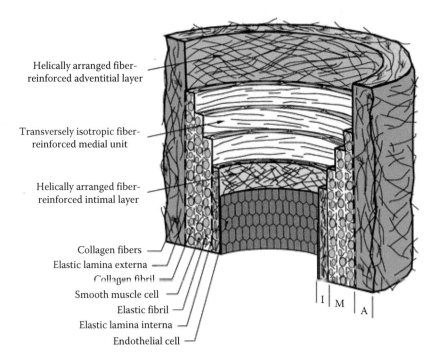

FIGURE 16.1 Arterial anatomy with distinct intimal (I), medial (M), and aventitial (A) layers; major cellular and ECM constituents are labeled for each layer. The intima is mainly composed of endothelial cells along with a type IV collagen basal membrane. The medial layer consists preferentially of circumferentially aligned smooth muscles that are interspersed with a network of elastic and collagen fibrils. The outer adventitial layer is predominantly composed of circumferentially aligned collagen bundles. (Gasser, T. C., R. W. Ogden, and G. A. Holzapfel. 2006. *J R Soc Interface* 3 (6): 17. Reproduced by permission of The Royal Society of Chemistry.)

16.3.2 Cardiac Tissue Structure and Composition

As depicted in Figure 16.2, cardiac muscle tissue is present within the heart along with other tissue types. All of the tissues within the heart are supported by an ECM, which is composed of macromolecules including hyaluronan, proteoglycans, collagens (mainly types I and III), elastin, fibrilin, tenascin, fibronectins, and laminins (Lockhart et al. 2011).

Myocytes are the major cellular constituent of the heart accounting for approximately 75% of the cardiac tissue volume. The primary function of cardiac myocytes or cardiomyocytes is to produce mechanical tension within the cardiac tissue. Additionally, innervation of the tissues provides the ability for contraction stimulation. Regulated by innervation, cardiac contractions are initiated by pacemaker cells that are mostly concentrated in the sinoatrial and atrioventricular nodes of the heart. The cardiomyocytes are enclosed by the sarcolemma, a lipid membrane, which functions as a semipermeable barrier that facilitates, in particular, ion transport to propagate action potentials, allowing involuntary muscle contractions.

Cells and Tissue Structures in Cardiovascular 3D Tissue Systems

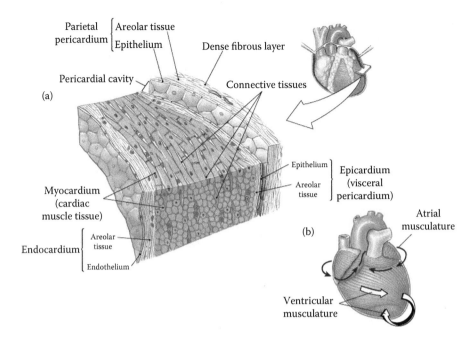

FIGURE 16.2 Cardiac anatomical illustration of the heart. (a) The different zones include the endocardium, myocardium, and epicardium. The myocardium is the major tissue of the heart and consists predominately of cardiomyocytes with interspersed connective tissue. (b) Macroscopic view of the heart. Arrows indicate contractile directionality due to cardiac muscle. Functionality depends on cardiac contraction to achieve ejection while passive relaxation results in filling. (Credit: Martini, F.H., M.J. Timmons, R.B. Tallitsch. *Human Anatomy*, 7th ed., New York, NY: Pearson Education, Inc. Copyright 2012. Reprinted by permission of Pearson Education, Inc., New York, NY)

Fibroblasts are the other major cells within the cardiac tissue. Fibroblasts provide structural support and maintain the integrity of the ECM for the cardiac tissue. In addition to ECM maintenance, fibroblasts also contribute to the cardiac development and passive mechanical properties, cell signaling, and electromechanical function in both healthy and diseased myocardium (Camelliti et al. 2005). During tissue damage, fibroblasts promote inflammation as well as fibrosis.

Other cells of the cardiac tissue include endothelial, vascular smooth muscle cells, and neural cells. Endothelial and vascular smooth muscle cells are especially associated with the vascularization of the heart, that is, formation of coronary vessels. The presence of neural cells is associated with the innervated regions of myocardium within the cardiac tissue to ensure that its contractile nature is maintained (Chen and Chen 2009).

16.3.3 Scaffolds for Cardiovascular Tissue Models

For cardiovascular *in vitro* models, multidimensional cultures are more appropriate to approximate the biological tissue. In 3D cardiovascular models, the ECM can be simulated using scaffolds. Indeed, 3D scaffolds promote mechanical support, provide physical and biological cues for cellular differentiation and, when seeded with appropriate cells, favor 3D organization observed in functional tissues (Gobin et al. 2016). The scaffolds used are generally porous to permit cellular adhesion and nutrient transport, and are biodegradable to allow their replacement by tissue over time. The materials used in scaffolds are mostly composed of natural or synthetic polymers. General scaffold considerations/requirements to keep in mind when selecting a specific material include biocompatibility, biodegradability, mechanical properties, scaffold architecture, and manufacturing (O'Brien 2011).

16.3.3.1 Scaffolds for Cardiac Tissue Development

For applications associated with cardiac tissue engineering and development, specific considerations such as the mechanical and electrical scaffold requirements are often critical. Furthermore, the scaffold must be biocompatible with all the tissue components of the myocardium. The scaffold must also be capable of adopting the specific properties of the cardiac tissue.

In the heart, cardiomyocytes contract to ensure its mechanical function, that is, blood flow. Tissue stiffness varies between healthy and diseased myocardium. Variation in tissue stiffness must be mimicked by scaffold stiffness. Thus, using a scaffold with stiffness similar to that of the healthy myocardial tissue is preferred in applications of tissue modeling and engineering. Indeed, using scaffolds with stiffness significantly different than the normal contractile heart tissue may impede the function of the tissue itself and/or surrounding tissues since the scaffold stiffness has been shown to influence cell differentiation (Discher et al. 2005).

In addition to mechanical stiffness, elasticity and tensile stress are additional properties that must be considered when selecting a proper scaffold. Elasticity refers to the ability of the myocardium to return to an undeformed state with no permanent deformations after relaxation and contraction. Tensile strength refers to the ability of the myocardium to stretch without rupturing. These properties, similar to stiffness, are integral in the process of myocardial contraction. Thus, to develop a functional tissue model that approximates these conditions, it is imperative to acknowledge that the scaffold accounts for the specific mechanical factors of the cardiac environment such as tensile stress and wide pressure ranges depending on the specific area of the heart.

Electrical conductance is another functional aspect of the heart that must be addressed in the scaffold design for a myocardial tissue construct. Signal transmission via electrical current is vital for myocardial function due to its role in synchronizing cardiomyocyte contraction. Synchronicity of cardiomyocyte contraction is a determining factor in the efficiency of cardiac output; disturbance of synchronicity may lead to more serious problems, such as arrhythmias. Due to the dependence of the functional output of the tissue model on the programming and synchronization of cardiomyocyte contractions, scaffolds should permit conduction to ensure that myocytes respond to electrical signals, which can be accomplished through the incorporation of electrically conductive nanowires within the scaffolds. It is important to note, however, that the incorporation of nanowires may be bypassed if an electrical syncytium is present (Kaiser and Coulombe 2015).

16.3.3.2 Scaffolds for Blood Vessel Development

When developing a tissue model for blood vessels, the material that is being used should be durable and capable of withstanding similar physiological hemodynamic forces while maintaining its structural integrity. To ensure that these mechanical properties are reproduced, the scaffold must facilitate preferential cellular alignment during culture. This alignment should mimic the circumferential orientation of the majority of cells of the artery. In addition, the overall arterial architecture should also be considered when determining the scaffold fabrication methods. The anatomical shape of a regenerated tissue depends on the scaffold initial structure. Thus, the development of arterial models should employ fabrication techniques that result in the production of tubular structures (Hu et al. 2008).

16.3.3.3 Culture Conditions for 3D Vascular Tissue Models

When recapitulating tissue development, the conditions encountered in the *in vivo* environment should be mimicked. Specific conditions encountered by both vasculature tissue and cardiac tissue include the mechanical strain associated with contraction and dilation mechanisms and various shear stresses due to fluid flow dynamics. Common ways to introduce mechanical stimuli include the use of specific bioreactors, such as a rotating wall vessel (RWV). RWVs provide dynamic laminar flow, produce levels of shear stress for both vascular and cardiac tissues, and reduce nutrient and waste diffusional limitations. The culture of cardiac tissue constructs within RWVs resulted in the development of elongated cells capable of spontaneous contraction (Martin et al. 2004). Additional modes of mechanical stimulation can be achieved through actual stretching or uniform compression as well as cyclical strain (Shachar et al. 2012; Lu and Ravens 2013).

When considering cardiac tissue models, electrical stimulation of the cardiomyocytes is another condition that is relevant and necessary for the tissue function and development. Applying electrical stimulation increases cellular differentiation and aids in synchronizing contractions and enhancing the overall contractile properties of the tissue (Radisic et al. 2007). Electrical stimulation is also supportive for structural development. Radisic and coworkers demonstrated that cardiac constructs supplemented with electrical stimulation, mimicking those of the native developed myofibers, aligned in the direction of the electrical field lines (Radisic et al. 2004).

16.4 APPROACHES TO CARDIOVASCULAR 3D TISSUE SYSTEMS

Although synthetic scaffold-based tissue reconstruction is used heavily in biomedical engineering, limitations still exist with synthetic scaffolds. Specifically, these limitations are associated with mismatched mechanical properties for tissue strength, deformability, elasticity, and compliance.

16.4.1 DECELLULARIZED SCAFFOLDS

To overcome some of these challenges, methods such as organ decellularization have been used. Decellularization, a technique used by tissue engineers during the process of tissue regeneration, is characterized by the removal of all cellular and nuclear content. Most decellularization processes are able to preserve the organ's ECM composition, biological activity, and a large degree of the associated mechanical integrity. Decellularized scaffolds have been used in tissue regeneration including *in vivo* applications, for example, decellularized tubular elastin scaffolds derived from porcine carotid arteries have been used in arterial remodeling (Chuang et al. 2009).

16.4.1.1 Tubular Scaffolds for Vessel Modeling

The use of tubular elastin scaffolds by Chuang and coworkers was motivated by the impaired function observed with artificial vascular grafts when used in arteries of small diameter (~5–6 mm). Mechanically, arteries consist of a concentric layer of elastin associated with collagen, whereas functionally elastin, a key component of the arterial ECM, provides elasticity to vessels to accommodate blood flow and pressure variations (Chuang et al. 2009).

To mimic arteries, Chuang and coworkers used decellularized porcine carotid arteries (~5 mm in diameter), obtained following alkaline extraction and treatment with penta-galloyl glucose to hinder elastin degradation (Chuang et al. 2009). The obtained decellularized scaffold maintained its cylindrical, 3D shape while promoting the attachment and growth of fibroblasts and endothelial cells *in vitro*. Moreover, the decellularized scaffolds showed a resistance to high burst pressures and decreased degradation rates for elastin *in vivo* (Chuang et al. 2009).

16.4.1.2 Myocardial Tissue Patches for Cardiac Tissue Engineering

Patients who have suffered from myocardial infarction are at risk of developing severe cardiomyopathy despite current treatments (Wang et al. 2010). Patch technology has been investigated as a method to repair damaged or diseased portions of the heart. Initially, patches were manufactured from synthetic materials like Dacron and tissue-derived components, such as chemically treated pericardium. Unfortunately, these patches resulted in inflammatory responses, mismatched mechanical properties, and thrombosis (Wang et al. 2010).

To address this issue, Wang and colleagues explored the use of a tissue-engineered solution for patch synthesis. Natural scaffolds in tissue engineering may be useful in providing specific cues to influence tissue formation. Especially, the group aimed to determine if myocardium scaffolds could preserve specific mechanical, ultrastructural, and compositional instructions to promote cardiac tissue differentiation (Wang et al. 2010).

To test this hypothesis, Wang and colleagues used sections of pig myocardium that were decellularized to achieve an ECM of the tissue to function as a natural scaffold for the seeding of bone marrow mononuclear cells. They observed complete decellularization after ~2.5 weeks and cellular infiltration and proliferation of differentiated peripheral blood mononuclear cells (PBMC) into cardiomyocytes. Mechanical characterization indicated that the decellularized scaffold alone was stiffer than the cardiac tissue; however, the cellularization of the scaffold led to mechanical properties similar to those observed in the cardiac tissue (Wang et al. 2010).

16.4.2 CELL SHEET ENGINEERING

Cell transplantation therapy has been used to treat damaged cardiac tissue following myocardial infarction. Direct injections of autologous myofibroblasts have shown limited success to restore function to the damaged tissue clinically (Shimizu et al. 2002). Tissue engineering approaches using 3D tissue transplants of biodegradable scaffolds and cells have been proposed as alternatives to direct injections for restoration of muscle function (Shimizu et al. 2002). However, scaffold degradation often leads to fibrosis (Shimizu et al. 2003). Alternatively, cell sheet engineering without scaffolds may be used to prevent inflammatory responses (Masuda et al. 2008).

Cell sheet engineering is a novel technique developed by Okano and colleagues (Yamato and Okano 2004). This technique involves the use of thermoresponsive cell culture substrates (Yamada et al. 1990). Viable cell sheets are obtained by culturing cells on temperature-responsive culture surfaces. The temperature-responsive polymer coating on the surface is poly(N-isopropylacrylamide) (PIPAAm) (Shimizu et al. 2002). The coating is applied to the surface via electron beam exposure, rendering the surface slightly hydrophobic and ensuring cell adhesion at 37°C. The surface reverses to hydrophilic below 32°C due to rapid hydration swelling of the grafted PIPAAm and detachment of cells (Okano et al. 1993).

The novelty of this technique is that unlike conventional trypsinization, where a proteolytic enzyme is used to degrade cell adhesion molecules for detachment of cells from the surface, this new technique maintains cell adhesion molecules as well as cell-to-cell junctions and receptor proteins (Yamato and Okano 2004), as shown in Figure 16.3 Native cardiac muscle cells are dense with gap junctions to allow electrical transmission (Yang et al. 2005).

Aspirating detached cell sheets and transferring them to another culture dish are used to fabricate 3D cell sheet constructs. The aspirated sheet is placed at the center of the dish and spread out manually using the pipet tip. The sheet is allowed to reattach for 30 min (Shimizu et al. 2002). Another sheet is layered on top of the first cell sheet in the same manner. Up to four sheets can be layered on each other with ensured viability and electrical stimulation between sheets (Yamato and Okano 2004).

A study by Shimizu and coworkers (Shimizu et al. 2002) examined the use of cell sheet engineering as a 3D tissue system for cardiovascular applications *in vitro*. In this *in vitro* study, cell sheet bilayers of neonatal rat cardiomyocytes exhibit synchronized pulsing crucial for transplanted tissue success. Histological analysis of the bilayer constructs confirms adhesion between the cell sheets. Evaluation by transmission electron microscopy shows the presence of myofilaments, Z-lines, and desmosines in bilayered constructs.

Each bilayered cell sheet eclectically communicated with other layered sheets. Manual electrical stimulation was applied to the upper sheet (up to 2.5 Hz) and the stimulation was detected in the lower sheet (Shimizu et al. 2002; Shimizu et al. 2002). In control experiments, the addition of a layer of collagen (70-μm thick) between the two cardiomyocytes cell sheets inhibited electrical stimulation between the two sheets.

Cell sheet engineering was also examined *in vivo* using rat cardiomyocytes cell sheets transplanted subcutaneously in nude mice. The transplanted sheets attached within 5 min (Yang et al. 2005). After three weeks, transplanted cell sheet grafts demonstrated synchronized beating, and neovascularization was confirmed histologically (Yamato and Okano 2004). Cell survival was observed following cell sheet transplantation for up to 1 year and for a maximum thickness of 80 μm or three cell sheets (Yang et al. 2007).

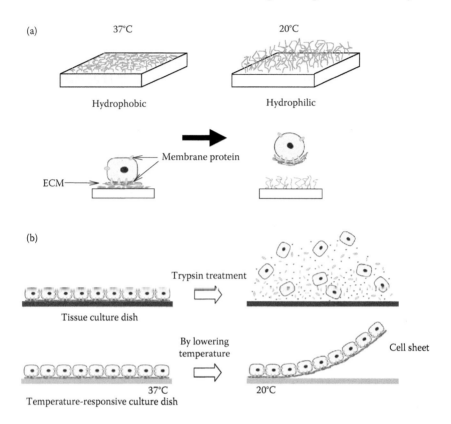

FIGURE 16.3 Harvesting of cell sheets in cell sheet engineering. (a) Cells attach to thermoresponsive substrate in hydrophobic state at 37°C and spontaneously detach from substrate as it becomes hydrophilic at 20°C with cell-to-cell junctions and adhesion molecules intact. (b) Conventional methods of cell harvesting use trypsin for enzymatic digestion to cleave adhesion proteins and cause cells to lift off culture substrate. The use of thermoresponsive culture substrates allows the cells to detach in sheets with adhesion proteins intact. (Reprinted from Masuda, S. et al., Cell sheet engineering for heart tissue repair, 60 (2):277–85, Copyright 2008, with permission from Elsevier.)

Dr. Okano's group used cell sheet engineering to treat damaged cardiac muscle following myocardial infarction, and the transplantation of cell sheets improved functionality of infarcted tissue of rat hearts (Yang et al. 2007). Polysurgery has been used *in vivo* to construct thicker cell sheet tissue transplants. Multistep transplantation at 1–2 day intervals for 10 separate transplantations has allowed the construction of cell sheets up to ~1 mm in thickness (30 sheets). Future work on this technology includes large animal testing using autologous myofibroblasts and fabrication of organ-like structures. Myocardial tubes have been fabricated by wrapping six cell sheets around a resected rat aorta with the capability of providing independent support as a graft replacement (Yang et al. 2007).

16.5 CONCLUSION AND PERSPECTIVE

There is a great need for 3D cardiovascular tissue systems. The ideal system would mimic the architecture of the cardiac or vessel system including the extracellular matrix and cells native to the tissues. Decellularized scaffolds properly mimic the architecture and matrix of arterial and cardiac tissues as a 3D test system. The most advanced 3D tissue system for cardiovascular application is cell sheet engineering. Cell sheet engineering allows the inclusion of native cells, communication between cell sheets, and electrical stimulation. Cell sheet engineering shows the most promise for advancing the field of cardiovascular 3D tissue systems.

REFERENCES

Akins, R. E. Jr., D. Rockwood, K. G. Robinson, D. Sandusky, J. Rabolt, and C. Pizarro. 2010. Three-dimensional culture alters primary cardiac cell phenotype. *Tissue Eng Part A* no. 16 (2):629–41.

Camelliti, P., T. K. Borg, and P. Kohl. 2005. Structural and functional characterisation of cardiac fibroblasts. *Cardiovasc Res* no. 65 (1):40–51.

Chen, C. Y., C. J. Ke, K. C. Yen, H. C. Hsieh, J. S. Sun, and F. H. Lin. 2015. 3D porous calcium-alginate scaffolds cell culture system improved human osteoblast cell clusters for cell therapy. *Theranostics* no. 5 (6):643–55.

Chen, L. S. and P. S. Chen. 2009. Nerve sprouting and cardiac arrhythmias. In D. P. Zipes and J. Jalife (Eds.) *Cardiac Electrophysiology: From Cell to Bedside* (381–90). Philadelphia: Saunders.

Chuang, T. H., C. Stabler, A. Simionescu, and D. T. Simionescu. 2009. Polyphenol-stabilized tubular elastin scaffolds for tissue engineered vascular grafts. *Tissue Eng Part A* no. 15 (10):2837–51.

Clark, J. M. and S. Glagov. 1979. Structural integration of the arterial wall. I. Relationships and attachments of medial smooth muscle cells in normally distended and hyperdistended aortas. *Lab Investig* no. 40 (5):587–602.

de Lange, W. J., L. F. Hegge, A. C. Grimes, C. W. Tong, T. M. Brost, R. L. Moss, and J. C. Ralphe. 2011. Neonatal mouse-derived engineered cardiac tissue: A novel model system for studying genetic heart disease. *Circ Res* no. 109 (1):8–19.

Discher, D. E., P. Janmey, and Y. L. Wang. 2005. Tissue cells feel and respond to the stiffness of their substrate. *Science* no. 310 (5751):1139–43.

Donoghue, P. S., T. Sun, N. Gadegaard, M. O. Riehle, and S. C. Barnett. 2014. Development of a novel 3D culture system for screening features of a complex implantable device for CNS repair. *Mol Pharm* no. 11 (7):2143–50.

Fan, X., R. Zou, Z. Zhao, P. Yang, Y. Li, and J. Song. 2009. Tensile strain induces integrin beta1 and ILK expression higher and faster in 3D cultured rat skeletal myoblasts than in 2D cultures. *Tissue Cell* no. 41 (4):266–70.

Gasser, T. C., R. W. Ogden, and G. A. Holzapfel. 2006. Hyperelastic modelling of arterial layers with distributed collagen fibre orientations. *J R Soc Interface* no. 3 (6):15–35.

Gobin, A. S., D. A. Taylor E. Chau, and L. C. Sampaio. 2016. Organogenesis. In E. Perin, L. Miller, D. Taylor, and J. Willerson (Eds.) *Stem Cell and Gene Therapy for Cardiovascular Disease* (349–73). Boston: Academic Press, Chapter 28.

Hu, X., H. Shen, F. Yang, J. Bei, and S. Wang. 2008. Preparation and cell affinity of microtubular orientation-structured PLGA(70/30) blood vessel scaffold. *Biomaterials* no. 29 (21):3128–36.

Jin, G., G. H. Yang, and G. Kim. 2015. Tissue engineering bioreactor systems for applying physical and electrical stimulations to cells. *J Biomed Mater Res B: Appl Biomater* no. 103 (4):935–48.

Kaiser, N. J. and K. L. Coulombe. 2015. Physiologically inspired cardiac scaffolds for tailored *in vivo* function and heart regeneration. *Biomed Mater* no. 10 (3):034003.

Lockhart, M., E. Wirrig, A. Phelps, and A. Wessels. 2011. Extracellular matrix and heart development. *Birth Defects Res A: Clin Mol Teratol* no. 91 (6):535–50.

Lu, L. and U. Ravens. 2013. The use of a novel cardiac bioreactor system in investigating fibroblast physiology and its perspectives. *Organogenesis* no. 9 (2):82–6.

Martin, I., D. Wendt, and M. Heberer. 2004. The role of bioreactors in tissue engineering. *Trends Biotechnol* no. 22 (2):80–6.

Martini, F. H., M. J. Timmons, and R. B. Tallitsch. 2012. The cardiovascular system: The heart. In F. H. Martini, M. J. Timmons, R. B. Tallitsch (Eds.) *Human Anatomy*, 7th ed., New York: Pearson Education, Inc.

Masuda, S., T. Shimizu, M. Yamato, and T. Okano. 2008. Cell sheet engineering for heart tissue repair. *Adv Drug Deliv Rev* no. 60 (2):277–85.

Nugent, H. M. and E. R. Edelman. 2003. Tissue engineering therapy for cardiovascular disease. *Circ Res* no. 92 (10):1068–78.

O'Brien, F. J. 2011. Biomaterials & scaffolds for tissue engineering. *Materials Today* no. 14 (3):88–95.

Okano, T., N. Yamada, H. Sakai, and Y. Sakurai. 1993. A novel recovery system for cultured cells using plasma-treated polystyrene dishes grafted with poly(N-isopropylacrylamide). *J Biomed Mater Res* no. 27 (10):1243–51.

Pontes Soares, C., V. Midlej, M. E. de Oliveira, M. Benchimol, M. L. Costa, and C. Mermelstein. 2012. 2D and 3D-organized cardiac cells shows differences in cellular morphology, adhesion junctions, presence of myofibrils and protein expression. *PLoS One* no. 7 (5):e38147.

Radisic, M., H. Park, S. Gerecht, C. Cannizzaro, R. Langer, and G. Vunjak-Novakovic. 2007. Biomimetic approach to cardiac tissue engineering. *Philos Trans R Soc Lond B: Biol Sci* no. 362 (1484):1357–68.

Radisic, M., H. Park, H. Shing, T. Consi, F. J. Schoen, R. Langer, L. E. Freed, and G. Vunjak-Novakovic. 2004. Functional assembly of engineered myocardium by electrical stimulation of cardiac myocytes cultured on scaffolds. *Proc Natl Acad Sci USA* no. 101 (52):18129–34.

Sakaguchi, K., T. Shimizu, and T. Okano. 2015. Construction of three-dimensional vascularized cardiac tissue with cell sheet engineering. *J Control Release* no. 205:83–8.

Shachar, M., N. Benishti, and S. Cohen. 2012. Effects of mechanical stimulation induced by compression and medium perfusion on cardiac tissue engineering. *Biotechnol Progress* no. 28 (6):1551–9.

Shimizu, T., M. Yamato, T. Akutsu, T. Shibata, Y. Isoi, A. Kikuchi, M. Umezu, and T. Okano. 2002. Electrically communicating three-dimensional cardiac tissue mimic fabricated by layered cultured cardiomyocyte sheets. *J Biomed Mater Res* no. 60 (1):110–7.

Shimizu, T., M. Yamato, Y. Isoi, T. Akutsu, T. Setomaru, K. Abe, A. Kikuchi, M. Umezu, and T. Okano. 2002. Fabrication of pulsatile cardiac tissue grafts using a novel 3-dimensional cell sheet manipulation technique and temperature-responsive cell culture surfaces. *Circ Res* no. 90 (3):e40.

Shimizu, T., M. Yamato, A. Kikuchi, and T. Okano. 2003. Cell sheet engineering for myocardial tissue reconstruction. *Biomaterials* no. 24 (13):2309–16.

Tung, L. and J. R. Borderies. 1992. Analysis of electric field stimulation of single cardiac muscle cells. *Biophys J* no. 63 (2):371–86.

Vunjak-Novakovic, G., N. Tandon, A. Godier, R. Maidhof, A. Marsano, T. P. Martens, and M. Radisic. 2010. Challenges in cardiac tissue engineering. *Tissue Eng Part B: Rev* no. 16 (2):169–87.

Wang, B., A. Borazjani, M. Tahai, A. L. Curry, D. T. Simionescu, J. Guan, F. To, S. H. Elder, and J. Liao. 2010. Fabrication of cardiac patch with decellularized porcine myocardial scaffold and bone marrow mononuclear cells. *J Biomed Mater Res A* no. 94 (4):1100–10.

Yamada, N., T. Okano, H. Sakai, F. Karikusa, Y. Sawasaki, and Y. Sakurai. 1990. Thermo-responsive polymeric surfaces; control of attachment and detachment of cultured cells. *Die Makromol Chem: Rapid Commun* no. 11 (11):571–6.

Yamato, M. and T. Okano. 2004. Cell sheet engineering. *Mater Today* no. 7 (5):42–7.

Yang, J., M. Yamato, C. Kohno, A. Nishimoto, H. Sekine, F. Fukai, and T. Okano. 2005. Cell sheet engineering: recreating tissues without biodegradable scaffolds. *Biomaterials* no. 26 (33):6415–22.

Yang, J., M. Yamato, T. Shimizu, H. Sekine, K. Ohashi, M. Kanzaki, T. Ohki, K. Nishida, and T. Okano. 2007. Reconstruction of functional tissues with cell sheet engineering. *Biomaterials* no. 28 (34):5033–43.

Zou, Y. and Y. Zhang. 2012. The biomechanical function of arterial elastin in solutes. *J Biomech Eng* no. 134 (7):1–6.

17 Signaling and Architectural Cues Necessary for 3D Diabetic Tissue Models

Rosalyn D. Abbott and David L. Kaplan

CONTENTS

17.1 Introduction 299
17.2 Pancreas 301
    17.2.1 Recapitulating Proper Cell Signaling within the Pancreas 301
    17.2.2 Architectural Cues within the Pancreas 305
    17.2.3 Pancreatic-Specific Diabetic Cues 305
17.3 Liver 306
    17.3.1 Recapitulating Proper Cell Signaling within the Liver 306
    17.3.2 Architectural Cues within the Liver 307
    17.3.3 Liver-Specific Diabetic Cues 308
17.4 Skeletal Muscle 308
    17.4.1 Recapitulating Proper Cell Signaling within the Skeletal Muscle 308
    17.4.2 Architectural Cues within the Skeletal Muscle 309
    17.4.3 Muscle-Specific Diabetic Cues 310
17.5 Adipose 310
    17.5.1 Recapitulating Proper Cell Signaling within the Adipose Tissue 310
    17.5.2 Architectural Cues within the Adipose Tissue 312
    17.5.3 Adipose-Specific Diabetic Cues 312
17.6 Conclusion and Perspective 312
Acknowledgments 313
References 313

17.1 INTRODUCTION

Diabetes mellitus is an overarching term for a group of metabolic diseases defined by high blood glucose levels (hyperglycemia) caused by deficiencies in either insulin secretion or insulin action, or a combination of both (Loghmani 2005). Pancreatic β-cells secrete insulin in response to changes in the extracellular glucose concentration to maintain blood glucose levels within narrow limits. Insulin regulates the uptake of glucose by skeletal muscle and white adipose tissues (throughout referred to as adipose tissue) and the use and production of glucose by the liver, despite daily fluxes in glucose caused by meals, fasting, or intense exercise (Figure 17.1) (Leibiger, Leibiger, and Berggren 2008). There are two main types of diabetes: Type I and type II that will be discussed in this chapter; however, there are other types of diabetes, including gestational diabetes and surgically induced diabetes that share common features of type I and type II diabetes that will not be discussed.

Type I diabetes, historically referred to as juvenile diabetes or insulin-dependent diabetes, most commonly develops at an early age; however, can also develop in adults. In type I diabetes, the body's immune system attacks the pancreatic β-cells that secrete insulin, creating an insulin deficiency throughout the body. Daily insulin injections are required to control blood glucose levels. Type I diabetes usually involves either a genetic predisposition or is triggered by environmental cues such as an infection or other stresses (Leslie and Delli Castelli 2004; Loghmani 2005). Type II diabetes, historically referred to as adult-onset diabetes or noninsulin-dependent diabetes, can affect people at any age, even children. Type II diabetes is usually diagnosed when patients become insulin resistant—a condition that occurs when liver, skeletal muscle, and adipose tissues do not respond effectively to insulin stimulation. As a result, the body requires more insulin to regulate glucose properly. Initially, the pancreas increases insulin secretion to counter the decreased responsiveness of the tissues; however, over time the pancreas function declines and does not produce enough insulin (for instance after meals) and treatment is required. People who are more likely to develop type II diabetes are: Inactive, overweight, have a genetic predisposition, or have another condition associated with insulin resistance (for example, polycystic ovary syndrome) (Loghmani 2005).

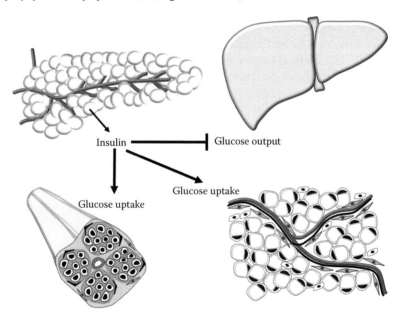

FIGURE 17.1 In healthy states, insulin secreted by β-cells in the pancreas stimulates the liver to stop glucose output, and the skeletal muscle and adipose tissue to uptake glucose.

While each type of diabetes has unique symptoms and etiology, the generalizations may not be strictly associated with each type. For instance, it is not uncommon for patients with type I diabetes to be insulin resistant, or patients with type II diabetes to require insulin injections. Over time, regardless of the cause, chronic hyperglycemia leads to severe health problems, including dehydration, nausea, vomiting, increased urination, ketoacidosis, visual impairment, blindness, kidney disease, nerve damage, impaired wound healing (which leads to amputations), cardiovascular disease, and stroke (Loghmani 2005; Amer et al. 2014).

While there are numerous diabetic animal models for studying different disease etiologies, they often do not correlate with the human disease (Perel et al. 2007). With the high risk of diabetic health-related problems and an increasing amount of diabetic cases reported, human *in vitro* tissue models of the disease pathology are needed to improve relevance to the human situation. While *in vitro* models do not duplicate *in vivo* interactions, they provide an additional avenue for studying human-specific disease etiologies. In this way, *in vitro* tissue models of diabetes are useful in a multitude of applications. In the drug-development process, they can be used to test new compounds that have not historically been used for the treatment of diabetes. *In vitro* models can also be used to test pharmacokinetics and toxicity of compounds that have shown promise as a treatment. These tissues can also be used to advance our current understanding of disease mechanisms to inform preventative actions.

This chapter will discuss approaches for *in vitro* tissue models (Table 17.1) related to type I and type II *Diabetes mellitus* focusing on the main organs affected by the feedback loop between the pancreas, liver, skeletal muscle, and adipose tissue (Reed and Scribner 1999; Kahn 2000; Amer et al. 2014). To create diabetic tissue models *in vitro* of each organ system, healthy physiology must first be recapitulated as a baseline. Organogenesis is highly regulated by many distinct cues to ensure that each cell type has proper intracellular and intercellular signaling. Proper architectural cues are also very important since the extracellular matrix (ECM) transmits signals to the cytoskeleton through integrins that initiate signaling cascades that affect the genetic expression (Juliano and Haskill 1993). Therefore, cell signaling, architecture, and diabetic cues will be discussed as applicable to each organ, respectively.

17.2 PANCREAS

The pancreas is a versatile gland that has exocrine and endocrine functions, which primarily control digestion and metabolism (Greggio et al. 2015). In particular, it rapidly senses blood glucose levels by secreting insulin, which is disrupted in diabetic patients. Therefore, to recreate baseline functionality, before creating a diabetic model, viable cells need to form cell aggregates that release insulin in response to changes in glucose levels (Amer et al. 2014).

17.2.1 Recapitulating Proper Cell Signaling within the Pancreas

In the pancreas (Figure 17.2), the acinar and ductal cells are responsible for exocrine functions, while the hormone-producing cells, β-, α-, δ-, and pp-cells, are responsible for the endocrine functions (Greggio et al. 2015). For diabetes models, the most

TABLE 17.1
Examples of Diabetic *In Vitro* Cell and Tissue Models

Organ	Type	Diabetic Stimulus	Outcome	Cell Type and Culture Condition
Pancreas	I	T cell coculture	↓ β-cell insulin secretion	Coculture of mouse pancreatic islets with fetal thymus lobes (Wilson and DeLuca 1997)
		Activated macrophage coculture	Islet cell lysis	Coculture of rat macrophages with islets (Appels et al. 1989; Burkart et al. 1992)
	II	Hyperglycemia	↓ β-cell function and viability	Mouse islets (Efanova et al. 1998; Waanders et al. 2009)
		Hyperlipidemia	↑ Mitochondrial stress regulator	Rat islets (Ling et al. 1996; Khaldi et al. 2004; Bensellam et al. 2009)
			↓ Glucose-stimulated insulin secretion	Mouse islets (Waanders et al. 2009)
Liver	I	Hyperglycemia	Decreased the concentration of IGF-I, but increased the concentration of IGF-II	Rat islets and mouse MIN6 pancreatic β-cells (Wang et al. 2007)
			↓ IGF-I, ↑ IGF-II	Rat hepatocytes (Han, Kang, and Park 2006)
	II	Insulin and fructose	↓ Glucose uptake, ↑ glucose accumulation within the culture medium and ↑ intracellular lipid accumulation	Human Chang liver cells (Williams et al. 2013)
		Hyperlipidemia	Palmitate-induced gluconeogenesis	H4IIE rat hepatocytes (Lee et al. 2011)
	Both	Hyperglycemia	↑ Lipid accumulation, ↑ mitochondria dysfunction, and ↑ oxygen species	Rat hepatocytes in hollow fiber based organoid culture (Lu et al. 2012)

(Continued)

TABLE 17.1 (Continued)
Examples of Diabetic *In Vitro* Cell and Tissue Models

Organ	Type	Diabetic Stimulus	Outcome	Cell Type and Culture Condition
Muscle	II	Hyperlipidemia	↑ Lipid accumulation, ↑ inflammation and ↓ insulin signaling	Human myotubes (Abildgaard et al. 2014)
		Inflammatory cytokines	↓ Insulin signaling, ↓ glucose uptake and ↑ inflammatory signaling	Primary human skeletal muscle cells (Sell et al. 2006; Lambernd et al. 2012)
		Chemerin	↓ Insulin signaling, ↓ glucose uptake and ↑ inflammatory signaling	Primary human skeletal muscle cells (Sell et al. 2009; Lambernd et al. 2012)
		Conditioned media from adipocytes	↓ Insulin signaling, ↓ glucose uptake, ↑ inflammatory signaling ↑ Reactive oxygen species and ↑ nitric oxide	Primary human skeletal muscle cells (Dietze-Schroeder et al. 2005; Sell et al. 2008; Lambernd et al. 2012)
		Adipocyte coculture	↓ Insulin-stimulated glucose uptake	Primary human skeletal muscle cells (Dietze et al. 2002; Dietze-Schroeder et al. 2005)
Adipose	II	Conditioned media from THP-1 cells	↑ IL-6, IL-8 and MCP-1, ↓ Insulin-stimulated glucose uptake	Human differentiated Simpson–Golabi–Behmel syndrome preadipocytes (Keuper et al. 2011; Kotnik et al. 2013; Zagotta et al. 2015)
		Macrophage coculture	↓ Insulin-stimulated glucose uptake	Human differentiated Simpson–Golabi–Behmel syndrome preadipocytes (Wentworth et al. 2010)
		Dioxin	↓ Insulin-stimulated glucose uptake	3T3-L1 mouse adipocytes (Hsu et al. 2010)
		Fatty acids	Altered cytokine secretion	3T3-L1 mouse adipocytes (Schaeffler et al. 2009)

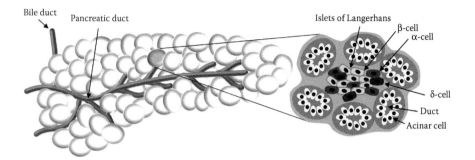

FIGURE 17.2 Schematic structure of the pancreas. Within the lobes of the pancreas the β-cells, α-cells, and δ-cells form the islets of Langerhans, which are adjacent to acinar cells and ducts.

relevant cell types are β- and α-cells, since the β-cells lower blood glucose levels by secreting insulin, while the α-cells increase blood glucose levels by secreting glucagon (Peyser et al. 2014). The β-cells and α-cells, together with somatostatin-producing δ-cells, pancreatic polypeptide producing pp-cells, and ghrelin producing cells, form the islets of Langerhans (Stendahl et al. 2009). Islets comprise 1%–2% of the total adult human pancreatic volume, with approximately one million islets scattered within the exocrine pancreas (Carroll 1992). Islets are extensively vascularized by fenestrated endothelial networks and innervated by sympathetic, parasympathetic, and sensory nerves (Carroll 1992; Brunicardi et al. 1996; Ahren 2000). The unique multicellular connections within the pancreas necessitate the synchronization of a multitude of signals to obtain the appropriate function of the β-cell under basal and glucose-stimulated conditions. Examples of known paracrine effects on the secretion of insulin by β-cells include the stimulatory effect of glucagon secreted by α-cells and the inhibitory effect of somatostatin by δ-cells.

To create proper cell–cell signaling, many approaches have been employed. Isolated islets are an attractive option for studying disease processes since the tissue contains the relevant cell types required for proper signaling in the appropriate matrix (Navarro-Alvarez et al. 2008). However, *in vitro* the isolated tissues rapidly lose mass, viability, and functions (Korbutt et al. 2004). Alternatively, primary cells have been separated from the tissue by enzymatic digestion, expanded, and used to create *in vitro* cell and tissue models. However, the expansion of dissociated pancreatic primary cells in 2D is challenging, and the cells can only be maintained for the short term in small numbers (Sugiyama et al. 2007; Furuyama et al. 2011). To enhance the capacity for the long-term culture, suspension in 3D enables maintenance for a few weeks (Paraskevas et al. 2000; Blauer et al. 2011; Houbracken et al. 2011). As another alternative, embryonic pancreatic multipotent progenitors have also been differentiated to create models *in vitro* (Greggio et al. 2013; Sugiyama et al. 2013). In the presence of growth factors, and grown within Matrigel®, progenitor cells can self-organize into different structures, including spheres composed of pancreatic progenitors and differentiated cells in "mini-pancreas" models and organoids (Greggio et al. 2015). Induced pluripotent stem cells have also been used in a similar manner to embryonic stem cells (Zhang et al. 2009). The most frequently used pancreatic cell lines are not human, however: RINm5F (rat), INS-1 (mouse), b-TC (mouse), and MIN6 (rat), with only MIN6 cells having the capability to release insulin in response to glucose stimulation (Amer et al. 2014).

17.2.2 ARCHITECTURAL CUES WITHIN THE PANCREAS

Adult human islets are partially encapsulated by fibroblasts, which secrete fibrillar collagen (Stendahl et al. 2009). Additional matrix proteins comprising the peri-insular basement membrane surround the islets, including laminin, nonfibrillar collagen, nidogen, entactin, and fibronectin (Van Deijnen et al. 1994; Jiang et al. 1999). ECM–β-cell interactions activate NF-κB signaling and the production of cytokines, which is required for proper glucose-stimulated insulin secretion (Hammar et al. 2005; Ribaux et al. 2007). The cellular orientations within the matrix are very important. Apico-basal (Kesavan et al. 2009) and planar polarities (Cortijo et al. 2012) are required for an appropriate endocrine cell function. In particular, planar cell polarity has been shown to be essential for pancreatic β-cell differentiation and glucose homeostasis (Cortijo et al. 2012). To recreate the 3D environment *in vitro* many platforms have been used, including suspension cultures, porous scaffolds (polylactide, polylactide-*co*-glycolide acid, with recombinant growth factors or ECM modification), microwell or micropatterning technologies (to control aggregation), different hydrogels or cell sheets (Shimizu et al. 2009; Amer et al. 2014).

17.2.3 PANCREATIC-SPECIFIC DIABETIC CUES

Type I and type II diabetes affect the normal functioning capacity of the pancreas in different ways. In type I diabetes, an autoimmune disorder causes T lymphocytes (T cells) to activate against and destroy pancreatic β-cells, decreasing the overall capacity of the pancreas to respond to changes in glucose levels by secreting insulin (Castano and Eisenbarth 1990; Amer et al. 2014). To model this affect *in vitro*, T cells have been cocultured with pancreatic tissue to suppress overall insulin secretion (Wilson and DeLuca 1997). Other toxic products (interleukin I, oxygen radicals, and nitric oxide) secreted by macrophages are also thought to destroy β-cells and have been incorporated in coculture models as well (Appels et al. 1989; Burkart et al. 1992).

In type II diabetes, the pancreas is forced to increase insulin secretion to counter the decreased responsiveness of the liver, skeletal muscle, and adipose tissues. In addition, glucose-stimulated insulin secretion is diminished (Cerasi 1995; Buchanan 2003), caused by moderate decreases in β-cell mass, as well as the functional impairment of the remaining β-cells (Kahn 2000; Butler et al. 2003). Functional alterations in β-cells are preceded and likely caused by chronic hyperglycemia and hyperlipidemia (Grill and Bjorklund 2001; Poitout and Robertson 2002). Therefore, elevated glucose levels of 10 mmol/L or higher (Ling et al. 1996; Efanova et al. 1998; Khaldi et al. 2004; Bensellam et al. 2009; Waanders et al. 2009) and high fat content (Wang et al. 2007; Waanders et al. 2009) have been used *in vitro* to negatively affect the β-cell function. However, it should be noted that *in vitro* glucose is required for β-cell survival and function (2–10 mmol/L) (Hoorens et al. 1996; Van de Casteele et al. 2003; Elouil et al. 2007; Bensellam et al. 2009).

Current pancreatic *in vitro* models of type I and type II diabetes focus on the endocrine cells in the pancreas, since they are the regulators of blood glucose levels. However, by doing so, these models largely ignore the exocrine pancreas which is a large quantity of the tissue mass and likely contributes to cell signaling in disease processes. In the future, it will be necessary to explore whether the exocrine cells interact and alter normal endocrine functioning in diabetes.

17.3 LIVER

The liver is a multifunctional organ that has diverse roles from detoxifying blood to producing and secreting blood and bile components, and to metabolizing proteins, steroids, fat, vitamins, iron, and glucose (LeCluyse et al. 2012). In particular, the liver has a fundamental role in regulating blood glucose levels (within 3.9–6.1 mM) (Sherwin 1980; Davidson et al. 2015). After a meal, insulin is secreted by β-cells in the pancreas and the liver responds by (1) storing excess glucose as glycogen and (2) inhibiting glucose production. During fasting, in response to glucagon secreted by pancreatic α-cells, the liver releases glucose by breaking down glycogen and synthesizing new glucose from precursors such as lactate and glucogenic amino acids via gluconeogenesis. In diabetic states, however, the homeostatic regulation of glucose is altered. Therefore, to recreate baseline liver functionality, before creating a diabetic tissue model, viable cells need to regulate glucose levels in response to insulin.

17.3.1 RECAPITULATING PROPER CELL SIGNALING WITHIN THE LIVER

In the liver, there are two classifications of cells: parenchymal cells and nonparenchymal cells. Parenchymal hepatocytes comprise approximately 60% of the cell population and approximately 80% of the liver's volume (Kmiec 2001; LeCluyse et al. 2012). Hepatocytes are highly differentiated epithelial cells responsible for most of the synthetic and metabolic functions of the liver (Ohashi and Okano 2014). The remaining 40% of the cell population, the nonparenchymal cells, are found in the sinusoidal compartment of the tissue and are only 6.5% of the total liver volume (Kmiec 2001; LeCluyse et al. 2012)—ECM comprises the rest of the liver volume (Figure 17.3). Nonparenchymal cells are a combination of bile duct epithelial cells, sinusoidal endothelial cells, stellate cells, Kupffer cells (resident macrophages), and intrahepatic lymphocytes (pit cells) (Kmiec 2001; LeCluyse et al. 2012).

Commonly used hepatic cells are primary animal hepatocytes, hepatocellular carcinoma (HepG2) cell lines, and human primary hepatocytes (Hoganson et al. 2008). While hepatocytes are most commonly incorporated into cell and tissue models alone (Wu et al. 1999; Dash et al. 2009; Tuschl et al. 2009; Wen et al. 2009; Lu et al. 2012), nonparenchymal cells support hepatic growth and function, and have been shown to affect glucose output in the liver (Kmiec 2001). Coculture of endothelial cells with hepatocytes improves hepatocyte-specific functions (Guguen-Guillouzo et al. 1983; Harimoto et al. 2002; Yamada et al. 2012) and can create sinusoidal surfaces (Salerno et al. 2011). In addition, sinusoidal endothelial cells, Kupffer cells, and stellate cells may exacerbate insulin resistance in hepatocytes by

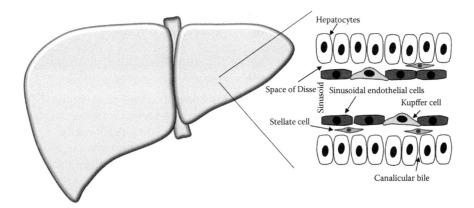

FIGURE 17.3 Schematic structure of the liver and a sinusoid. Hepatocytes are polarized cells with their basolateral domain interfacing with the sinusoidal endothelial cells and the apical domains midway between the lateral domains contacting neighboring hepatocytes (canalicular bile). Endothelial lined sinusoids bind Kupffer cells, while the stellate cells are located in the space of Disse.

increasing oxidative stress and secreting inflammatory cytokines that attract further inflammatory infiltration and a fibrogenic response (Leclercq et al. 2007).

17.3.2 Architectural Cues within the Liver

The liver has a complex architecture that consists of three different acinar zones that have distinct cells, solute concentrations, oxygen tension, and gene expression (LeCluyse et al. 2012). Matrix composition is different depending on the zone and is found between the hepatocytes and the endothelial cells in a region known as the space of Disse. Depending on the zone, the matrix can consist of fibrillar collagens (types I and III), laminins, vimentin, hyaluronans, and proteoglycans, with matrix around the central vein predominantly comprised of type IV and VI collagens, syndecans 1 and 4, and no hyaluronans or laminins (Reid et al. 1992). Additionally, the cyto-architecture in the liver is very important for the cellular function. Hepatocytes are polarized cells with functionally different domains—the baso-lateral domains (interface with the sinusoidal microvasculature on opposite sides of the single cell layers) and the apical domains midway between the lateral domains (canalicular bile, contacting neighboring hepatocytes) (LeCluyse et al. 2012).

Hepatocytes, like other cells, are influenced by their surrounding architecture. Monolayer *in vitro* cell models have been conventionally used for metabolic drug-screening studies due to their ease of setup (Dash et al. 2009), however they rapidly lose liver-specific functions (Brandon et al. 2003) and change their metabolic patterns after three days of culture (Bissell et al. 1978). Further complexity has been added to the 2D configuration with collagen sandwich cultures improving the physiological relevance for long-term studies (Tuschl et al. 2009). However, even with the added complexity, cells do not respond to insulin stimulation appropriately (Hansson et al. 2004). To further enhance relevance, 3D cultures of hepatocytes have been established that preserve liver-specific functions and glucose metabolism better than monolayer cultures (Wu et al. 1999; Wen et al. 2009; Lu et al. 2012).

17.3.3 LIVER-SPECIFIC DIABETIC CUES

Insulin resistance affects the liver in the prediabetic and diabetic state of type II diabetes, where hepatocytes fail to respond (or have a reduced response) to normal circulating insulin levels with glucose storage (Kahn and Flier 2000). Additionally, there is impaired suppression of hepatic glucose production, both of which result in systemic hyperglycemia (Leclercq et al. 2007). Insulin also regulates fat synthesis and storage in the liver; therefore, lipids accumulate within the liver, interfering with insulin signaling and contributing to insulin resistance (Samuel et al. 2010). To model these effects, *in vitro* insulin supplemented with fructose has been used to create an insulin resistance model where there was a decrease in insulin-stimulated glucose uptake, an increase in glucose accumulation in the media, and an increase in intra cellular lipid accumulation (Williams et al. 2013). Additionally, hyperlipidemia was also used to create a type II diabetic model that resulted in palmitate-induced gluconeogenesis (Lee et al. 2011). Untreated type I diabetes also results in hyperglycemia in the liver. Therefore, the effect of hyperglycemia has been used to simulate a type I diabetic state (Han et al. 2006) as well as a general diabetic disease state (Lu et al. 2012).

17.4 SKELETAL MUSCLE

Skeletal muscle is a metabolically active tissue that generates and transmits contractile forces. At rest, skeletal muscle energy demand is met by breaking down fatty acids and the cells have limited permeability to glucose (due to low levels of glucose transporter type 4 (GLUT4) in the plasma membrane) (Cheng et al. 2014). In response to insulin, however, GLUT4 is transported from intracellular vesicles to the plasma membrane, enabling glucose to enter myofibers (it should be noted that moderate to heavy exercise can also cause GLUT4 translocation, independent of insulin) (Cheng et al. 2014). In this way, insulin stimulates glucose transport in skeletal muscle and adipose tissue, with 80% of the human body's glucose uptake occurring in the skeletal muscle (Ferrannini et al. 1988). However, in diabetic patients, insulin levels and glucose uptake are altered. Therefore, to recreate baseline skeletal muscle functionality, before creating a diabetic tissue model, viable cells need to transport glucose in response to insulin.

17.4.1 RECAPITULATING PROPER CELL SIGNALING WITHIN THE SKELETAL MUSCLE

Skeletal muscle is composed of multiple parallel, striated multinucleated myofibers (Figure 17.4). Each multinucleated myofiber functions as a single cell and can extend the whole length of the muscle (Yan et al. 2007). Located at the periphery of the myofibers are satellite cells, whose function is to repair and replace damaged cells (Yan et al. 2007). Skeletal muscle also has an extensive neurovascular network that forms an organized branching pattern throughout myofibers for blood supply and innervation (Dennis and Kosnik 2000).

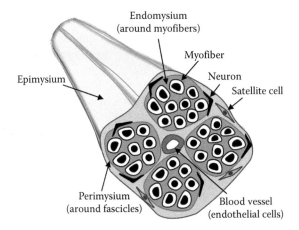

FIGURE 17.4 Schematic structure of skeletal muscle. Skeletal muscle is composed of multiple parallel, striated multinucleated myofibers that can extend the whole length of the muscle. Located at the periphery of the myofibers are satellite cells and an extensive neuro-vascular network that forms an organized branching pattern throughout myofibers for blood supply and innervation. Myofibers are the bulk of skeletal muscle tissue, and are dispersed in ECM: the endomysium (around individual myofibers), the perimysium (around fascicles) and the epimysium (around the entire muscle).

In vitro multinucleated myotubes are immature myofibers. The most common cell types used to create myotubes are human satellite cells, mouse C2C12, primary myoblasts from mice and humans, and L6 rat myoblasts (Cittadella Vigodarzere and Mantero 2014). Embryonic stem cells and induced pluripotent stem cells can also be differentiated into myotubes, but further work is needed to produce sufficient numbers of cells to generate contractile myofibers (Cheng et al. 2014). As in other tissues, cocultures that attempt to recapitulate the innervation and vascularization of the skeletal muscle significantly enhance functionality (Cheng et al. 2014).

17.4.2 Architectural Cues within the Skeletal Muscle

Connective tissue, consisting of mostly collagen, tethers adjacent myofibers together. Myofibers are the bulk of skeletal muscle tissue, and are dispersed in ECM which connects them to tendon junctions through three fibrous layers: The endomysium (around individual myofibers), the perimysium (around fascicles), and the epimysium (around the entire muscle) (Cittadella Vigodarzere and Mantero 2014). Therefore, scaffold-free muscle bundles, termed myooids, have been used in some cases to form models *in vitro* (Cheng et al. 2014). In these systems, fibroblasts synthesize the structurally supporting ECM. However, scaffolds are also commonly used including synthetic (polylactide-*co*-glycolide), natural (collagen, fibrin, hyaluronan-based hydrogel, Matrigel®), and acellular muscle ECM (Longo et al. 2012; Cittadella Vigodarzere and Mantero 2014).

17.4.3 Muscle-Specific Diabetic Cues

In skeletal muscle, type II diabetes predominately manifests as decreased insulin-mediated glucose uptake (Leclercq et al. 2007). Insulin resistance is thought to be caused by an increase in inflammatory cytokines (Steinberg et al. 2006) circulating lipids (Roden et al. 2000), accumulation of toxic lipid metabolites within the tissue (Skovbro et al. 2008), and oxidative stress which leads to the accumulation of reactive oxygen species (Urakawa et al. 2003; Yuzefovych et al. 2010). Therefore, inflammatory cytokines (Sell et al. 2006; Lambernd et al. 2012) and hyperlipidemia (Abildgaard et al. 2014) have been used to evaluate increases in lipid accumulation, inflammatory signaling, and insulin-mediated glucose uptake *in vitro*. Additionally, bi-directional crosstalk between skeletal muscle and adipose tissue is implicated in the cascade of events leading to impaired responsiveness to insulin, preconditioning patients to type II diabetes (Trayhurn et al. 2011; Bakke et al. 2012). Therefore, conditioned media and coculture with adipose tissue have been used to create insulin resistance, decreased glucose uptake, and increased inflammatory signaling, oxygen species, and nitric oxide release in skeletal muscle cultures (Dietze et al. 2002; Dietze-Schroeder et al. 2005; Sell et al. 2008; Lambernd et al. 2012). Finally, since most of the body's glucose uptake occurs in skeletal muscle, myotubes have been used as an *in vitro* model to test the effect of different diabetic treatments on insulin-stimulated glucose uptake. Treatments for improving responsiveness to insulin in this system have ranged from chromium and zinc (C2C12 mouse cells [Miranda and Dey 2004]) to cinnamic acid (L6 rat cells [Lakshmi et al. 2009]).

17.5 ADIPOSE

Adipose tissue is an endocrine organ that secretes cytokines that regulate appetite, insulin sensitivity, angiogenesis, blood pressure, and immune responses (Maury and Brichard 2010). In addition, adipose tissue releases fatty acids into the circulation, which is oxidized by peripheral tissues (mainly the skeletal muscle). Similar to skeletal muscle, insulin stimulation causes GLUT4 translocation to the plasma membrane resulting in glucose uptake. In diabetic states, glucose uptake is altered within the adipose tissue as well. Therefore, to recreate baseline adipose tissue functionality, before creating a diabetic model, viable cells need to uptake glucose in response to insulin.

17.5.1 Recapitulating Proper Cell Signaling within the Adipose Tissue

Adipose tissue is primarily composed of tightly packed, spherical adipocytes that have a unilocular morphology—a single large lipid droplet that fills almost the entire cellular volume—(Wronska and Kmiec 2012) (Figure 17.5). Adipocytes vary in size depending on their lipid content, with large cells having a higher metabolic activity (Wronska and Kmiec 2012). In addition to adipocytes, adipose tissue is highly vascularized and is innervated predominantly by the sympathetic nervous system (Wronska and Kmiec 2012). The stromal vascular fraction contains the other resident

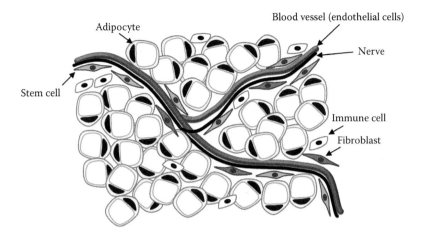

FIGURE 17.5 Schematic structure of adipose tissue. Adipose tissue is primarily composed of tightly packed, spherical adipocytes that have a unilocular morphology (a single large lipid droplet that fills almost the entire cellular volume). The stromal vascular fraction contains the other resident cell types of adipose tissue, including: stem cells, endothelial cells, fibroblasts, vascular smooth muscle cells, neurons and immune cells.

cell types of adipose tissue, including stem cells, endothelial cells, fibroblasts, vascular smooth muscle cells, and immune cells (Wronska and Kmiec 2012).

In vitro cell and tissue models use a variety of approaches to culture adipocyte-like cells. Animal cell lines (mainly murine 3T3-L1 and 3T3-F442A) have been extensively used in cultures, and they undergo adipogenesis; however, they lack the characteristic unilocular morphology of adipocytes (Serlachius and Andersson 2004). Cell suspension cultures have also been used, and they involve floating adipocytes in a culture medium. However, this technique is only a short-term solution, as the floating cells are not exposed to adequate nutrition and lyse within a week of culture (Zhang et al. 2000). Another technique, referred to as "ceiling cultures" also takes advantage of the adipocyte buoyancy, and it involves filling a culture flask completely with the medium to allow the cells to attach to the ceiling of the flask. Although the attached cells proliferate and exhibit some functional characteristics, they have a fibroblast-like morphology and lack the characteristic unilocular lipid droplet (Sugihara et al. 1986, 1987). The most common method of generating adipose tissue involves differentiating human adipose-derived stem cells in 2D or 3D systems. This method requires lengthy culture times (>3 weeks) to differentiate the stem cells into adipocytes, and in the absence of perfusion, do not contain the unilocular lipid droplet (Gerlach et al. 2012). To enhance physiological relevance, endothelial cells have been incorporated with differentiated stem cells (Kang et al. 2009; Choi, Gimble, Vunjak-Novakovic et al. 2010; Bellas et al. 2013; Haug et al. 2015), demonstrating improved adipogenic outcomes. In addition, endothelial cells have a key role in the control of the inflammatory process associated with type II diabetes (Sengenes et al. 2007).

17.5.2 ARCHITECTURAL CUES WITHIN THE ADIPOSE TISSUE

Adipocytes, themselves, are key stromal components of adipose tissue. They are surrounded by ECM comprised of collagen (I, III, IV), proteoglycans and elastin (Wronska and Kmiec 2012). Like other cells, adipocytes behave differently in 2D versus 3D environments (Cukierman et al. 2002). In particular, 3D culture systems improve differentiation potential (Stacey et al. 2009; Girandon et al. 2011) and increase secretion (Stacey et al. 2009) and production (Grayson et al. 2004) of adipogenic proteins and gene expression patterns (Chun et al. 2006). Therefore, adipocytes have been cultured in a multitude of different scaffolds, including synthetic scaffolds (polylactide, polyglycolide), natural scaffolds (collagen, fibrin, gelatin, hyaluronan-based hydrogel, Matrigel®, silk), and adipose derived ECM (Choi, Gimble, Lee et al. 2010).

17.5.3 ADIPOSE-SPECIFIC DIABETIC CUES

Similar to skeletal muscle, in the adipose tissue, type II diabetes predominately manifests as decreased insulin-mediated uptake of glucose (Leclercq et al. 2007). In addition, the tissue also releases fatty acids, reactive oxygen species, tumor necrosis factor alpha (TNFα), and other adipo-cytokines, which impair insulin action in the skeletal muscle and liver (Leclercq et al. 2007). Therefore, both inflammation (Hsu et al. 2010; Wentworth et al. 2010; Keuper et al. 2011; Kotnik et al. 2013; Zagotta et al. 2015) and hyperlipidemia (Schaeffler et al. 2009) have been studied for their effect on the adipose tissue and secreted factors.

17.6 CONCLUSION AND PERSPECTIVE

The complex etiology of type I and II diabetes requires complex tissue models of disease mechanisms to predict therapeutic and preventative actions. In the future, combining the current models in coculture systems will provide a more systemic view of the bidirectional crosstalk that occurs between tissues. "Organ on a chip" models allow complex cellular interactions to be explored between tissues, with very low tissue mass. As an example, a three-way-connected culture of hepatocytes, adipose tissue, and endothelial cells has been created to evaluate hyperglycemic effects (Iori et al. 2012). Additionally, more tissue models investigating the distinct responses of different tissues to the same stimuli (Han et al. 2006; Nowis et al. 2014) will inform specific roles of individual tissues in the cascade of events that leads to type I and type II diabetes. This will be required for understanding which molecular mechanisms are responsible for the many diabetes-associated subphenotypes, such as the nonobese with increased liver fat or the obese with low plasma adiponectin (Stumvoll 2004). For these types of studies, nondestructive modes of analyses will be required to follow the same tissue model throughout culture, such as using endogenous contrasts to assess metabolism (Georgakoudi and Quinn 2012). Ultimately, all human models will be required to better predict human disease processes and treatments.

ACKNOWLEDGMENTS

The authors would like to thank the National Institutes of Health (NIH) Tissue Engineering Resource Center (P41 EB002520) for supporting our tissue engineering studies.

REFERENCES

Abildgaard, J., D. C. Henstridge, A. T. Pedersen, K. G. Langley, C. Scheele, B. K. Pedersen, and B. Lindegaard. 2014. In vitro palmitate treatment of myotubes from postmenopausal women leads to ceramide accumulation, inflammation and affected insulin signaling. *PLoS One* no. 9 (7):e101555.

Ahren, B. 2000. Autonomic regulation of islet hormone secretion—implications for health and disease. *Diabetologia* no. 43 (4):393–410.

Amer, L. D., M. J. Mahoney, and S. J. Bryant. 2014. Tissue engineering approaches to cell-based type 1 diabetes therapy. *Tissue Eng Part B: Rev* no. 20 (5):455–67.

Appels, B., V. Burkart, G. Kantwerk-Funke, J. Funda, V. Kolb-Bachofen, and H. Kolb. 1989. Spontaneous cytotoxicity of macrophages against pancreatic islet cells. *J Immunol* no. 142 (11):3803–08.

Bakke, S. S., C. Moro, N. Nikolic, N. P. Hessvik, P. M. Badin, L. Lauvhaug, K. Fredriksson et al. 2012. Palmitic acid follows a different metabolic pathway than oleic acid in human skeletal muscle cells; lower lipolysis rate despite an increased level of adipose triglyceride lipase. *Biochim Biophys Acta* no. 1821 (10):1323–33.

Bellas, E., K. G. Marra, and D. L. Kaplan. 2013. Sustainable three-dimensional tissue model of human adipose tissue. *Tissue Eng Part C: Methods* no. 19 (10):745–54.

Bensellam, M., L. Van Lommel, L. Overbergh, F. C. Schuit, and J. C. Jonas. 2009. Cluster analysis of rat pancreatic islet gene mRNA levels after culture in low-, intermediate- and high-glucose concentrations. *Diabetologia* no. 52 (3):463–76.

Bissell, D. M., G. A. Levine, and M. J. Bissell. 1978. Glucose metabolism by adult hepatocytes in primary culture and by cell lines from rat liver. *Am J Physiol* no. 234 (3):C122–30.

Blauer, M., I. Nordback, J. Sand, and J. Laukkarinen. 2011. A novel explant outgrowth culture model for mouse pancreatic acinar cells with long-term maintenance of secretory phenotype. *Eur J Cell Biol* no. 90 (12):1052–60.

Brandon, E. F., C. D. Raap, I. Meijerman, J. H. Beijnen, and J. H. Schellens. 2003. An update on in vitro test methods in human hepatic drug biotransformation research: Pros and cons. *Toxicol Appl Pharmacol* no. 189 (3):233–46.

Brunicardi, F. C., J. Stagner, S. Bonner-Weir, H. Wayland, R. Kleinman, E. Livingston, P. Guth et al. 1996. Microcirculation of the islets of Langerhans. Long Beach Veterans Administration Regional Medical Education Center Symposium. *Diabetes* no. 45 (4):385–92.

Buchanan, T. A. 2003. Pancreatic beta-cell loss and preservation in type 2 diabetes. *Clin Ther* no. 25 (Suppl. B):B32–B46.

Burkart, V., Y. Imai, B. Kallmann, and H. Kolb. 1992. Cyclosporin A protects pancreatic islet cells from nitric oxide-dependent macrophage cytotoxicity. *FEBS Lett* no. 313 (1):56–58.

Butler, A. E., J. Janson, S. Bonner-Weir, R. Ritzel, R. A. Rizza, and P. C. Butler. 2003. Beta-cell deficit and increased beta-cell apoptosis in humans with type 2 diabetes. *Diabetes* no. 52 (1):102–10.

Carroll, P. B. 1992. Anatomy and physiology of islets of Langerhans. In *Pancreatic Islet Cell Transplantation*, 7–18, edited by C. Ricordi, and R. G. Landes. Austin, TX: R. G. Landes Co.

Castano, L. and G. S. Eisenbarth. 1990. Type-I diabetes: A chronic autoimmune disease of human, mouse, and rat. *Annu Rev Immunol* no. 8:647–79.

Cerasi, E. 1995. Insulin deficiency and insulin resistance in the pathogenesis of NIDDM: Is a divorce possible? *Diabetologia* no. 38 (8):992–97.

Cheng, C. S., B. N. Davis, L. Madden, N. Bursac, and G. A. Truskey. 2014. Physiology and metabolism of tissue-engineered skeletal muscle. *Exp Biol Med (Maywood)* no. 239 (9):1203–14.

Choi, J. H., J. M. Gimble, K. Lee, K. G. Marra, J. P. Rubin, J. J. Yoo, G. Vunjak-Novakovic, and D. L. Kaplan. 2010. Adipose tissue engineering for soft tissue regeneration. *Tissue Eng Part B: Rev* no. 16 (4):413–26.

Choi, J. H., J. M. Gimble, G. Vunjak-Novakovic, and D. L. Kaplan. 2010. Effects of hyperinsulinemia on lipolytic function of three-dimensional adipocyte/endothelial co-cultures. *Tissue Eng Part C: Methods* no. 16 (5):1157–65.

Chun, T. H., K. B. Hotary, F. Sabeh, A. R. Saltiel, E. D. Allen, and S. J. Weiss. 2006. A pericellular collagenase directs the 3-dimensional development of white adipose tissue. *Cell* no. 125 (3):577–91.

Cittadella Vigodarzere, G. and S. Mantero. 2014. Skeletal muscle tissue engineering: Strategies for volumetric constructs. *Front Physiol* no. 5:362, doi: 10.3389/fphys.2014.00362.

Cortijo, C., M. Gouzi, F. Tissir, and A. Grapin-Botton. 2012. Planar cell polarity controls pancreatic beta cell differentiation and glucose homeostasis. *Cell Rep* no. 2 (6):1593–606.

Cukierman, E., R. Pankov, and K. M. Yamada. 2002. Cell interactions with three-dimensional matrices. *Curr Opin Cell Biol* no. 14 (5):633–39.

Dash, A., W. Inman, K. Hoffmaster, S. Sevidal, J. Kelly, R. S. Obach, L. G. Griffith, and S. R. Tannenbaum. 2009. Liver tissue engineering in the evaluation of drug safety. *Expert Opin Drug Metab Toxicol* no. 5 (10):1159–74.

Davidson, M. D. M. Lehrer, and S. R. Khetani. 2015. Hormone and drug-mediated modulation of glucose metabolism in a microscale model of the human liver. *Tissue Eng Part C: Methods* no. 21 (7):716–25.

Dennis, R. G. and P. E. Kosnik 2nd. 2000. Excitability and isometric contractile properties of mammalian skeletal muscle constructs engineered *in vitro*. *In vitro Cell Dev Biol Anim* no. 36 (5):327–35.

Dietze, D., M. Koenen, K. Rohrig, H. Horikoshi, H. Hauner, and J. Eckel. 2002. Impairment of insulin signaling in human skeletal muscle cells by co-culture with human adipocytes. *Diabetes* no. 51 (8):2369–76.

Dietze-Schroeder, D., H. Sell, M. Uhlig, M. Koenen, and J. Eckel. 2005. Autocrine action of adiponectin on human fat cells prevents the release of insulin resistance-inducing factors. *Diabetes* no. 54 (7):2003–11.

Efanova, I. B., S. V. Zaitsev, B. Zhivotovsky, M. Kohler, S. Efendic, S. Orrenius, and P. O. Berggren. 1998. Glucose and tolbutamide induce apoptosis in pancreatic beta-cells. A process dependent on intracellular Ca^{2+} concentration. *J Biol Chem* no. 273 (50):33501–07.

Elouil, H., M. Bensellam, Y. Guiot, D. Vander Mierde, S. M. Pascal, F. C. Schuit, and J. C. Jonas. 2007. Acute nutrient regulation of the unfolded protein response and integrated stress response in cultured rat pancreatic islets. *Diabetologia* no. 50 (7):1442–52.

Ferrannini, E., D. C. Simonson, L. D. Katz, G. Reichard Jr., S. Bevilacqua, E. J. Barrett, M. Olsson, and R. A. DeFronzo. 1988. The disposal of an oral glucose load in patients with non-insulin-dependent diabetes. *Metabolism* no. 37 (1):79–85.

Furuyama, K., Y. Kawaguchi, H. Akiyama, M. Horiguchi, S. Kodama, T. Kuhara, S. Hosokawa et al. 2011. Continuous cell supply from a Sox9-expressing progenitor zone in adult liver, exocrine pancreas and intestine. *Nat Genet* no. 43 (1):34–41.

Georgakoudi, I. and K. P. Quinn. 2012. Optical imaging using endogenous contrast to assess metabolic state. *Annu Rev Biomed Eng* no. 14:351–67.

Gerlach, J. C., Y. C. Lin, C. A. Brayfield, D. M. Minteer, H. Li, J. P. Rubin, and K. G. Marra. 2012. Adipogenesis of human adipose-derived stem cells within three-dimensional hollow fiber-based bioreactors. *Tissue Eng Part C: Methods* no. 18 (1):54–61.

Girandon, L., N. Kregar-Velikonja, K. Bozikov, and A. Barlic. 2011. *In vitro* models for adipose tissue engineering with adipose-derived stem cells using different scaffolds of natural origin. *Folia Biol (Praha)* no. 57 (2):47–56.

Grayson, W. L., T. Ma, and B. Bunnell. 2004. Human mesenchymal stem cells tissue development in 3D PET matrices. *Biotechnol Prog* no. 20 (3):905–12.

Greggio, C., F. De Franceschi, M. Figueiredo-Larsen, S. Gobaa, A. Ranga, H. Semb, M. Lutolf, and A. Grapin-Botton. 2013. Artificial three-dimensional niches deconstruct pancreas development *in vitro*. *Development* no. 140 (21):4452–62.

Greggio, C., F. De Franceschi, and A. Grapin-Botton. 2015. Concise reviews: *In vitro*-produced pancreas organogenesis models in three dimensions: Self-organization from few stem cells or progenitors. *Stem Cells* no. 33 (1):8–14.

Grill, V. and A. Bjorklund. 2001. Overstimulation and beta-cell function. *Diabetes* no. 50 (Suppl. 1):S122–S124.

Guguen-Guillouzo, C., B. Clement, G. Baffet, C. Beaumont, E. Morel-Chany, D. Glaise, and A. Guillouzo. 1983. Maintenance and reversibility of active albumin secretion by adult rat hepatocytes co-cultured with another liver epithelial cell type. *Exp Cell Res* no. 143 (1):47–54.

Hammar, E. B., J. C. Irminger, K. Rickenbach, G. Parnaud, P. Ribaux, D. Bosco, D. G. Rouiller, and P. A. Halban. 2005. Activation of NF-kappaB by extracellular matrix is involved in spreading and glucose-stimulated insulin secretion of pancreatic beta cells. *J Biol Chem* no. 280 (34):30630–37.

Han, H. J., C. W. Kang, and S. H. Park. 2006. Tissue-specific regulation of insulin-like growth factors and insulin-like growth factor binding proteins in male diabetic rats *in vivo* and *in vitro*. *Clin Exp Pharmacol Physiol* no. 33 (12):1172–79.

Hansson, P. K., A. K. Asztely, J. C. Clapham, and S. A. Schreyer. 2004. Glucose and fatty acid metabolism in McA-RH7777 hepatoma cells vs. rat primary hepatocytes: Responsiveness to nutrient availability. *Biochim Biophys Acta* no. 1684 (1–3):54–62.

Harimoto, M., M. Yamato, M. Hirose, C. Takahashi, Y. Isoi, A. Kikuchi, and T. Okano. 2002. Novel approach for achieving double-layered cell sheets co-culture: Overlaying endothelial cell sheets onto monolayer hepatocytes utilizing temperature-responsive culture dishes. *J Biomed Mater Res* no. 62 (3):464–70.

Haug, V., N. Torio-Padron, G. B. Stark, G. Finkenzeller, and S. Strassburg. 2015. Comparison between endothelial progenitor cells and human umbilical vein endothelial cells on neovascularization in an adipogenesis mouse model. *Microvasc Res* no. 97:159–66.

Hoganson, D. M., H. I. Pryor 2nd, and J. P. Vacanti. 2008. Tissue engineering and organ structure: A vascularized approach to liver and lung. *Pediatr Res* no. 63 (5):520–26.

Hoorens, A., M. Van de Casteele, G. Kloppel, and D. Pipeleers. 1996. Glucose promotes survival of rat pancreatic beta cells by activating synthesis of proteins which suppress a constitutive apoptotic program. *J Clin Invest* no. 98 (7):1568–74.

Houbracken, I., E. de Waele, J. Lardon, Z. Ling, H. Heimberg, I. Rooman, and L. Bouwens. 2011. Lineage tracing evidence for transdifferentiation of acinar to duct cells and plasticity of human pancreas. *Gastroenterology* no. 141 (2):731–41, 741.e1–4.

Hsu, H. F., T. C. Tsou, H. R. Chao, Y. T. Kuo, F. Y. Tsai, and S. C. Yeh. 2010. Effects of 2,3,7,8-tetrachlorodibenzo-p-dioxin on adipogenic differentiation and insulin-induced glucose uptake in 3T3-L1 cells. *J Hazard Mater* no. 182 (1–3):649–55.

Iori, E., B. Vinci, E. Murphy, M. C. Marescotti, A. Avogaro, and A. Ahluwalia. 2012. Glucose and fatty acid metabolism in a 3 tissue *in-vitro* model challenged with normo- and hyperglycaemia. *PLoS One* no. 7 (4):e34704.

Jiang, F. X., D. S. Cram, H. J. DeAizpurua, and L. C. Harrison. 1999. Laminin-1 promotes differentiation of fetal mouse pancreatic beta-cells. *Diabetes* no. 48 (4):722–30.

Juliano, R. L. and S. Haskill. 1993. Signal transduction from the extracellular matrix. *J Cell Biol* no. 120 (3):577–85.

Kahn, B. B. and J. S. Flier. 2000. Obesity and insulin resistance. *J Clin Invest* no. 106 (4):473–81.

Kahn, S. E. 2000. The importance of the beta-cell in the pathogenesis of type 2 diabetes mellitus. *Am J Med* no. 108 (Suppl. 6a):2s–8s.

Kang, J. H., J. M. Gimble, and D. L. Kaplan. 2009. In vitro 3D model for human vascularized adipose tissue. *Tissue Eng Part A* no. 15 (8):2227–36.

Kesavan, G., F. W. Sand, T. U. Greiner, J. K. Johansson, S. Kobberup, X. Wu, C. Brakebusch, and H. Semb. 2009. Cdc42-mediated tubulogenesis controls cell specification. *Cell* no. 139 (4):791–801.

Keuper, M., M. Bluher, M. R. Schon, P. Moller, A. Dzyakanchuk, K. Amrein, K. M. Debatin, M. Wabitsch, and P. Fischer-Posovszky. 2011. An inflammatory micro-environment promotes human adipocyte apoptosis. *Mol Cell Endocrinol* no. 339 (1–2):105–13.

Khaldi, M. Z., Y. Guiot, P. Gilon, J. C. Henquin, and J. C. Jonas. 2004. Increased glucose sensitivity of both triggering and amplifying pathways of insulin secretion in rat islets cultured for 1 wk in high glucose. *Am J Physiol Endocrinol Metab* no. 287 (2):E207–E217.

Kmiec, Z. 2001. Cooperation of liver cells in health and disease. *Adv Anat Embryol Cell Biol* no. 161:Iii–xiii, 1–151.

Korbutt, G. S., A. G. Mallett, Z. Ao, M. Flashner, and R. V. Rajotte. 2004. Improved survival of microencapsulated islets during *in vitro* culture and enhanced metabolic function following transplantation. *Diabetologia* no. 47 (10):1810–18.

Kotnik, P., M. Keuper, M. Wabitsch, and P. Fischer-Posovszky. 2013. Interleukin-1beta downregulates RBP4 secretion in human adipocytes. *PLoS One* no. 8 (2):e57796.

Lakshmi, B. S., S. Sujatha, S. Anand, K. N. Sangeetha, R. B. Narayanan, C. Katiyar, A. Kanaujia et al. 2009. Cinnamic acid, from the bark of *Cinnamomum cassia*, regulates glucose transport via activation of GLUT4 on L6 myotubes in a phosphatidylinositol 3-kinase-independent manner. *J Diabetes* no. 1 (2):99–106.

Lambernd, S., A. Taube, A. Schober, B. Platzbecker, S. W. Gorgens, R. Schlich, K. Jeruschke, J. Weiss, K. Eckardt, and J. Eckel. 2012. Contractile activity of human skeletal muscle cells prevents insulin resistance by inhibiting pro-inflammatory signalling pathways. *Diabetologia* no. 55 (4):1128–39.

Leclercq, I. A., A. Da Silva Morais, B. Schroyen, N. Van Hul, and A. Geerts. 2007. Insulin resistance in hepatocytes and sinusoidal liver cells: Mechanisms and consequences. *J Hepatol* no. 47 (1):142–56.

LeCluyse, E. L., R. P. Witek, M. E. Andersen, and M. J. Powers. 2012. Organotypic liver culture models: Meeting current challenges in toxicity testing. *Crit Rev Toxicol* no. 42 (6):501–48.

Lee, K. T., T. W. Jung, H. J. Lee, S. G. Kim, Y. S. Shin, and W. K. Whang. 2011. The antidiabetic effect of ginsenoside Rb2 via activation of AMPK. *Arch Pharm Res* no. 34 (7):1201–08.

Leibiger, I. B., B. Leibiger, and P. O. Berggren. 2008. Insulin signaling in the pancreatic betacell. *Annu Rev Nutr* no. 28:233–51.

Leslie, R. D. and M. Delli Castelli. 2004. Age-dependent influences on the origins of autoimmune diabetes: Evidence and implications. *Diabetes* no. 53 (12):3033–40.

Ling, Z., R. Kiekens, T. Mahler, F. C. Schuit, M. Pipeleers-Marichal, A. Sener, G. Kloppel, W. J. Malaisse, and D. G. Pipeleers. 1996. Effects of chronically elevated glucose levels on the functional properties of rat pancreatic beta-cells. *Diabetes* no. 45 (12):1774–82.

Loghmani, E. 2005. Diabetes mellitis: Type 1 and type 2. In *Guidelines for Adolescent Nutrition Services*, 167–82, edited by J. Stang, and M. Story. Minneapolis: University of Minnesota.

Longo, U. G., M. Loppini, A. Berton, F. Spiezia, N. Maffulli, and V. Denaro. 2012. Tissue engineered strategies for skeletal muscle injury. *Stem Cells Int* no. 2012:175038.

Lu, Y., G. Zhang, C. Shen, K. Uygun, M. L. Yarmush, and Q. Meng. 2012. A novel 3D liver organoid system for elucidation of hepatic glucose metabolism. *Biotechnol Bioeng* no. 109 (2):595–604.

Maury, E. and S. M. Brichard. 2010. Adipokine dysregulation, adipose tissue inflammation and metabolic syndrome. *Mol Cell Endocrinol* no. 314 (1):1–16.

Miranda, E. R. and C. S. Dey. 2004. Effect of chromium and zinc on insulin signaling in skeletal muscle cells. *Biol Trace Elem Res* no. 101 (1):19–36.

Navarro-Alvarez, N., J. D. Rivas-Carrillo, A. Soto-Gutierrez, T. Yuasa, T. Okitsu, H. Noguchi, S. Matsumoto, J. Takei, N. Tanaka, and N. Kobayashi. 2008. Reestablishment of microenvironment is necessary to maintain *in vitro* and *in vivo* human islet function. *Cell Transplant* no. 17 (1–2):111–19.

Nowis, D., A. Malenda, K. Furs, B. Oleszczak, R. Sadowski, J. Chlebowska, M. Firczuk et al. 2014. Statins impair glucose uptake in human cells. *BMJ Open Diabetes Res Care* no. 2 (1):e000017.

Ohashi, K. and T. Okano. 2014. Functional tissue engineering of the liver and islets. *Anat Rec (Hoboken)* no. 297 (1):73–82.

Paraskevas, S., D. Maysinger, R. Wang, T. P. Duguid, and L. Rosenberg. 2000. Cell loss in isolated human islets occurs by apoptosis. *Pancreas* no. 20 (3):270–76.

Perel, P., I. Roberts, E. Sena, P. Wheble, C. Briscoe, P. Sandercock, M. Macleod, L. E. Mignini, P. Jayaram, and K. S. Khan. 2007. Comparison of treatment effects between animal experiments and clinical trials: Systematic review. *BMJ* no. 334 (7586):197.

Peyser, T., E. Dassau, M. Breton, and J. S. Skyler. 2014. The artificial pancreas: Current status and future prospects in the management of diabetes. *Ann N Y Acad Sci* no. 1311:102–23.

Poitout, V. and R. P. Robertson. 2002. Minireview: Secondary beta-cell failure in type 2 diabetes—a convergence of glucotoxicity and lipotoxicity. *Endocrinology* no. 143 (2):339–42.

Reed, M. J. and K. A. Scribner. 1999. *In-vivo* and *in-vitro* models of type 2 diabetes in pharmaceutical drug discovery. *Diabetes Obes Metab* no. 1 (2):75–86.

Reid, L. M., A. S. Fiorino, S. H. Sigal, S. Brill, and P. A. Holst. 1992. Extracellular matrix gradients in the space of Disse: Relevance to liver biology. *Hepatology* no. 15 (6):1198–203.

Ribaux, P., J. A. Ehses, N. Lin-Marq, F. Carrozzino, M. Boni-Schnetzler, E. Hammar, J. C. Irminger, M. Y. Donath, and P. A. Halban. 2007. Induction of CXCL1 by extracellular matrix and autocrine enhancement by interleukin-1 in rat pancreatic beta-cells. *Endocrinology* no. 148 (11):5582–90.

Roden, M., H. Stingl, V. Chandramouli, W. C. Schumann, A. Hofer, B. R. Landau, P. Nowotny, W. Waldhausl, and G. I. Shulman. 2000. Effects of free fatty acid elevation on postabsorptive endogenous glucose production and gluconeogenesis in humans. *Diabetes* no. 49 (5):701–07.

Salerno, S., C. Campana, S. Morelli, E. Drioli, and L. De Bartolo. 2011. Human hepatocytes and endothelial cells in organotypic membrane systems. *Biomaterials* no. 32 (34):8848–59.

Samuel, V. T., K. F. Petersen, and G. I. Shulman. 2010. Lipid-induced insulin resistance: Unravelling the mechanism. *Lancet* no. 375 (9733):2267–77.

Schaeffler, A., P. Gross, R. Buettner, C. Bollheimer, C. Buechler, M. Neumeier, A. Kopp, J. Schoelmerich, and W. Falk. 2009. Fatty acid-induced induction of Toll-like receptor-4/nuclear factor-kappaB pathway in adipocytes links nutritional signalling with innate immunity. *Immunology* no. 126 (2):233–45.

Sell, H., D. Dietze-Schroeder, U. Kaiser, and J. Eckel. 2006. Monocyte chemotactic protein-1 is a potential player in the negative cross-talk between adipose tissue and skeletal muscle. *Endocrinology* no. 147 (5):2458–67.

Sell, H., K. Eckardt, A. Taube, D. Tews, M. Gurgui, G. Van Echten-Deckert, and J. Eckel. 2008. Skeletal muscle insulin resistance induced by adipocyte-conditioned medium: Underlying mechanisms and reversibility. *Am J Physiol Endocrinol Metab* no. 294 (6):E1070–77.

Sell, H., J. Laurencikiene, A. Taube, K. Eckardt, A. Cramer, A. Horrighs, P. Arner, and J. Eckel. 2009. Chemerin is a novel adipocyte-derived factor inducing insulin resistance in primary human skeletal muscle cells. *Diabetes* no. 58 (12):2731–40.

Sengenes, C., A. Miranville, K. Lolmede, C. A. Curat, and A. Bouloumie. 2007. The role of endothelial cells in inflamed adipose tissue. *J Intern Med* no. 262 (4):415–21.

Serlachius, M. and L. C. Andersson. 2004. Upregulated expression of stanniocalcin-1 during adipogenesis. *Exp Cell Res* no. 296 (2):256–64.

Sherwin, R. S. 1980. Role of the liver in glucose homeostasis. *Diabetes Care* no. 3 (2):261–65.

Shimizu, H., K. Ohashi, R. Utoh, K. Ise, M. Gotoh, M. Yamato, and T. Okano. 2009. Bioengineering of a functional sheet of islet cells for the treatment of diabetes mellitus. *Biomaterials* no. 30 (30):5943–49.

Skovbro, M., M. Baranowski, C. Skov-Jensen, A. Flint, F. Dela, J. Gorski, and J. W. Helge. 2008. Human skeletal muscle ceramide content is not a major factor in muscle insulin sensitivity. *Diabetologia* no. 51 (7):1253–60.

Stacey, D. H., S. E. Hanson, G. Lahvis, K. A. Gutowski, and K. S. Masters. 2009. In vitro adipogenic differentiation of preadipocytes varies with differentiation stimulus, culture dimensionality, and scaffold composition. *Tissue Eng Part A* no. 15 (11):3389–99.

Steinberg, G. R., B. J. Michell, B. J. van Denderen, M. J. Watt, A. L. Carey, B. C. Fam, S. Andrikopoulos et al. 2006. Tumor necrosis factor alpha-induced skeletal muscle insulin resistance involves suppression of AMP-kinase signaling. *Cell Metab* no. 4 (6):465–74.

Stendahl, J. C., D. B. Kaufman, and S. I. Stupp. 2009. Extracellular matrix in pancreatic islets: Relevance to scaffold design and transplantation. *Cell Transplant* no. 18 (1):1–12.

Stumvoll, M. 2004. Control of glycaemia: From molecules to men. Minkowski Lecture 2003. *Diabetologia* no. 47 (5):770–81.

Sugihara, H., N. Yonemitsu, S. Miyabara, and S. Toda. 1987. Proliferation of unilocular fat cells in the primary culture. *J Lipid Res* no. 28 (9):1038–45.

Sugihara, H., N. Yonemitsu, S. Miyabara, and K. Yun. 1986. Primary cultures of unilocular fat cells: Characteristics of growth *in vitro* and changes in differentiation properties. *Differentiation* no. 31 (1):42–49.

Sugiyama, T., C. M. Benitez, A. Ghodasara, L. Liu, G. W. McLean, J. Lee, T. A. Blauwkamp et al. 2013. Reconstituting pancreas development from purified progenitor cells reveals genes essential for islet differentiation. *Proc Natl Acad Sci USA* no. 110 (31):12691–96.

Sugiyama, T., R. T. Rodriguez, G. W. McLean, and S. K. Kim. 2007. Conserved markers of fetal pancreatic epithelium permit prospective isolation of islet progenitor cells by FACS. *Proc Natl Acad Sci U S A* no. 104 (1):175–80.

Trayhurn, P., C. A. Drevon, and J. Eckel. 2011. Secreted proteins from adipose tissue and skeletal muscle—adipokines, myokines and adipose/muscle cross-talk. *Arch Physiol Biochem* no. 117 (2):47–56.

Tuschl, G., J. Hrach, Y. Walter, P. G. Hewitt, and S. O. Mueller. 2009. Serum-free collagen sandwich cultures of adult rat hepatocytes maintain liver-like properties long term: A valuable model for *in vitro* toxicity and drug-drug interaction studies. *Chem Biol Interact* no. 181 (1):124–37.

Urakawa, H., A. Katsuki, Y. Sumida, E. C. Gabazza, S. Murashima, K. Morioka, N. Maruyama et al. 2003. Oxidative stress is associated with adiposity and insulin resistance in men. *J Clin Endocrinol Metab* no. 88 (10):4673–76.

Van de Casteele, M., B. A. Kefas, Y. Cai, H. Heimberg, D. K. Scott, J. C. Henquin, D. Pipeleers, and J. C. Jonas. 2003. Prolonged culture in low glucose induces apoptosis of rat pancreatic beta-cells through induction of c-myc. *Biochem Biophys Res Commun* no. 312 (4):937–44.

Van Deijnen, J. H., P. T. Van Suylichem, G. H. Wolters, and R. Van Schilfgaarde. 1994. Distribution of collagens type I, type III and type V in the pancreas of rat, dog, pig and man. *Cell Tissue Res* no. 277 (1):115–21.

Waanders, L. F., K. Chwalek, M. Monetti, C. Kumar, E. Lammert, and M. Mann. 2009. Quantitative proteomic analysis of single pancreatic islets. *Proc Natl Acad Sci USA* no. 106 (45):18902–07.

Wang, X., L. Zhou, G. Li, T. Luo, Y. Gu, L. Qian, X. Fu, F. Li, J. Li, and M. Luo. 2007. Palmitate activates AMP-activated protein kinase and regulates insulin secretion from beta cells. *Biochem Biophys Res Commun* no. 352 (2):463–68.

Wen, Y. A., D. Liu, Y. Y. Xiao, D. Luo, Y. F. Dong, and L. P. Zhang. 2009. Enhanced glucose synthesis in three-dimensional hepatocyte collagen matrix. *Toxicol In Vitro* no. 23 (4):744–47.

Wentworth, J. M., G. Naselli, W. A. Brown, L. Doyle, B. Phipson, G. K. Smyth, M. Wabitsch, P. E. O'Brien, and L. C. Harrison. 2010. Pro-inflammatory CD11c+CD206+ adipose tissue macrophages are associated with insulin resistance in human obesity. *Diabetes* no. 59 (7):1648–56.

Williams, S., S. Roux, T. Koekemoer, M. van de Venter, and G. Dealtry. 2013. Sutherlandia frutescens prevents changes in diabetes-related gene expression in a fructose-induced insulin resistant cell model. *J Ethnopharmacol* no. 146 (2):482–89.

Wilson, S. S. and D. DeLuca. 1997. NOD fetal thymus organ culture: An *in vitro* model for the development of T cells involved in IDDM. *J Autoimmun* no. 10 (5):461–72.

Wronska, A. and Z. Kmiec. 2012. Structural and biochemical characteristics of various white adipose tissue depots. *Acta Physiol (Oxf)* no. 205 (2):194–208.

Wu, F. J., J. R. Friend, R. P. Remmel, F. B. Cerra, and W. S. Hu. 1999. Enhanced cytochrome P450 IA1 activity of self-assembled rat hepatocyte spheroids. *Cell Transplant* no. 8 (3):233–46.

Yamada, M., R. Utoh, K. Ohashi, K. Tatsumi, M. Yamato, T. Okano, and M. Seki. 2012. Controlled formation of heterotypic hepatic micro-organoids in anisotropic hydrogel microfibers for long-term preservation of liver-specific functions. *Biomaterials* no. 33 (33):8304–15.

Yan, W., S. George, U. Fotadar, N. Tyhovych, A. Kamer, M. J. Yost, R. L. Price, C. R. Haggart, J. W. Holmes, and L. Terracio. 2007. Tissue engineering of skeletal muscle. *Tissue Eng* no. 13 (11):2781–90.

Yuzefovych, L., G. Wilson, and L. Rachek. 2010. Different effects of oleate vs. palmitate on mitochondrial function, apoptosis, and insulin signaling in L6 skeletal muscle cells: Role of oxidative stress. *Am J Physiol Endocrinol Metab* no. 299 (6):E1096–105.

Zagotta, I., E. Y. Dimova, K. M. Debatin, M. Wabitsch, T. Kietzmann, and P. Fischer-Posovszky. 2015. Obesity and inflammation: Reduced cytokine expression due to resveratrol in a human *in vitro* model of inflamed adipose tissue. *Front Pharmacol* no. 6:79.

Zhang, D., W. Jiang, M. Liu, X. Sui, X. Yin, S. Chen, Y. Shi, and H. Deng. 2009. Highly efficient differentiation of human ES cells and iPS cells into mature pancreatic insulin-producing cells. *Cell Res* no. 19 (4):429–38.

Zhang, H. H., S. Kumar, A. H. Barnett, and M. C. Eggo. 2000. Ceiling culture of mature human adipocytes: Use in studies of adipocyte functions. *J Endocrinol* no. 164 (2):119–28.

18 Optimizing 3D Models of Engineered Skeletal Muscle

Megan E. Kondash, Brittany N. J. Davis, and George A. Truskey

CONTENTS

18.1 Introduction 322
18.2 Cell Source 322
    18.2.1 Cell Lines.. 322
    18.2.2 Primary Cells.. 324
        18.2.2.1 Primary Satellite Cells and Myoblasts............................... 324
        18.2.2.2 Impact of Fibroblasts on Myogenic Cells in Engineered Muscle.. 326
        18.2.2.3 iPSC-Derived Myoblasts.. 326
    18.2.3 Species of Cell Donor 327
18.3 Scaffolding and Extracellular Matrix... 328
    18.3.1 Decellularized Scaffolds.. 330
    18.3.2 Hydrogel Scaffolds 330
        18.3.2.1 Natural Biopolymer Hydrogels 331
        18.3.2.2 Synthetic Hydrogels 333
18.4 Promoting Maturation and Function 333
    18.4.1 Force Production.. 334
        18.4.1.1 Optimizing Formulation Parameters 335
        18.4.1.2 Effect of Convection in Culture Media on Skeletal Muscle Maturation 335
        18.4.1.3 Mechanical Stimulation 336
        18.4.1.4 Electrical Stimulation 336
    18.4.2 Expanding the Relevance of the Engineered Muscle Model............ 337
        18.4.2.1 Innervation.. 337
        18.4.2.2 Vascularization 337
        18.4.2.3 Metabolism 338
18.5 Conclusion and Perspective 341
References.. 341

18.1 INTRODUCTION

Engineered skeletal muscle tissue can be designed and optimized for the replacement of damaged or diseased skeletal muscle tissue, or serve as an *in vitro* model of both healthy and disease state skeletal muscle. Such *in vitro* models can be used to screen drug responses and address basic science questions that are difficult to address *in vivo*. Although the endpoints of these two applications are distinct, the design parameters overlap, as both objectives benefit from an engineered tissue that most closely mimics the physiological conditions and functions of skeletal muscle *in vivo*.

In the realm of producing a functional regenerative tool, engineered skeletal muscle must incorporate into the existing muscle upon implantation, promote vascularization, produce significant contractile forces, respond to mechanical and electrical stimuli, and exhibit a physiological metabolic profile. Muscle loss due to traumatic injuries, sarcopenia, congenital defects, or diseases such as muscular dystrophy, a progressive degenerative genetic disease resulting in irretrievable loss of muscle mass, motivates the fabrication of such engineered muscle to replace the lost or damaged tissue. *In vitro*, engineered muscle bundles can be used to examine the safety and efficacy of pharmaceuticals or allow for in-depth and noninvasive investigation into the basic function of skeletal muscle in a 3-dimensional (3D) environment. The drug discovery and testing process for treatment of skeletal muscle-associated diseases including sarcopenia, the age-related loss of muscle mass, type 2 diabetes, and neurodegenerative muscular diseases, could benefit from an *in vitro* human tissue model (Truskey et al. 2013). For such applications, engineered muscle must mimic its *in vivo* counterpart both phenotypically and functionally. This chapter discusses relevant biological considerations for the creation of engineered muscle, including cell source, scaffold, or extracellular matrix (ECM) composition, and identifying and improving markers of *in vitro* muscle function such as force production and metabolism.

18.2 CELL SOURCE

Skeletal muscle tissue *in vivo* is composed of multinucleated, striated muscle fibers, or myofibers, which are in turn composed of organized contractile protein structures known as myofibrils. Satellite cells, located on the periphery of skeletal muscle fibers, are self-renewing Pax7 positive stem cells capable of asymmetric division, allowing them to produce myoblasts while simultaneously repopulating the satellite cell niche (Brack and Rando 2012). During the muscle repair process *in vivo*, myoblasts, the proliferative but fate-committed progeny of satellite cells (Campion 1984), fuse with damaged myofibers. Several sources of myogenic cells are used to produce engineered skeletal muscle, including rodent cell lines, rodent and human primary cells, and induced pluripotent stem cells (iPSCs) (Figure 18.1). These cell sources vary in their ability to accurately recapitulate the function of native human muscle tissue.

18.2.1 Cell Lines

Cell lines that have been immortalized offer a nearly limitless cell source, and produce experimental results that are not affected by donor variability or cell

Optimizing 3D Models of Engineered Skeletal Muscle

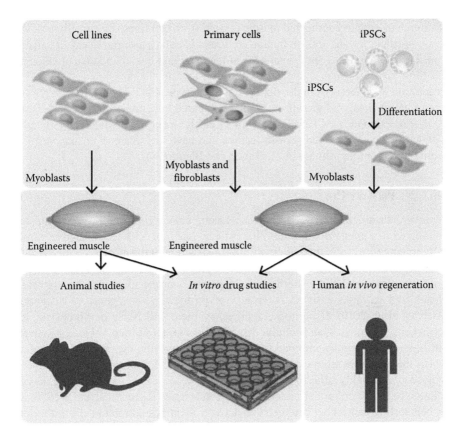

FIGURE 18.1 Engineered muscle can be fabricated from either cells lines, unsorted primary cells, or differentiated iPSCs. This engineered muscle can then be used for animal studies, *in vitro* drug studies, or human *in vivo* muscle regeneration.

senescence. Although cell lines offer a stable, well-characterized, readily available source of cells, they often behave differently than primary cells, impacting the function of the engineered skeletal muscle. Two cell lines commonly used to form engineered skeletal muscle are the C2C12 mouse myoblast line (Dennis et al. 2001) and the L6 rat myoblast cell line (Chen et al. 2015). 3D skeletal muscle constructs made without a hydrogel or polymer, called myoids, and derived from C2C12 cells, demonstrate significantly different force production kinetics than myoids constructed with primary cells from adult mouse muscle (Dennis et al. 2001). Myoids made from the mouse cell line are less excitable and exhibit approximately four times lower specific force production than myoids made from primary adult cells, and they had a half-relaxation time an order of magnitude higher than that seen in myoids made using primary adult cells (Dennis et al. 2001). Engineered skeletal muscle formed using C2C12 cells do not exhibit the tetanus force traces seen in normally functioning skeletal muscle as a response to increased frequency of electrical stimulation, and peak force does not increase with increased frequency of stimulation (Rhim et al. 2010). These differences in force kinetics suggest dysfunction in calcium handling in engineered muscle formed from cell lines, specifically a slower decay of calcium transients. In human cultured myotubes, a slower decay of calcium transients is associated with functional immaturity and low abundance of calcium-handling proteins when compared with adult muscle fibers (Olsson et al. 2015). In addition to differences in developmental phenotype, C2C12 cells differ in regulation of metabolism and growth rate when compared to primary cells (Dennis et al. 2001). For example, C2C12 cells grow more easily in culture than do primary cells, without the need for added growth factors, and have the potential for uncontrolled proliferation, unlike primary cells (Rando and Blau 1994).

18.2.2 Primary Cells

Primary cells are obtained directly from skeletal muscle tissue of the donor, and are not altered in a manner that immortalizes them. Satellite cells are isolated by physically freeing them from their niche within the structure of the muscle via mechanical and enzymatic disruption of the surrounding ECM and muscle fibers (Danoviz and Yablonka-Reuveni 2012). Alternatively, explanted muscle tissue can be dissected, plated, and cultured until an outgrowth of proliferative myogenic cells appears (Merrick et al. 2010). Using these approaches, there will likely be fibroblasts, red blood cells, adipocytes, and cellular debris present (Danoviz and Yablonka-Reuveni 2012). Isolations can be enriched for satellite cells by using the preplate method, in which the cell suspension or explanted tissue is plated for a brief period of time to remove more quickly adhering cell types such as fibroblasts before removing the cell solution to be plated on the intended culture substrate (Richler and Yaffe 1970), or by cell sorting using flow cytometry to actively identify and retain cells with satellite cell-like morphologies (Yablonka-Reuveni 1988; Baroffio et al. 1993) or specific combinations of cell markers (Pasut et al. 2012; Liu et al. 2015).

The isolated cells can either be used immediately to form engineered skeletal muscle or cultured and expanded in monolayer culture before being used for the engineered skeletal muscle. However, during *in vitro* culture satellite cells do not remain quiescent, instead entering into the cell cycle as proliferative muscle precursors (Montarras et al. 2005). Expansion of primary cells is limited, because as the cells reach their limit of population doublings, they become senescent and do not differentiate as efficiently. For example, primary cells obtained from two human skeletal muscle biopsies began losing their capacity for differentiation after seven population doublings (Owens et al. 2013). Despite their relatively short lifetime in culture, primary cells are preferred over genetically abnormal immortalized cell lines because they better retain a physiological phenotype, offering a more suitable model of *in vivo* function.

18.2.2.1 Primary Satellite Cells and Myoblasts

In native muscle tissue, satellite cells are the primary cell type responsible for muscle regeneration. They are normally quiescent and are identifiable both by their positioning close to myofibers, in a niche between the basal lamina and sarcolemma of the fiber, and expression of Pax7. Activation of satellite cells can be caused by injury, mechanical stretch, or secreted growth factors, and is marked by initiation of proliferation and the coexpression of Pax7 and MyoD (Le Grand and Rudnicki 2007). Once the cells have been activated to a proliferative state they can either commit to a differentiated fate, downregulating Pax7 and upregulating myogenin (MyoG) expression until they undergo fusion to form MyoG$^+$ myotubes expressing differentiation markers such as myosin heavy chain, incorporate into an existing myotube, or continue to self-renew, eventually downregulating MyoD expression and repopulating the stem cell niche as Pax7$^+$ cells (Edom et al. 1994; Le Grand and Rudnicki 2007; Fishman et al. 2013).

Despite the tendency of satellite cells to differentiate in culture, engineered 3D skeletal muscle bundles fabricated using primary rat satellite cells that were adherently cultured *in vitro* for 36 h after isolation retained a higher density of satellite cells in the mature engineered muscle than did engineered muscle fabricated using freshly isolated satellite cells (Juhas and Bursac 2014). Similarly as a result of the adherent culture period, once in the engineered muscle, MyoD$^+$ and MyoG$^+$ cells that had been adherently cultured, a population that includes recently fused myoblasts or myoblasts on the verge of fusion, differentiated more quickly to a mature MyoG$^+$ myofiber phenotype than their freshly isolated counterparts. These myofibers formed stem cell niches in which the remaining Pax7$^+$ satellite cell population was retained (Figure 18.2), reminiscent of similar niches found in muscle *in vivo*. In addition, the capacity of the adherently cultured cells for more rapid differentiation resulted in higher contractile force production due to increased robustness of

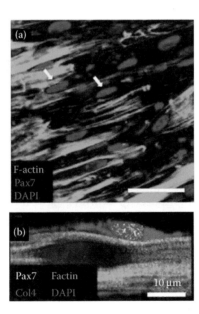

FIGURE 18.2 (a) The presence of Pax7$^+$ cells in engineered muscle formed from human primary cells is indicated by the white arrows. (Reprinted from Madden, L. et al. 2015. *eLife* no. 4:e04885.) (b) In engineered muscle formed from primary rat cells, immunostaining shows a Pax7$^+$ cell adjacent to the myofiber sarcolemma. (Reprinted from Juhas, M. et al. 2014. *Proc Natl Acad Sci USA* no. 111 (15):5508–13. With permission.)

contractile elements (Juhas and Bursac 2014). Together, these results indicate that the use of adherently cultured cells may be preferable to freshly isolated satellite cells in engineered muscle.

18.2.2.2 Impact of Fibroblasts on Myogenic Cells in Engineered Muscle

During isolation of primary myogenic cells, fibroblasts are present in the isolated cell population. The number of fibroblasts is reduced by a brief preplating process, which takes advantage of the more rapid adhesion of fibroblasts than myoblasts to uncoated surfaces, and serves to decrease the final amount of fibroblasts present in the isolation (Richler and Yaffe 1970). However, a cell population that is composed of myogenic cells with some fibroblasts is desirable for the formation of engineered skeletal muscle. Attempts to form myooids using only C2C12 cells failed, as the cells never delaminated from the culture surface, instead forming a monolayer of differentiated and undifferentiated cells. Only once the C2C12 cells were cultured with a fibroblast cell line did myooids form, likely aided by the ECM produced by the fibroblasts (Dennis et al. 2001).

In addition, fibroblasts are necessary for the formation of a continuous basal lamina structure around differentiating myotubes. Fibroblasts deposit type IV collagen and laminin, two of the main components of the basal lamina structure (Kuhl et al. 1984). *In vivo*, the basal lamina is important for its role in muscle structure and strength and as a crucial component of myogenesis and signaling (Sanes 2003). In fibrin-based engineered skeletal muscle, fibroblasts contribute to the formation of a fibroblast-rich exterior, which resembles the connective tissue layer that surrounds muscles in native tissue (Juhas et al. 2014). Fibroblasts also play an important role in fibrin degradation and gel compaction over time (De Jesus and Sander 2014), contributing to the passive forces present within the bundle structure.

18.2.2.3 iPSC-Derived Myoblasts

Fibroblasts and other terminally differentiated cells that have been induced to dedifferentiate to a pluripotent state (iPSCs) offer a promising source of cells for engineered skeletal muscle. iPSCs can be expanded to achieve high cell numbers and can then be differentiated to a myogenic lineage following overexpression of MYOD. In monolayer culture, these myogenic cells are able to fuse into multinucleated, myosin heavy chain (MHC) positive myotubes capable of visible contractions in response to an electrical stimulus (Tanaka et al. 2013). The appeal of iPSCs is the possibility of patient-specific cells obtained with a minimally invasive procedure such as a skin biopsy (Takahashi et al. 2007), or peripheral blood draw (Staerk et al. 2010). For engineered skeletal muscle that is to be implanted, using the patient's own cells to produce the muscle tissue bypasses most of the adverse immune responses that transplants induce. Induced pluripotent cells can be generated from patients with varied genetic backgrounds, establishing the response to both normal and disease genetic variants. For example, iPSCs have been generated from fibroblasts of patients with Duchenne's muscular dystrophy, and the differentiated myogenic cells retain the muscular dystrophy phenotype, which is responsive to treatment *in vitro* (Abujarour et al. 2014). Although one advantage of iPSCs is their ability to differentiate into multiple lineages, it also represents a risk for implanted tissues using these cells. If cells are not sorted properly, and undifferentiated iPSCs are inadvertently delivered *in vivo*, they have the potential to proliferate and form teratomas (Herberts et al. 2011).

Dedifferentiation of primary cells to produce iPSCs involves the simultaneous induced expression of several transcription factors, such as Oct4, c-Myc, Sox2, and Klf4, which alter gene expression such that the cells gain pluripotency potential similar to that of embryonic stem cells (Takahashi et al. 2007). However, this process tends to result in excess mutations and epigenetic instability in iPSC populations, independent of the technique used to produce the iPSCs and originating from both the reprogramming process and subsequent selection and expansion of the reprogrammed cells (Gore et al. 2011; Lister et al. 2011). This genomic instability in turn contributes to tumorigenesis potential (Mayshar et al. 2010). The risks associated with iPSCs may be mitigated by using small molecules (Hou et al. 2013) or nonintegrating methods (Schlaeger et al. 2015) to induce dedifferentiation.

iPSC-derived myogenic cells show promising regenerative potential in animal studies (Filareto et al. 2013), but for the purposes of engineered muscle, the challenge remains to produce an iPSC-derived cell population functionally equivalent to isolated primary cells *in vitro*. The process of deriving myogenic cells from iPSCs requires directed differentiation involving cell sorting for enrichment, induced expression of exogenous genes such as Pax7, or treatment with small molecules in order to produce a mature phenotype (Abujarour and Valamehr 2015). Although iPSC-based engineered skeletal muscles do not offer a risk-free option for regenerative medicine, they do show exciting potential for uses in drug screening.

18.2.3 Species of Cell Donor

Commonly, the cell source for engineered skeletal muscle *in vitro* has been rodent cells, as they are simple to obtain and sufficient for first-pass, preliminary studies to detect overt toxicity. Rodent cells offer value as a way to optimize the engineered muscle fabrication process, but are not acceptable for translational studies. Human myoblasts are available commercially, and these cells behave comparably to freshly isolated primary cells (Madden et al. 2015). However, if a source of tissue is available, cells can be isolated, expanded, and frozen for future use. Importantly, for regenerative purposes, it is possible to isolate a patient's own cells for use in the engineered muscle, although in the absence of iPSC technology the isolation would require an invasive procedure to obtain the tissue.

Rodents and other species do not provide an entirely accurate model of human function. For example, there is a poor correlation between the expression of mouse and human genes following an acute inflammatory stress, which can have an impact on liver-specific drug metabolism (Seok et al. 2013). Further, there are known immunological signaling pathway discrepancies between the two species (Mestas and Hughes 2004). Interspecies differences in function play a role in the appearance of unexpected side effects of drugs during clinical trials. In the case of some drugs, animal models have failed to predict drug-induced mitochondrial toxicity that occurs once the drug is in clinical trials (Dykens and Will 2007). A specific example of the potential for varied drug responses across species is evident in the screening process of cerivastatin. Cerivastatin is a synthetic statin that is structurally distinct from previously approved "natural" fermentation-derived statins produced as secondary metabolites of fungi (Furberg and Pitt 2001; Manzoni and Rollini 2002). In preclinical animal trials, cerivastatin exhibited widely variable species-dependent side effects that were largely attributed to interspecies differences in metabolism of the drug. Despite a high sensitivity of dogs to the drug, it was determined to be safe for humans at therapeutic levels (von Keutz and Schluter 1998). Once in the market, cerivastatin caused rhabdomyolysis, severe or fatal breakdown of skeletal muscle tissue, in a small percentage of patients (Furberg and Pitt 2001), potentially due to statin-induced ubiquinone deficiency in the muscle leading to defects in cellular respiration (von Keutz and Schluter 1998). Rhabdomyolysis was notably observed in patients who were concurrently undergoing treatment with gemfibrozil, which increases the plasma concentration of cerivastatin (Backman et al. 2002), or in those receiving the highest approved dose of cerivastatin (Staffa et al. 2002). This incident underlines the species-dependent response that a drug may elicit, drug–drug interactions, and the resulting uncertainty about which results to apply to potential human responses, strengthening the argument for the use of human cells for screening studies. When engineered human myobundles were cultured with either cerivastatin or lovastatin (a statin that has not caused safety concerns and remains on the market), the engineered muscle exhibited toxicity to cerivastatin at doses 100× less than those at which lovastatin toxicity was observed, a result that is in accord with clinical reports (Madden et al. 2015). Importantly, engineered human muscle provides a drug screening platform that enables testing of drugs and drug interactions on the same patient, to determine which treatment regimens will yield the highest safety and efficacy for that particular patient.

18.3 SCAFFOLDING AND EXTRACELLULAR MATRIX

Engineered skeletal muscle can be fabricated either in the absence or presence of a scaffold. Engineered muscle fabricated with no additional scaffolding is composed purely of cells and their own ECM. The myogenic cells grow to confluence, at which point they typically begin to fuse, and the resultant spontaneous contractions cause them to delaminate from the hydrophobic culture surface (Baker et al. 2003) (Figure 18.3). The cells in these scaffold-free constructs achieve the aligned structure necessary for proper muscle function by exerting passive tension on artificial tendons located on either end of the culture area (Strohman et al. 1990; Dennis et al. 2001). This method, which is used to produce the myooids described earlier, relies solely on the ECM produced by the myoblasts and fibroblasts to provide the structure of the muscle. Myogenic cells in culture secrete ECM proteins such as collagen (Beach et al. 1985; Gillies and Lieber 2011), but fibroblasts are likely responsible for the bulk of the ECM proteins that provide the structural support in myooids (Dennis et al. 2001). However, many protocols for the formation of 3D engineered muscle use a scaffold, such as a hydrogel structure or a decellularized scaffold (Figure 18.3). A scaffold provides mechanical support and offers a 3D environment for differentiation to occur, in contrast to the differentiation in monolayer culture required for formation of scaffold-free myooids. In addition, a scaffold allows control over the dimensions and physical properties of the matrix in which the cells grow, offering a tunable engineered muscle system.

Optimizing 3D Models of Engineered Skeletal Muscle

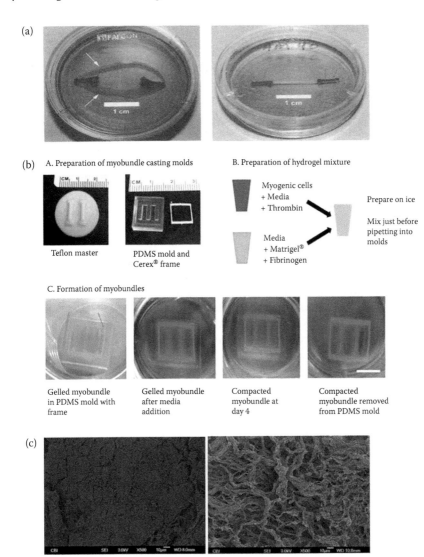

FIGURE 18.3 (a) Formation of myooids using a scaffold-free system in which the differentiating cells detach from the culture surface and form a cylinder of cells suspended between the two anchors. (With kind permission from Springer Science+Business Media: *In Vitro Cell Dev Biol Anim*, Excitability and isometric contractile properties of mammalian skeletal muscle constructs engineered *in vitro*, no. 36, 2000, 327–35, Dennis, R. G., and P. E. Kosnik, 2nd., 3, Copyright Society for *In Vitro* Biology.) (b) Formation of engineered muscle using a hydrogel-based system. (Reprinted from Madden, L. et al. 2015. *eLife* no. 4:e04885.) (c) Skeletal muscle tissue prior to decellularization (left), and the decellularized ECM product (right). (Reprinted from *Biomaterials*, 33 (10), Wolf, M. T. et al., Biologic scaffold composed of skeletal muscle extracellular matrix, 2916–25, Copyright 2012, with permission from Elsevier.)

18.3.1 DECELLULARIZED SCAFFOLDS

Decellularized skeletal muscle scaffolds conserve the structural elements of the tissue's ECM, neural pathways, and blood vessels, facilitating tissue organization with repopulated native cells, either via seeding *in vitro* or ingrowth of cells *in vivo* (Porzionato et al. 2015). Once completely decellularized, the tissue is unlikely to provoke an immune response, as the remaining ECM proteins are highly conserved (Porzionato et al. 2015). Some disruption of the ECM structure occurs during the decellularization process (Crapo et al. 2011), but human skeletal muscle tissue decellularized using a trypsin–EDTA incubation followed by incubation in a Triton X-NH_4OH mixture for 72 h with constant agitation retained their collagen and elastic fiber structure, as well as proteoglycans and glycosaminoglycans (Porzionato et al. 2015). In addition, decellularized skeletal muscle scaffolds retain the basal lamina structure, and upon implantation in an *in vivo* injury model, are populated by regenerating myofibers formed from myogenic cells that migrated into the scaffold and differentiated (Perniconi et al. 2011). Other advantages of decellularized scaffolds include the opportunity for more rapid vascularization and innervation of the scaffold upon implantation due to the presence of the preformed vasculature and neural network architecture. Decellularized scaffolds seeded with C2C12 myoblasts and differentiated for 3 weeks *in vitro* were capable of producing forces (Borschel et al. 2004), but the specific forces are substantially lower than for C2C12 myooids (Dennis et al. 2001) or engineered muscle formed using a hydrogel scaffold and C2C12 cells (Khodabukus and Baar 2015), and well below forces that would be considered physiological. The low forces were attributed in part to the lack of vascularization within the engineered muscle. Nutrient supply to cells, which relies on diffusion within the nonvascularized engineered tissue, limits the size of the tissues, which in turn limits the force production by the engineered muscle (Borschel et al. 2004). The density, degree of alignment, and extent of maturation of the myofibers also play a role in force production. The myoblasts seeded within the decellularized scaffold differentiated into multinucleated myotubes with contractile structures that resembled but did not appear to entirely recapitulate the tightly packed organizational structure of contractile elements in native tissue (Borschel et al. 2004).

18.3.2 HYDROGEL SCAFFOLDS

In native tissue, the ECM provides structural support and signals that direct cell fate decisions (Lutolf and Hubbell 2005). The ECM consists primarily of collagen and elastic fibrils that are highly hydrated due to the presence of glycosaminoglycans (Lutolf and Hubbell 2005). Unlike a decellularized scaffold, the ECM provided by a hydrogel does not offer the advantage of a preformed local architecture, but a hydrogel mimics the behavior of the natural ECM, maintaining the overall geometry of the engineered muscle while allowing myoblasts to freely proliferate within the gel. Upon differentiation and maturation in a hydrogel scaffold, the cells remodel the hydrogel components and replace it with their own ECM (Fedorovich et al. 2007), a process which together with cell-mediated hydrogel compaction can ultimately produce engineered muscle with a higher cell density than that originally seeded.

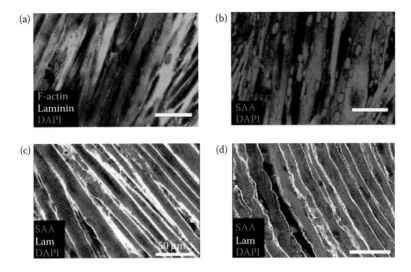

FIGURE 18.4 (a, b) Immunostaining of human engineered muscle depicts aligned, striated myofibers surrounded by laminin. (Reprinted from Madden, L. et al. 2015. *eLife* no. 4:e04885.) (c) Immunostaining of engineered muscle formed from primary rat cells depicts aligned, striated myofibers surrounded by laminin. (Reprinted from Juhas, M. et al. 2014. *Proc Natl Acad Sci USA* no. 111 (15):5508–13. With permission.) (d) Immunostaining of rat native muscle shows similar features to rat engineered muscle. (Reprinted from Juhas, M. et al. 2014. *Proc Natl Acad Sci USA* no. 111 (15):5508–13. With permission.)

When the cells in a hydrogel-based engineered muscle generate stress on the gel, compacting it, the hydrogel must be fixed in place at the ends to resist these stresses. The resulting uniaxial stress within the gel promotes myofiber alignment (Shansky et al. 1997) (Figure 18.4). Myofiber alignment results in parallel contractile units that exert directed force in response to an electrical stimulus. Different methods have been used to maintain the geometry of the engineered muscle; for example, the organoids described earlier were seeded so that they attach to wire screens on either end of the culture area (Shansky et al. 1997). Other methods of maintaining the engineered muscle geometry include attachment around steel pins (Lee and Vandenburgh 2013), silk sutures (Huang et al. 2005), fixed Velcro (Rhim et al. 2007), and nylon frames (Bian et al. 2012). Alternatively, alignment within the 3D hydrogel structure has been achieved by prealigning differentiating myoblasts on micropatterned substrates, and then suspending the prealigned myotubes within a gel (Lam et al. 2009). The hydrogel structure can be formed using either natural biopolymers or synthetic polymers or a combination of the two.

18.3.2.1 Natural Biopolymer Hydrogels

Fibrin, collagen, and Matrigel®, a mixture of structural proteins secreted by mouse sarcoma cells, are purified natural biopolymers derived from tissues and used to create hydrogel-based engineered skeletal muscle. These biopolymers promote cellular growth in part because these components provide the cells with a matrix composition that mimics that of native ECM.

The ECM provided by Matrigel® contains cell adhesion ligands (Meng et al. 2010) to which the differentiating myoblasts can attach (Swasdison and Mayne 1992), allowing the cells to differentiate in three dimensions within the matrix (Bian and Bursac 2009). However, the composition of Matrigel® is not clearly defined, leading to uncertainty about how variations in Matrigel® lot impact engineered muscle function, and Matrigel® contains xenogenic components that would be recognized by a human immune system as foreign, eliciting an unwanted immune response upon implantation and precluding use in humans.

In vitro, Matrigel® is commonly combined with either collagen or fibrin in hydrogel scaffolds. In collagen–Matrigel® gels, C2C12 myoblasts differentiated to form striated, multinucleated fibers with paxillin localizing to the ends of the fibers. This expression of paxillin, which is a protein specific to the myotendinous junction, indicates the possibility of an early stage junction forming between the myotubes and the cell-produced collagen I fibrils in the gel (Rhim et al. 2007). For engineered muscle to be used regeneratively, it will need to be able to form such connections in the native muscle. However, engineered muscle made using collagen–Matrigel® gels can only sustain small numbers of cells since they tend to compact quickly and rupture (Bian and Bursac 2009).

Alternatively, engineered skeletal muscle tissue has been prepared using fibrin-based gels, which form when thrombin cleaves fibrinogen, resulting in polymeric fibrin networks. These gels allow the cells to proliferate and self-organize, as well as produce their own ECM. Fibrin is highly bioactive; it contains the cell adhesion motif RGD, which promotes cell attachment, and the cleavage products produced during the transition from fibrinogen to fibrin act as mitogens, regulating proliferation of surrounding cells (Herrick et al. 1999). In smooth muscle and tendon engineered tissue systems, fibrin gels promote cell–ECM production to a greater extent than do collagen gels (Grassl et al. 2002; Breidenbach et al. 2015), perhaps due to the fact that fibrin binds growth factors such as fibroblast growth factor (FGF) and insulin growth factor (IGF), leading to increased protein synthesis (Martino et al. 2013). Fibrin contains a heparin-binding domain that gives it this ability to bind growth factors and sequester them within the engineered construct (Martino et al. 2013). IGF is known to promote skeletal muscle hypertrophy through stimulation of both proliferation and differentiation pathways; in fact, myoblast differentiation is stimulated in part by autocrine secretion of IGF, an effect that can be enhanced by introducing exogenous IGF (Florini et al. 1996). FGF plays a role in increasing the number of proliferative satellite cells in rats, contributing to an enhanced injury response (Yablonka-Reuveni et al. 1999). FGF-6 is specifically expressed in muscle and induces proliferation of cultured myoblasts while inhibiting differentiation, allowing for expansion of the undifferentiated cell population (Bentzinger et al. 2010). In FGF-6 knockout mice, regenerative potential following injury was limited and damaged tissue exhibited fibrosis not seen in wild-type mice (Floss et al. 1997). Although in a separate FGF-6 knockout model, regeneration following injury was not affected by the lack of FGF-6 (Fiore et al. 2000), injection of recombinant human FGF-6 into injured muscle of wild type mice accelerated the regenerative process (Armand et al. 2003). FGF-2 is present in the basement membrane of adult muscle and promotes satellite cell replication in murine models of muscular dystrophy (Lefaucheur and Sebille 1995).

As the cells mature, they remodel the fibrin matrix, eventually degrading much of the original fibrin and replacing it with their own ECM (Lam et al. 2009). Unlike engineered muscle bundles formed using a collagen–Matrigel® mixture, bundles formed using fibrin-based gels are capable of lasting for significant time periods in culture (up to at least 5 weeks) without deteriorating and rupturing (Hinds et al. 2011). This effect is likely due either to an improvement in mechanical strength due to the increased ECM produced in fibrin gels, or the higher compliance of fibrin fibers compared to collagen, allowing the matrix to better resist the force of spontaneous myofiber contractions (Bian and Bursac 2009).

18.3.2.2 Synthetic Hydrogels

Synthetic polymers can be synthesized in a highly reproducible manner (Fernandes et al. 2012), and they offer a tighter degree of control over the properties of the engineered tissue than do purified tissue-derived biopolymers (Rizzi et al. 2012), as they can be tuned to achieve desired mechanical properties and functionalized to engage in defined interactions with cells (Seliktar 2012). Due to the importance of the ECM in regulating myogenesis (Velleman 1999), functionalization of synthetic polymers to enable those cell fate-directing interactions is essential. Poly(ethylene glycol) (PEG) is a synthetic, biocompatible polymer that can be photocrosslinked to form a hydrogel and can be made bioactive by modification with small peptide sequences to promote cell adhesion and migration, growth factors to direct cellular processes such as differentiation, and linkages with cleavage sequences to enable control over enzyme-mediated hydrogel degradation (Drury and Mooney 2003; Lutolf and Hubbell 2005; Seliktar 2012). For example, C2C12 cells encapsulated in PEG-maleimide hydrogels functionalized with RGD adhesion sequences differentiated to form multinucleated cells capable of causing a 20% decrease in the hydrogel length upon addition of a contractile agent, demonstrating the feasibility of engineered skeletal muscle fabricated using a synthetic polymer (Salimath and Garcia 2014).

Hydrogels formed using a combination of synthetic and natural polymers make use of the best of both worlds. PEG can be combined with fibrinogen (Almany and Seliktar 2005; Fuoco et al. 2012, 2015) or collagen (Sargeant et al. 2012) to form a hybrid polymer that retains the inherent cell-signaling benefits of natural polymer hydrogels without the necessity of synthesizing the bioactive peptide sequences, with the added consistency and tunability of synthetic polymer hydrogels (Zhu and Marchant 2011). Such hydrogels are capable of supporting myogenic cell adhesion and differentiation to contractile myofibers both *in vitro* and *in vivo* (Fuoco et al. 2012, 2015), and their potential for injection followed by *in situ* crosslinking makes them ideal for regenerative purposes.

18.4 PROMOTING MATURATION AND FUNCTION

Although gene and protein expression analysis offer information about the similarities between the engineered tissue and the *in vivo* tissue, such observations do not build a complete story. In skeletal muscle, force production has been identified as a crucial functional characteristic of the muscle tissue *in vivo* that must be recapitulated *in vitro* for both regenerative and drug screening purposes. The metabolic profile of the engineered muscle is also critical when considering aspects of muscle function such as drug metabolism.

18.4.1 Force Production

Native muscle responds to a single electrical stimulus with a single contraction, producing a twitch force. When repeated electrical stimuli grow temporally closer together, the muscle engages in a sustained contraction, producing a tetanus force (Figure 18.5). In rats, maximum tetanic specific force (force normalized by cross-sectional area) *in vivo* reaches a magnitude of approximately 250 kN/m^2 (Urbanchek et al. 2001; Mendias et al. 2006), with a unitless tetanus to twitch ratio in adult rat skeletal muscle of 3.5–5 (Close 1972; Huang et al. 2005). In addition, native muscle demonstrates a length–tension curve, with contractile forces increasing as the muscle is stretched until the muscle produces peak force when myosin and actin fibers optimally overlap. Stretching above the maximum level results in declining forces as the overlap of contractile elements begins to interfere with force production (Close 1972). Engineered muscle is capable of recapitulating the force–length curve, as well as the production of twitch and tetanus forces matching adult muscle tetanus to twitch ratios (Dennis and Kosnik 2000; Huang et al. 2005), but falls short of the standard set by *in vivo* muscle when it comes to the magnitude of specific force (force/cross-sectional area) production. Prior to force optimization, most engineered muscle formed using rodent cells yields specific forces with a magnitude of approximately 1%–8% of the magnitude produced by their native, adult muscle counterparts (Dennis et al. 2001; Liao and Zhou 2009; Hinds et al. 2011; Yamamoto et al. 2011). Due to the importance of high active force production for both regenerative and drug screening purposes, considerable effort has been invested in optimizing engineered muscle to produce improved forces. There are some circumstances inherent to the *in vivo* muscle environment, such as innervation and vascularization, that impact the function of native muscle and remain largely elusive for *in vitro* culture, as discussed in a later section. However, the formulation and culture conditions of the engineered

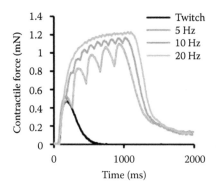

FIGURE 18.5 Engineered muscle formed from human primary cells demonstrates a characteristic single twitch force and summation of twitch forces leading to tetanus as stimulation frequency increases. (Reprinted from Madden, L. et al. 2015. *eLife* no. 4:e04885.)

muscle can be altered to overcome some shortcomings of *in vitro* culture, leading to engineered muscle capable of producing higher, more physiologically relevant forces.

18.4.1.1 Optimizing Formulation Parameters

The absence of the native organization of muscle and the lack of maturity of muscle fibers *in vitro* are likely the major causes of the low forces seen in engineered skeletal muscle, as unoptimized engineered muscle is typically characterized by thin, incompletely matured fibers surrounded by excessive amounts of ECM and an acellular core (Powell et al. 2002). By varying the matrix composition, and in turn the cell–matrix interactions, it is possible to enhance the maturation of the fibers within the engineered muscle and improve the function. Engineered skeletal muscle formed by suspending primary neonatal rat myoblasts in a fibrin gel produced approximately threefold higher contractile forces than those formed using the same cell density in a collagen gel, suggesting that the interactions of the cells with specific matrix proteins may have a substantial impact on the force production of the muscle (Hinds et al. 2011). When the same investigators formed engineered muscle with increasing fibrinogen and increasing Matrigel® concentrations, they saw increased protein:DNA ratios and increased myotube diameter, indicative of more robust fibers. These bundles with the largest myotube diameter also produced the highest active force. Fibrin hydrogel-based self-assembled rat engineered skeletal muscle produced specific forces of 36.3 kN/m^2, which is a considerable improvement upon the forces achieved by fibrin-free self-assembled rat engineered skeletal muscle, which produced specific forces of 2.9 kN/m^2 (Huang et al. 2005).

The size of the engineered muscle influences its force production; a thicker tissue will inherently produce larger absolute forces, which is ideal for regenerative purposes. However, in the absence of vascularization, the tissue thickness is constrained by the diffusion of nutrients and oxygen, so larger engineered muscle tissues produce a lower specific force because the center is either devoid of cells or contains necrotic cells (Dennis and Kosnik 2000; Liao and Zhou 2009). The open pore structure of hydrogels is ideal for promoting diffusion, but even within such a structure, cells must be within 100–200 μm of the nutrient and oxygen source to remain viable (Lovett et al. 2009). A further limitation includes the relatively low solubility of oxygen in aqueous solutions such as culture media (Allen et al. 2001). Decreasing the thickness of the engineered muscle can reduce the nutrient and oxygen gradients within the tissue (Cheng et al. 2014), and decrease the relative volume of the acellular region, an ideal solution for the use of engineered muscle in the drug testing process. Other proposed methods for decreasing the acellular region while maintaining a clinically relevant size of the tissue include mixing of the culture media (Juhas and Bursac 2014), perfusion of media over the engineered tissue (Chromiak et al. 1998), or vascularization.

18.4.1.2 Effect of Convection in Culture Media on Skeletal Muscle Maturation

Typically, tissue engineered muscles are cultured under static conditions, with no fluid flow or bulk motion around the bundles. This can lead to a nutrient gradient within the media, resulting in a lack of oxygen and nutrients directly surrounding and within the engineered muscle. In the absence of a vascular system to deliver oxygen and nutrients directly to the cells, other methods such as perfusion of the media (Salehi-Nik et al. 2013) or media mixing can be used to overcome diffusion limitations and ensure that there is sufficient transport to the interior of engineered muscle. The introduction of dynamic culture conditions, in which muscle bundles are rocked during culture at 24 rocks per minute with a ±30° tilt, aims to diminish the gradient within the bundle and culture media and allow for improved mass transport of oxygen and nutrients within the engineered muscle environment (Juhas and Bursac 2014). Static controls in this experiment showed only a thin layer of viable myofibers along the exterior of the muscle bundle, with a generally acellular core, indicative of cell migration toward a more nutrient-rich environment. Dynamic culture of the fibrin-based engineered muscle formed using rat myogenic cells increased the total cross-sectional area of the tissue occupied by viable myofibers from approximately 0.18 mm^2 in static controls to approximately 0.63 mm^2 (Juhas and Bursac 2014). In the same study, the diameter of myofibers in dynamically cultured engineered muscle increased, and the muscles themselves produced 6–7-fold higher forces than those cultured in static conditions, indicating progress toward a more physiologically relevant tissue structure.

18.4.1.3 Mechanical Stimulation

In an attempt to produce engineered skeletal muscle that is highly aligned, mimicking the alignment of muscle fibers *in vivo*, some groups have applied unidirectional stretch to differentiating engineered muscle. In two-dimensional (2D) studies, uniaxial strain induced directional differentiation of mouse myoblasts to form cross-striated fibers (Pennisi et al. 2011). These externally applied forces mimic those forces experienced by muscles *in vivo*, which affect protein synthesis (Goldspink et al. 1995) and muscle morphology in postdevelopment muscle adaptations. When human skeletal muscle cells in a collagen–Matrigel® construct were cyclically stretched over the course of differentiation, the resulting engineered muscle contained larger fibers with a mean diameter 12% greater than those of the unstretched controls (Powell et al. 2002). The stretch regimen used in these experiments began one week postcasting, and consisted of three stretch/relaxation cycles followed by about 28 min of static conditions, with stretches occurring at a 5% strain for 2 days, followed by 10% strain for 2 days, and 15% strain for 4 days. Although active force production was not measured in these experiments, the increase in both fiber diameter and fiber area indicates an improvement in the physiological structure of the engineered muscle that could translate to higher force production.

18.4.1.4 Electrical Stimulation

Since native muscle is constantly receiving electrical signals from motor neurons, and upon denervation, skeletal muscle undergoes atrophy (Wilson and Harris 1993), electrical stimulation of engineered muscle in *in vitro* cultures more closely mimics the conditions seen by native muscle. When engineered skeletal muscles formed from fibrin gels containing C2C12 cells were chronically electrically stimulated (4×0.1 ms pulses at 2.5 V/mm delivered over the course of 400 ms with 3.6 s recovery for 7 days), the tetanus or twitch force was two times higher than unstimulated muscle, consistent with a more mature fiber phenotype (Donnelly et al. 2010). Electrical stimulation can also produce fiber type switching, which has important implications for the metabolic state of the engineered muscle (Khodabukus et al. 2015).

18.4.2 EXPANDING THE RELEVANCE OF THE ENGINEERED MUSCLE MODEL

To be fully representative of native muscle tissue, engineered muscle will need to incorporate the complex tissue interactions that are present in native muscle, including innervation and vascularization. These are well-established goals for any engineered tissue, but they have been difficult to achieve *in vitro*, in the absence of the complex environmental and signaling cues present *in vivo*.

18.4.2.1 Innervation

In vivo muscle forms neuromuscular junctions with motor neurons, at which they receive their electrical input from the neurons. Denervation of skeletal muscle results in changes in protein expression, leading to atrophy and decreases in force production, as well as fiber type switching resulting in metabolic changes in skeletal muscle (Block et al. 1991; Coderre et al. 1992). When skeletal muscle is denervated, a group of myogenic factors involved in muscle development, including MyoD and myogenin, are upregulated and accompanied by a significant decrease in myofiber cross-sectional area (Voytik et al. 1993; Chen et al. 2011). This upregulation of myogenin directly regulates the expression of atrophy-associated genes that have been connected with losses in muscle mass (Macpherson et al. 2011). Electrical stimulation of engineered skeletal muscle may offer an alternative to innervation, but cannot completely recapitulate the *in vivo* environment. To more fully mimic the native environment of muscle, neuromuscular junctions have been formed *in vitro*, in both 2D and 3D culture systems. In 2D, functional neuromuscular junctions have been formed using a variety of cell species combinations, including more recently, human stem-cell derived motoneurons and human skeletal muscle cells: the ideal cell source for use as a drug screening platform. This neuromuscular junction model demonstrated striated skeletal muscle cells capable of firing action potentials in response to motoneuron stimulus, resulting in cell contraction (Guo et al. 2011).

Neuromuscular junction formation was achieved in fibrin-based tissue engineered muscle using rat motor neurons and myoblasts. These innervated engineered muscles demonstrated a high percentage of striated fibers, indicating increased fiber maturation, as well as an increase in active force production when compared with engineered muscle cultured using only myoblasts (Martin et al. 2015). This result presents an opportunity for not only increasing the extent of biomimicry of skeletal muscle, but also expanding the functional aspects of skeletal muscle that can be examined *in vitro* to include the neuromuscular junction.

18.4.2.2 Vascularization

Most engineered tissues have been designed with the hope that the body will vascularize the engineered muscle upon implantation. However, this has been difficult to achieve in skeletal muscle due to the dense nature of the tissue and the high level of vascularization *in vivo* (Levenberg et al. 2005). In addition, for applications in drug screening, the engineered tissues must be complete and functional in their *in vitro* environment. Vascularization offers advantages in terms of enabling the study of muscle–vasculature interactions, and also addresses the challenges of oxygen and nutrient diffusion limitations within tissue engineered muscle. Although fully vascularized engineered skeletal muscle has not yet been produced *in vitro*, there are some preimplantation approaches that have achieved more rapid vascularization once the engineered muscle is implanted. One approach is to form engineered muscle using cells that have been retrovirally transduced such that they produce the angiogenesis growth factor vascular endothelial growth factor (VEGF). Upon implantation, they promote capillary bed formation both internally as well as in nearby tissue (Lu et al. 2001). In another preimplantation approach, endothelial cells, fibroblasts, and myoblasts were cocultured on a porous scaffold. The endothelial cells self-organized to form tubular networks that, after implantation, contained red blood cells, indicating that they had anastomosed with the *in vivo* vasculature (Levenberg et al. 2005). However, functionally vascularized *in vitro* engineered skeletal muscle remains elusive.

18.4.2.3 Metabolism

The metabolic state of engineered skeletal muscle is a significant indicator of the suitability of engineered muscle as a replacement for or supplementation of *in vivo* drug studies. Recapitulating the metabolic milieu found *in vivo* is of the utmost importance when the engineered muscle is used to test the effects of pharmaceuticals, when changes in metabolism can indicate drug toxicity. In addition, because skeletal muscle is a large contributor to the insulin-mediated glucose uptake response, the muscles must accurately simulate that process if they are to be used to screen drugs for Type 2 diabetes. Skeletal muscle accounts for 75% of glucose uptake post insulin stimulation (e.g., following a meal) (Baron et al. 1988). Much of our knowledge about insulin-mediated uptake in skeletal muscle thus far has been obtained from *in vitro* experiments done with monolayer cultures, but there are indications that skeletal muscle cultured in a 2D system may not accurately represent intact skeletal muscle in the body. The increase in glucose uptake in response to insulin is typically diminished *in vitro* when compared to adult skeletal muscle *in vivo*. In humans, *in vivo* insulin-mediated glucose uptake rates are typically 6–8-fold higher than basal uptake rates (DeFronzo et al. 1981; Bonadonna et al. 1990), whereas *in vitro* insulin stimulation of cultured human myotubes typically only results in a 1.3–3-fold increase in uptake rates (Sarabia et al. 1990; Sarabia et al. 1992; Ciaraldi et al. 1995, 2005; Henry et al. 1995; Al-Khalili et al. 2003). Because the conditions experienced by a cell cultured in monolayer are devoid of many of the tissue-specific interactions seen *in vivo*, such as mechanical cues, biochemical cues, and cell–cell contact (Pampaloni et al. 2007), the 3D environment offered by tissue engineered skeletal muscle may result in a more physiological metabolic state than that of monolayer cultures.

Glucose enters skeletal muscle cells primarily via two glucose transporters, GLUT1 and GLUT4, that allow selective movement of glucose down its concentration gradient into the cell. GLUT1 is responsible for constitutive, basal glucose uptake in skeletal muscle, whereas GLUT4 is responsible for insulin-stimulated glucose uptake. However, the ratio of GLUT1 to GLUT4 expression increases when cells are taken from a 3D physiological environment and plated in a 2D culture system, causing a change in the metabolic behavior of cells cultured *in vitro*. *In vivo*, rat muscle has a GLUT1/GLUT4 protein ratio value that varies from 0.1 to 0.6 (Sarabia et al. 1992; Kraegen et al. 1993), whereas rat constructs *in vitro* showed a GLUT1/GLUT4 protein ratio of 6.3:1 (Baker et al. 2003). *In vivo*, human muscle was found to have a GLUT1:GLUT4 total cell mRNA expression ratio of 0.6:1 (Stuart et al. 2000), whereas total cell mRNA expression levels in myotubes *in vitro* showed a ratio of 12:1 (Al-Khalili et al. 2003). The high GLUT1 content seen in cultured cells contributes to a high basal uptake rate that dilutes the insulin responsive glucose uptake by the relatively less abundant GLUT4 transporters.

This change in the GLUT1:GLUT4 ratio appears to be consistent with studies of denervated muscle. Protein expression analysis of transected muscles from mice reveals significantly decreased levels of GLUT4, whereas GLUT1 protein expression was significantly increased (Callahan et al. 2015). This study also found decreases in insulin responsiveness of the transected muscles at early time points, which is consistent with previous studies that found a decrease in insulin response following denervation of rat muscle with corresponding decreases in GLUT4 protein levels and increases in GLUT1 protein levels (Block et al. 1991; Coderre et al. 1992). In addition, *ex vivo* muscle fibers cultured after removal from human muscle tissue show decreased insulin responses when compared with the insulin response seen in human muscle *in vivo* (DeFronzo et al. 1981; Dohm et al. 1988; Andreasson et al. 1991; Bonadonna et al. 1993; Zierath et al. 1994, 1996). Thus, denervation of skeletal muscle cells may be one factor that skews the GLUT1:GLUT4 ratio *in vitro*, resulting in a decreased insulin response.

Culture conditions that expose skeletal muscle cells to supraphysiological levels of nutrients or hormones can also have an impact on the function of insulin-mediated glucose uptake. Human skeletal muscle myotubes cultured in hyperglycemic conditions (20 mM glucose) produce a 40% decrease in basal glucose uptake and complete absence of an insulin response (Aas et al. 2011). In animal models, skeletal muscle GLUT4 protein levels are depressed in hyperglycemic conditions (Klip et al. 1994). In contrast, culturing control human cells in hyperglycemic conditions (10 and 20 mM) did not decrease insulin responsiveness in differentiated human myotubes, unless hyperglycemic conditions were combined with hyperinsulinemia (Ciaraldi et al. 1995).

Supraphysiological insulin levels stimulate proliferation and differentiation of myoblasts (Ewton et al. 1994). However, in hyperinsulinemia conditions (30 μM), differentiating human skeletal muscle myoblasts exhibited increased membrane-specific GLUT1 expression corresponding to a doubling of the basal glucose uptake rate, while also decreasing insulin-stimulated transport by 30%–40%, yielding an undiscernible insulin response (Ciaraldi et al. 1995). In the same study, cells grown in media containing only 22 pM insulin for both growth and differentiation periods showed a nearly threefold insulin-mediated increase in glucose uptake.

Glucose and fatty acids are both potential substrates for oxidative metabolism, and there is competition between the two as fuel sources in skeletal muscle. Studies on human leg skeletal muscle indicate that glucose oxidation accounts for 76% of oxygen consumption in hyperinsulinemic conditions, but upon addition of free fatty acids, that percentage drops to 53%, indicating a shift to fatty acid substrates (Kelley et al. 1993). In humans, high levels of free fatty acids in the plasma and increased intramuscular lipids are associated with insulin resistance, leading to decreased glucose disposal (Schwenk et al. 2010). However, saturated and unsaturated fatty acids may have distinct effects on insulin-stimulated glucose disposal, with saturated fatty acids such as palmitate primarily responsible for the reduction of the insulin response (Dimopoulos et al. 2006). In contrast, unsaturated fatty acids such as oleate are capable of rescuing the insulin response following palmitate-induced insulin resistance (Coll et al. 2008). In addition, unsaturated fatty acids stimulate differentiation in L6 myotubes (Hurley et al. 2006). Typical skeletal muscle cell culture conditions are devoid of fatty acids, but the addition of physiological ratios of saturated and unsaturated fatty acids could serve a valuable role in recreating the energy sources available to muscle *in vivo*.

Together, these results indicate that tissue engineered skeletal muscle culture conditions have the potential to exert a significant effect on both basal and insulin-stimulated uptake and must be optimized to allow for maximal differentiation potential while not shifting the metabolic pathways to a nonphysiological state.

18.4.2.3.1 Fiber Type Switching

Mature skeletal muscle consists of four primary mature fiber types distinguished by the primary expressed form of myosin heavy chain; type 1 fibers, which are characterized by slow twitch kinetics and the presence of oxidative enzymes, and three forms of type 2 fibers characterized by fast twitch kinetics and the presence of more glycolytic enzymes. Fast twitch fibers express higher levels of GLUT1 and lower levels of GLUT4 than their slow twitch counterparts (Daugaard et al. 2000; Gaster et al. 2000). Interestingly, skeletal muscle cultured *in vitro* had a much higher percentage of fast twitch fibers, as identified by expression of fast twitch associated myosin heavy chain proteins, than the tissue from which it was isolated (Gaster et al. 2001), and cultured myotubes typically express more immature embryonic and perinatal myosin heavy chain isoforms (Cheng et al. 2014). If myotubes *in vitro* have a tendency to differentiate into fast twitch fibers, this may partially explain the lower expression levels of GLUT4 than their counterpart muscle *in vivo*.

Skeletal muscle fibers *in vivo* demonstrate some plasticity, with the capacity to switch fiber type in response to training, though the effect is subtle (Booth and Thomason 1991; Scott et al. 2001). Fast to slow fiber type switching is more dramatic *in vitro* (Booth and Thomason 1991), and can be accomplished *in vitro* by electrical stimulation (Kubis et al. 2002; Khodabukus et al. 2015) and modification of culture conditions (Kubis et al. 2002; Hanke et al. 2008). Engineered muscle formed with C2C12 cells and electrically stimulated at a frequency of 10 Hz and an active time of 60% responded in a duration-dependent manner to contraction durations of at least 6 s with a switch to slower adult MHC isoforms. A contraction duration of 0.6 s did not produce changes in expression of fast MHC isoforms, indicating that the duration of contraction is an important factor in the regulation of MHC protein expression. The fast-to-slow transition is additionally characterized by slower twitch kinetics and higher expression of GLUT4 and metabolic proteins associated with promoting a slow twitch fiber type (Khodabukus et al. 2015). In this case, inducing fiber type switching to produce cultures enriched with slow twitch fibers could elicit an insulin response more in line with that seen *in vivo*, due to increased GLUT4 expression.

18.5 CONCLUSION AND PERSPECTIVE

The ideal physiologically relevant tissue engineered skeletal muscle consists structurally of aligned, dense, mature myofibers and exhibits high force production and metabolic responses similar to those in native muscle, with the capacity for innervation and vascularization. These engineered muscles can be used for both regenerative and toxicological and drug screening purposes. When constructing such a system, human cells are necessary to produce a clinically relevant product, which must be weighed against the advantage of ease of culture of cell lines. The ability of scaffolding material to produce more functional muscle has been thoroughly investigated, nutrient and oxygen transport issues have been addressed via dynamic culture, and external manipulation of the engineered muscle via mechanical and electrical stimulation have proved effective at producing a more mature muscle. Despite the vast progress achieved over the past few decades, we must continue to develop and characterize these engineered tissues. Producing engineered muscle that matches the metabolic profile of native muscle would ensure accurate results from drug screening, and incorporation of vasculature and innervation would both improve the physiological relevance of the muscle for drug screening uses, as well as ease their incorporation into the body for regenerative purposes.

REFERENCES

Aas, V., N. P. Hessvik, M. Wettergreen, A. W. Hvammen, S. Hallen, G. H. Thoresen, and A. C. Rustan. 2011. Chronic hyperglycemia reduces substrate oxidation and impairs metabolic switching of human myotubes. *Biochim Biophys Acta* no. 1812 (1):94–105.

Abujarour, R., M. Bennett, B. Valamehr, T. T. Lee, M. Robinson, D. Robbins, T. Le, K. Lai, and P. Flynn. 2014. Myogenic differentiation of muscular dystrophy-specific induced pluripotent stem cells for use in drug discovery. *Stem Cells Transl Med* no. 3 (2):149–60.

Abujarour, R. and B. Valamehr. 2015. Generation of skeletal muscle cells from pluripotent stem cells: Advances and challenges. *Front Cell Dev Biol* no. 3:29.

Al-Khalili, L., A. V. Chibalin, K. Kannisto, B. B. Zhang, J. Permert, G. D. Holman, E. Ehrenborg, V. D. Ding, J. R. Zierath, and A. Krook. 2003. Insulin action in cultured human skeletal muscle cells during differentiation: Assessment of cell surface GLUT4 and GLUT1 content. *Cell Mol Life Sci* no. 60 (5):991–8.

Allen, C. B., B. K. Schneider, and C. W. White. 2001. Limitations to oxygen diffusion and equilibration in *in vitro* cell exposure systems in hyperoxia and hypoxia. *Am J Physiol: Lung Cell Mol Physiol* no. 281 (4):L1021–7.

Almany, L. and D. Seliktar. 2005. Biosynthetic hydrogel scaffolds made from fibrinogen and polyethylene glycol for 3D cell cultures. *Biomaterials* no. 26 (15):2467–77.

Andreasson, K., D. Galuska, A. Thorne, T. Sonnenfeld, and H. Wallberg-Henriksson. 1991. Decreased insulin-stimulated 3–0-methylglucose transport in *in vitro* incubated muscle strips from type II diabetic subjects. *Acta Physiol Scand* no. 142 (2):255–60.

Armand, A. S., T. Launay, C. Pariset, B. Della Gaspera, F. Charbonnier, and C. Chanoine. 2003. Injection of FGF6 accelerates regeneration of the soleus muscle in adult mice. *Biochim Biophys Acta* no. 1642 (1–2):97–105.

Backman, J. T., C. Kyrklund, M. Neuvonen, and P. J. Neuvonen. 2002. Gemfibrozil greatly increases plasma concentrations of cerivastatin. *Clin Pharmacol Ther* no. 72 (6):685–91.

Baker, E. L., R. G. Dennis, and L. M. Larkin. 2003. Glucose transporter content and glucose uptake in skeletal muscle constructs engineered *in vitro*. *In Vitro Cell Dev Biol Anim* no. 39 (10):434–9.

Baroffio, A., J. P. Aubry, A. Kaelin, R. M. Krause, M. Hamann, and C. R. Bader. 1993. Purification of human muscle satellite cells by flow cytometry. *Muscle Nerve* no. 16 (5):498–505.

Baron, A. D., G. Brechtel, P. Wallace, and S. V. Edelman. 1988. Rates and tissue sites of non-insulin- and insulin-mediated glucose uptake in humans. *Am J Physiol* no. 255 (6 Pt 1):E769–74.

Beach, R. L., J. S. Rao, and B. W. Festoff. 1985. Extracellular-matrix synthesis by skeletal muscle in culture. Major secreted collagenous proteins of clonal myoblasts. *Biochem J* no. 225 (3):619–27.

Bentzinger, C. F., J. von Maltzahn, and M. A. Rudnicki. 2010. Extrinsic regulation of satellite cell specification. *Stem Cell Res Ther* no. 1 (3):27.

Bian, W. and N. Bursac. 2009. Engineered skeletal muscle tissue networks with controllable architecture. *Biomaterials* no. 30 (7):1401–12.

Bian, W., M. Juhas, T. W. Pfeiler, and N. Bursac. 2012. Local tissue geometry determines contractile force generation of engineered muscle networks. *Tissue Eng Part A* no. 18 (9–10):957–67.

Block, N. E., D. R. Menick, K. A. Robinson, and M. G. Buse. 1991. Effect of denervation on the expression of two glucose transporter isoforms in rat hindlimb muscle. *J Clin Invest* no. 88 (5):1546–52.

Bonadonna, R. C., S. Del Prato, M. P. Saccomani, E. Bonora, G. Gulli, E. Ferrannini, D. Bier, C. Cobelli, and R. A. DeFronzo. 1993. Transmembrane glucose transport in skeletal muscle of patients with non-insulin-dependent diabetes. *J Clin Invest* no. 92 (1):486–94.

Bonadonna, R. C., L. Groop, N. Kraemer, E. Ferrannini, S. Del Prato, and R. A. DeFronzo. 1990. Obesity and insulin resistance in humans: A dose-response study. *Metabolism* no. 39 (5):452–9.

Booth, F. W. and D. B. Thomason. 1991. Molecular and cellular adaptation of muscle in response to exercise: Perspectives of various models. *Physiol Rev* no. 71 (2):541–85.

Borschel, G. H., R. G. Dennis, and W. M. Kuzon, Jr. 2004. Contractile skeletal muscle tissue-engineered on an acellular scaffold. *Plast Reconstr Surg* no. 113 (2):595–602; discussion 603-4.

Brack, A. S. and T. A. Rando. 2012. Tissue-specific stem cells: Lessons from the skeletal muscle satellite cell. *Cell Stem Cell* no. 10 (5):504–14.

Breidenbach, A. P., N. A. Dyment, Y. Lu, M. Rao, J. T. Shearn, D. W. Rowe, K. E. Kadler, and D. L. Butler. 2015. Fibrin gels exhibit improved biological, structural, and mechanical properties compared with collagen gels in cell-based tendon tissue-engineered constructs. *Tissue Eng Part A* no. 21 (3–4):438–50.

Callahan, Z. J., M. Oxendine, J. L. Wheatley, C. Menke, E. A. Cassell, A. Bartos, P. C. Geiger, and P. J. Schaeffer. 2015. Compensatory responses of the insulin signaling pathway restore muscle glucose uptake following long-term denervation. *Physiol Rep* no. 3 (4):1–12.

Campion, D. R. 1984. The muscle satellite cell: A review. *Int Rev Cytol* no. 87:225–51.

Chen, L., H. W. Huang, S. H. Gu, L. Xu, Y. D. Gu, and J. G. Xu. 2011. The study of myogenin expression in denervated human skeletal muscles. *J Int Med Res* no. 39 (2):378–87.

Chen, S., T. Nakamoto, N. Kawazoe, and G. Chen. 2015. Engineering multi-layered skeletal muscle tissue by using 3D microgrooved collagen scaffolds. *Biomaterials* no. 73:23–31.

Cheng, C. S., B. N. Davis, L. Madden, N. Bursac, and G. A. Truskey. 2014. Physiology and metabolism of tissue-engineered skeletal muscle. *Exp Biol Med (Maywood)* no. 239 (9):1203–14.

Chromiak, J. A., J. Shansky, C. Perrone, and H. H. Vandenburgh. 1998. Bioreactor perfusion system for the long-term maintenance of tissue-engineered skeletal muscle organoids. *In Vitro Cell Dev Biol Anim* no. 34 (9):694–703.

Ciaraldi, T. P., L. Abrams, S. Nikoulina, S. Mudaliar, and R. R. Henry. 1995. Glucose transport in cultured human skeletal muscle cells. Regulation by insulin and glucose in nondiabetic and non-insulin-dependent diabetes mellitus subjects. *J Clin Invest* no. 96 (6):2820–7.

Ciaraldi, T. P., S. A. Phillips, L. Carter, V. Aroda, S. Mudaliar, and R. R. Henry. 2005. Effects of the rapid-acting insulin analog glulisine on cultured human skeletal muscle cells: Comparisons with insulin and insulin-like growth factor I. *J Clin Endocrinol Metab* no. 90 (10):5551–8.

Close, R. I. 1972. Dynamic properties of mammalian skeletal muscles. *Physiol Rev* no. 52 (1):129–97.

Coderre, L., M. M. Monfar, K. S. Chen, S. J. Heydrick, T. G. Kurowski, N. B. Ruderman, and P. F. Pilch. 1992. Alteration in the expression of GLUT-1 and GLUT-4 protein and messenger RNA levels in denervated rat muscles. *Endocrinology* no. 131 (4):1821–5.

Coll, T., E. Eyre, R. Rodriguez-Calvo, X. Palomer, R. M. Sanchez, M. Merlos, J. C. Laguna, and M. Vazquez-Carrera. 2008. Oleate reverses palmitate-induced insulin resistance and inflammation in skeletal muscle cells. *J Biol Chem* no. 283 (17):11107–16.

Crapo, P. M., T. W. Gilbert, and S. F. Badylak. 2011. An overview of tissue and whole organ decellularization processes. *Biomaterials* no. 32 (12):3233–43.

Danoviz, M. E. and Z. Yablonka-Reuveni. 2012. Skeletal muscle satellite cells: Background and methods for isolation and analysis in a primary culture system. *Methods Mol Biol* no. 798:21–52.

Daugaard, J. R., J. N. Nielsen, S. Kristiansen, J. L. Andersen, M. Hargreaves, and E. A. Richter. 2000. Fiber type-specific expression of GLUT4 in human skeletal muscle: Influence of exercise training. *Diabetes* no. 49 (7):1092–5.

DeFronzo, R. A., E. Jacot, E. Jequier, E. Maeder, J. Wahren, and J. P. Felber. 1981. The effect of insulin on the disposal of intravenous glucose. Results from indirect calorimetry and hepatic and femoral venous catheterization. *Diabetes* no. 30 (12):1000–7.

De Jesus, A. M. and E. A. Sander. 2014. Observing and quantifying fibroblast-mediated fibrin gel compaction. *J Vis Exp* (83):e50918.

Dennis, R. G. and P. E. Kosnik, 2nd, 2000. Excitability and isometric contractile properties of mammalian skeletal muscle constructs engineered *in vitro*. *In Vitro Cell Dev Biol Anim* no. 36 (5):327–35.

Dennis, R. G., P. E. Kosnik, 2nd, M. E. Gilbert, and J. A. Faulkner. 2001. Excitability and contractility of skeletal muscle engineered from primary cultures and cell lines. *Am J Physiol Cell Physiol* no. 280 (2):C288–95.

Dimopoulos, N., M. Watson, K. Sakamoto, and H. S. Hundal. 2006. Differential effects of palmitate and palmitoleate on insulin action and glucose utilization in rat L6 skeletal muscle cells. *Biochem J* no. 399 (3):473–81.

Dohm, G. L., E. B. Tapscott, W. J. Pories, D. J. Dabbs, E. G. Flickinger, D. Meelheim, T. Fushiki, S. M. Atkinson, C. W. Elton, and J. F. Caro. 1988. An *in vitro* human muscle preparation suitable for metabolic studies. Decreased insulin stimulation of glucose transport in muscle from morbidly obese and diabetic subjects. *J Clin Invest* no. 82 (2):486–94.

Donnelly, K., A. Khodabukus, A. Philp, L. Deldicque, R. G. Dennis, and K. Baar. 2010. A novel bioreactor for stimulating skeletal muscle *in vitro*. *Tissue Eng Part C Methods* no. 16 (4):711–8.

Drury, J. L. and D. J. Mooney. 2003. Hydrogels for tissue engineering: Scaffold design variables and applications. *Biomaterials* no. 24 (24):4337–51.

Dykens, J. A. and Y. Will. 2007. The significance of mitochondrial toxicity testing in drug development. *Drug Discov Today* no. 12 (17–18):777–85.

Edom, F., V. Mouly, J. P. Barbet, M. Y. Fiszman, and G. S. Butler-Browne. 1994. Clones of human satellite cells can express *in vitro* both fast and slow myosin heavy chains. *Dev Biol* no. 164 (1):219–29.

Ewton, D. Z., S. L. Roof, K. A. Magri, F. J. McWade, and J. R. Florini. 1994. IGF-II is more active than IGF-I in stimulating L6A1 myogenesis: Greater mitogenic actions of IGF-I delay differentiation. *J Cell Physiol* no. 161 (2):277–84.

Fedorovich, N. E., J. Alblas, J. R. de Wijn, W. E. Hennink, A. J. Verbout, and W. J. Dhert. 2007. Hydrogels as extracellular matrices for skeletal tissue engineering: State-of-the-art and novel application in organ printing. *Tissue Eng* no. 13 (8):1905–25.

Fernandes, S., S. Kuklok, J. McGonigle, H. Reinecke, and C. E. Murry. 2012. Synthetic matrices to serve as niches for muscle cell transplantation. *Cells Tissues Organs* no. 195 (1–2):48–59.

Filareto, A., S. Parker, R. Darabi, L. Borges, M. Iacovino, T. Schaaf, T. Mayerhofer et al. 2013. An ex vivo gene therapy approach to treat muscular dystrophy using inducible pluripotent stem cells. *Nat Commun* no. 4:1549.

Fiore, F., A. Sebille, and D. Birnbaum. 2000. Skeletal muscle regeneration is not impaired in Fgf6$^{-/-}$ mutant mice. *Biochem Biophys Res Commun* no. 272 (1):138–43.

Fishman, J. M., A. Tyraskis, P. Maghsoudlou, L. Urbani, G. Totonelli, M. A. Birchall, and P. De Coppi. 2013. Skeletal muscle tissue engineering: Which cell to use? *Tissue Eng Part B Rev* no. 19 (6):503–15.

Florini, J. R., D. Z. Ewton, and S. A. Coolican. 1996. Growth hormone and the insulin-like growth factor system in myogenesis. *Endocr Rev* no. 17 (5):481–517.

Floss, T., H. H. Arnold, and T. Braun. 1997. A role for FGF-6 in skeletal muscle regeneration. *Genes Dev* no. 11 (16):2040–51.

Fuoco, C., R. Rizzi, A. Biondo, E. Longa, A. Mascaro, K. Shapira-Schweitzer, O. Kossovar et al. 2015. *In vivo* generation of a mature and functional artificial skeletal muscle. *EMBO Mol Med* no. 7 (4):411–22.

Fuoco, C., M. L. Salvatori, A. Biondo, K. Shapira-Schweitzer, S. Santoleri, S. Antonini, S. Bernardini et al. 2012. Injectable polyethylene glycol-fibrinogen hydrogel adjuvant improves survival and differentiation of transplanted mesoangioblasts in acute and chronic skeletal-muscle degeneration. *Skelet Muscle* no. 2 (1):24.

Furberg, C. D. and B. Pitt. 2001. Withdrawal of cerivastatin from the world market. *Curr Control Trials Cardiovasc Med* no. 2 (5):205–7.

Gaster, M., S. R. Kristensen, H. Beck-Nielsen, and H. D. Schroder. 2001. A cellular model system of differentiated human myotubes. *APMIS* no. 109 (11):735–44.

Gaster, M., P. Poulsen, A. Handberg, H. D. Schroder, and H. Beck-Nielsen. 2000. Direct evidence of fiber type-dependent GLUT-4 expression in human skeletal muscle. *Am J Physiol: Endocrinol Metab* no. 278 (5):E910–6.

Gillies, A. R. and R. L. Lieber. 2011. Structure and function of the skeletal muscle extracellular matrix. *Muscle Nerve* no. 44 (3):318–31.

Goldspink, D. F., V. M. Cox, S. K. Smith, L. A. Eaves, N. J. Osbaldeston, D. M. Lee, and D. Mantle. 1995. Muscle growth in response to mechanical stimuli. *Am J Physiol* no. 268 (2 Pt 1):E288–97.

Gore, A., Z. Li, H. L. Fung, J. E. Young, S. Agarwal, J. Antosiewicz-Bourget, I. Canto et al. 2011. Somatic coding mutations in human induced pluripotent stem cells. *Nature* no. 471 (7336):63–7.

Grassl, E. D., T. R. Oegema, and R. T. Tranquillo. 2002. Fibrin as an alternative biopolymer to type-I collagen for the fabrication of a media equivalent. *J Biomed Mater Res* no. 60 (4):607–12.

Guo, X., M. Gonzalez, M. Stancescu, H. H. Vandenburgh, and J. J. Hickman. 2011. Neuromuscular junction formation between human stem cell-derived motoneurons and human skeletal muscle in a defined system. *Biomaterials* no. 32 (36):9602–11.

Hanke, N., J. D. Meissner, R. J. Scheibe, V. Endeward, G. Gros, and H. P. Kubis. 2008. Metabolic transformation of rabbit skeletal muscle cells in primary culture in response to low glucose. *Biochim Biophys Acta* no. 1783 (5):813–25.

Henry, R. R., L. Abrams, S. Nikoulina, and T. P. Ciaraldi. 1995. Insulin action and glucose metabolism in nondiabetic control and NIDDM subjects. Comparison using human skeletal muscle cell cultures. *Diabetes* no. 44 (8):936–46.

Herberts, C. A., M. S. Kwa, and H. P. Hermsen. 2011. Risk factors in the development of stem cell therapy. *J Transl Med* no. 9:29.

Herrick, S., O. Blanc-Brude, A. Gray, and G. Laurent. 1999. Fibrinogen. *Int J Biochem Cell Biol* no. 31 (7):741–6.

Hinds, S., W. Bian, R. G. Dennis, and N. Bursac. 2011. The role of extracellular matrix composition in structure and function of bioengineered skeletal muscle. *Biomaterials* no. 32 (14):3575–83.

Hou, P., Y. Li, X. Zhang, C. Liu, J. Guan, H. Li, T. Zhao et al. 2013. Pluripotent stem cells induced from mouse somatic cells by small-molecule compounds. *Science* no. 341 (6146):651–4.

Huang, Y. C., R. G. Dennis, L. Larkin, and K. Baar. 2005. Rapid formation of functional muscle *in vitro* using fibrin gels. *J Appl Physiol (1985)* no. 98 (2):706–13.

Hurley, M. S., C. Flux, A. M. Salter, and J. M. Brameld. 2006. Effects of fatty acids on skeletal muscle cell differentiation *in vitro*. *Br J Nutr* no. 95 (3):623–30.

Juhas, M. and N. Bursac. 2014. Roles of adherent myogenic cells and dynamic culture in engineered muscle function and maintenance of satellite cells. *Biomaterials* no. 35 (35):9438–46.

Juhas, M., G. C. Engelmayr, Jr., A. N. Fontanella, G. M. Palmer, and N. Bursac. 2014. Biomimetic engineered muscle with capacity for vascular integration and functional maturation *in vivo*. *Proc Natl Acad Sci USA* no. 111 (15):5508–13.

Kelley, D. E., M. Mokan, J. A. Simoneau, and L. J. Mandarino. 1993. Interaction between glucose and free fatty acid metabolism in human skeletal muscle. *J Clin Invest* no. 92 (1):91–8.

Khodabukus, A. and K. Baar. 2015. Glucose concentration and streptomycin alter *in vitro* muscle function and metabolism. *J Cell Physiol* no. 230 (6):1226–34.

Khodabukus, A., L. M. Baehr, S. C. Bodine, and K. Baar. 2015. Role of contraction duration in inducing fast-to-slow contractile and metabolic protein and functional changes in engineered muscle. *J Cell Physiol* no. 230 (10):2489–97.

Klip, A., T. Tsakiridis, A. Marette, and P. A. Ortiz. 1994. Regulation of expression of glucose transporters by glucose: A review of studies *in vivo* and in cell cultures. *FASEB J* no. 8 (1):43–53.

Kraegen, E. W., J. A. Sowden, M. B. Halstead, P. W. Clark, K. J. Rodnick, D. J. Chisholm, and D. E. James. 1993. Glucose transporters and *in vivo* glucose uptake in skeletal and cardiac muscle: Fasting, insulin stimulation and immunoisolation studies of GLUT1 and GLUT4. *Biochem J* no. 295 (Pt 1):287–93.

Kubis, H. P., R. J. Scheibe, J. D. Meissner, G. Hornung, and G. Gros. 2002. Fast-to-slow transformation and nuclear import/export kinetics of the transcription factor NFATc1 during electrostimulation of rabbit muscle cells in culture. *J Physiol* no. 541 (Pt 3):835–47.

Kuhl, U., M. Ocalan, R. Timpl, R. Mayne, E. Hay, and K. von der Mark. 1984. Role of muscle fibroblasts in the deposition of type-IV collagen in the basal lamina of myotubes. *Differentiation* no. 28 (2):164–72.

Lam, M. T., Y. C. Huang, R. K. Birla, and S. Takayama. 2009. Microfeature guided skeletal muscle tissue engineering for highly organized 3-dimensional free-standing constructs. *Biomaterials* no. 30 (6):1150–5.

Lee, P. H. and H. H. Vandenburgh. 2013. Skeletal muscle atrophy in bioengineered skeletal muscle: A new model system. *Tissue Eng Part A* no. 19 (19–20):2147–55.

Lefaucheur, J. P. and A. Sebille. 1995. Basic fibroblast growth factor promotes *in vivo* muscle regeneration in murine muscular dystrophy. *Neurosci Lett* no. 202 (1–2):121–4.

Le Grand, F. and M. A. Rudnicki. 2007. Skeletal muscle satellite cells and adult myogenesis. *Curr Opin Cell Biol* no. 19 (6):628–33.

Levenberg, S., J. Rouwkema, M. Macdonald, E. S. Garfein, D. S. Kohane, D. C. Darland, R. Marini et al. 2005. Engineering vascularized skeletal muscle tissue. *Nat Biotechnol* no. 23 (7):879–84.

Liao, H. and G. Q. Zhou. 2009. Development and progress of engineering of skeletal muscle tissue. *Tissue Eng Part B Rev* no. 15 (3):319–31.

Lister, R., M. Pelizzola, Y. S. Kida, R. D. Hawkins, J. R. Nery, G. Hon, J. Antosiewicz-Bourget et al. 2011. Hotspots of aberrant epigenomic reprogramming in human induced pluripotent stem cells. *Nature* no. 471 (7336):68–73.

Liu, L., T. H. Cheung, G. W. Charville, and T. A. Rando. 2015. Isolation of skeletal muscle stem cells by fluorescence-activated cell sorting. *Nat Protoc* no. 10 (10):1612–24.

Lovett, M., K. Lee, A. Edwards, and D. L. Kaplan. 2009. Vascularization strategies for tissue engineering. *Tissue Eng Part B Rev* no. 15 (3):353–70.

Lu, Y., J. Shansky, M. Del Tatto, P. Ferland, X. Wang, and H. Vandenburgh. 2001. Recombinant vascular endothelial growth factor secreted from tissue-engineered bioartificial muscles promotes localized angiogenesis. *Circulation* no. 104 (5):594–9.

Lutolf, M. P. and J. A. Hubbell. 2005. Synthetic biomaterials as instructive extracellular microenvironments for morphogenesis in tissue engineering. *Nat Biotechnol* no. 23 (1):47–55.

Macpherson, P. C., X. Wang, and D. Goldman. 2011. Myogenin regulates denervation-dependent muscle atrophy in mouse soleus muscle. *J Cell Biochem* no. 112 (8):2149–59.

Madden, L., M. Juhas, W. E. Kraus, G. A. Truskey, and N. Bursac. 2015. Bioengineered human myobundles mimic clinical responses of skeletal muscle to drugs. *eLife* no. 4:e04885.

Manzoni, M. and M. Rollini. 2002. Biosynthesis and biotechnological production of statins by filamentous fungi and application of these cholesterol-lowering drugs. *Appl Microbiol Biotechnol* no. 58 (5):555–64.

Martin, N. R., S. L. Passey, D. J. Player, V. Mudera, K. Baar, L. Greensmith, and M. P. Lewis. 2015. Neuromuscular Junction Formation in Tissue-Engineered Skeletal Muscle Augments Contractile Function and Improves Cytoskeletal Organization. *Tissue Eng Part A* no. 21 (19–20):2595–604.

Martino, M. M., P. S. Briquez, A. Ranga, M. P. Lutolf, and J. A. Hubbell. 2013. Heparin-binding domain of fibrin(ogen) binds growth factors and promotes tissue repair when incorporated within a synthetic matrix. *Proc Natl Acad Sci U S A* no. 110 (12):4563–8.

Mayshar, Y., U. Ben-David, N. Lavon, J. C. Biancotti, B. Yakir, A. T. Clark, K. Plath, W. E. Lowry, and N. Benvenisty. 2010. Identification and classification of chromosomal aberrations in human induced pluripotent stem cells. *Cell Stem Cell* no. 7 (4):521–31.

Mendias, C. L., J. E. Marcin, D. R. Calerdon, and J. A. Faulkner. 2006. Contractile properties of EDL and soleus muscles of myostatin-deficient mice. *J Appl Physiol (1985)* no. 101 (3):898–905.

Meng, Y., S. Eshghi, Y. J. Li, R. Schmidt, D. V. Schaffer, and K. E. Healy. 2010. Characterization of integrin engagement during defined human embryonic stem cell culture. *FASEB J* no. 24 (4):1056–65.

Merrick, D., H. C. Chen, D. Larner, and J. Smith. 2010. Adult and embryonic skeletal muscle microexplant culture and isolation of skeletal muscle stem cells. *J Vis Exp* (43):e2051. doi: 10.3791/2051.

Mestas, J. and C. C. Hughes. 2004. Of mice and not men: Differences between mouse and human immunology. *J Immunol* no. 172 (5):2731–8.

Montarras, D., J. Morgan, C. Collins, F. Relaix, S. Zaffran, A. Cumano, T. Partridge, and M. Buckingham. 2005. Direct isolation of satellite cells for skeletal muscle regeneration. *Science* no. 309 (5743):2064–7.

Olsson, K., A. J. Cheng, S. Alam, M. Al-Ameri, E. Rullman, H. Westerblad, J. T. Lanner, J. D. Bruton, and T. Gustafsson. 2015. Intracellular Ca(2+)-handling differs markedly between intact human muscle fibers and myotubes. *Skelet Muscle* no. 5:26.

Owens, J., K. Moreira, and G. Bain. 2013. Characterization of primary human skeletal muscle cells from multiple commercial sources. *In Vitro Cell Dev Biol Anim* no. 49 (9):695–705.

Pampaloni, F., E. G. Reynaud, and E. H. Stelzer. 2007. The third dimension bridges the gap between cell culture and live tissue. *Nat Rev Mol Cell Biol* no. 8 (10):839–45.

Pasut, A., P. Oleynik, and M. A. Rudnicki. 2012. Isolation of muscle stem cells by fluorescence activated cell sorting cytometry. *Methods Mol Biol* no. 798:53–64.

Pennisi, C. P., C. G. Olesen, M. de Zee, J. Rasmussen, and V. Zachar. 2011. Uniaxial cyclic strain drives assembly and differentiation of skeletal myocytes. *Tissue Eng Part A* no. 17 (19–20):2543–50.

Perniconi, B., A. Costa, P. Aulino, L. Teodori, S. Adamo, and D. Coletti. 2011. The promyogenic environment provided by whole organ scale acellular scaffolds from skeletal muscle. *Biomaterials* no. 32 (31):7870–82.

Porzionato, A., M. M. Sfriso, A. Pontini, V. Macchi, L. Petrelli, P. G. Pavan, A. N. Natali, F. Bassetto, V. Vindigni, and R. De Caro. 2015. Decellularized human skeletal muscle as biologic scaffold for reconstructive surgery. *Int J Mol Sci* no. 16 (7):14808–31.

Powell, C. A., B. L. Smiley, J. Mills, and H. H. Vandenburgh. 2002. Mechanical stimulation improves tissue-engineered human skeletal muscle. *Am J Physiol: Cell Physiol* no. 283 (5):C1557–65.

Rando, T. A. and H. M. Blau. 1994. Primary mouse myoblast purification, characterization, and transplantation for cell-mediated gene therapy. *J Cell Biol* no. 125 (6):1275–87.

Rhim, C., C. S. Cheng, W. E. Kraus, and G. A. Truskey. 2010. Effect of microRNA modulation on bioartificial muscle function. *Tissue Eng Part A* no. 16 (12):3589–97.

Rhim, C., D. A. Lowell, M. C. Reedy, D. H. Slentz, S. J. Zhang, W. E. Kraus, and G. A. Truskey. 2007. Morphology and ultrastructure of differentiating three-dimensional mammalian skeletal muscle in a collagen gel. *Muscle Nerve* no. 36 (1):71–80.

Richler, C. and D. Yaffe. 1970. The *in vitro* cultivation and differentiation capacities of myogenic cell lines. *Dev Biol* no. 23 (1):1–22.

Rizzi, R., C. Bearzi, A. Mauretti, S. Bernardini, S. Cannata, and C. Gargioli. 2012. Tissue engineering for skeletal muscle regeneration. *Muscles Ligaments Tendons J* no. 2 (3):230–4.

Salehi-Nik, N., G. Amoabediny, B. Pouran, H. Tabesh, M. A. Shokrgozar, N. Haghighipour, N. Khatibi, F. Anisi, K. Mottaghy, and B. Zandieh-Doulabi. 2013. Engineering parameters in bioreactor's design: A critical aspect in tissue engineering. *Biomed Res Int* no. 2013:762132.

Salimath, A. S. and A. J. Garcia. 2014. Biofunctional hydrogels for skeletal muscle constructs. *J Tissue Eng Regen Med* 10:967–76.

Sanes, J. R. 2003. The basement membrane/basal lamina of skeletal muscle. *J Biol Chem* no. 278 (15):12601–4.

Sarabia, V., L. Lam, E. Burdett, L. A. Leiter, and A. Klip. 1992. Glucose transport in human skeletal muscle cells in culture. Stimulation by insulin and metformin. *J Clin Invest* no. 90 (4):1386–95.

Sarabia, V., T. Ramlal, and A. Klip. 1990. Glucose uptake in human and animal muscle cells in culture. *Biochem Cell Biol* no. 68 (2):536–42.

Sargeant, T. D., A. P. Desai, S. Banerjee, A. Agawu, and J. B. Stopek. 2012. An *in situ* forming collagen-PEG hydrogel for tissue regeneration. *Acta Biomater* no. 8 (1):124–32.

Schlaeger, T. M., L. Daheron, T. R. Brickler, S. Entwisle, K. Chan, A. Cianci, A. DeVine et al. 2015. A comparison of non-integrating reprogramming methods. *Nat Biotechnol* no. 33 (1):58–63.

Schwenk, R. W., G. P. Holloway, J. J. Luiken, A. Bonen, and J. F. Glatz. 2010. Fatty acid transport across the cell membrane: Regulation by fatty acid transporters. *Prostaglandins Leukot Essent Fatty Acids* no. 82 (4–6):149–54.

Scott, W., J. Stevens, and S. A. Binder-Macleod. 2001. Human skeletal muscle fiber type classifications. *Phys Ther* no. 81 (11):1810–6.

Seliktar, D. 2012. Designing cell-compatible hydrogels for biomedical applications. *Science* no. 336 (6085):1124–8.

Seok, J., H. S. Warren, A. G. Cuenca, M. N. Mindrinos, H. V. Baker, W. Xu, D. R. Richards et al. 2013. Genomic responses in mouse models poorly mimic human inflammatory diseases. *Proc Natl Acad Sci USA* no. 110 (9):3507–12.

Shansky, J., M. Del Tatto, J. Chromiak, and H. Vandenburgh. 1997. A simplified method for tissue engineering skeletal muscle organoids *in vitro*. *In Vitro Cell Dev Biol Anim* no. 33 (9):659–61.

Staerk, J., M. M. Dawlaty, Q. Gao, D. Maetzel, J. Hanna, C. A. Sommer, G. Mostoslavsky, and R. Jaenisch. 2010. Reprogramming of human peripheral blood cells to induced pluripotent stem cells. *Cell Stem Cell* no. 7 (1):20–4.

Staffa, J. A., J. Chang, and L. Green. 2002. Cerivastatin and reports of fatal rhabdomyolysis. *N Engl J Med* no. 346 (7):539–40.

Strohman, R. C., E. Bayne, D. Spector, T. Obinata, J. Micou-Eastwood, and A. Maniotis. 1990. Myogenesis and histogenesis of skeletal muscle on flexible membranes *in vitro*. *In Vitro Cell Dev Biol* no. 26 (2):201–8.

Stuart, C. A., G. Wen, W. C. Gustafson, and E. A. Thompson. 2000. Comparison of GLUT1, GLUT3, and GLUT4 mRNA and the subcellular distribution of their proteins in normal human muscle. *Metabolism* no. 49 (12):1604–9.

Swasdison, S. and R. Mayne. 1992. Formation of highly organized skeletal muscle fibers *in vitro*. Comparison with muscle development *in vivo*. *J Cell Sci* no. 102 (Pt 3):643–52.

Takahashi, K., K. Tanabe, M. Ohnuki, M. Narita, T. Ichisaka, K. Tomoda, and S. Yamanaka. 2007. Induction of pluripotent stem cells from adult human fibroblasts by defined factors. *Cell* no. 131 (5):861–72.

Tanaka, A., K. Woltjen, K. Miyake, A. Hotta, M. Ikeya, T. Yamamoto, T. Nishino et al. 2013. Efficient and reproducible myogenic differentiation from human iPS cells: Prospects for modeling Miyoshi Myopathy *in vitro*. *PLoS One* no. 8 (4):e61540.

Truskey, G. A., H. E. Achneck, N. Bursac, H. Chan, C. S. Cheng, C. Fernandez, S. Hong et al. 2013. Design considerations for an integrated microphysiological muscle tissue for drug and tissue toxicity testing. *Stem Cell Res Ther* no. 4 (Suppl 1):S10.

Urbanchek, M. G., E. B. Picken, L. K. Kalliainen, and W. M. Kuzon, Jr. 2001. Specific force deficit in skeletal muscles of old rats is partially explained by the existence of denervated muscle fibers. *J Gerontol A Biol Sci Med Sci* no. 56 (5):B191–7.

Velleman, S. G. 1999. The role of the extracellular matrix in skeletal muscle development. *Poult Sci* no. 78 (5):778–84.

von Keutz, E. and G. Schluter. 1998. Preclinical safety evaluation of cerivastatin, a novel HMG-CoA reductase inhibitor. *Am J Cardiol* no. 82 (4b):11j–7j.

Voytik, S. L., M. Przyborski, S. F. Badylak, and S. F. Konieczny. 1993. Differential expression of muscle regulatory factor genes in normal and denervated adult rat hindlimb muscles. *Dev Dyn* no. 198 (3):214–24.

Wilson, S. J. and A. J. Harris. 1993. Formation of myotubes in aneural rat muscles. *Dev Biol* no. 156 (2):509–18.

Wolf, M. T., K. A. Daly, J. E. Reing, and S. F. Badylak. 2012. Biologic scaffold composed of skeletal muscle extracellular matrix. *Biomaterials* no. 33 (10):2916–25.

Yablonka-Reuveni, Z. 1988. Discrimination of myogenic and nonmyogenic cells from embryonic skeletal muscle by 90 degrees light scattering. *Cytometry* no. 9 (2):121–5.

Yablonka-Reuveni, Z., R. Seger, and A. J. Rivera. 1999. Fibroblast growth factor promotes recruitment of skeletal muscle satellite cells in young and old rats. *J Histochem Cytochem* no. 47 (1):23–42.

Yamamoto, Y., A. Ito, H. Fujita, E. Nagamori, Y. Kawabe, and M. Kamihira. 2011. Functional evaluation of artificial skeletal muscle tissue constructs fabricated by a magnetic force-based tissue engineering technique. *Tissue Eng Part A* no. 17 (1–2):107–14.

Zhu, J. and R. E. Marchant. 2011. Design properties of hydrogel tissue-engineering scaffolds. *Expert Rev Med Devices* no. 8 (5):607–26.

Zierath, J. R., D. Galuska, L. A. Nolte, A. Thorne, J. S. Kristensen, and H. Wallberg-Henriksson. 1994. Effects of glycaemia on glucose transport in isolated skeletal muscle from patients with NIDDM: *In vitro* reversal of muscular insulin resistance. *Diabetologia* no. 37 (3):270–7.

Zierath, J. R., L. He, A. Guma, E. Odegoard Wahlstrom, A. Klip, and H. Wallberg-Henriksson. 1996. Insulin action on glucose transport and plasma membrane GLUT4 content in skeletal muscle from patients with NIDDM. *Diabetologia* no. 39 (10):1180–9.

19 Recapitulating the Microenvironment of Glioblastoma Multiforme Using 3D Tissue Culture Models

Meghan Logun, Steven Stice, and Lohitash Karumbaiah

CONTENTS

19.1	Introduction	351
19.2	Glioblastomas	352
19.3	The Brain Extracellular Matrix (ECM)	353
19.4	Tumor Cell Invasion	355
19.5	Angiogenesis	356
19.6	The Cancer Stem Cell Hypothesis	358
19.7	GBM Treatment Paradigms	359
19.8	Current 2D and 3D Models of Brain Tumor Invasion	361
19.9	Future Design of 3D Models to Study Brain Tumor Invasion	364
19.10	Conclusion and Perspective	367
References		367

19.1 INTRODUCTION

In the realm of malignant cancers, brain tumors are among the most destructive (Ostrom et al. 2014). Brain tumors account for approximately 3% of new cancer cases in adults and almost 25% of new cancers found in children (Butowski 2015). Brain cancers are unique from other bodily neoplasms, notably in location and behavior. While cancers grow and metastasize from the original organ or tissue once malignant, primary brain tumors remain confined to the central nervous system (CNS) where they continue to grow and expand (Kleihues and Sobin 2000). Eventually, brain tumors outgrow the limited space in the brain and disturb other precious structures, thus rendering cognitive and motor processes damaged.

Brain tumors can arise from different types of cells in the brain and spinal cord. Roughly, one-third of these are gliomas, tumors originating from support cells known as glial cells (Ostrom et al. 2014). Disruption to the p53 and Rb signaling pathways is common in high-grade gliomas, which allows cells to evade apoptosis or growth inhibition (Collins 1999; Rasheed et al. 1999; Rathore et al. 1999). Aberrant cells could also avoid growth restrictions due to overactive telomerase activity or from alterations in the Ras growth factor mediation pathway (Feldkamp et al. 1999; Sano et al. 1998). Gliomas are commonly classified as either astrocytic or oligodendroglial (Ostrom et al. 2014). Astrocytomas specifically arise from the star-shaped astrocytes that contribute to connective tissue and blood–brain barrier (BBB) for the protection of the brain, and they are graded by both the degree of abnormality in tissue (I-IV) and the rate of growth (low grade or high grade) (Huttner 2012; Marquet et al. 2007; Romeike 2007). A grade I glioma would be considered benign and treated with surgical resection, but a grade III glioma or higher would be considered malignant. These anaplastic tumors typically express heightened mitotic activity and include cells of various shapes and sizes, but do not show signs of necrosis or vascularization (Castillo et al. 2000). The most malignant form of astrocytoma is glioblastoma multiforme (GBM, grade IV), which is distinguished by the presence of necrosis and blood vessel formation around the tumor.

19.2 GLIOBLASTOMAS

GBM accounts for the majority of malignant gliomas diagnosed in the United States, most commonly in men ages 45–65 (Ostrom et al. 2014). *De novo* GBM (primary tumors) are more common and expand more rapidly than the secondary GBM, which begin as low or mid-grade astrocytomas before transforming into their more malignant counterparts (Biernat et al. 1997). Glioma cells invade in a path through the brain referred to as "Scherer's structures," moving from the brain parenchyma and following existing blood vessels across white matter tracts outward, toward the subarachnoid space in the meninges of the brain (Cuddapah et al. 2014). Ultimately, this spread of individual cells allows the tumor to penetrate essential brain regions and form multiple GBM masses, referred to as "multicentric GBM" (Batzdorf and Malamud 1963). As a result, multiple resection surgeries are often required to remove the infiltrating and recurring cell masses, which ultimately leads to disability, and eventually the death of the patient.

GBM has a large number of proliferating cells at all times, and this proliferation is supplemented by local blood supply. Due to a rapid cell turnover, there is usually a collection of necrotic cells in the center of the tumor mass, which is another signal of high-grade GBM rather than mid-grade astrocytoma (Barker et al. 1996). Due to the rapid growth of these brain cancers, the most common physical symptoms include a build-up of pressure within the brain cavity along with other impairments in brain areas that control coordination and processing. GBM is extremely difficult to treat depending on the location or size of the tumor mass, and complete surgical resection is rarely successful due to nonuniform boundaries, cellular heterogeneity, and attachments to critical brain areas (Figure 19.1). Chemotherapy treatments can be used within treatment plans alone, post-surgery, or concurrently with radiation therapy depending on the best method to approach the type and location of the tumor. Unfortunately, gliomas have the tendency to recur locally after treatment or resection, making these tumors extremely hard to treat (Wakimoto et al. 2009) (Figure 19.1).

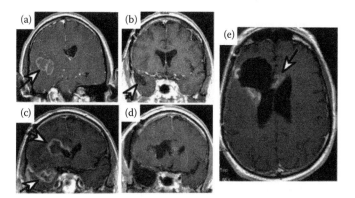

FIGURE 19.1 MRI scans of a GBM patient showing recurrence of the tumor after tumor resection. (a) Pre-surgery scan. (b) Post-surgery scan after gross total resection and radiation therapy, no tumor to be seen. (c) Six months after surgery and therapy, tumor returned at resection margin and with a second tumor mass at the Sylvian fissure of frontal lobe. (d) Scan after another resection, this time removing both tumor bodies. (e) Scan demonstrating recurrence at the resection margin and with migration across the corpus callosum. (Reprinted from previous publication Holland, E. C. 2000. *Proc Natl Acad Sci USA* no. 97 (12):6242–44, Copyright [2000], with permission National Academy of Sciences, USA.)

19.3 THE BRAIN EXTRACELLULAR MATRIX (ECM)

The brain microenvironment is a tightly controlled milieu of glia, cytokines, chemokines, catecholamines, and growth factors in which cells migrate, proliferate, and differentiate (Entschladen et al. 2005). The ECM of the CNS constitutes approximately 10%–20% of total brain volume (Nicholson and Sykova 1998). These extracellular components provide support to the brain cells and a means of communication between cells (Ou and Hosseinkhani 2014). Brain ECM can be divided into three components: The basement membrane, the perineuronal nets, and the neural interstitial matrix (Figure 19.2). The basement membrane is a region of tissue between cerebral blood vessels and the rest of the brain's connective tissue. This membrane connects with astrocytes to form the BBB (Lau et al. 2013). The basal lamina is the layer of ECM secreted by epithelial cells composed of type IV collagen, fibronectin, and laminin (Lau et al. 2013). Tight junctions between the basement membrane to pericytes and astrocytes control the BBB, preventing the passage of macromolecules. The presence of pericytes around blood vessels is thought to regulate endothelial cell proliferation and survival (Hellstrom et al. 2001). Outside of the basement membrane are the perineuronal nets which protect interneuron synapses and neuroplasticity and become more rigid over time postdevelopment (Hensch 2005). Perineuronal nets are composed of chondroitin-sulfate proteoglycans (CSPGs), tenascin R, and hyaluronan, and they form large cartilaginous agglomerates around neuron cell bodies (Deepa et al. 2006; Koppe et al. 1997). The remaining components of brain ECM make up the interstitial matrix, including CSPGs, tenascin R, and fibrous proteins (Figure 19.2). In healthy brain parenchyma, hyaluronic acid and CSPGs make up the majority of ECM along with laminin, collagen IV, and fibronectin (Giordana et al.

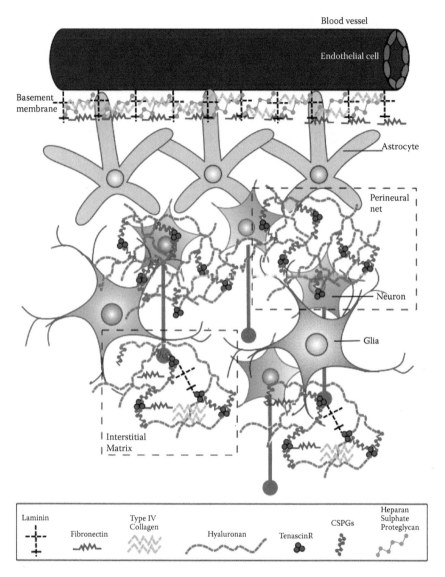

FIGURE 19.2 Components of the brain ECM. The ECM has three main elements: the basement membrane that lines blood vessels and astrocytic feet, the dense perineuronal nets around neurons, and the looser interstitial matrix. (Adapted from previous publication Lau, L. W. et al. 2013. *Nat Rev Neurosci* no. 14 (10):722–29.)

1985; Rutka et al. 1988). CSPGs are negatively charged glycosylated proteins vital to the brain ECM, with the hyaluronic acid-binding group of lecticans being particularly abundant in brain tissues (Ruoslahti 1996). Hyaluronic acid is a long unsulfated glycosaminoglycan (GAG) that noncovalently recruits other GAGs and proteoglycans for attachment, and has been implicated in cell proliferation and cytoskeletal reorganization (Bourguignon et al. 1997; Oliferenko et al. 2000; Toole 2001). Brain

ECM molecules play a tightly controlled role in cell migration through development, and aberrant ECM can directly promote cancer cell metastasis and contribute to abnormal angiogenesis (Cox and Erler 2011).

The ECM around GBM becomes dense with more fibrillar collagens than healthy brain ECM, especially around the basement membrane of surrounding blood vessels (Huijbers et al. 2010). Healthy brain tissue has a relatively soft ECM (elastic modulus of 0.5–1 kPa) with areas of increased rigidity around white matter tracts (Miller et al. 2000). Gliomas have been found to prefer tissue with increased stiffness and are known to degrade unwanted ECM components to better suit their needs (Ulrich et al. 2009). This remodeling can be accomplished by the secretion of matrix metalloproteinases (MMPs), which are enzymes involved in tissue modification and are known to be employed by glioma cells (Wiranowska et al. 2000). Cathepsin B and urokinase plasminogen activator proteases have also been more recently implicated in the glioma expression and contribute to the breakdown of neural connective tissue (Lakka and Rao 2008; Rao 2003). MMPs are also involved in growth factor signaling, inflammation response, apoptosis, angiogenesis, and the formation of the tumor metastatic niche (Kessenbrock et al. 2010). ECM turnover begins with the activation of MMP-2, MMP-9, and membrane type I metalloproteinase 1 (MT1-MMP) (Forsyth et al. 1999). These MMPs degrade surrounding ECM, destroying the natural organization of the matrix and boundaries of healthy brain tissue (Koul et al. 2001). GBM invades preferentially along white matter tracts, using MMPs to proteolytically degrade ECM collagen, laminin, and fibronectin in their path (Artym et al. 2006).

19.4 TUMOR CELL INVASION

Malignant tumors are dynamic, and the individual tumor cells are constantly adapting to the environment depending on where they are located around the peritumoral rim (Berens and Giese 1999). The onset of GBM invasion is marked by excessive proliferation in cell number and volume. GBM tumors are marked by a necrotic core and vascular hyperplasia, both indicating accelerated growth and poor prognosis for the patient (Daumas-Duport et al. 1988). This accelerated tumor growth eventually leads to hypoxia and the formation of pseudopalisades. Pseudopalisades are hypercellular regions surrounding necrotic foci and secrete proangiogenic factors required for the formation of new vasculature to feed the growing needs of the tumor (Brat et al. 2002, 2004). Rapid growth creates an increasingly hypoxic tumor environment due to constraints on local blood supply, prompting a metabolic change toward glycolysis within the tumor cells and enhancing tumor cell invasion (Keunen et al. 2011). Necrotic and hypoxic regions cluster in the GBM core and around the tumoral rim, while angiogenic areas form on the periphery (Brat and Van Meir 2001; Straume et al. 2002). Late stage gliomas consist of a necrotic core on the inside with angiogenic glomeruloid bodies on the periphery, which triggers a shift toward enabling outward growth and migration away from the central tumor core.

The microvascular hyperplasia on the tumor edge enables outward growth by individual migrating cells. Conventionally, individual tumor cells leave the primary tumor and enter blood vessels to move and give rise to new tumor masses in distant organs (Friedl and Wolf 2003). *De novo* brain tumors invade diffusely as single cells, preferring to move along blood vessels and white matter tracts but not invading into the blood vessel walls (Esiri 2000). At this stage, tumor cells down regulate proliferation and resist apoptosis to devote resources toward migration from the center mass, even changing morphology if necessary to facilitate movement (Giese et al. 2003; Lauffenburger and Horwitz 1996).

Chemotactic cues stimulate the projection of the cell membrane, driving local actin polymerization to form focal contacts in the ECM of tissue. Fortification of focal contacts leads to attachment to ECM molecules, but lessened adhesion pushes migration onward (Palecek et al. 1997; Yamaguchi et al. 2005). Chemical stimulants have varying effects on downstream signaling cascades, including receptor tyrosine kinase activation, which has direct effects on focal adhesion kinase (FAK) complex formation (Steeg 2006). FAK is necessary for stable focal contacts between cells and ECM and acts as the effector to couple integrin–ECM interactions with intracellular signaling (Wang et al. 2000). Once the cell responds to pro-migratory environmental signals, it will lose its cell contacts and begin movement through the surrounding connective tissue (Thiery 2002). Connective tissue cancers, including GBM, participate in mesenchymal movement to disperse from the primary tumor mass (Friedl and Wolf 2003; Paulus et al. 1996). Classic mesenchymal migration involves the polarization of the cell membrane in the direction of movement, splitting the cell into leading and trailing edges (Zhong et al. 2010). The cell's leading pseudopodium will remodel focal adhesions and secrete MMPs to degrade local ECM components, while the trailing edge of the cell will detach remaining focal adhesions (Demuth and Berens 2004; Friedl and Wolf 2003; Zhong et al. 2010). Cell movement leaves a trail of deficits through ECM, as the tumor cell body gains in momentum and volume (Friedl and Wolf 2003). Tumor cell invasion is marked by a change in the cadherin expression and recruitment of proteases to clear a path through the ECM for the cells to move (Friedl and Wolf 2003). Degradation of ECM results in proteases releasing local growth factors and chemokines that stimulate cell motility and invasion (Folgueras et al. 2004).

19.5 ANGIOGENESIS

The growth of CNS tumors within the brain requires a steady supply of oxygen and nutrients found in the blood stream. The best way for a rapidly growing tumor to avail of this energy source is to create its own (Bao et al. 2006b). Malignant gliomas recruit native blood vessels, causing the expression of angiogenesis regulator angiopoietin-2 by the endothelial cells to trigger cellular apoptosis and hypoxic conditions in the brain (Fischer et al. 2005). Invasive gliomas display excessive angiogenesis along with an increased expression of vascular endothelial growth factors (VEGFs) that work to increase blood vessel formation (Bao et al. 2006b; Plate et al. 1992, 1994) (Figure 19.3). VEGFs are proteins expressed by cells that bind to transmembrane receptors on endothelial cells to encourage cell proliferation, migration, and viability (Hatva et al. 1995). VEGF-encoding genes are upregulated by transcription factors such as hypoxia inducible factor-1 (HIF-1), which is activated under low-oxygen conditions for the cells (Zagzag et al. 2000). GBM pseudopalisades express high levels of VEGF and HIF-1 and -2 (Brat et al. 2004; Shweiki et al. 1992; Zagzag

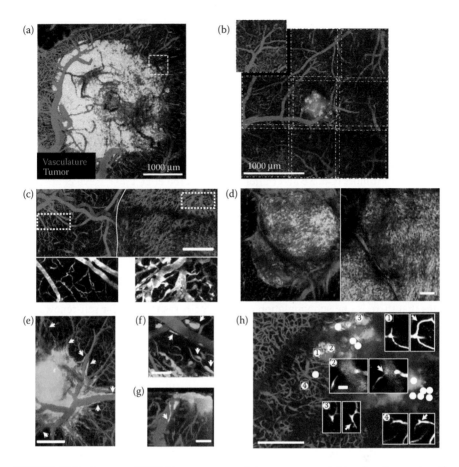

FIGURE 19.3 Images of GBM tumor xenograft in a mouse model to view tumor growth and angiogenesis. (a) Gross image of tumor under 20× Water Immersion objective. (b) Stitched images used for quantifications within the study. (c) Images showing distinction between healthy vasculature on the left and the swollen blood vessels within tumor tissue on the right. (d) Average vascular density (red) and tumor cell density (green) before and after a 10-day interval. Images from a 25 μm horizontal section of tumor. (e,f) Horizontal mean projection images demonstrating perivascular invasion (arrows). (g) Sagittal 3D projection displaying tumor cells (arrows) migrating into deeper brain regions along a large blood vessel. (h) Mean projection of the area of interest scanned for vascular changes every day. Any changes (white dots) were found within a 150 μm radius from tumor margins. Insets contain examples of microvascular changes (arrows). Scale bars, (a,b): 1 mm; (c,d,h): 300 μm; (f,g): 50 μm; (h insets): 25 μm. (Reprinted with permission from previous publication Ricard, C. et al. 2013. *PLoS One* no. 8 (9):e72655.)

et al. 2008). Pseudopalisading cells contribute to tumor proliferation and angiogenesis through the production of VEGF and directly influence GBM malignancy.

The progression of GBM is difficult to treat or halt through aggressive surgery, radiotherapy, or chemotherapy due in part to the abnormal structure of blood vessels built to feed the tumor (Jain et al. 2007) (Figure 19.3). A low-oxygen environment with high interstitial fluid pressure casts influence toward an aggressively malignant tumor, so certain cancer treatments that attack the cells individually may not be as effective at reducing the tumor as desired (Jain et al. 2007). Looking for treatments that inhibit angiogenesis hold molecular promise, targeting the blood vessels that provide the tumor mass with nutrients and oxygen to grow (Kirsch et al. 2000). However, intratumoral heterogeneity makes targeting any one aspect of GBM very difficult. GBM has marked genomic variability across the tumor mass, expressing fluctuating antigenic signals and growth rates (Bonavia et al. 2011; Furnari et al. 2007; Yung et al. 1982). This observed heterogeneity may be the result of cancer stem cells (CSCs), and their aberrant differentiation creating the mosaic of malignancy seen in brain tumors (Clarke and Fuller 2006; Dalerba et al. 2007; Reya et al. 2001).

19.6 THE CANCER STEM CELL HYPOTHESIS

There are unique properties bestowed upon stem cells: self-renewal, differentiation potential, and extensive proliferation capability (Jordan et al. 2006). Somatic stem cells in a healthy body self-renew and proliferate to repair damaged or aging tissue, using immortal properties to keep tissue fully functional. The theory of CSCs states that there is one subpopulation of tumor cells responsible for self-renewal and tumorigenesis (Visvader and Lindeman 2008). CSCs are similar to normal stem cells, expressing comparable markers and performing the same functions for the tumor. Self-renewal in particular, is useful to cancer cells to facilitate oncogenesis and invasion through the host tissues (Soltysova et al. 2005). CSCs continue to asymmetrically divide, creating a population of more self-renewing CSCs and another population of tumor somatic cells that differentiate into the hallmark heterogeneous tumor mass (Soltysova et al. 2005). CNS CSCs have the ability to form neurospheres, centers of self-renewal for the tumor.

Various studies have attempted to provide evidence of the CSC hypothesis under laboratory conditions without conclusive results, lending to the controversial nature of these ideas (Rosen and Jordan 2009). The induction of a tumor commonly used in rodent models is not adequate to compare it to a human tumor because of fundamental differences in microenvironment and immune response (Rosen and Jordan 2009). A lack of *in vivo* methods to study CSCs is apparent in the debate between the intrinsic and extrinsic models. The intrinsic model suggests that there are certain cancer cells within the tumor which possess stem-cell-like qualities that contribute to the genetic heterogeneity, and the extrinsic model postulates that all tumor cells have equal capabilities but they react in response to the environment to create heterogeneity (Rosen and Jordan 2009). Xenotransplantation studies in mice have demonstrated that the microenvironment and experimental conditions play a role in the propagation of CSCs; however, results from transplantation studies can vary depending on the strain of cancer used and demonstrate that not all cancers need a population of CSCs to grow (Cho and Clarke 2008; Visvader and Lindeman 2008; Zhang et al. 2008). CSCs are found to express genetics similar to neural stem cells, specifically in regard to cell-membrane protein CD133 (Singh et al. 2003, 2004). CD133 is a glycoprotein found in cellular protrusions and has been associated with various progenitor cells and, interestingly, certain cancer cells (Corbeil et al. 2000;

Horn et al. 1999; Sanai et al. 2005; Singh et al. 2003). GBM CSCs have also been found with the abilities to self-renew, differentiate into neurons or glia, and reform spheres after differentiation has begun (Yuan et al. 2004).

Unique aspects of GBM include a high level of cellular heterogeneity and differentiation throughout the tumor, hosting a multitude of different genetic mutations that pose great challenges to targeted cancer treatments (Tabatabai and Weller 2011). The environment and the tumor's needs, beginning with the creation of the tumor perivascular niche, directly affect CSC activity. Stem cells typically take up residence in areas dense with blood vessels, and here these cells switch between self-renewal and cell differentiation among the nutrient-rich vascular niche (Yang and Wechsler-Reya 2007). Brain CSCs form these vascular niches and stay close to capillary structures, secreting proangiogenic factors including VEGFs to rapidly add mass to the growing tumor body (Bao et al. 2006b; Calabrese et al. 2007). Just as the vasculature around the tumor is important, the ECM interactions are also implicated in maintaining that balance between the renewal and maturation of the stem cells. The stem cell niche usually provides inhibitory signals for proliferation and differentiation to prevent tumorigenesis, but mutations in niche elements or in stem cells break that regulatory check on proliferation and allow CSCs to develop self-sufficient properties (Li and Neaves 2006). CSCs inhabit perivascular regions of the tumor where there is enrichment by Notch bioligands and other ECM proteins. These elements work together to remodel the local ECM and vasculature (Bao et al. 2006b; Calabrese et al. 2007; Zhu et al. 2011). GBMs have the ability to remodel their ECMs, adding another dimension to the complexity of invading tumor masses. ECM remodeling contributes to CSC survival, allowing the tumor cells to react to the lack of factors or nutrients needed for self-renewal.

Macrophages and microglia are the primary response mechanisms of the immune system when tissue homeostasis is thrown off balance. The presence of foreign agents immediately prompts the immune cells to begin eliminating the invaders and damaged tissue (de Visser et al. 2006). Chronic inflammation, however, has been implicated in fostering an innate tumorigenic environment because the constantly active immune cells regulate local cell proliferation and can suppress the native antitumor response (de Visser et al. 2006). CSCs also take measures to evade the body's immune response by mediating immunosuppression and forming tumorigenic neurospheres (Galli et al. 2004; Sanai et al. 2005). The ability of GBM to alter immunosuppression poses a massive threat to potential therapies.

19.7 GBM TREATMENT PARADIGMS

Though treatment depends on the type, size, and location of the tumor, the standard of care for patients of GBM has remained constant over years: The first approach is complete surgical resection followed by radiation and chemotherapy to eradicate cells and damage tumor cell DNA (Holland 2000). Various MRIs are done on GBM patients to enhance the view of the tumor, but even these detailed images cannot capture every single cell, and recurrence can be seen as early as six months post-surgery (Holland 2000). Even with the best possible surgical performance and the requisite therapeutic measures afterward, the mean survival of a GBM patient is between a few months to one year (Jelsma and Bucy 1967). Current therapies are too limited to treat the invading cells left behind after resection.

One issue in treating GBM with conventional therapies is the heterogeneous cellular structure of the tumor—an approach that might be successful with treating one subset of cells might not treat another (Holland 2000). Radiation or chemotherapy is commonly used in combination with gross total or subtotal resection where possible, but radiation or chemotherapeutics alone have not proven to effectively reduce the tumor (Meis et al. 1991; Stewart 2002). CSCs expressing high levels of CD133 contribute toward radioresistance by increasing the cellular repair mechanisms for DNA damage, rendering radiation therapies ineffective, and increasing chance of recurrence for the patient (Bao et al. 2006a). The CSC hypothesis credits individual populations of CSCs as the reason for the vast genetic heterogeneity among the tumor cells, but targeting those populations is difficult to do using traditional therapeutic methods. Radiation and chemotherapy are effective at targeting the tumor mass on the larger scale, but when some cancer cells and CSCs are left behind, those individuals go on to reform another tumor with increased resistance capabilities (Cho et al. 2013a). Gamma knife radiosurgery (GKS) is a noninvasive, high-dose radiation therapy technique that targets the tumor when the affected brain area is too delicate or too hard to reach with standard neurosurgery, or if a less invasive approach is needed for the patient (Shamisa et al. 2013). GKS has immediate promising results, but has the potential to promote radiation-induced neoplasia (Elsamadicy et al. 2015; Shamisa et al. 2013).

Anti-angiogenic approaches target VEGF-signaling pathways, and patients usually experience reduced fluid build-up and intracranial pressure (Bergers and Hanahan 2008; Verhoeff et al. 2009). These treatments are founded on the paradigm that the tumor cannot continue growing without the support system of a constant blood supply (Fidler and Ellis 2004; Jain et al. 2007). Though extensive vascularization is a hallmark of GBM and anti-angiogenic drugs seem to reduce the tumor, GBM can circumvent this therapy and continue to show cell migration deeper into the brain from the primary tumor (Verhoeff et al. 2009). Combining anti-angiogenic treatments with chemotherapy drugs has conflicting effects on GBM; tumors create a personalized version of the BBB that contributes to chemotherapeutic resistance, but chemotherapy drugs cannot cross that BBB efficiently without the vasculature around the tumor (Regina et al. 2001; Verhoeff et al. 2009). Chemotherapy has alkylating agents crossing the BBB to induce apoptosis of the alien cells, but tumors can block this action through activity of DNA repair enzyme O-methylguanine-DNA methyltransferase (MGMT), or by upregulating epidermal growth factor receptors to disturb the normal apoptosis response in cells with DNA damage (Sarkaria et al. 2008). Newer strategies look to combine chemotherapeutics with other small molecule drugs to halt tumor invasion and increase patient prognosis (Munson et al. 2012). The addition of a drug targeting cell invasion could lead to a combinatorial treatment for GBM that increases patient survival and stops cell invasion.

Though the cellular mechanisms of cancer growth are certainly important to dissect, the tumor niche is another avenue of research to help elucidate a role for the observed alterations in cell behavior (Lu et al. 2012). The tumor ECM is an active participant in the devolution of normal cell signaling and healthy ECM dynamics (Lu et al. 2012). Certain ECM components can become overexpressed in cancerous tissue, and any changes to ECM biochemical makeup and cytoarchitecture can contribute to tumor growth. With the ECM being invaluable to the cancer niche, research targeting the relationship between abnormal ECM and tumor progression can lead to new courses of action in fighting brain cancers. A three-dimensional (3D) model of the healthy brain ECM could be used to explore how gliomas remodel and move through the substrate to create that distinct tumor niche.

19.8 CURRENT 2D AND 3D MODELS OF BRAIN TUMOR INVASION

In vivo models can provide a living 3D environment for the tumor, the most commonly used technique being the human xenograft (Nyga et al. 2011; Richmond and Su 2008). The advantage of xenograft models is the natural stromal cell interactions with the tumor cells as the tumors grow. However, monitoring their progress can be difficult without sacrificing the animal along the way. GBM xenografts are commonly placed subcutaneously in either heterotopic or orthotopic placement on the animal (Giannini et al. 2005). Xenograft models are useful in providing rapid tumor formation and development, but using cell lines can purport different behavioral phenotypes than seen in actual GBM tumors due to alteration by cell culture conditions (Fomchenko and Holland 2006). The formation of spontaneous tumors in genetically engineered mice (GEM) is another *in vivo* option, and is desirable because of the imitation of natural tumor behaviors such as angiogenesis and invasion (Fomchenko and Holland 2006; Huse and Holland 2009). The cons of GEM models of brain cancers include reproducibility, genetic heterogeneity, and variability of development among the induced tumors. This approach does produce biological information on brain tumors but is difficult to use with goals of testing therapeutics (Huse and Holland 2009).

Cell-based *in vitro* methods traditionally evaluate cellular behavior and response to functionalized 2D surfaces, and have proven helpful in work concerning cells of the brain and CNS (Hopkins et al. 2015). With respect to cancer research, 2D models are extremely useful for looking at cell proliferation or invasion, quantifying focal adhesions, and examining molecular relationships. Two-dimensional gel electrophoresis and mass spectrometry techniques are useful in identifying protein expression phenotypes of cancer cells (Lage 2004). Two-dimensional systems offer insights through comparing a controlled environmental factor to the observed cellular response, but unfortunately cannot assess cell–cell interactions or cell response to extracellular cues (Figure 19.4). Cells grown in 2D form flat monolayers to the one adherent surface and are more likely to be killed by lower doses of chemotherapeutics or radiation methods, making the efficacy of novel cancer-fighting drugs hard to evaluate *in vitro* (Desoize and Jardillier 2000).

Tumor spheroids are 3D structures of cancer cells used to mimic the multicellular, solid tumors seen *in vivo*. Previously, spontaneous aggregation was used to create rough tumor cell spheroids for cancer studies. However, research with metastatic cancer cell lines has shown that the aggregation of tumor cells to each other and to other cells (homotypic and heterotypic aggregation, respectively) is unique to early malignant tumors (Glinsky et al. 2000; Kim 2005; Langlois et al. 1979).

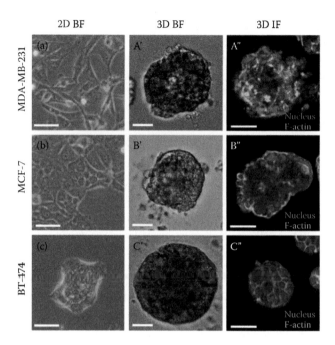

FIGURE 19.4 A challenge of 2D cell culture: creating conditions for realistic cell morphology. When cells are forced to move through ECM conditions, they more closely replicate behavior *in vivo* instead of simply adhering to the surface they are given in 2D cell culture methods. This panel shows three different breast cancer cell lines and their behavior in 2D and 3D culture methods, respectively. (Reprinted with permission from previous publication Lovitt, C. J. et al. 2014. *Biology (Basel)* no. 3 (2):345–67.)

To encourage the cells to form spheroids independently, the liquid overlay culture techniques can be used to promote spontaneous homotypic aggregation. Spheroids made in liquid overlay conditions do retain cellular differentiation processes, but altered cell adhesion behavior has been noted due to the nature of the basement membrane (Kim 2005). Liquid overlay is a widely used technique for creating 3D tumor aggregates and looking at cell differentiation, but spinner flasks, the hanging drop method, or gyratory shakers are also used to create large multicellular spheroids in liquid media (Kim 2005). If working with a tumor cell line that does not readily aggregate in culture, microcarrier beads are useful tools to form spheroids with more sensitive cell lines (Clark and Hirtenstein 1981; Jessup et al. 1997). Microcarrier beads assist in the flow of nutrients across nearby cells, and the manipulation of the beads allows the researcher to choose the cell density per unit volume to control proliferation and spheroid seed volume. The beads can be adhered to each other to create larger spheroids if desired, and since these are well mixed into the culture media, environmental conditions can be manipulated. Tumor spheroids are great models of looking at intercellular signaling and behavior, but cells not encapsulated in a 3D substrate lack those important interactions with outside growth factors that also play a role in cell fate (Wang et al. 1998). Cell spheroid techniques go farther in looking at cellular interactions and endogenous ECM effects, but do not take into account the exogenous ECM factors produced by surrounding stromal cells (Kim 2005). To study tumor cell behavior and contribute to potential therapeutics, a brain-mimetic 3D tissue model would yield an incredible insight into the molecular behavior of cancer and its interactions with stromal elements.

Current commonly used 3D models for brain tissue involve creating tumor spheroids and then encasing them into a designed polymer scaffold or hydrogel to study cell–ECM interactions (Charoen et al. 2014). This technique allows the researcher to account for cell type and size of the tissue, as well as enables the cells' primary interactions to be with each other to reinforce the tissue (Charoen et al. 2014) (Figure 19.4). There are several natural scaffold materials used in cancer research, including laminin, fibrin, and collagen-based options, among others (Chwalek et al. 2014; Pedron et al. 2013). These materials can also be enriched with signaling molecules and other bioligands to further specify a cellular response in the tumor tissue from the ECM (Figure 19.4). Different drug delivery methods can be assessed through polymer scaffold models, showing a potential for treatments through the tumor response in a particular environment (Charoen et al. 2014).

Matrigel® and collagen studies with GBM yield information on cell migration, but natural materials have issues with batch variability, degradability, and mechanical property adjustments (Ananthanarayanan et al. 2011; Chwalek et al. 2014). Matrigel®, which is made from a laminin-dense basement membrane, does not allow for gelation or network structure to be closely controlled and thus reproducibility is limited in creating a matrix for *ex vivo* studies (Chwalek et al. 2014; Pedron et al. 2013). Collagen-based matrices are lacking other connective tissue elements and can be difficult to control for crosslinking (Yamada and Cukierman 2007). The synthetic scaffolds, in contrast, do offer more control over mechanical and biochemical properties, as well as allow for the addition of certain peptides to test ligand function in tumor progression (Chwalek et al. 2014). Synthetic scaffolds can also be manipulated by degradability and growth factor delivery as controlled variables in tumor studies (Chwalek et al. 2011, 2014; Silva et al. 2009). GBM tumors are able to remodel the brain ECM and synthesize certain protein elements to aid in invasion through the area, and so matrices containing brain ECM-like constituents are needed (Pedron et al. 2013). A challenge from the biomaterials standpoint is the need for a controllable system in lab condition that is also biocompatible with the brain tumor cells. These issues are applied on all scales, down to the molecular level of how a chemical in a 3D construct could affect intercellular signaling of a tumor cell. GBM cell morphology, movement, and proliferation have been shown to be dependent on the mechanical properties of the matrix, and thus variables including rigidity and ligand functionality should be carefully chosen to accurately mimic biological tissue (Ananthanarayanan et al. 2011). Tissue microenvironment is essential to the function and development of healthy cells, and changes in that environment can cause aberrant cell behavior like that seen in tumor cell proliferation and progression (Ronnov-Jessen et al. 1996).

Since 2D models cannot adequately replicate the tumor microenvironment and animal studies are labor intensive, a 3D model that closely mimics the tumor microenvironment could lead to a universally accepted test standard for brain tumor studies. Cells grown in a 2D monolayer exhibit a uniform proliferation across all cells, but a 3D matrix will promote zones of proliferation among a tumor spheroid as well as induce a cell morphology analogous to the parent tissue (Lin and Chang 2008; Lee et al. 2013). Two-dimensional monolayer cultures and animal studies fall short during drug development studies due to the presentation of unrealistic cell culture conditions and due to fundamental differences between human and animal metabolisms, respectively (Figure 19.4). Chemotherapeutics are more likely to succeed in 2D cultures than with tumor spheroid cultures assuming equal permeation of the drug into both matrices, due to the spheroid being protected by the layers of cells similar to a true tumor (Perche and Torchilin 2012; Rangarajan et al. 2004) (Figure 19.4). Three-dimensional cultures can replicate the cellular heterogeneity and multicellular structure that contribute to cancer mechanisms of drug resistance (Loessner et al. 2010). Variety in cell proliferation and gene expression translates into a myriad of cell morphologies, ECM interactions, and drug resistance abilities in realistic 3D assays (Bellis et al. 2013; Longati et al. 2013; Luca et al. 2013).

19.9 FUTURE DESIGN OF 3D MODELS TO STUDY BRAIN TUMOR INVASION

The molecular interactions that define and shape tumor growth are largely influenced by the tumor microenvironment. Yet, a challenge to *in vivo* models remains the design and application of a 3D tissue system that adequately encapsulates the heterogeneity of signals prevailing in this milieu. The vast majority of currently available 3D brain tumor models do not adequately mimic the diversity of elements prevailing in the tumor microenvironment. Engineering such a model can be done in a top-down or bottom-up approach; top-down referring to bulk fabrication and then modification of a scaffold to suit the experimental design, while bottom-up builds up a scaffold piece by piece to obtain a desired microenvironmental condition (Todhunter et al. 2015; Wu et al. 2012). Care should be taken when choosing materials, depending on the nature of the biological components and the tissue that is being emulated. The chosen scaffold should take into account mechanical architecture, porosity, and biomolecular interactions with the biological components. For brain mimetic tissue, the component materials should be able to emulate the heterogenic interstitial matrix with the proper nutrient and gas exchange, hydration, temperature, and pH for cells to grow and thrive. Micro- and nanofibrillar polymers can be used in 3D cell culture, but synthetic fibers can cause a varying cellular responses when compared to natural components (Lutolf and Hubbell 2005). Natural ECM-based hydrogels consisting of GAGs and or collagen provide realistic mechanical stresses for encapsulated cells to react accordingly (Lutolf and Hubbell 2005). Natural ECMs can provide true-to-form tissue dynamics with the inclusion of biological ligands and growth factors (Lutolf and Hubbell 2005).

Creating a gradient within a 3D matrix can be accomplished in porous scaffolds, such as hydrogels (DeLong et al. 2005; Wong et al. 2008; Wu et al. 2012). Hydrogels containing natural ECM components are beneficial in examining tumor invasiveness because variables such as gel pore size, bioligand inclusion, and gradients can be altered to fit the needs of the study. A hydrogel matrix that allows for selective functionalization can be networked with the relevant macromolecules to create a working biomaterial which can be used to test glioma invasion and progression (Pedron et al.

2013). Brain mimetic hydrogel models are desirable for their high water content, allowing close replication to tissue conditions (Wang et al. 2014). Hydrogels can also be adapted to account for elasticity and pore size, which directly affect cell motility (Ananthanarayanan et al. 2011). Hydrogel systems with mechanical gradients can elucidate a relationship between mechanotaxic cell migration and the environment (Rao et al. 2012). Increased hydrogel stiffness has been observed to cause GBM cells *in vitro* to change to a bipolar morphology, displaying cell sensitivity to environmental conditions (Rao et al. 2012). By incorporating fluid flow into 3D tumor modeling, hydrogels have the potential to better represent the interactions that take place between tumor cells and ECM. Cell behavior is also reflective of matrix composition, making it imperative that a model of brain tumor behavior includes the essential ECM molecules (Rao et al. 2013a). GBM behavior is sensitive to biomimetic material, and thus factors including hydrogel composition, mechanical properties, and topography should be taken into account in the design of a 3D model.

One roadblock to a successful *in vitro* model of brain cancers is the issue of creating realistic angiogenesis in culture. Basic tumor–ECM interactions are quantifiable by current 3D models, but beyond that are the tumor–vasculature interactions which also characterize invasiveness of the cancer cells (Chwalek et al. 2014). During tumorigenesis, the cells undergo an activation of neoangiogenesis characterized by the production of MMPs and the remodeling of local ECM (Fang et al. 2000; Moses 1997; Stetler-Stevenson 1999). As tumor cells migrate, they remodel local ECM along their path to promote survival and proliferation, and this changes the interstitial flow of the ECM. In cancerous tissue, interstitial fluid can build up and greatly increase the pressure in the brain area (Boucher et al. 1990). Glioma cells have been shown to migrate along paths of interstitial flow, which aids growth factor movement around the tumor (Munson et al. 2013; Qazi et al. 2011).

GBM cells migrate in a directed pathway through brain matter to infiltrate diffusely, most commonly along white matter tracts in the brain (Louis 2006). Functionalized hydrogels can be enriched with nanofibers to emulate the realistic topography of real brain tissue and the characteristic white matter that GBM cells follow (Rao et al. 2013b). Incorporating nanofibers into gels can replicate white matter to guide tumor cells through the model, or even toward drug-laden areas for testing of potential therapeutics (Jain et al. 2014).

Microfluidics has opened the doors for the "organs-on-chips," cell culture devices made with circulating chambers for cells to move through based on their preference to the selected testing conditions. Organs-on-chips have massive implications for preclinical drug testing and applications for testing the tumor cell niche. This mechanically active environment is difficult to replicate. Incorporating microfluidics allows for the manipulation of dynamic fluids in a scaffold, and can be directly implanted within hydrogels to shuttle macromolecules throughout the material (Huh et al. 2011). These devices use microfluidic channels lined with the cells of interest to realistically model the desired organ system. Microfluidics can create laminar flow through the microchannels to create interstitial flow similar to true physiological conditions, and when combined with a 3D cell culture substrate can also replicate cell–ECM interactions (Ma et al. 2013) (Figure 19.5). Microfluidics are being increasingly used in neuroscience to study neuron and neural stem cell behavior

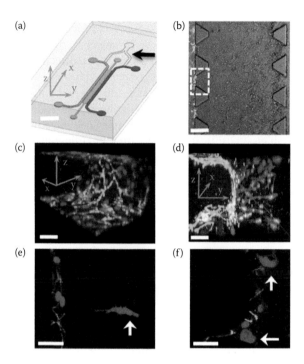

FIGURE 19.5 Microfluidic tumor–vascular interface model. (a) Endothelial channel (green), tumor channel (red), and 3D ECM (dark gray) between the two channels. Channels are 500 μm wide, 20 mm in length, and 120 μm in height. Black arrow shows the y-junction. (Scale bar: 2 mm). (b) Phase contrast image showing the fibrosarcoma cells (HT1080, red) invading through the ECM (gray) toward the endothelium (MVEC, green). A single 3D ECM hydrogel matrix region is outlined with the white dashed square. (Scale bar: 300 μm.) (c) VE-cadherin and DAPI staining to show confluency of the endothelial monolayer on the 3D ECM (outlined with white square in b). (d) Three-dimensional rendering of a confocal z-stack of a single region showing the tumor cells invading in 3D and adhering to the endothelium. (Scale bar: 30 μm.) (e) HT1080 cell (white arrow) invading in 3D toward endothelium. (Scale bar: 30 μm.) (f) HT1080 cells in contact with the endothelial monolayer. In (c)–(f), all scale bars are 30 μm. Green, VE-cadherin: blue, DAPI: red, HT1080-mCherry, x-, y-, z-coordinate indication is appropriately adjusted in A, C, D. (Reprinted with permission from previous publication Zervantonakis, I. K. et al. 2012. *Proc Natl Acad Sci USA* no. 109 (34):13515–20.)

(Wang et al. 2009). The BBB can also be replicated on a microfluidics chip to evaluate drug progression through the tight junctions or to model degenerative conditions (Griep et al. 2013). Fluid flow in the brain is faster along paths of least resistance, such as along white matter tracks in the brain, creating an attractive path for tumor cells to follow (Geer and Grossman 1997). A microfluidics platform can combine surface-bound and 3D elements to accurately replicate disease conditions and cellular response (Cho et al. 2013b). Interstitial flow could also be redistributing chemotactic cues, drawing tumor cells along flow pathways toward lymphatics, nerves, and white matter (Fleury et al. 2006). Ideally, microfluidics will contribute to GBM biology and therapy research in a biomimetic environment.

The vast majority of preclinical cancer treatments do not produce results in the latter stages of clinical trials in human patients, wasting time and resources without concrete progress. Two-dimensional culture mechanisms and animal models cannot accurately test out novel therapies before trials with humans. Though both of these methods are useful, a 3D model can augment our knowledge of cancer biology and weed out inconsequential drug candidates by providing a realistic, controllable laboratory model of human cancers. To develop a model of the tumor microenvironment, multiple key elements have to be accounted for: bioligand gradients, hypoxia and oxygen conditions, interstitial flow, and angiogenesis. By integrating the complex network of factors and advanced imaging techniques, a 3D model of cancer can improve the impact of preclinical drug testing.

19.10 CONCLUSION AND PERSPECTIVE

The development of 3D models to study GBM progression has tremendous implications for our understanding of malignant brain tumors and for converging upon clinically translatable therapeutic interventions. Over recent years, many strides have been made toward fighting other cancers; yet, median survival for GBM has not strayed from the average of one year. Brain cancers pose an uncommon challenge because of the devastatingly invasive nature and resistance to the standard therapeutic options, and these issues are rooted in the knowledge of the genetic and molecular heterogeneity in such cancers. Moving toward a more complete understanding of brain tumor, biology will pave the path toward finding the ideal molecular targets to efficiently fight these cancers. Hydrogels, interstitial flow, chemokine gradients, and other parameters that are characteristic of the brain tumor microenvironment are critical design elements that need to be incorporated into futuristic designs of 3D brain tumor models. Such models would produce invaluable evidence as to why malignant tumors progress as they do through brain tissue, and likely lead to the formulation of therapeutic strategies to halt tumor progression in GBM patients.

REFERENCES

Ananthanarayanan, B., Y. Kim, and S. Kumar. 2011. Elucidating the mechanobiology of malignant brain tumors using a brain matrix-mimetic hyaluronic acid hydrogel platform. *Biomaterials* no. 32 (31):7913–23.

Artym, V. V., Y. Zhang, F. Seillier-Moiseiwitsch, K. M. Yamada, and S. C. Mueller. 2006. Dynamic interactions of cortactin and membrane type 1 matrix metalloproteinase at invadopodia: Defining the stages of invadopodia formation and function. *Cancer Res* no. 66 (6):3034–43.

Bao, S., Q. Wu, R. E. McLendon, Y. Hao, Q. Shi, A. B. Hjelmeland, M. W. Dewhirst, D. D. Bigner, and J. N. Rich. 2006a. Glioma stem cells promote radioresistance by preferential activation of the DNA damage response. *Nature* no. 444 (7120):756–60.

Bao, S., Q. Wu, S. Sathornsumetee, Y. Hao, Z. Li, A. B. Hjelmeland, Q. Shi, R. E. McLendon, D. D. Bigner, and J. N. Rich. 2006b. Stem cell-like glioma cells promote tumor angiogenesis through vascular endothelial growth factor. *Cancer Res* no. 66 (16):7843–48.

Barker, F. G., 2nd, R. L. Davis, S. M. Chang, and M. D. Prados. 1996. Necrosis as a prognostic factor in glioblastoma multiforme. *Cancer* no. 77 (6):1161–66.

Batzdorf, U. and N. Malamud. 1963. The problem of multicentric gliomas. *J Neurosurg* no. 20:122–36.

Bellis, A. D., B. P. Bernabe, M. S. Weiss, S. Shin, S. Weng, L. J. Broadbelt, and L. D. Shea. 2013. Dynamic transcription factor activity profiling in 2D and 3D cell cultures. *Biotechnol Bioeng* no. 110 (2):563–72.

Berens, M. E. and A. Giese. 1999. "…those left behind." Biology and oncology of invasive glioma cells. *Neoplasia* no. 1 (3):208–19.

Bergers, G. and D. Hanahan. 2008. Modes of resistance to anti-angiogenic therapy. *Nat Rev Cancer* no. 8 (8):592–603.

Biernat, W., Y. Tohma, Y. Yonekawa, P. Kleihues, and H. Ohgaki. 1997. Alterations of cell cycle regulatory genes in primary (*de novo*) and secondary glioblastomas. *Acta Neuropathol* no. 94 (4):303–09.

Bonavia, R., M. M. Inda, W. K. Cavenee, and F. B. Furnari. 2011. Heterogeneity maintenance in glioblastoma: A social network. *Cancer Res* no. 71 (12):4055–60.

Boucher, Y., L. T. Baxter, and R. K. Jain. 1990. Interstitial pressure gradients in tissue-isolated and subcutaneous tumors: Implications for therapy. *Cancer Res* no. 50 (15):4478–84.

Bourguignon, L. Y., H. Zhu, A. Chu, N. Iida, L. Zhang, and M. C. Hung. 1997. Interaction between the adhesion receptor, CD44, and the oncogene product, p185HER2, promotes human ovarian tumor cell activation. *J Biol Chem* no. 272 (44):27913–18.

Brat, D. J., A. A. Castellano-Sanchez, S. B. Hunter, M. Pecot, C. Cohen, E. H. Hammond, S. N. Devi, B. Kaur, and E. G. Van Meir. 2004. Pseudopalisades in glioblastoma are hypoxic, express extracellular matrix proteases, and are formed by an actively migrating cell population. *Cancer Res* no. 64 (3):920–27.

Brat, D. J., A. Castellano-Sanchez, B. Kaur, and E. G. Van Meir. 2002. Genetic and biologic progression in astrocytomas and their relation to angiogenic dysregulation. *Adv Anat Pathol* no. 9 (1):24–36.

Brat, D. J. and E. G. Van Meir. 2001. Glomeruloid microvascular proliferation orchestrated by VPF/VEGF: A new world of angiogenesis research. *Am J Pathol* no. 158 (3):789–96.

Butowski, N. A. 2015. Epidemiology and diagnosis of brain tumors. *Continuum (Minneap Minn)* no. 21 (2 Neuro-oncology):301–13.

Calabrese, C., H. Poppleton, M. Kocak, T. L. Hogg, C. Fuller, B. Hamner, E. Y. Oh et al. 2007. A perivascular niche for brain tumor stem cells. *Cancer Cell* no. 11 (1):69–82.

Castillo, M., J. K. Smith, and L. Kwock. 2000. Correlation of myo-inositol levels and grading of cerebral astrocytomas. *AJNR Am J Neuroradiol* no. 21 (9):1645–49.

Charoen, K. M., B. Fallica, Y. L. Colson, M. H. Zaman, and M. W. Grinstaff. 2014. Embedded multicellular spheroids as a biomimetic 3D cancer model for evaluating drug and drug-device combinations. *Biomaterials* no. 35 (7):2264–71.

Cho, D. Y., S. Z. Lin, W. K. Yang, H. C. Lee, D. M. Hsu, H. L. Lin, C. C. Chen, C. L. Liu, W. Y. Lee, and L. H. Ho. 2013a. Targeting cancer stem cells for treatment of glioblastoma multiforme. *Cell Transplant* no. 22 (4):731–39.

Cho, H., T. Hashimoto, E. Wong, Y. Hori, L. B. Wood, L. Zhao, K. M. Haigis, B. T. Hyman, and D. Irimia. 2013b. Microfluidic chemotaxis platform for differentiating the roles of soluble and bound amyloid-beta on microglial accumulation. *Sci Rep* no. 3:1823.

Cho, R. W. and M. F. Clarke. 2008. Recent advances in cancer stem cells. *Curr Opin Genet Dev* no. 18 (1):48–53.

Chwalek, K., L. J. Bray, and C. Werner. 2014. Tissue-engineered 3D tumor angiogenesis models: Potential technologies for anti-cancer drug discovery. *Adv Drug Deliv Rev* no. 79–80:30–39.

Chwalek, K., K. R. Levental, M. V. Tsurkan, A. Zieris, U. Freudenberg, and C. Werner. 2011. Two-tier hydrogel degradation to boost endothelial cell morphogenesis. *Biomaterials* no. 32 (36):9649–57.

Clark, J. M. and M. D. Hirtenstein. 1981. Optimizing culture conditions for the production of animal cells in microcarrier culture. *Ann N Y Acad Sci* no. 369:33–46.

Clarke, M. F. and M. Fuller. 2006. Stem cells and cancer: Two faces of eve. *Cell* no. 124 (6):1111–15.

Collins, V. P. 1999. Progression as exemplified by human astrocytic tumors. *Semin Cancer Biol* no. 9 (4):267–76.

Corbeil, D., K. Roper, A. Hellwig, M. Tavian, S. Miraglia, S. M. Watt, P. J. Simmons, B. Peault, D. W. Buck, and W. B. Huttner. 2000. The human AC133 hematopoietic stem cell antigen is also expressed in epithelial cells and targeted to plasma membrane protrusions. *J Biol Chem* no. 275 (8):5512–20.

Cox, T. R. and J. T. Erler. 2011. Remodeling and homeostasis of the extracellular matrix: Implications for fibrotic diseases and cancer. *Dis Model Mech* no. 4 (2):165–78.

Cuddapah, V. A., S. Robel, S. Watkins, and H. Sontheimer. 2014. A neurocentric perspective on glioma invasion. *Nat Rev Neurosci* no. 15 (7):455–65.

Dalerba, P., R. W. Cho, and M. F. Clarke. 2007. Cancer stem cells: Models and concepts. *Annu Rev Med* no. 58:267–84.

Daumas-Duport, C., B. Scheithauer, J. O'Fallon, and P. Kelly. 1988. Grading of astrocytomas. A simple and reproducible method. *Cancer* no. 62 (10):2152–65.

de Visser, K. E., A. Eichten, and L. M. Coussens. 2006. Paradoxical roles of the immune system during cancer development. *Nat Rev Cancer* no. 6 (1):24–37.

Deepa, S. S., D. Carulli, C. Galtrey, K. Rhodes, J. Fukuda, T. Mikami, K. Sugahara, and J. W. Fawcett. 2006. Composition of perineuronal net extracellular matrix in rat brain: A different disaccharide composition for the net-associated proteoglycans. *J Biol Chem* no. 281 (26):17789–800.

DeLong, S. A., J. J. Moon, and J. L. West. 2005. Covalently immobilized gradients of bFGF on hydrogel scaffolds for directed cell migration. *Biomaterials* no. 26 (16):3227–34.

Demuth, T. and M. E. Berens. 2004. Molecular mechanisms of glioma cell migration and invasion. *J Neurooncol* no. 70 (2):217–28.

Desoize, B. and J. Jardillier. 2000. Multicellular resistance: A paradigm for clinical resistance? *Crit Rev Oncol Hematol* no. 36 (2–3):193–207.

Elsamadicy, A. A., R. Babu, J. P. Kirkpatrick, and D. C. Adamson. 2015. Radiation-induced malignant gliomas: A current review. *World Neurosurg* no. 83 (4):530–42.

Entschladen, F., T. L. Drell, K. Lang, J. Joseph, and K. S. Zaenker. 2005. Neurotransmitters and chemokines regulate tumor cell migration: Potential for a new pharmacological approach to inhibit invasion and metastasis development. *Curr Pharm Des* no. 11 (3):403–11.

Esiri, M. 2000. Russell and Rubinstein's pathology of tumors of the nervous system. Sixth edition. *J Neurol Neurosurg Psychiatry* no. 68 (4):538d.

Fang, J., Y. Shing, D. Wiederschain, L. Yan, C. Butterfield, G. Jackson, J. Harper, G. Tamvakopoulos, and M. A. Moses. 2000. Matrix metalloproteinase-2 is required for the switch to the angiogenic phenotype in a tumor model. *Proc Natl Acad Sci USA* no. 97 (8):3884–89.

Feldkamp, M. M., P. Lala, N. Lau, L. Roncari, and A. Guha. 1999. Expression of activated epidermal growth factor receptors, Ras-guanosine triphosphate, and mitogen-activated protein kinase in human glioblastoma multiforme specimens. *Neurosurgery* no. 45 (6):1442–53.

Fidler, I. J. and L. M. Ellis. 2004. Neoplastic angiogenesis—not all blood vessels are created equal. *N Engl J Med* no. 351 (3):215–16.

Fischer, I., J. P. Gagner, M. Law, E. W. Newcomb, and D. Zagzag. 2005. Angiogenesis in gliomas: Biology and molecular pathophysiology. *Brain Pathol* no. 15 (4):297–310.

Fleury, M. E., K. C. Boardman, and M. A. Swartz. 2006. Autologous morphogen gradients by subtle interstitial flow and matrix interactions. *Biophys J* no. 91 (1):113–21.

Folgueras, A. R., A. M. Pendas, L. M. Sanchez, and C. Lopez-Otin. 2004. Matrix metalloproteinases in cancer: From new functions to improved inhibition strategies. *Int J Dev Biol* no. 48 (5–6):411–24.

Fomchenko, E. I. and E. C. Holland. 2006. Mouse models of brain tumors and their applications in preclinical trials. *Clin Cancer Res* no. 12 (18):5288–97.

Forsyth, P. A., H. Wong, T. D. Laing, N. B. Rewcastle, D. G. Morris, H. Muzik, K. J. Leco et al. 1999. Gelatinase-A (MMP-2), gelatinase-B (MMP-9) and membrane type matrix metalloproteinase-1 (MT1-MMP) are involved in different aspects of the pathophysiology of malignant gliomas. *Br J Cancer* no. 79 (11–12):1828–35.

Friedl, P. and K. Wolf. 2003. Tumour-cell invasion and migration: Diversity and escape mechanisms. *Nat Rev Cancer* no. 3 (5):362–74.

Furnari, F. B., T. Fenton, R. M. Bachoo, A. Mukasa, J. M. Stommel, A. Stegh, W. C. Hahn et al. 2007. Malignant astrocytic glioma: Genetics, biology, and paths to treatment. *Genes Dev* no. 21 (21):2683–710.

Galli, R., E. Binda, U. Orfanelli, B. Cipelletti, A. Gritti, S. De Vitis, R. Fiocco, C. Foroni, F. Dimeco, and A. Vescovi. 2004. Isolation and characterization of tumorigenic, stem-like neural precursors from human glioblastoma. *Cancer Res* no. 64 (19):7011–21.

Geer, C. P. and S. A. Grossman. 1997. Interstitial fluid flow along white matter tracts: A potentially important mechanism for the dissemination of primary brain tumors. *J Neurooncol* no. 32 (3):193–201.

Giannini, C., J. N. Sarkaria, A. Saito, J. H. Uhm, E. Galanis, B. L. Carlson, M. A. Schroeder, and C. D. James. 2005. Patient tumor EGFR and PDGFRA gene amplifications retained in an invasive intracranial xenograft model of glioblastoma multiforme. *Neuro Oncol* no. 7 (2):164–76.

Giese, A., R. Bjerkvig, M. E. Berens, and M. Westphal. 2003. Cost of migration: Invasion of malignant gliomas and implications for treatment. *J Clin Oncol* no. 21 (8):1624–36.

Giordana, M. T., I. Germano, G. Giaccone, A. Mauro, A. Migheli, and D. Schiffer. 1985. The distribution of laminin in human brain tumors: An immunohistochemical study. *Acta Neuropathol* no. 67 (1–2):51–57.

Glinsky, V. V., M. E. Huflejt, G. V. Glinsky, S. L. Deutscher, and T. P. Quinn. 2000. Effects of Thomsen-Friedenreich antigen-specific peptide P-30 on beta-galactoside-mediated homotypic aggregation and adhesion to the endothelium of MDA-MB-435 human breast carcinoma cells. *Cancer Res* no. 60 (10):2584–88.

Griep, L. M., F. Wolbers, B. de Wagenaar, P. M. ter Braak, B. B. Weksler, I. A. Romero, P. O. Couraud, I. Vermes, A. D. van der Meer, and A. van den Berg. 2013. BBB on chip: Microfluidic platform to mechanically and biochemically modulate blood-brain barrier function. *Biomed Microdevices* no. 15 (1):145–50.

Hatva, E., A. Kaipainen, P. Mentula, J. Jaaskelainen, A. Paetau, M. Haltia, and K. Alitalo. 1995. Expression of endothelial cell-specific receptor tyrosine kinases and growth factors in human brain tumors. *Am J Pathol* no. 146 (2):368–78.

Hellstrom, M., H. Gerhardt, M. Kalen, X. Li, U. Eriksson, H. Wolburg, and C. Betsholtz. 2001. Lack of pericytes leads to endothelial hyperplasia and abnormal vascular morphogenesis. *J Cell Biol* no. 153 (3):543–53.

Hensch, T. K. 2005. Critical period plasticity in local cortical circuits. *Nat Rev Neurosci* no. 6 (11):877–88.

Holland, E. C. 2000. Glioblastoma multiforme: The terminator. *Proc Natl Acad Sci USA* no. 97 (12):6242–44.

Hopkins, A. M., E. DeSimone, K. Chwalek, and D. L. Kaplan. 2015. 3D *in vitro* modeling of the central nervous system. *Prog Neurobiol* no. 125:1–25.

Horn, P. A., H. Tesch, P. Staib, D. Kube, V. Diehl, and D. Voliotis. 1999. Expression of AC133, a novel hematopoietic precursor antigen, on acute myeloid leukemia cells. *Blood* no. 93 (4):1435–37.

Huh, D., G. A. Hamilton, and D. E. Ingber. 2011. From 3D cell culture to organs-on-chips. *Trends Cell Biol* no. 21 (12):745–54.

Huijbers, I. J., M. Iravani, S. Popov, D. Robertson, S. Al-Sarraj, C. Jones, and C. M. Isacke. 2010. A role for fibrillar collagen deposition and the collagen internalization receptor endo180 in glioma invasion. *PLoS One* no. 5 (3):e9808.

Huse, J. T. and E. C. Holland. 2009. Genetically engineered mouse models of brain cancer and the promise of preclinical testing. *Brain Pathol* no. 19 (1):132–43.

Huttner, A. 2012. Overview of primary brain tumors: Pathologic classification, epidemiology, molecular biology, and prognostic markers. *Hematol Oncol Clin North Am* no. 26 (4):715–32.

Jain, A., M. Betancur, G. D. Patel, C. M. Valmikinathan, V. J. Mukhatyar, A. Vakharia, S. B. Pai, B. Brahma, T. J. MacDonald, and R. V. Bellamkonda. 2014. Guiding intracortical brain tumour cells to an extracortical cytotoxic hydrogel using aligned polymeric nanofibres. *Nat Mater* no. 13 (3):308–16.

Jain, R. K., E. di Tomaso, D. G. Duda, J. S. Loeffler, A. G. Sorensen, and T. T. Batchelor. 2007. Angiogenesis in brain tumours. *Nat Rev Neurosci* no. 8 (8):610–22.

Jelsma, R. and P. C. Bucy. 1967. The treatment of glioblastoma multiforme of the brain. *J Neurosurg* no. 27 (5):388–400.

Jessup, J. M., D. Brown, W. Fitzgerald, R. D. Ford, A. Nachman, T. J. Goodwin, and G. Spaulding. 1997. Induction of carcinoembryonic antigen expression in a three-dimensional culture system. *In Vitro Cell Dev Biol Anim* no. 33 (5):352–57.

Jordan, C. T., M. L. Guzman, and M. Noble. 2006. Cancer stem cells. *N Engl J Med* no. 355 (12):1253–61.

Kessenbrock, K., V. Plaks, and Z. Werb. 2010. Matrix metalloproteinases: Regulators of the tumor microenvironment. *Cell* no. 141 (1):52–67.

Keunen, O., M. Johansson, A. Oudin, M. Sanzey, S. A. Rahim, F. Fack, F. Thorsen et al. 2011. Anti-VEGF treatment reduces blood supply and increases tumor cell invasion in glioblastoma. *Proc Natl Acad Sci USA* no. 108 (9):3749–54.

Kim, J. B. 2005. Three-dimensional tissue culture models in cancer biology. *Semin Cancer Biol* no. 15 (5):365–77.

Kirsch, M., G. Schackert, and P. M. Black. 2000. Anti-angiogenic treatment strategies for malignant brain tumors. *J Neurooncol* no. 50 (1–2):149–63.

Kleihues, P. and L. H. Sobin. 2000. World Health Organization classification of tumors. *Cancer* no. 88 (12):2887.

Koppe, G., G. Bruckner, W. Hartig, B. Delpech, and V. Bigl. 1997. Characterization of proteoglycan-containing perineuronal nets by enzymatic treatments of rat brain sections. *Histochem J* no. 29 (1):11–20.

Koul, D., R. Parthasarathy, R. Shen, M. A. Davies, S. A. Jasser, S. K. Chintala, J. S. Rao et al. 2001. Suppression of matrix metalloproteinase-2 gene expression and invasion in human glioma cells by MMAC/PTEN. *Oncogene* no. 20 (46):6669–78.

Lage, H. 2004. Proteomics in cancer cell research: An analysis of therapy resistance. *Pathol Res Pract* no. 200 (2):105–17.

Lakka, S. S. and J. S. Rao. 2008. Antiangiogenic therapy in brain tumors. *Expert Rev Neurother* no. 8 (10):1457–73.

Langlois, A. J., W. D. Holder, Jr., J. D. Iglehart, W. A. Nelson-Rees, S. A. Wells, Jr., and D. P. Bolognesi. 1979. Morphological and biochemical properties of a new human breast cancer cell line. *Cancer Res* no. 39 (7 Pt 1):2604–13.

Lau, L. W., R. Cua, M. B. Keough, S. Haylock-Jacobs, and V. W. Yong. 2013. Pathophysiology of the brain extracellular matrix: A new target for remyelination. *Nat Rev Neurosci* no. 14 (10):722–29.

Lauffenburger, D. A. and A. F. Horwitz. 1996. Cell migration: A physically integrated molecular process. *Cell* no. 84 (3):359–69.

Lee, J. M., P. Mhawech-Fauceglia, N. Lee, L. C. Parsanian, Y. G. Lin, S. A. Gayther, and K. Lawrenson. 2013. A three-dimensional microenvironment alters protein expression and chemosensitivity of epithelial ovarian cancer cells *in vitro*. *Lab Invest* no. 93 (5):528–42.

Li, L. and W. B. Neaves. 2006. Normal stem cells and cancer stem cells: The niche matters. *Cancer Res* no. 66 (9):4553–57.

Lin, R. Z. and H. Y. Chang. 2008. Recent advances in three-dimensional multicellular spheroid culture for biomedical research. *Biotechnol J* no. 3 (9–10):1172–84.

Loessner, D., K. S. Stok, M. P. Lutolf, D. W. Hutmacher, J. A. Clements, and S. C. Rizzi. 2010. Bioengineered 3D platform to explore cell–ECM interactions and drug resistance of epithelial ovarian cancer cells. *Biomaterials* no. 31 (32):8494–506.

Longati, P., X. Jia, J. Eimer, A. Wagman, M. R. Witt, S. Rehnmark, C. Verbeke, R. Toftgard, M. Lohr, and R. L. Heuchel. 2013. 3D pancreatic carcinoma spheroids induce a matrix-rich, chemoresistant phenotype offering a better model for drug testing. *BMC Cancer* no. 13:95.

Louis, D. N. 2006. Molecular pathology of malignant gliomas. *Annu Rev Pathol* no. 1:97–117.

Lovitt, C. J., T. B. Shelper, and V. M. Avery. 2014. Advanced cell culture techniques for cancer drug discovery. *Biology (Basel)* no. 3 (2):345–67.

Lu, P., V. M. Weaver, and Z. Werb. 2012. The extracellular matrix: A dynamic niche in cancer progression. *J Cell Biol* no. 196 (4):395–406.

Luca, A. C., S. Mersch, R. Deenen, S. Schmidt, I. Messner, K. L. Schafer, S. E. Baldus, W. Huckenbeck, R. P. Piekorz, W. T. Knoefel, A. Krieg, and N. H. Stoecklein. 2013. Impact of the 3D microenvironment on phenotype, gene expression, and EGFR inhibition of colorectal cancer cell lines. *PLoS One* no. 8 (3):e59689.

Lutolf, M. P. and J. A. Hubbell. 2005. Synthetic biomaterials as instructive extracellular microenvironments for morphogenesis in tissue engineering. *Nat Biotechnol* no. 23 (1):47–55.

Ma, H., H. Xu, and J. Qin. 2013. Biomimetic tumor microenvironment on a microfluidic platform. *Biomicrofluidics* no. 7 (1):11501.

Marquet, G., O. Dameron, S. Saikali, J. Mosser, and A. Burgun. 2007. Grading glioma tumors using OWL-DL and NCI thesaurus. *AMIA Annu Symp Proc* no. 2007:508–12.

Meis, J. M., K. L. Martz, and J. S. Nelson. 1991. Mixed glioblastoma multiforme and sarcoma. A clinicopathologic study of 26 radiation therapy oncology group cases. *Cancer* no. 67 (9):2342–49.

Miller, K., K. Chinzei, G. Orssengo, and P. Bednarz. 2000. Mechanical properties of brain tissue *in-vivo*: Experiment and computer simulation. *J Biomech* no. 33 (11):1369–76.

Moses, M. A. 1997. The regulation of neovascularization of matrix metalloproteinases and their inhibitors. *Stem Cells* no. 15 (3):180–89.

Munson, J. M., R. V. Bellamkonda, and M. A. Swartz. 2013. Interstitial flow in a 3D microenvironment increases glioma invasion by a CXCR4-dependent mechanism. *Cancer Res* no. 73 (5):1536–46.

Munson, J. M., L. Fried, S. A. Rowson, M. Y. Bonner, L. Karumbaiah, B. Diaz, S. A. Courtneidge et al. 2012. Anti-invasive adjuvant therapy with imipramine blue enhances chemotherapeutic efficacy against glioma. *Sci Transl Med* no. 4 (127):127ra36.

Nicholson, C. and E. Sykova. 1998. Extracellular space structure revealed by diffusion analysis. *Trends Neurosci* no. 21 (5):207–15.

Nyga, A., U. Cheema, and M. Loizidou. 2011. 3D tumour models: Novel *in vitro* approaches to cancer studies. *J Cell Commun Signal* no. 5 (3):239–48.

Oliferenko, S., I. Kaverina, J. V. Small, and L. A. Huber. 2000. Hyaluronic acid (HA) binding to CD44 activates Rac1 and induces lamellipodia outgrowth. *J Cell Biol* no. 148 (6):1159–64.

Ostrom, Q. T., H. Gittleman, P. Liao, C. Rouse, Y. Chen, J. Dowling, Y. Wolinsky, C. Kruchko, and J. Barnholtz-Sloan. 2014. CBTRUS statistical report: Primary brain and central nervous system tumors diagnosed in the United States in 2007–2011. *Neuro Oncol* no. 16 (Suppl 4):iv1–63.

Ou, K. L. and H. Hosseinkhani. 2014. Development of 3D *in vitro* technology for medical applications. *Int J Mol Sci* no. 15 (10):17938–62.

Palecek, S. P., J. C. Loftus, M. H. Ginsberg, D. A. Lauffenburger, and A. F. Horwitz. 1997. Integrin-ligand binding properties govern cell migration speed through cell-substratum adhesiveness. *Nature* no. 385 (6616):537–40.

Paulus, W., I. Baur, A. S. Beutler, and S. A. Reeves. 1996. Diffuse brain invasion of glioma cells requires beta 1 integrins. *Lab Invest* no. 75 (6):819–26.

Pedron, S., E. Becka, and B. A. Harley. 2013. Regulation of glioma cell phenotype in 3D matrices by hyaluronic acid. *Biomaterials* no. 34 (30):7408–17.

Perche, F. and V. P. Torchilin. 2012. Cancer cell spheroids as a model to evaluate chemotherapy protocols. *Cancer Biol Ther* no. 13 (12):1205–13.

Plate, K. H., G. Breier, H. A. Weich, H. D. Mennel, and W. Risau. 1994. Vascular endothelial growth factor and glioma angiogenesis: Coordinate induction of VEGF receptors, distribution of VEGF protein and possible *in vivo* regulatory mechanisms. *Int J Cancer* no. 59 (4):520–29.

Plate, K. H., G. Breier, H. A. Weich, and W. Risau. 1992. Vascular endothelial growth factor is a potential tumour angiogenesis factor in human gliomas *in vivo*. *Nature* no. 359 (6398):845–48.

Qazi, H., Z. D. Shi, and J. M. Tarbell. 2011. Fluid shear stress regulates the invasive potential of glioma cells via modulation of migratory activity and matrix metalloproteinase expression. *PLoS One* no. 6 (5):e20348.

Rangarajan, A., S. J. Hong, A. Gifford, and R. A. Weinberg. 2004. Species- and cell type-specific requirements for cellular transformation. *Cancer Cell* no. 6 (2):171–83.

Rao, J. S. 2003. Molecular mechanisms of glioma invasiveness: The role of proteases. *Nat Rev Cancer* no. 3 (7):489–501.

Rao, S. S., S. Bentil, J. DeJesus, J. Larison, A. Hissong, R. Dupaix, A. Sarkar, and J. O. Winter. 2012. Inherent interfacial mechanical gradients in 3D hydrogels influence tumor cell behaviors. *PLoS One* no. 7 (4):e35852.

Rao, S. S., J. Dejesus, A. R. Short, J. J. Otero, A. Sarkar, and J. O. Winter. 2013a. Glioblastoma behaviors in three-dimensional collagen–hyaluronan composite hydrogels. *ACS Appl Mater Interfaces* no. 5 (19):9276–84.

Rao, S. S., M. T. Nelson, R. Xue, J. K. DeJesus, M. S. Viapiano, J. J. Lannutti, A. Sarkar, and J. O. Winter. 2013b. Mimicking white matter tract topography using core-shell electrospun nanofibers to examine migration of malignant brain tumors. *Biomaterials* no. 34 (21):5181–90.

Rasheed, B. K., R. N. Wiltshire, S. H. Bigner, and D. D. Bigner. 1999. Molecular pathogenesis of malignant gliomas. *Curr Opin Oncol* no. 11 (3):162–67.

Rathore, A., P. Kamarajan, M. Mathur, S. Sinha, and C. Sarkar. 1999. Simultaneous alterations of retinoblastoma and p53 protein expression in astrocytic tumors. *Pathol Oncol Res* no. 5 (1):21–27.

Regina, A., M. Demeule, A. Laplante, J. Jodoin, C. Dagenais, F. Berthelet, A. Moghrabi, and R. Beliveau. 2001. Multidrug resistance in brain tumors: Roles of the blood–brain barrier. *Cancer Metastasis Rev* no. 20 (1–2):13–25.

Reya, T., S. J. Morrison, M. F. Clarke, and I. L. Weissman. 2001. Stem cells, cancer, and cancer stem cells. *Nature* no. 414 (6859):105–11.

Ricard, C., F. Stanchi, T. Rodriguez, M. C. Amoureux, G. Rougon, and F. Debarbieux. 2013. Dynamic quantitative intravital imaging of glioblastoma progression reveals a lack of correlation between tumor growth and blood vessel density. *PLoS One* no. 8 (9):e72655.

Richmond, A. and Y. Su. 2008. Mouse xenograft models vs GEM models for human cancer therapeutics. *Dis Model Mech* no. 1 (2–3):78–82.

Romeike, B. F. 2007. Classification and documentation of diffuse gliomas. *Radiologe* no. 47 (6):530–35.

Ronnov-Jessen, L., O. W. Petersen, and M. J. Bissell. 1996. Cellular changes involved in conversion of normal to malignant breast: Importance of the stromal reaction. *Physiol Rev* no. 76 (1):69–125.

Rosen, J. M. and C. T. Jordan. 2009. The increasing complexity of the cancer stem cell paradigm. *Science* no. 324 (5935):1670–73.

Ruoslahti, E. 1996. Brain extracellular matrix. *Glycobiology* no. 6 (5):489–92.

Rutka, J. T., G. Apodaca, R. Stern, and M. Rosenblum. 1988. The extracellular matrix of the central and peripheral nervous systems: Structure and function. *J Neurosurg* no. 69 (2):155–70.

Sanai, N., A. Alvarez-Buylla, and M. S. Berger. 2005. Neural stem cells and the origin of gliomas. *N Engl J Med* no. 353 (8):811–22.

Sano, T., A. Asai, K. Mishima, T. Fujimaki, and T. Kirino. 1998. Telomerase activity in 144 brain tumours. *Br J Cancer* no. 77 (10):1633–37.

Sarkaria, J. N., G. J. Kitange, C. D. James, R. Plummer, H. Calvert, M. Weller, and W. Wick. 2008. Mechanisms of chemoresistance to alkylating agents in malignant glioma. *Clin Cancer Res* no. 14 (10):2900–08.

Shamisa, A., M. Bance, S. Nag, C. Tator, S. Wong, G. Noren, and A. Guha. 2013. Glioblastoma multiforme occurring in a patient treated with gamma knife surgery: Case report and review of the literature. *J Neurosurg* no. 119 (Suppl):816–21.

Shweiki, D., A. Itin, D. Soffer, and E. Keshet. 1992. Vascular endothelial growth factor induced by hypoxia may mediate hypoxia-initiated angiogenesis. *Nature* no. 359 (6398):843–45.

Silva, A. K., C. Richard, M. Bessodes, D. Scherman, and O. W. Merten. 2009. Growth factor delivery approaches in hydrogels. *Biomacromolecules* no. 10 (1):9–18.

Singh, S. K., I. D. Clarke, M. Terasaki, V. E. Bonn, C. Hawkins, J. Squire, and P. B. Dirks. 2003. Identification of a cancer stem cell in human brain tumors. *Cancer Res* no. 63 (18):5821–28.

Singh, S. K., C. Hawkins, I. D. Clarke, J. A. Squire, J. Bayani, T. Hide, R. M. Henkelman, M. D. Cusimano, and P. B. Dirks. 2004. Identification of human brain tumour initiating cells. *Nature* no. 432 (7015):396–401.

Soltysova, A., V. Altanerova, and C. Altaner. 2005. Cancer stem cells. *Neoplasma* no. 52 (6):435–40.

Steeg, P. S. 2006. Tumor metastasis: Mechanistic insights and clinical challenges. *Nat Med* no. 12 (8):895–904.

Stetler-Stevenson, W. G. 1999. Matrix metalloproteinases in angiogenesis: A moving target for therapeutic intervention. *J Clin Invest* no. 103 (9):1237–41.

Stewart, L. A. 2002. Chemotherapy in adult high-grade glioma: A systematic review and meta-analysis of individual patient data from 12 randomised trials. *Lancet* no. 359 (9311):1011–18.

Straume, O., P. O. Chappuis, H. B. Salvesen, O. J. Halvorsen, S. A. Haukaas, J. R. Goffin, L. R. Begin, W. D. Foulkes, and L. A. Akslen. 2002. Prognostic importance of glomeruloid microvascular proliferation indicates an aggressive angiogenic phenotype in human cancers. *Cancer Res* no. 62 (23):6808–11.

Tabatabai, G. and M. Weller. 2011. Glioblastoma stem cells. *Cell Tissue Res* no. 343 (3):459–65.

Thiery, J. P. 2002. Epithelial-mesenchymal transitions in tumour progression. *Nat Rev Cancer* no. 2 (6):442–54.

Todhunter, M. E., N. Y. Jee, A. J. Hughes, M. C. Coyle, A. Cerchiari, J. Farlow, J. C. Garbe, M. A. LaBarge, T. A. Desai, and Z. J. Gartner. 2015. Programmed synthesis of three-dimensional tissues. *Nat Methods* no. 12 (10):975–81.

Toole, B. P. 2001. Hyaluronan in morphogenesis. *Semin Cell Dev Biol* no. 12 (2):79–87.

Ulrich, T. A., E. M. de Juan Pardo, and S. Kumar. 2009. The mechanical rigidity of the extracellular matrix regulates the structure, motility, and proliferation of glioma cells. *Cancer Res* no. 69 (10):4167–74.

Verhoeff, J. J., O. van Tellingen, A. Claes, L. J. Stalpers, M. E. van Linde, D. J. Richel, W. P. Leenders, and W. R. van Furth. 2009. Concerns about anti-angiogenic treatment in patients with glioblastoma multiforme. *BMC Cancer* no. 9:444.

Visvader, J. E. and G. J. Lindeman. 2008. Cancer stem cells in solid tumours: Accumulating evidence and unresolved questions. *Nat Rev Cancer* no. 8 (10):755–68.

Wakimoto, H., S. Kesari, C. J. Farrell, W. T. Curry, Jr., C. Zaupa, M. Aghi, T. Kuroda et al. 2009. Human glioblastoma-derived cancer stem cells: Establishment of invasive glioma models and treatment with oncolytic herpes simplex virus vectors. *Cancer Res* no. 69 (8):3472–81.

Wang, C., X. Tong, and F. Yang. 2014. Bioengineered 3D brain tumor model to elucidate the effects of matrix stiffness on glioblastoma cell behavior using PEG-based hydrogels. *Mol Pharm* no. 11 (7):2115–25.

Wang, D., J. R. Grammer, C. S. Cobbs, J. E. Stewart, Jr., Z. Liu, R. Rhoden, T. P. Hecker, Q. Ding, and C. L. Gladson. 2000. p125 focal adhesion kinase promotes malignant astrocytoma cell proliferation *in vivo*. *J Cell Sci* no. 113 (Pt 23):4221–30.

Wang, F., V. M. Weaver, O. W. Petersen, C. A. Larabell, S. Dedhar, P. Briand, R. Lupu, and M. J. Bissell. 1998. Reciprocal interactions between beta1-integrin and epidermal growth factor receptor in three-dimensional basement membrane breast cultures: A different perspective in epithelial biology. *Proc Natl Acad Sci USA* no. 95 (25):14821–26.

Wang, J., L. Ren, L. Li, W. Liu, J. Zhou, W. Yu, D. Tong, and S. Chen. 2009. Microfluidics: A new cosset for neurobiology. *Lab Chip* no. 9 (5):644–52.

Wiranowska, M., A. M. Rojiani, P. E. Gottschall, L. C. Moscinski, J. Johnson, and S. Saporta. 2000. CD44 expression and MMP-2 secretion by mouse glioma cells: Effect of interferon and anti-CD44 antibody. *Anticancer Res* no. 20 (6b):4301–06.

Wong, A. P., R. Perez-Castillejos, J. Christopher Love, and G. M. Whitesides. 2008. Partitioning microfluidic channels with hydrogel to construct tunable 3-D cellular microenvironments. *Biomaterials* no. 29 (12):1853–61.

Wu, J., Z. Mao, H. Tan, L. Han, T. Ren, and C. Gao. 2012. Gradient biomaterials and their influences on cell migration. *Interface Focus* no. 2 (3):337–55.

Yamada, K. M. and E. Cukierman. 2007. Modeling tissue morphogenesis and cancer in 3D. *Cell* no. 130 (4):601–10.

Yamaguchi, H., J. Wyckoff, and J. Condeelis. 2005. Cell migration in tumors. *Curr Opin Cell Biol* no. 17 (5):559–64.

Yang, Z. J. and R. J. Wechsler-Reya. 2007. Hit 'em where they live: Targeting the cancer stem cell niche. *Cancer Cell* no. 11 (1):3–5.

Yuan, X., J. Curtin, Y. Xiong, G. Liu, S. Waschsmann-Hogiu, D. L. Farkas, K. L. Black, and J. S. Yu. 2004. Isolation of cancer stem cells from adult glioblastoma multiforme. *Oncogene* no. 23 (58):9392–400.

Yung, W. K., J. R. Shapiro, and W. R. Shapiro. 1982. Heterogeneous chemosensitivities of subpopulations of human glioma cells in culture. *Cancer Res* no. 42 (3):992–98.

Zagzag, D., M. Esencay, O. Mendez, H. Yee, I. Smirnova, Y. Huang, L. Chiriboga, E. Lukyanov, M. Liu, and E. W. Newcomb. 2008. Hypoxia- and vascular endothelial growth factor-induced stromal cell-derived factor-1alpha/CXCR4 expression in glioblastomas: One plausible explanation of Scherer's structures. *Am J Pathol* no. 173 (2):545–60.

Zagzag, D., D. R. Friedlander, B. Margolis, M. Grumet, G. L. Semenza, H. Zhong, J. W. Simons, J. Holash, S. J. Wiegand, and G. D. Yancopoulos. 2000. Molecular events implicated in brain tumor angiogenesis and invasion. *Pediatr Neurosurg* no. 33 (1):49–55.

Zervantonakis, I. K., S. K. Hughes-Alford, J. L. Charest, J. S. Condeelis, F. B. Gertler, and R. D. Kamm. 2012. Three-dimensional microfluidic model for tumor cell intravasation and endothelial barrier function. *Proc Natl Acad Sci USA* no. 109 (34):13515–20.

Zhang, M., F. Behbod, R. L. Atkinson, M. D. Landis, F. Kittrell, D. Edwards, D. Medina et al. 2008. Identification of tumor-initiating cells in a p53-null mouse model of breast cancer. *Cancer Res* no. 68 (12):4674–82.

Zhong, J., A. Paul, S. J. Kellie, and G. M. O'Neill. 2010. Mesenchymal migration as a therapeutic target in glioblastoma. *J Oncol* no. 2010:430142.

Zhu, T. S., M. A. Costello, C. E. Talsma, C. G. Flack, J. G. Crowley, L. L. Hamm, X. He et al. 2011. Endothelial cells create a stem cell niche in glioblastoma by providing NOTCH ligands that nurture self-renewal of cancer stem-like cells. *Cancer Res* no. 71 (18):6061–72.

Section IV

Business Considerations

EDITOR'S NOTE ON BUSINESS CONSIDERATIONS

The final step in developing a successful 3D tissue-based test system is its translation into a commercially viable product. While information regarding the path of Food and Drug Administration (FDA) designation for a biomedical product is more widely accessible, the additional steps necessary to achieve insurance coverage and reimbursement codes are not as clear. Indeed, a successful biomedical product must achieve both regulatory designation (e.g. clearance, approval) and must clear preparatory steps for commercialization (coverage, coding, and reimbursement), as illustrated in Figure S1.

Currently, the various ways a specific 3D tissue test system may be used dictate specific activities and requirements within the FDA designation process. First, a 3D tissue test system used to determine a health state of a patient as an *in vitro* diagnostic (IVD) is regulated according to the code of federal regulations 21CFR809.3 that states "In vitro diagnostic products are those reagents, instruments, and systems intended for use in the diagnosis of disease or other conditions, including a determination of the state of health, in order to cure, mitigate, treat, or prevent disease or its sequelae. Such products are intended for use in the collection, preparation, and examination of specimens taken from the human body. These products are *devices* as defined in section 201(h) of the Federal Food, Drug, and Cosmetic Act (the act), and may also be biological products subject to section 351 of the Public Health Service Act" (Food and Drug Administration 2016a). The standard FDA requirements for IVD determination will depend on the rarity of the disease addressed, whether there is an unmet need for the test, and the risk associated in using the results from the test. Alternatively, a specific 3D tissue test system may improve the effective use of a given therapeutic. In this case, the 3D test system would be considered as necessary for the proper use of the therapeutic as a companion diagnostic or more fully as an

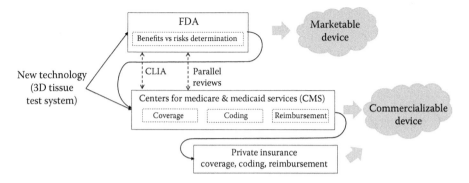

FIGURE S1 Path to translation. The FDA path (top) highlights the designation by the regulatory agency. The "coverage, coding, and reimbursement" path (middle) highlights that a service or device must be "effective" as well as "cost effective" for expenses related to use to be reimbursed by insurance companies.

in vitro companion diagnostic. Such a companion diagnostic is used by a health care professional to (i) decide if a patient may benefit from the therapeutic, (ii) evaluate if a patient may be at higher risk using the therapeutic, and (iii) monitor response to therapeutic to advise further treatment levels (Food and Drug Administration 2016b). These two use scenarios describe a process in which one company or laboratory manufactures the devices and a second laboratory uses those devices for testing.

A laboratory-developed test (LDT) is a third use scenario in which an IVD test is designed, manufactured, and used within a single laboratory (Food and Drug Administration 2015). That is, a laboratory has designed and manufactured a test for internal use only. Such a test may be designed as a local replacement for an FDA-cleared or approved IVD test. For example, a hospital lab may run its own vitamin D assay, even though there is an FDA-cleared test for vitamin D currently on the market (Food and Drug Administration 2015). Due to the increasing complexity of testing, the evolving philosophy and regulation are that LDTs should be regulated as devices.

Clinical Laboratory Improvement Amendments (CLIA) establish quality standards for laboratories to ensure the accuracy, reliability, and timeliness of the patient's test results. Three federal agencies are responsible for CLIA: The FDA, the Centers for Medicare and Medicaid Services (CMS), and the Center for Disease Control (CDC) (Department of Health and Human Services 2015; Food and Drug Administration 2014). The CMS issues laboratory certificates, conducts inspections, and enforces regulatory compliance. The FDA develops rules and guidance for CLIA complexity categorization that define certification and inspection requirements. The CDC develops technical standards and laboratory practice guidelines, including standards and guidelines for cytology. The CDC also manages the Clinical Laboratory Improvement Advisory Committee (CLIAC).

Regulatory designation is the first step along the continuum toward coverage and reimbursement decisions crucial for a product to fair favorably in the marketplace. For the vast majority of products, gaining coverage—and then appropriate coding and reimbursement—from major insurers is an essential next step. The CMS must independently determine (i) the clinical utility, that is, does the test output improve patient outcomes? and (ii) the economic utility, that is, are patient outcomes worth the cost of the test?

Because the landscape is evolving toward the regulation of diagnostic tests as devices, Chapter 20 details the path of devices through the insurance and billing environment and bridges the gap in knowledge between approval and commercial viability. The authors use examples of medical devices to highlight the challenging paths through the current regulatory environment. The successful translation of *in vitro* test systems research into products will require navigation through similar regulatory paths.

At this time, the CMS is in the process of implementing clinical laboratory payment reforms passed by Congress in 2014. This legislation, that is, the Protecting Access to Medicare Act of 2014, provides new rules for coding, coverage, and payment of advance diagnostic laboratory tests (ADLTs). ADLTs include tests that analyze "biomarkers of deoxyribonucleic acid, ribonucleic acid, or proteins combined with a unique algorithm to yield a single patient-specific result." Medicare will tie payment rates for ADLTs to the average of private payer rates. In addition, Medicare will determine these rates by surveying clinical laboratories.

The information and recommendations provided in this chapter, though specific to medical devices, provide readers with key information to understand the complex processes of Medicare coverage and payment policies. Since both ADLTs and medical devices are coded through the same systems (Current Procedural Terminology [CPT] and Healthcare Common Procedure Coding System [HCPCS]), some of the processes described in the following also apply to ADLTs. These processes will continue to evolve for ADLTs as CMS releases additional guidance in the coming years.

REFERENCES

Department of Health and Human Services. Clinical Laboratory Improvement Amendments (CLIA) and Medicare Laboratory Services, 2015. Available from https://www.cms.gov/Outreach-and-Education/Medicare-Learning-Network-MLN/MLNProducts/Downloads/CLIABrochure.pdf

Food and Drug Administration. Clinical Laboratory Improvement Amendments (CLIA), 2014. Available from http://www.fda.gov/MedicalDevices/DeviceRegulationandGuidance/IVDRegulatoryAssistance/ucm124105.htm

Food and Drug Administration. Laboratory Developed Tests, 2015. Available from http://www.fda.gov/MedicalDevices/ProductsandMedicalProcedures/InVitroDiagnostics/ucm407296.htm

Food and Drug Administration. CFR: Code of Federal Regulations Title 21, 2016a. Available from http://www.accessdata.fda.gov/scripts/cdrh/cfdocs/cfcfr/CFRSearch.cfm?FR=809.3

Food and Drug Administration. Companion Diagnostics, 2016b. Available from http://www.fda.gov/MedicalDevices/ProductsandMedicalProcedures/InVitroDiagnostics/ucm407297.htm

20 Bringing Regenerative Medicine to Patients
The Coverage, Coding, and Reimbursement Processes

Khin-Kyemon Aung, Scott Levy,[*] and Sujata K. Bhatia

CONTENTS

20.1 Introduction 381
20.2 Coverage 382
    20.2.1 Local Coverage Determination (LCD) 383
    20.2.2 National Coverage Determination 387
20.3 Future Directions in Coverage 387
    20.3.1 FDA–CMS Parallel Review 387
    20.3.2 Coverage with Evidence Development 388
    20.3.3 Commercial Insurance Coverage 389
20.4 Payment 390
    20.4.1 Codes and Payment for Physicians and Devices 390
    20.4.2 Medicare Payment to Hospitals 392
    20.4.3 Coding-Enhanced Price Competition 393
    20.4.4 Seeking a New CPT Code 394
    20.4.5 Seeking a New HCPCS Code 395
    20.4.6 Special Payments for New-Technologies 395
    20.4.7 Downstream Impact on Other Payers 396
    20.4.8 Leaving Fee-For-Service System 396
20.5 Conclusion and Perspective 397
References 397

20.1 INTRODUCTION

After the Food and Drug Administration (FDA) approves or clears a new device, theoretically, manufacturers have full access to U.S. markets and can start selling their products directly to consumers. In reality though, clearing the FDA is only the first step along the continuum of coverage and reimbursement decisions necessary

---

[*] Khin-Kyemon Aung and Scott Levy equally contributed to this work and both serve as first authors.

for a product to fair favorably in the marketplace. For the vast majority of products, gaining coverage—and then appropriate coding and reimbursement—from major insurers is an essential next step.

The importance of coverage, coding, and reimbursement is underscored by the company Organogenesis' experience in the early-2000s. In 1998, Organogenesis became the first company to earn FDA approval for a mass-produced product with living human cells—a skin substitute called Apligraf® used for healing ulcers such as diabetic foot ulcers and chronic venous leg ulcers. Given that Organogenesis was one of the only companies with FDA approval for a skin substitute at the time, it quickly cornered the market. Nevertheless, by 2002, the company had filed for Chapter 11 bankruptcy. A number of reasons have been attributed to Organogenesis' collapse, primarily a poor business model and poor communication between the leadership of the company, investors, and customers (Bouchie 2002). However, restrictive reimbursement policies have also been implicated (Bouchie 2002).

According to an article on the Organogenesis' bankruptcy filing, the Centers for Medicare & Medicaid Services (CMS) was partially to blame for the bankruptcy with its "stringent limitations, restricting reimbursement for the products for use on only the most severe wounds and for a limited number of units per patient" (Bouchie 2002). Although FDA approval is imperative for manufacturers to gain access to U.S. markets, securing favorable Medicare coverage from CMS, coding, and reimbursement is critical for strong market performance. In other words, much to the dismay of many biotechnology companies, FDA approval is not enough.

Coverage refers to a payer's decision on whether a product is eligible for payment and the circumstances under which the product will be reimbursed. Coding refers to how products are billed by a provider, and reimbursement refers to the scheme under which a product will be paid and the amount that will be paid. Favorable decisions at each of these three junctures help manufacturers facilitate broader use of their product.

This chapter focuses on Medicare coverage and payment policy. Medicare is one of the largest public insurers in the United States and covers more than 50 million lives of individuals aged 65 years or more as well as younger Americans with a disability or with end-stage renal disease. The CMS is a federal agency that makes decisions on coverage, coding, and reimbursement for Medicare and Medicaid, which is a state-based public insurance program for low-income families, children, pregnant women, and individuals with disabilities. Given the vast number of lives that are covered under Medicare, CMS has considerable influence on the national payer market and much of the content discussed here applies broadly to state Medicaid programs and commercial insurers.

20.2 COVERAGE

Since its founding in 1965, Medicare has only covered items and services that are deemed "reasonable and necessary." This concept is not clearly defined, and many have criticized the definition as ambiguous. In addition to meeting the criteria of "reasonable and necessary," new technologies applying for coverage must also fall within the scope of defined Medicare benefit categories, which are groupings that Medicare uses to classify items and services for coverage. Examples of Medicare benefit categories include inpatient hospital services and home health services (a complete list of benefit categories can be found in Table 20.1). Medicare also explicitly does not cover some items and services, such as cosmetic surgery, hearing aids, and personal comfort items.

CMS makes coverage decisions on a local and national level, and its final decision applies to both traditional Medicare and Medicare Advantage. Traditional Medicare is a fee-for-service program where the federal government pays directly for healthcare services. Medicare Advantage, on the other hand, is a program that allows Medicare beneficiaries to receive their care through private insurers contracting with CMS. CMS pays health insurers capitated, or fixed, predetermined rates. In turn, these health insurers privately contract with providers.

Not every new product requires or receives a formal coverage decision. Innovations that incrementally improve upon previous technologies and are billed under some of Medicare's payment schemes—such as the inpatient and outpatient prospective payment systems, which will be discussed in greater detail below—usually do not need a separate coverage determination.

20.2.1 Local Coverage Determination (LCD)

CMS develops local coverage policies for Medicare Parts A (inpatient services) and B (outpatient services) through the use of 12 private Medicare Administrative Contractors (MACs). These contractors primarily process Medicare claims, but also develop coverage policies within their own respective jurisdictions if no applicable national coverage decision is available. MAC jurisdiction varies from 2 to 10 states or U.S. territories. Table 20.2 lists the current MAC jurisdictions for Medicare Parts A and B. CMS is planning on consolidating the number of MACs to 10 in the future, and there are separate MAC jurisdictions for durable medical equipment and home health and hospice. Companies that want to sell their products in multiple MAC jurisdictions will need approval from each of the associated MACs.

When a MAC identifies a new item or service that does not have a coverage determination, the MAC first tries to adapt an existing LCD. If an existing one cannot be modified for the specific item, service, or situation, then the MAC will develop a new LCD. MACs review clinical data—published studies in peer-reviewed journals and data from randomized clinical trials—and gather opinions from medical experts in the field or medical associations—to determine whether a product is reasonable and necessary. Their decisions dictate the clinical circumstances under which an item or service is deemed reasonable and necessary (and thus eligible for reimbursement) as well. In some cases, the MAC will post a draft LCD for public comment for a minimum of 45 days and schedule meetings open to the public. After the comment period closes, the MAC considers all the evidence and comments gathered before issuing a final version of the LCD on its website. Under Medicare guidelines, the MAC must then provide a notice period of at least 45 calendar days before the LCD can go into effect.

It is important to note that devices that do not have an LCD can still be reimbursed. MACs can make case-by-case decisions on whether or not to pay for procedures using that device. Unfortunately, MACs take longer to process these bills. In addition, they are also more likely to reject these claims than a claim in compliance with an LCD. In most cases, it is in the best interest of device companies to receive an LCD.

TABLE 20.1
List of Medicare Benefit Categories

Column 1	Column 2	Column 3	Column 4
Ambulance services	Diagnostic services in outpatient hospital	Institutional Dialysis services and supplies	Post-hospital extended care services
Ambulatory surgical center facility services	Diagnostic tests (other)	Leg, arm, back, and neck braces (orthotics)	Post-institutional home health services
Antigens	Diagnostic x-ray tests	Medical nutrition therapy services	Prostate cancer screening tests
Artificial legs, arms, and eyes	Drugs and biologicals	Nurse practitioner services	Prosthetic devices
Audiology services	Durable medical equipment	Optometrist services	Qualified psychologist services
Blood clotting factors for hemophilia patients	Erythropoietin for dialysis patients	Oral anticancer drugs	Religious nonmedical health care institution
Bone mass measurement	Extended care services	Oral antiemetic drugs	Rural health clinic services
Certified nurse-midwife services	Eyeglasses after cataract surgery	Orthotics and prosthetics	Screening for glaucoma
Certified registered nurse anesthetist services	Federally qualified health center services	Osteoporosis Drug	Screening Mammography
Chiropractor services	Hepatitis B vaccine and administration	Outpatient hospital services incident to a physician's service	Screening pap smear
Clinical nurse specialist services	Home dialysis supplies and equipment	Outpatient occupational therapy services	Screening pelvic exam
Clinical social worker services	Home health services	Outpatient physical therapy services	Self-care home dialysis support services
Colorectal cancer screening tests	Hospice care	Outpatient speech language pathology services	Shoes for patients with diabetes
Comprehensive outpatient rehabilitation facility (CORF) services	Immunosuppressive drugs	Partial hospitalization services	Skilled nursing facility
Critical access hospital services	Incident to a physician's professional service	Physician assistant services	Splints, casts, other devices used for reduction of fractures and dislocations
Dentist services	Influenza vaccine and administration	Physicians' services	Surgical dressings
Diabetes outpatient self-management training	Inpatient hospital services	Pneumococcal vaccine and administration	Transplantation services for ESRD-entitled beneficiaries
Diagnostic laboratory tests	Inpatient psychiatric hospital services	Podiatrist services	X-ray, radium, and radioactive isotope therapy

TABLE 20.2
MAC Jurisdictions for Medicare Parts A and B

MAC Name	MAC Jurisdiction	States within Jurisdiction
Wisconsin Physicians Service Insurance Corporation	5	Iowa, Kansas, Missouri, Nebraska
National Government Services, Inc.	6	Illinois, Minnesota, Wisconsin
Wisconsin Physicians Service Insurance Corporation	8	Indiana, Michigan
CGS Administrators, LLC	15	Kentucky, Ohio
Noridian Healthcare Solutions, LLC	E	California, Hawaii, Nevada, American Somoa, Guam, Northern Mariana Islands
Noridian Healthcare Solutions, LLC	F	Alaska, Arizona, Idaho, Montana, North Dakota, Oregon, South Dakota, Utah, Washington, Wyoming
Novitas Solutions, Inc.	H	Arkansas, Colorado, New Mexico, Oklahoma, Texas, Louisiana, Mississippi
Cahaba Government Benefit Administrators, LLC	J	Alabama, Georgia, Tennessee
National Government Services, Inc.	K	Connecticut, New York, Maine, Massachusetts, New Hampshire, Rhode Island, Vermont
Novitas Solutions, Inc.	L	Delaware, District of Columbia, Maryland, New Jersey, Pennsylvania (includes Part B for counties of Arlington and Fairfax in Virginia and the city of Alexandria in Virginia)
Palmetto GBA, LLC	M	North Carolina, South Carolina, Virginia, West Virginia (excludes Part B for the counties of Arlington and Fairfax in Virginia and the city of Alexandria in Virginia)
First Coast Service Options, Inc.	N	Florida, Puerto Rico, U.S. Virgin Islands

Source: Adapted from Centers for Medicare & Medicaid Services. 2015. Medicare administrative contractors (MACs). MACs by State. Available at https://www.cms.gov/Medicare/Medicare-Contracting/Medicare-Administrative-Contractors/Downloads/MACs-by-State-April-2015.pdf.

Each LCD provides information about the date the coverage determination will go into effect, the description of the covered services, the diagnoses codes for which the product can be used and reimbursed (see Table 20.3), and the distinct coverage area. Since the coverage policy created by each MAC only applies to providers within the contractor's jurisdiction, there can be wide variation in coverage between geographic areas, and beneficiaries in different parts of the country can have uneven access to new medical technologies.

These discrepancies in coverage have been widely reported and remain a concern for some federal agencies and stakeholders. In an analysis of 2011 data, the Office of Inspector General found that LCDs inconsistently prohibited or limited coverage across states (Office of Inspector General, 2014). Per their report, there were "at least 2

TABLE 20.3
Billing Codes by Provider

Providers	Description	Example
Physicians and other medical professionals		
ICD-10-CM	Identifies the patient's medical diagnoses	L89.112 (stage 2 pressure ulcer on the right upper back)
CPT	Identifies a medical service provided by billing professional	15271 (application of high cost skin substitute to trunk, arms, or legs)
HCPCS	Identifies a device, treatment, or supply	Q4101 (Apligraf)
Inpatient hospital stays (facility payment)		
ICD-10-CM	Identifies the patient's medical diagnoses	
ICD-10-PCS	Describe the patient's medical or surgical treatment plan	0HB6XZZ (excision of back skin, external approach)
MS-DRG	Episode-based payment for inpatient hospital stays	570 (skin debridement with major complications or comorbidities)
Outpatient hospital visits (facility payment)		
ICD-10-CM	Identifies the patient's medical diagnoses	L89.112 (stage 2 pressure ulcer on the right upper back)
CPT	Identifies a medical service provided by billing professional	15271 (application of high cost skin substitute to trunk, arms, or legs)
HCPCS	Identifies a device, treatment, or supply	Q4101 (Apligraf)
APC	Service-based payment for outpatient hospital services	0328 (level III skin repair)

different coverage policies for 59% of the procedure codes subject to LCDs" and "all but two of these procedure codes were subject to one or more LCDs that limited coverage in some, but not all States. These findings led to OIG's recommendation that CMS require MACs to develop a single set of coverage policies" (Office of Inspector General, 2014).

Other governmental entities have reached similar conclusions in the past. In 2001, the Medicare Payment Advisory Commission, which advises Congress on Medicare policy, recommended that Medicare eliminate LCDs due to the disparities that arise (Medicare Payment Advisory Commission 2001). In 2003, the Government Accountability Office, another congressional advisory entity, suggested replacing MAC-issued LCDs with national coverage decisions (US Governement Accountability Office 2003). Researchers have also expressed concerns about the decentralized coverage process, questioning whether LCDs lead to disparities in access, varying quality standards across states, lower thresholds for evidence, and duplicative effort (Foote 2003). Congress attempted to address these issues through Section 731 of the 2003 Medicare Modernization Act, which included provisions for CMS to more systematically determine which LCDs should be adopted nationally. Device, biologic, and pharmaceutical corporations have resisted calls to abandon the LCD process, asserting that the LCD process allows manufacturers and patients to gain quicker access to the market and technologies, respectively.

20.2.2 NATIONAL COVERAGE DETERMINATION

An alternative approach to LCDs is to seek coverage for products via national coverage determinations (NCDs). Similar to the local determination, NCDs provide guidance on the conditions under which a product or service is or is not covered. The advantage of an NCD is that a favorable coverage decision applies to all Medicare patients across the country. For the most part, NCDs trump existing individual LCD parameters, though MACs can add more coverage criteria as long as they do not contradict the NCD.

CMS or third parties, such as medical device companies, may formally request an NCD. CMS actively reviews current LCDs to determine whether an NCD is necessary. Once CMS begins to review an NCD, the agency must respond with a preliminary decision within 6 months of receipt, unless CMS needs an external review of the NCD request. It takes up to 90 days for a preliminary NCD to be finalized and another 6 months for CMS to fully implement any necessary coding and payment changes. CMS uses internal agency expertise for most coverage decisions. However, when the technology under review is highly controversial or may have a large impact on the Medicare program and its beneficiaries, the agency sometimes calls upon the Medicare Evidence Development and Coverage Advisory Committee (MEDCAC), which provides independent and expert advice on the quality of the technology's evidence.

Studies show that the level of evidence needed to achieve an NCD has increased over time (Chambers et al. 2015). Over the past 50 years, CMS has only issued about 300 NCDs despite thousands of new drugs, biologics, devices, and therapeutics coming to the market. With the passage of the Affordable Care Act, there has been an enhanced focus on improving patient experiences of care and the health of communities while reducing costs. Modifications to the coverage process could be a policy lever through which these goals can be achieved, and researchers have suggested a variety of ways that coverage determinations could be improved.

One intriguing idea is a statutory change allowing CMS to approve or deny coverage for items based on the comparative clinical effectiveness of the new technology compared to analogous technologies that are already covered (Tunis et al. 2011; Pearson and Bach 2010). Another suggestion is to have MEDCAC systematically identify high-value technologies that are covered locally now, but should be covered nationally in the future (Tunis et al. 2011). Others suggest more tightly linking coverage decisions with reimbursement levels and allowing CMS to more explicitly consider cost-effectiveness in making their coverage decisions (Tunis et al. 2011). Manufacturers should closely monitor potential changes by CMS in the coming years.

20.3 FUTURE DIRECTIONS IN COVERAGE

20.3.1 FDA–CMS PARALLEL REVIEW

The FDA and CMS use separate criteria and request different types of clinical evidence when making their respective decisions. Whereas "safe and effective" is the threshold for FDA approval or clearance, CMS covers only what is "reasonable and necessary." The independent processes can lead to delays and discrepancies between the FDA and CMS, causing additional hurdles and concerns for drug and device manufacturers. Because Medicare coverage decisions can have a large influence nationally, the consequences of a delayed or negative Medicare coverage decision extend beyond being locked out of the Medicare market.

To address these potential discrepancies and reduce the time between CMS and FDA decisions, CMS and the FDA launched a 2-year pilot parallel review process. A more efficient review process could not only benefit manufacturers, but also benefit patients, as they would have quicker access to the most cutting edge technologies and therapies on the market.

Though parallel review is appealing in principle, trade associations as well as large device manufacturers and pharmaceutical companies have expressed strong reservations about the project. Critics argue that the process could actually place additional burden on applicants with little returns. Since the majority of new products are already covered by LCDs, manufacturers argued that parallel review was unnecessary. In 2011, during the public comment phase of the parallel review process, Biotechnology Innovation Organization, the largest biotechnology trade group in the country, wrote strongly against the pilot stating that "developing a new parallel review process potentially resulting in more NCDs for drugs and biologics is not necessary because… local contractors often are best placed to assess the reasonableness and necessity for their respective and unique constituents, and more NCDs are not necessarily better" (Emmett and Todd 2011).

Another concern is that the all-or-nothing approach of an NCD could actually have the consequence of limiting access in case of a negative decision. Johnson & Johnson asserted that "many new treatments should be available for use by physicians, as is currently the case, before a decision is made to standardize coverage nationally" (DeSantis and Buto 2011). Genentech questioned one of the rationales for the pilot, claiming that the current approval process has actually not "resulted in significant delays in post-approval coverage" (Morris 2011).

Despite the critical initial feedback, the pilot was extended for two more years in 2013. In August 2014, CMS and FDA jointly announced the FDA approval and national coverage determination of Cologuard®, a noninvasive colorectal screening test that detects potentially cancerous growths through the use of DNA screenings. It marked the first joint announcement and CMS leadership hailed the joint decision as a case of "unprecedented collaboration…[that] will provide timely access for Medicare beneficiaries" (Food and Drug Administration 2014). Deputy Director Nancy Stade of the FDA's Center for Devices and Radiological Health added that parallel review cut "as many as six months from the time from study initiative to coverage" (Food and Drug Administration 2014). Kevin Conroy, CEO of Exact Sciences, thanked CMS and the FDA, praising the decision as *a major milestone* (Exact Sciences Corp. 2014). In late 2016, the parallel review program was extended indefinitely.

20.3.2 Coverage with Evidence Development

CMS often has low-quality or insufficient evidence available at the onset of the NCD process to come to a final coverage decision. In these situations, CMS is placed in a difficult position: deny coverage, which could stymie innovation and hamper patients' access to potentially beneficial new technologies, or approve coverage with little insight into the product's ultimate effectiveness. Between 1999 and 2007, CMS issued a favorable decision in 60% of the cases it took on, even though the evidence supporting the technology was usually considered to be of "poor or fair quality" at best (Neumann et al. 2008).

To better handle these situations, CMS developed a process to cover certain items and services on the condition that the manufacturers will gather additional data on the clinical benefits. This process, known as coverage with evidence development (CED), serves two purposes: it allows manufacturers to have additional time to collect data that could better inform a final coverage decision and allows patients to benefit from experimental technologies and procedures.

Under the terms of the CED, Medicare will only reimburse drugs, biologics, and devices if the patients receiving them are enrolled in a clinical trial or study. The study results must be reported to CMS for use in a future coverage assessment. Coverage via CED is temporary, and a CED cycle is completed once CMS reviews the application again and comes to a final national coverage decision. At that time, CMS can decide to deny or approve coverage of the product.

There are a number of operational and ethical complexities to CED that industry representatives and researchers have voiced. Biomedical and pharmaceutical companies have expressed concerns that the CED process will result in higher evidentiary thresholds, place extra burdens on manufacturers, and will be used by MACs in LCDs, not only by CMS in NCDs. Researchers have also chimed in, questioning whether CEDs will allow payers to indefinitely delay making coverage decisions. CMS issued revised guidance on CED in November 2014; however, the new guidance still remains ambiguous as to whether CEDs can be applied on the local level (Centers for Medicare & Medicaid Services 2014).

CED remains a critical vehicle through which new technologies can gain national coverage, and it will continue to impact the regenerative medicine industry for years to come. Currently, there are several CEDs that may be of particular interest to the regenerative medicine community, including allogeneic hematopoietic stem cell transplants for indications such as myelodysplastic syndrome, multiple myeloma, sickle cell disease, and myelofibrosis. These CEDs, for the first time, offer consistent coverage of bone marrow transplants for these four indications, as researchers gather data about stem cell transplant recipients' and donors' recovery times and long-term outcomes. Under CED, there is an opportunity for manufacturers to work closely with CMS to reach a favorable coverage decision and to bring their product to market earlier than under traditional pathways.

20.3.3 Commercial Insurance Coverage

Each private payer makes its own decisions on which items and services to cover. Given CMS' influence nationally though, it is often assumed that private payers typically follow the agency's lead on coverage determinations. However, recent analyses show that CMS national coverage determinations and private payer coverage policies were only consistent with each other approximately 50% of the time (Chambers et al. 2015). CMS was more restrictive in its coverage decision 25% of the time, and for the remaining 25% of the time, CMS was less restrictive (Chambers et al. 2015).

This underscores the complicated nature of gaining coverage in both public and private insurance markets. Given the importance and complexity of gaining coverage, many companies hire law firms or consulting firms that specialize in navigating the regulatory process.

20.4 PAYMENT

The next step after gaining coverage is securing proper reimbursement. A new device first needs a standardized shorthand, known as a code, for payers and providers to describe the device and related treatments in medical bills. Medicare then sets reimbursement rates on a code-by-code basis paying different amounts for care provided in different clinical settings. There are several ways that a device manufacturer can affect the codes used to bill for its device and consequently the reimbursement paid for the device and related treatments. Although coding may seem like nothing more than a mundane and byzantine component of the United States' paperwork-intensive healthcare system, coding can actually dictate a device's reimbursement rate, utilization, and profitability.

20.4.1 Codes and Payment for Physicians and Devices

Medical coding systems vary by the place of service and type of provider billing for the service, though some coding systems are used in multiple settings. Physicians and other medical professionals use five-digit numbers known as Current Procedural Terminology codes (CPT codes or simply CPTs[*]) to bill for the services they provide.[†] Each CPT corresponds to a defined medical treatment. For example, a physician applying a high cost skin substitute to a wounded arm would record CPT code 15271 on the medical bill. CPT codes do not, however, identify a specific company's device that must be used. Nevertheless, providers may only perform some procedures using certain types of devices. For example, in 2015, physicians could bill for code 15271 when using 1 of over 20 different skin substitute models. Irrespective of the skin substitute used, each physician would still bill Medicare using 15271 code.

Medicare reimburses for most, but not all, CPTs.[‡] For each CPT, the Medicare Physician Fee Schedule has an associated relative value unit (RVU), which is calculated by summing the estimated physician work, practice expense, and malpractice liability associated with each treatment.[§] The practice expense component is the most important component for device manufacturers as it generally includes the costs of the implantable biologics and devices used in a procedure. The RVU is then

---

[*] Please see Table 20.4 for a full listing of acronyms used in this chapter.
[†] We use "CPTs" as shorthand for Category I CPTs. Category II and III CPTs are used for performance measurement and experimental technologies, respectively. These two categories are not generally relevant for device manufacturers seeking codes that will lead to Medicare reimbursement.
[‡] Medicare does not reimburse a CPT code for different reasons, including the code not meeting CMS' "reasonable and necessary" requirement or not following under a defined benefit category.
[§] The work component is a function of the estimated practitioner time, skill, training, and intensity associated with providing the given service.

TABLE 20.4
Table of Acronyms

APC	Ambulatory Payment Classification
ASC	Ambulatory Surgical Center
CED	Coverage with Evidence Development
CMS	Centers for Medicare and Medicaid Services
CPT	Current Procedural Terminology
FDA	Food and Drug Administration
HCPCS	Healthcare Common Procedure Coding System
ICD-10-PCS	International Classification of Diseases, 10th Edition, Procedural Coding System
ICD-10-CM	International Classification of Diseases, 10th Edition, Clinical Modification
LCD	Local Coverage Determination
MAC	Medicare Administrative Contractor
MEDCAC	Medicare Evidence Development and Coverage Advisory Committee
MS-DRG	Medicare Severity Diagnosis Related Group
NCD	National Coverage Determination
NOC	Miscellaneous/Not Otherwise Classified
NTAP	New-Technology Add-On Payment
OIG	Office of Inspector General
RUC	Relative Value Unit Committee
RVU	Relative Value Unit

multiplied by the Medicare conversion factor, which is the same for each CPT. For example, in 2015, a physician billing CPT Code 15271 for services performed in an independent physician's office has a Medicare RVU of 4.0, which is then multiplied by the 2015 conversion factor ($35.93) for a total payment of $144.*

However, Medicare would pay $56 less to a physician performing that treatment in a facility (skilled nursing facility, ambulatory surgical center, inpatient or outpatient hospital). Medicare calculates the payment to the facility-based physician using the same work and malpractice liability components but a reduced practice expense component. This is because the facility is expected to cover some of the practice expenses, including the cost of implantable biologics and other devices associated with the procedure, and receive payment for those costs when it separately bills Medicare under the applicable facility payment system.

For medical professionals and facilities to successfully obtain reimbursement for their services, they must also include patient diagnoses in the bill. All providers use the same set of six-digit diagnoses codes known as International Classification of Diseases, 10th Edition, Clinical Modification (ICD-10-CM) codes. For example, ICD-10-CM code L89.112 refers to a stage 2 pressure ulcer on the right upper back.

When billing for treatments involving an implantable biologic or device, professionals as well as outpatient hospitals and ambulatory surgical centers (ASCs) are

---

* Medicare reimbursement rates for each CPT code can be found on Medicare's website at: https://www.cms.gov/apps/physician-fee-schedule/overview.aspx.

also supposed to list the code for the type of device used. Devices, supplies, and procedures that do not have their own CPT codes are listed using a standardized set of five-digit alphanumeric codes known as the Level II Healthcare Common Procedure Coding System (HCPCS).* For example, in addition to billing CPT Code 15271, the *procedure* for applying a skin substitute, an office-based physician would include the HCPCS in the bill for the *skin substitute* applied to the wound (e.g., Q4101—Apligraf®). Because the payment associated with the CPT code incorporates the cost of medical devices in the practice expense, Medicare does not separately pay for most devices. Consequently, a provider includes Q4101 (Apligraf®) in the billing, but Medicare only pays for 15271, which includes the cost of skin substitutes.

Although some kinds of devices, such as skin substitutes, tend to have separate HCPCS (pronounced "hickpicks") codes for each manufacturer's device model, HCPCS generally do not correspond to specific device models. Moreover, competing devices are often billed using the same HCPCS. Indeed, a new device must have a significant therapeutic distinction from existing devices in order to justify a new code. Similar to skin substitute manufacturers, manufacturers of new 3D tissue test systems will likely want to obtain a model-specific HCPCS. As discussed further below, model-specific HCPCS codes facilitate efforts to collect data on the device's efficacy and costs. These data play an important role in enabling 3D tissue test system manufacturers to argue for more favorable CPT coding and thus payment rates.

Payment for devices is typically built into the payment to the physician or facility for the billed procedure. For office-based procedures, the cost of devices and supplies is often packaged into the practice expense component of the procedure's RVU and thus payment, though Medicare will pay separately for some devices. For facility-based treatments, the cost is usually omitted from the practice expense component of the RVU and thus payment to the physician. Instead, the cost is included in payments to the Medicare facility as discussed further in the section below on separately billable codes.†

20.4.2 Medicare Payment to Hospitals

Medicare reimburses hospitals separately for inpatient stays and outpatient visits using the Inpatient Prospective Payment System (IPPS) and the Outpatient Prospective Payment System (OPPS), respectively.‡ The IPPS pays preset rates designed to reflect the expected facility costs associated with a patient's diagnoses, ICD-10-CMs, and ICD-10 Procedural Coding System (ICD-10-PCS), procedural codes that describe the patient's medical or surgical treatment plan.§ Using these

---

* CPT codes are also known as Level 1 HCPCS codes. However, in this chapter, we refer to HCPCS Level 2 codes as simply "HCPCS."
† A device being separately payable for physicians does not imply that it will be separately payable to a facility, or vice versa.
‡ Medicare pays other medical facilities, such as skilled nursing facilities, inpatient rehabilitation facilities, and long-term acute care hospitals, according to their own prospective payment systems. For more information on how Medicare pays these facilities, see http://medpac.gov/-documents-/payment-basics.
§ Unlike physicians and outpatient hospitals, inpatient hospital billing does not use CPT or HCPCS codes.

billing codes and a complicated grouping formula, Medicare assigns each patient to a Medicare severity diagnosis related group (MS-DRG), which is intended to be a comprehensive payment with almost no separate payments for additional treatments and tests.* With devices bundled into MS-DRGs (e.g., 570—Skin Debridement with Major Complications or Comorbidities), hospitals have a strong financial incentive to use low cost devices.

Outpatient hospitals bill Medicare using the CPT, HCPCS, and ICD-10-CM codes associated with the patient's treatment. Using these billing codes and preset rules, the OPPS assigns each patient to one or more Ambulatory Payment Classification (APC) groups, which represent the average facility cost for many treatments with similar clinical characteristics and costs. Irrespective of the underlying CPT code, all services within a given APC are reimbursed the same amount. For example, an outpatient hospital billing for any of 52 surgical CPTs pertaining to skin repair will receive a $1405 in payment for APC 0328 (Level III Skin Repair).

Like the IPPS's DRGs, the OPPS' APC groups include services, drugs, implantable devices, supplies, and other items. However, the OPPS does not package *all* relevant facility expenses into the APC, making separate payments for some drugs, devices, etc. in addition to the APC. Some separate payments are required by statute, whereas others result from the agency's policy judgment and the rulemaking process. For example, contrast agents. In 2008, CMS began limiting the number of separate payments and expanding the number of items and services that are packaged into APC groups. In 2014 and 2015, CMS enhanced the packaging of items, supplies, and services, particularly for device-dependent procedures. CMS believes that further packaging will continue to incentivize outpatient hospitals to provide care more efficiently. CMS is expected to continue expanding the set of packaged items in the coming years.

20.4.3 CODING-ENHANCED PRICE COMPETITION

The coding systems described above implicitly or explicitly bundle multiple services or treatment options into a single code. A physician billing a CPT code can often use one of several different devices, but the payment will be the same. Because reimbursement for APCs is set based on the average costs to facilities for those CPT codes in the APC, an outpatient hospital with an otherwise average cost structure might lose money if its surgeon uses a device that is more expensive than average for that APC. These coding practices can make low cost devices more financially attractive to providers than high cost devices billed under the same code. They also can make separately payable devices more attractive to providers. Given the connection between coding and price competition, coding decisions can significantly impact device pricing, provider utilization, and the return on investment for the device's manufacturer.

---

* Medicare makes separate payments for certain new technologies as discussed later on in this chapter. In addition, Medicare pays for other reasons, including medical education, providing care to uninsured patients, unpaid patient cost sharing, extremely expensive patients, etc. For a more comprehensive treatment, see MedPAC payment basics, http://medpac.gov/documents/payment-basics/hospital-acute-inpatient-services-payment-system-14.pdf?sfvrsn=0.

20.4.4 Seeking a New CPT Code

For many device manufacturers, including manufacturers of the 3D tissue test systems, a new CPT code is a financial boon. A new code is assigned a new reimbursement rate that reflects the cost of the new procedure. Consequently, if a physician can perform the procedure using only the manufacturer's new device, the reimbursement rate will reflect the cost of the manufacturer's device as well as the skill and time associated with the physician using it. With a new CPT code, the new device and existing devices will compete for provider utilization more on the basis of clinical efficacy and less on the basis of pricing.

In contrast, if physicians using the manufacturer's new device must bill an existing CPT code, which is already associated with other devices, reimbursement for that code reflects the average cost of the procedure and the other devices that can be used. If the manufacturer's device is more expensive than other devices associated with the procedure, the manufacturer is at a disadvantage. Of course, the opposite is true if the manufacturer's new device is assigned to an existing code associated with devices that are more expensive than the manufacturer's new device.

Obtaining a new CPT code takes at least 1 year and often takes even longer. Once the FDA has approved or cleared a device, the manufacturer and other related stakeholders can seek a new CPT code from the American Medical Association's (AMA) CPT Editorial Board, which is primarily composed of representatives from physician specialty societies. Once approved, the AMA's Relative Value Unit Committee (RUC), which is also largely composed of representatives from physician specialty societies, recommends the treatment and device's direct practice expenses and work expenses for the code's RVU. Although CMS makes the final decisions regarding RVU, CMS has historically accepted most of the RUC's recommendations on the work component (Laugesen et al. 2012). With seats at these exclusive tables, specialty societies often play a more direct role in these conversations than device manufacturers. Nonetheless, device manufacturers play an important role generating clinical data and peer-reviewed journal articles, demonstrating the treatment's clinical efficacy to the CPT Editorial Board and providing cost data to inform the RUC's recommendations (Alliance for Regenerative Medicine 2013).

The CPT Editorial Board has a list of criteria for creating a new code, designed to ensure that a new treatment or device is meaningfully different from existing treatments and devices and thus unable to be appropriately billed using existing codes. For example, a new code cannot be for "a fragmentation of an existing procedure or service not currently reportable as complete service by one or more existing codes" (American Medical Association 2016).

The CPT Editorial Board meets three times a year and adheres to a tight schedule with meetings in 2016 focused on changes that will take effect in 2018. Device manufacturers hoping to apply for a permanent CPT code immediately after FDA clearance must begin preparing their data and applications well in advance of deadlines. Close attention to the Editorial Board's calendar is essential.

Although there is no fee for requesting a coding change for CPT codes (or HCPCS codes), manufacturers may incur expenses writing their request and generating any data needed to show clinical efficacy. In addition, like the coverage process, some device manufacturers hire consulting firms to help them navigate coding.

20.4.5 Seeking a New HCPCS Code

A new HCPCS code, even if temporary, can also help a new device manufacturer, particularly if a new CPT code is delayed, denied, or not sought. A new HCPCS code enables providers and payers to specifically reference a company's device in bills, enabling CMS and others to collect data on the device's clinical efficacy and costs. Manufacturers often use these data in conversations with the CPT Editorial Board and CMS to demonstrate the unique features or efficacy of the device and thus the need for favorable coding or payment changes. A temporary HCPCS can also help a manufacturer enter the market without delay. Without a device-specific code or assignment to an existing code, providers may need to use "miscellaneous/not otherwise classified" (NOC) codes, which are often denied by commercial payers.

A device manufacturer can seek a HCPCS code from the CMS' HCPCS Workgroup, which is composed of representatives from CMS, other payers, providers, and other stakeholders. The Workgroup has a list of criteria for creating a new code, designed to ensure that a new treatment is meaningfully different from existing treatment options and thus unable to be appropriately billed using existing codes. Like CPT codes, a request for a new HCPCS can only begin after the FDA has approved or cleared a device. The HCPCS Workgroup's calendar is less rigid than the CPT Editorial Board's calendar, but failing to meet deadlines can still result in long delays.

20.4.6 Special Payments for New-Technologies

Because Medicare inpatient and outpatient payments are both calculated using claims data submitted in prior years, the DRG and APC payments, respectively, incorporate the pricing effects of new technology on a lagged basis. In order to provide access to new technology and to adequately account for its cost, both hospital payment systems have special payment options for new technologies that represent "substantial clinical improvement" over existing treatment options. As a result, device manufacturers seeking these add-on payments need robust data and findings demonstrating their device's clinical efficacy relative to other devices already in use.

New outpatient hospital technologies can receive 2–3 years of "pass-through status" under which the new device is unbundled from the billed APC and reimbursed at the hospital's sticker price for the device minus a discount. In other words, Medicare pays for the APC plus the pass-through payment for the device used minus the medical device expense built into the APC rate. New inpatient hospital treatments can receive a Medicare new-technology add-on payment (NTAP) for 1–3 years.

Although similar in some respects, the NTAP is both harder to obtain and less generous than pass-through status. From 2001 to 2015, CMS approved only 19 of 53 applications for NTAPs for new devices and treatments, but granted pass-through status to 18 skin substitutes alone over that same period (Hernandez et al. 2015). Unlike pass-through payments, the NTAP rate is such that a hospital will still face financial losses when using the new technology.

20.4.7 Downstream Impact on Other Payers

State Medicaid programs and commercial insurers use the same CPT and HCPCS codes that Medicare uses. As a result, coding changes can affect pricing for the device across for multiple payers. In addition, many commercial insurance plans tie payment to physicians and hospitals to a percent of the Medicare rates.

20.4.8 Leaving Fee-For-Service System

Although coding creates similar incentives for hospitals and physicians, in practice, these incentives are complicated by the many oddities of the medical device market. Perhaps the most striking feature of how hospitals purchase devices is that physicians select the implantable medical devices (which, tellingly, are also referred to as physician preference items) used in surgeries, but hospitals must foot the bill (Montgomery and Schneller 2007). Knowing this, medical device companies and their sales representatives try to build brand loyalty among physicians (Burns et al. 2009), offer physicians advice and guidance on using their devices (Montgomery and Schneller 2007), and use gag clauses to prohibit hospitals from disclosing the negotiated price for each device to their physicians (Montgomery and Schneller 2007). As a result, some hospitals try to limit physician contact with manufacturers at the hospital (Burns et al. 2009). Studies show that physicians are often distrustful of their hospital's purchasing manager (Burns et al. 2009), and are often unaware of the cost of various devices (Okike et al. 2014).

Given these and many other peculiarities of the device market, hospitals often have little control over device selection, little leverage in negotiations with manufacturers, and thus little choice but to pay manufacturers' requested rates. In the current fee-for-service system, in which providers are paid based on the number and type of services they provide, physicians can afford to ignore prices, especially when someone else (i.e., the hospital) is paying.

However, the Affordable Care Act creates new incentives for physicians to collaborate with their hospitals. The Act includes many provisions encouraging physicians and hospitals to leave the fee-for-service system and participate in alternative payment models, such as accountable care organizations (ACOs), that reward high quality, low cost care. Between 2011 and 2014, the percentage of healthcare payment paid under alternative payment models increased from 0% to 20% (Conway 2015). Physicians in these alternative payment models are assuming responsibility for the cost and quality of care and now have strong incentives to work with their hospitals. By pooling their market power, hospitals and physicians can use their increased leverage to negotiate for lower prices for devices. Although accountable care organizations have not yet focused on reducing surgical costs (Dupree et al. 2014), alternative payment models will likely lead to increased attention to spending on surgery and devices. Some hospitals and physicians in alternative payment methodologies are already strengthening their technical assessment committees, placing a greater emphasis on price and clinical effectiveness when selecting devices (Robinson 2012).

These changes will enhance the market power of providers relative to device manufacturers and place significant downward pressure on device industry prices. Device manufacturers producing breakthrough technologies and incremental improvements will fare best in this changing environment (Robinson 2012). Manufacturers with truly superior products will still have the monopolistic market power to demand high prices. With no viable substitute, providers will have little choice but to pay the high rates. Manufacturers producing lower cost versions of existing devices while maintaining quality may benefit from providers' increased price sensitivity and capture increased market share.

20.5 CONCLUSION AND PERSPECTIVE

There has been unprecedented change in the healthcare system over the past decade. Pathways to engage and collaborate with the FDA and CMS during the coverage decision-making process have newly emerged, and efforts to streamline historically complicated regulatory systems are underway. With Medicare increasingly bundling outpatient hospital payments and providers generally moving toward alternative payment models, the medical device industry will face more price sensitive and consolidated providers. Although putting pressure on the industry as a whole, these trends present tremendous opportunities for manufacturers who can strike the balance between innovation and value. In the coming decade, quality, efficiency, cost-effectiveness, and value will remain key themes. The following recommendations may be useful for innovators interested in pursuing coverage, coding, or reimbursement:

- Identify the intended population of the item or service, whether a coverage determination is needed, and which payers to approach about a coverage determination (if needed).
- Develop a payment strategy and engage with the FDA and CMS early on during the product development cycle, especially if Medicare is an intended payer.
- Determine the level of clinical evidence necessary to achieve a favorable coverage decision at either a local or national level as well as favorable coding decisions and, if applicable, special Medicare payments for new technologies.
- Explore parallel review and weigh the pros and cons of pursuing local versus national coverage determinations.
- Develop applications for new codes in advance of the FDA approving or clearing the device.
- Begin working with specialty societies related to your device before it goes before the CPT Editorial Board.

REFERENCES

Alliance for Regenerative Medicine. 2013. Alliance for regenerative medicine reimbursement portfolio. Available at http://alliancerm.org/sites/default/files/ARM_Reimbursement_ Portfolio_Oct_2013.pdf, 1–28.
American Medical Association. 2016. Applying for CPT® Codes. Available at http://www. ama-assn.org/ama/pub/physician-resources/solutions-managing-your-practice/coding-billing-insurance/cpt/applying-cpt-codes.page?

Bouchie, A. 2002. Tissue engineering firms go under. *Nat Biotechnol* no. 20 (12):1178–9.
Burns, L. R., M. G. Housman, R. E. Booth, Jr., and A. Koenig. 2009. Implant vendors and hospitals: competing influences over product choice by orthopedic surgeons. *Health Care Manage Rev* no. 34 (1):2–18.
Centers for Medicare & Medicaid Services. 2014. Guidance for the public, industry, and CMS staff: Coverage with evidence development. Available at https://www.cms.gov/medicare-coverage-database/details/medicare-coverage-document-details.aspx?MCDId=27.
Centers for Medicare & Medicaid Services. 2015. Medicare administrative contractors (MACs). MACs by State. Available at https://www.cms.gov/Medicare/Medicare-Contracting/Medicare-Administrative-Contractors/Downloads/MACs-by-State-April-2015.pdf
Chambers, J. D., M. Chenoweth, M. J. Cangelosi, J. Pyo, J. T. Cohen, and P. J. Neumann. 2015. Medicare is scrutinizing evidence more tightly for national coverage determinations. *Health Aff (Millwood)* no. 34 (2):253–60.
Chambers, J. D., M. Chenoweth, T. Thorat, and P. J. Neumann. 2015. Private payers disagree with Medicare over medical device coverage about half the time. *Health Aff (Millwood)* no. 34 (8):1376–82.
Conway, P. 2015. CMS innovation and health care delivery system reform. Available at https://www.qualityforum.org/Supporting.../Conway_Supporting_Document.aspx, 1–28.
DeSantis, P. and K. Buto. 2011. Comments on FDA/CMS Federal Register Notice – Docket No. FDA-2010-N-0308. Biotechnology Industry Organization (BIO) – Comment Johnson & Johnson – Comment, Available at http://www.regulations.gov/document?D=FDA-2010-N-0308-0039, 1–12.
Dupree, J. M., K. Patel, S. J. Singer, M. West, R. Wang, M. J. Zinner, and J. S. Weissman. 2014. Attention to surgeons and surgical care is largely missing from early medicare accountable care organizations. *Health Aff (Millwood)* no. 33 (6):972–9.
Emmett, A. J. and L. L. Todd. 2011. Comments on Parallel review of medical products, FDA-2010-N-0308. Biotechnology Industry Organization (BIO) – Comment. Available at http://www.regulations.gov/document?D=FDA-2010-N-0308-0038, 1–12.
Exact Sciences Corp. 2014. Exact Sciences Announces Final Payment Decision for Cologuard® from the Centers for Medicare & Medicaid Services. Available at http://www.exactsciences.com/about/latest-news/final-payment-decision-for-cologuard-from-cms
Food and Drug Administration. 2014. FDA approves first non-invasive DNA screening test for colorectal cancer. FDA News Release. Available at http://www.fda.gov/NewsEvents/Newsroom/PressAnnouncements/ucm409021.htm
Foote, S. B. 2003. Focus on locus: evolution of Medicare's local coverage policy. *Health Aff (Millwood)* no. 22 (4):137–46.
Hernandez, J., S. F. Machacz, and J. C. Robinson. 2015. US hospital payment adjustments for innovative technology lag behind those in Germany, France, and Japan. *Health Aff (Millwood)* no. 34 (2):261–70.
Laugesen, M. J., R. Wada, and E. M. Chen. 2012. In setting doctors' Medicare fees, CMS almost always accepts the relative value update panel's advice on work values. *Health Aff (Millwood)* no. 31 (5):965–72.
Medicare Payment Advisory Commission. 2001. Report to the Congress. Reducing Medicare complexity and regulatory burden. Available at http://www.medpac.gov/docs/default-source/contractor-reports/report-to-the-congress-reducing-medicare-complexity-and-regulatory-burden-december-2001-.pdf?sfvrsn=0, 1–69.
Montgomery, K. and E. S. Schneller. 2007. Hospitals' strategies for orchestrating selection of physician preference items. *Milbank Q* no. 85 (2):307–35.

Morris, E. L. 2011. Comments on Parallel review of medical products [FDA-2010-N-0308]. Biotechnology Industry Organization (BIO)—Comment. Available at http://www.regulations.gov/document?D=FDA-2010-N-0308-0033, 1–5.

Neumann, P. J., M. S. Kamae, and J. A. Palmer. 2008. Medicare's national coverage decisions for technologies, 1999–2007. *Health Aff (Millwood)* no. 27 (6):1620–31.

Office of Inspector General. 2014. Local coverage determinations create inconsistency in Medicare coverage, OEI-01-11-00500. Available at https://oig.hhs.gov/oei/reports/oei-01-11-00500.asp, 1–23.

Okike, K., R. V. O'Toole, A. N. Pollak, J. A. Bishop, C. M. McAndrew, S. Mehta, W. W. Cross, 3rd, G. E. Garrigues, M. B. Harris, and C. T. Lebrun. 2014. Survey finds few orthopedic surgeons know the costs of the devices they implant. *Health Aff (Millwood)* no. 33 (1):103–9.

Pearson, S. D. and P. B. Bach. 2010. How Medicare could use comparative effectiveness research in deciding on new coverage and reimbursement. *Health Aff (Millwood)* no. 29 (10):1796–804.

Robinson, J. C. 2012. Providers' payment and delivery system reforms hold both threats and opportunities for the drug and device industries. *Health Aff (Millwood)* no. 31 (9):2059–67.

Tunis, S. R., R. A. Berenson, S. E. Phurrough, and P. E. Mohr. 2011. Improving the quality and efficiency of the Medicare program through coverage policy. Available at http://healthreformgps.org/wp-content/uploads/Urban-Institute-Medicare-Coverage-August-2011.pdf, 1–21.

US Government Accountability Office. 2003. Medicare: Divided authority for policies on coverage of procedures and devices results in inequities, GAO-03-175. Available at http://www.gao.gov/products/GAO-03-175, 1–54.

Index

A

Accountable care organizations (ACOs), 396
Acini, 143
ACL, *see* Anterior cruciate ligament
ACOs, *see* Accountable care organizations
Activation Protein-1 (AP-1), 221
Additive manufacturing, 9
Adhesive cells, 203
Adipocyte, 77, 271; *see also* Nipple and breast construction
 -secreted factors, 148
Adipose tissue, 146, 299, 310; *see also* 3D diabetic tissue models
 adipose-specific diabetic cues, 312
 architectural cues within, 312
 ceiling cultures, 311
 recapitulating cell signaling within, 310
 structure of, 311
ADLTs, *see* Advance diagnostic laboratory tests
Advance diagnostic laboratory tests (ADLTs), 379
AFM, *see* Atomic force microscopy
Air impedance techniques, 204
Allografting, 126
AMA, *see* American Medical Association's
Ambulatory Payment Classification (APC), 391, 393
Ambulatory Surgical Center (ASC), 391
American Medical Association's (AMA), 394
American Type Culture Collection (ATCC), 77
Analysis of variances (ANOVA), 63
ANOVA, *see* Analysis of variances
Anterior cruciate ligament (ACL), 274
Anti-cancer molecules, 148
Anti-inflammatory cytokines, 219; *see also* Pro-and anti-inflammatory cytokines
AP-1, *see* Activation Protein-1
APC, *see* Ambulatory Payment Classification
Apico-basal markers, 272
Apligraf®, 382
Apoptosis, 217
Arteries, 198
ASC, *see* Ambulatory Surgical Center
ATCC, *see* American Type Culture Collection
Atherosclerosis, 199
Atomic force microscopy (AFM), 158
Autograft, 126

B

Basal media I (BMI), 77
Basement membrane (BM), 251
 proteins, 267, 272
BBB, *see* Blood–brain barrier
BCSCs, *see* Breast cancer stem cells
Bioengineered 3D tissue graft model, 241; *see also* Cell–cell communications
Bioengineered myocardial tissue grafts, 241
Biofabrication, 1, 9, 27; *see also* Layer-by-layer fabrication; Single layers combination; 3D biofabrication
 approaches, 11
 bio-loom design, 22
 bulk, 11–14
 droplet deposition system, 26
 drop-on-demand inkjet printers, 26
 expectations and errors in, 15
 extrusion and drawing process, 24
 on-demand vs. continuous process, 15
 quality, 15
 rapid prototyping, 9–11
 standard vs. twill weave, 22
 thermal inkjet printers, 26
 weaving process, 21
 woven scaffolds, 23
Bioprinting, 25
Bioreactor, 34, 51–53; *see also* Tissue stimulation
 aggregate component architecture for, 43–46
 combined parameter assessments, 48–49
 controls, 49–51
 design considerations, 36–37
 form factors, 40–41
 ideal responsibilities of, 34
 measurement parameters, 47–48
 operational modes, 45
 parameters and sensing methods, 46
 perfusion bioreactors, 38, 40
 research, 34–35
 rotating-wall, 38–40
 sensing and control in, 46
 stirred-flask, 37–38
 thematic, 37
Blood–brain barrier (BBB), 352
Blood vessel, 198–199; *see also* Cardiovascular system
BM, *see* Basement membrane
BMI, *see* Basal media I
BMP-2, *see* Bone morphogenetic protein-2
BMP8, *see* Bone morphogenic protein 8

401

Bone, 137
  graft implantation, 126
  scaffold, 128
  tissue regeneration and repair, 125
Bone engineering, 125, 137
  allografting, 126
  autograft, 126
  bone graft, 126–127
  bone scaffold, 128
  electrospinning nanofiber structures, 131–133
  fracture healing, 125–126
  hydrogels in, 135–137
  microsphere based scaffold development, 131
  phase separation, 133–134
  porogen leaching in, 129–131
  regenerative engineering, 127–129
  scaffold design and fabrication, 129
  synthetic polymeric nanofibers, 132
  3D model systems, 127
  3D printing bone scaffolds, 135
  vascularization, 132–133
Bone morphogenetic protein-2 (BMP-2), 136, 177
Bone morphogenic protein 8 (BMP8), 224
Bone-on-a-chip models, 183; *see also*
       Mineralized 3D culture systems
Bone sialoprotein (BSP), 173
Brain; *see also* Glioblastoma multiforme
  microenvironment, 353
  mimetic hydrogel models, 365
  tumor invasion, 361–364
  tumors, 351
Brain extracellular matrix, 353; *see also*
       Glioblastoma multiforme
  components of, 354
Breast, 142; *see also* Breast stem cell; Engineered
       composites; Engineered mammary
       tissue systems; Mammary gland;
       Nipple and breast construction
  acini, 143
  adipocyte-secreted factors, 148
  adipose tissue, 146
  cancer, 75, 250
  cancer development and tumor progression, 143–144
  cancer risk factors, 144
  carcinogenesis, 266
  duct of breast epithelium, 146
  lactation, 143
  mammary development and anatomy, 142–144
  mechanical properties, 145
  microenvironment, 146–148
  normal glandular basement membrane, 146
  structural components, 147
  structure of, 250
  tissue properties, 145

Breast cancer
  metastasis to bone, 170
  therapeutic progress in, 266
Breast cancer stem cells (BCSCs), 254; *see also*
       Breast stem cell
Breast metastasis suppressor 1 (BRMS1), 240
Breast microcalcifications, 171; *see also*
       Mineralized 3D culture systems
  classifications, 173
Breast stem cell, 249, 258
  breast cancer, 250
  cancer stem cell discoveries, 256
  CSCs, 250
  differences in cells, 251
  gel-based matrices, 251–253
  heterotypic 3D *in vitro* systems, 256–258
  mammospheres, 253–255
  Matrigel® systems, 252
  role of Notch1 in colony formation, 253
BRMS1, *see* Breast metastasis suppressor 1
BSP, *see* Bone sialoprotein
Bulk fabrication, 11–12; *see also* Biofabrication
Business consideration, 377; *see also* 3D tissue
       test system

C

CAD, *see* Computer-aided design
Calcium L-lactate (CL), 133
CAMs, *see* Cellular adhesion molecules
Cancer-promoting molecules, 148
Cancer stem cells (CSCs), 250; *see also* Breast
       stem cell
  hypothesis, 358–359
Cardiac tissue cells, 289; *see also* Cardiovascular
       3D tissue systems
Cardiomyocytes, 196
Cardiovascular 3D tissue systems, 285, 295
  approaches to, 291
  arterial anatomy, 288
  arterial composition, 287
  cardiac tissue, 288–289
  cell sheet engineering, 292, 293–294
  considerations for, 287
  culture conditions for 3D vascular tissue
       models, 291
  decellularized scaffolds, 291–292
  heart anatomy, 289
  limitations of, 286–287
  myocardial tissue patches, 292
  myocytes, 288
  scaffolds for blood vessel development, 291
  scaffolds for cardiac tissue development, 290
  scaffolds for cardiovascular tissue models, 289
  synchronicity of cardiomyocyte
       contraction, 290

Index

tubular scaffolds for vessel modeling, 292
Cardiovascular disease, 193
Cardiovascular system, 195; *see also* 3D cardiovascular tissue scaffolds
    arteries, 198
    ascending aorta, 198
    atherosclerosis, 199
    blood vessel, 198–199
    cardiomyocytes, 196
    H&E stained myocardium, 195
    heart valve, 196–198
    heart valves with trichrome, 197
    myocardium, 195–196
    valve disease, 197
    VIC, 196–197
Cardiovascular tissues, 41
CDC, *see* Center for Disease Control
cDNA, *see* Complementary DNA
CED, *see* Coverage with evidence development
Ceiling cultures, 311
Cell–biomaterial interactions, 20
Cell–cell communications, 233, 242
    deficiency in GJIC, 237
    gap junctional intercellular communication, 234–237
    gap junctions/connexins in 3D systems, 240–241
    gap junctions/connexins in cancer initiation and promotion, 237–240
    gap junctions/connexins in cancer progression, 240
    intercellular communication, 234
    loss of connexin, 238
    multicellular organisms, 234
    myocardial tissue grafts, 241
    scaffoldless 3D model, 241
    tumor formation, 237
    tumorigenesis stages, 238
Cell–mineral interactions, 176; *see also* Mineralized 3D culture systems
    cell-and tissue-based methods, 176–177
    cell-and tissue-derived mineralized matrices, 178
    collagen as substrates, 181–182
    mineralization of collagen fibrils, 182
    synthetic HA into scaffolds, 179, 177, 180–181
Cell processes, 141
Cell sheet engineering, 293–294; *see also* Cardiovascular 3D tissue systems
Cell transplantation therapy, 292
Cellular adhesion molecules (CAMs), 205
Cellular processes, 233
Cellular remodeling, 202
Center for Disease Control (CDC), 378

Centers for Medicare and Medicaid Services (CMS), 378, 382, 391
Central nervous system (CNS), 351
Cerivastatin, 327
Chemotaxis, 217
Chondroitin-sulfate proteoglycans (CSPGs), 353
CL, *see* Calcium L-lactate
CLIA, *see* Clinical Laboratory Improvement Amendments
CLIAC, *see* Clinical Laboratory Improvement Advisory Committee
Clinical Laboratory Improvement Advisory Committee (CLIAC), 378
Clinical Laboratory Improvement Amendments (CLIA), 378
CM, *see* Conditioned medium
CMOS, *see* Complementary metal-oxide-semiconductor
CMS, *see* Centers for Medicare and Medicaid Services
CNS, *see* Central nervous system
Coding, 382
Collagen, 181
Collagen-based matrices, 268
Complementary DNA (cDNA), 240
Complementary metal-oxide-semiconductor (CMOS), 35
Compression bioreactor, 42; *see also* Bioreactor
Computer-aided design (CAD), 14
Conditioned medium (CM), 222
Connective tissue, 309
Connexin (Cx), 235; *see also* Cell–cell communications; Gap junctions
    in cancer initiation and promotion, 237–240
    in cancer progression, 240
    domains, 235
    loss of, 238
    proteins, 236
    in 3D systems, 240–241
Coverage, 382, 389–390; *see also* Regenerative medicine
    billing codes by provider, 386
    with evidence development, 388–389
    FDA–CMS parallel review, 387–388
    future directions in, 387
    local coverage determination, 383–386
    MAC jurisdictions for Medicare Parts A and B, 385
    Medicare benefit categories, 383, 384
    Medicare Modernization Act, 386
    national coverage determination, 387
Coverage with evidence development (CED), 389, 391
CryoValve® SG Pulmonary Valve, 203
CSCs, *see* Cancer stem cells
CSPGs, *see* Chondroitin-sulfate proteoglycans

Current Procedural Terminology codes (CPT codes), 379, 390, 391, 392; *see also* Regenerative medicine
  coding-enhanced price competition, 393
  downstream impact on payers, 396
  leaving fee-for-service system, 396–397
  Medicare payment to hospitals, 392–393
  new CPT code, 394–395
  new HCPCS code, 395
  and payment, 390–392
  special payments for new-technologies, 395
Customized nipple implant, 84; *see also* Nipple and breast construction
Cx, *see* Connexin
Cytokines, 216; *see also* Pro-and anti-inflammatory cytokines

D

DCIS, *see* Ductal carcinoma *in situ*
DDT, *see* Dichlorodiphenyltrichloroethane
Decellularization, 291
Decellularized scaffolds, 330
Desmosomes, 234
DHA, *see* Docosahexaenoic acid
Diabetes mellitus, 299
  types, 300
Dichlorodiphenyltrichloroethane (DDT), 237
Differential scanning calorimetry (DSC), 110
Differentiation medium I (DMI), 77
Disc electrospinning, 204
DMBA (7,12-dimethylbenz(a) anthracene), 239
DMEM, *see* Dulbecco's Modified Eagle's Medium
DMI, *see* Differentiation medium I
Docosahexaenoic acid (DHA), 148
DPBS, *see* Dulbecco's phosphate buffer saline solution
Droplet deposition system, 26
Drop-on-demand inkjet printers, 26
DSC, *see* Differential scanning calorimetry
Ductal carcinoma *in situ* (DCIS), 144
Dulbecco's Modified Eagle's Medium (DMEM), 77, 95, 158
Dulbecco's phosphate buffer saline solution (DPBS), 77
Durotaxis, 206

E

EBM, *see* Endothelial cell basal media
E-cadherin, 239
ECM, *see* Extracellular matrix
ECs, *see* Endothelial cells
EDTA, *see* Ethylenediaminetetraacetic acid
EGF, *see* Epidermal growth factor
EGM, *see* Endothelial cell growth medium

EHS, *see* Engelbreth-Holm-Swarm
Eicosapentaenoic acid (EPA), 148
Elasticity, 290
Electromagnetic fields (EMFs), 35
Electrospinning, 12, 131, 202–203; *see also* Bone engineering
Electrospun nanofibers, 132
EMFs, *see* Electromagnetic fields
eMSCs, *see* Endometrial mesenchymal stem cells
EMT, *see* Epithelial to mesenchymal transitions
Endometrial mesenchymal stem cells (eMSCs), 120
Endothelial cell basal media (EBM), 76
Endothelial cell growth medium (EGM), 77
Endothelial cells (ECs), 76, 198
Endothelium, 195
Engelbreth-Holm-Swarm (EHS), 176
Engineered composites, 141, 160–161; *see also* Breast; Engineered mammary tissue systems
  atomic force microscopy setup, 158
  breast cancer cell response evaluation, 156–157
  chitosan–gelatin beads, 156
  evaluated for mechanical testing, 158
  fabrication and characterization, 157–159
  3D cell culture, 159–160
Engineered mammary tissue systems, 148; *see also* Breast; Engineered composites
  cell culture systems, 149
  drug evaluation, 155–156
  mammary tissue models, 149
  3D *in vitro* mammary models, 150–152
  tissue development and morphogenesis, 149, 153
  tumor cell metastasis and invasion, 154–155
  tumor formation and vascularization, 153–154
Engineered skeletal muscle tissue, 322, 341
  cell lines, 322–324
  cell source, 322
  convection effect in culture media, 335–336
  decellularized scaffolds, 330
  electrical stimulation, 336–337
  engineered muscle fabrication, 323
  engineered muscle from human primary cells, 334
  fiber type switching, 340–341
  fibroblast impact on myogenic cells, 326
  fibroblasts, 326
  force production, 333, 334–335
  formation of myooids, 329
  hydrogel scaffolds, 330–331
  immunostaining of human engineered muscle, 331
  innervation, 337
  iPSC-derived myoblasts, 326–327

Index

iPSC-derived myogenic cells, 327
Matrigel®, 332
mechanical stimulation, 336
metabolism, 338–340
myoblasts, 327
myofibrils, 322
natural biopolymer hydrogels, 331–333
neuromuscular junction formation, 337
optimizing formulation parameters, 335
Pax7+ cells in engineered muscle, 325
primary cells, 324
primary satellite cells and myoblasts, 324–326
promoting maturation and function, 333–334
scaffolding and extracellular matrix, 328–329
skeletal muscle tissue, 322
species of cell donor, 327–328
supraphysiological insulin levels, 339
synthetic hydrogels, 333
vascularization, 337–338
EPA, *see* Eicosapentaenoic acid
Epidermal growth factor (EGF), 250
Epithelial specific antigen (ESA), 256
Epithelial to mesenchymal transitions (EMT), 154
ER, *see* Estrogen receptor
ESA, *see* Epithelial specific antigen
Estrogen receptor (ER), 250
EthD-1, *see* Ethidium homodimer-1
Ethidium homodimer-1 (EthD-1), 78
Ethylenediaminetetraacetic acid (EDTA), 95
Extracellular matrix (ECM), 40, 92, 144, 250

F

FADD, *see* Fas-Associated Death Domain
FAK, *see* Focal adhesion kinase
Fas-Associated Death Domain (FADD), 220
FBR, *see* Foreign body response
FBS, *see* Fetal bovine serum
FDA, *see* U.S. Food and Drug Administration
FDM, *see* Fused deposition modeling
Female mammary gland, *see* Breast
Fetal bovine serum (FBS), 77, 95
FGF, *see* Fibroblast growth factor
Fibrin, 332; *see also* Engineered skeletal muscle tissue
  gel, 76
Fibroadenomas, 145
Fibroblast growth factor (FGF), 332
  FGF5, 224
Focal adhesion kinase (FAK), 356
Force production, 333; *see also* Engineered skeletal muscle tissue
Foreign body response (FBR), 25
Fourier transform infrared spectrometry (FTIR), 112
Fracture healing, 125–126; *see also* Bone engineering
FTIR, *see* Fourier transform infrared spectrometry
Fused deposition modeling (FDM), 14

G

GA-1000, *see* Gentamicin/amphoterecin
GAG, *see* Glycosaminoglycan
Gamma knife radiosurgery (GKS), 360
Gap junctional intercellular communication (GJIC), 234; *see also* Cell–cell communications
  lack in neoplastic cells, 239
Gap junctions, 234; *see also* Cell–cell communications
  channel gating, 236
  channels, 236
  connexon, 235
  kinetic routes of control, 236
  regional functions, 236–237
  structure of, 235
GBM, *see* Glioblastoma multiforme
GEM, *see* Genetically engineered mice
Genetically engineered mice (GEM), 361
Gentamicin/amphoterecin (GA-1000), 77
GJIC, *see* Gap junctional intercellular communication
GKS, *see* Gamma knife radiosurgery
Glial cells, 352
Glioblastoma multiforme (GBM), 351, 367
  angiogenesis, 356–358
  brain extracellular matrix, 353–355
  brain microenvironment, 353
  brain mimetic hydrogel models, 365
  brain tumor invasion, 361–364
  brain tumors, 351
  cancer stem cell hypothesis, 358–359
  cell-based *in vitro* methods, 361
  challenge of 2D cell culture, 362
  conventional therapies, 360
  future design of 3D models, 364–367
  glioblastomas, 352
  malignant tumors, 355
  microfluidics, 365
  microfluidic tumor–vascular interface model, 366
  MRI scans of GBM patient, 353
  multicentric, 352
  organs-on-chips, 365
  progression of, 357
  treatment paradigms, 359–361
  tumor cell invasion, 355–356
  tumor xenograft in mouse model, 357
Glioblastoma stem cells (GSCs), 254; *see also* Breast stem cell

Gliomas, 352; *see also* Glioblastoma multiforme
Glucose-stimulated insulin secretion (GSIS), 241
Glucose transporter type 4 (GLUT4), 308
GLUT4, *see* Glucose transporter type 4
Glycosaminoglycan (GAG), 354
Growth factors, 332
GSIS, *see* Glucose-stimulated insulin secretion

H

H&E, *see* Hematoxylin and eosin
HA, *see* Hydroxyapatite
HARV, *see* High aspect ratio vessel
HCPCS, *see* Healthcare Common Procedure Coding System
Healthcare Common Procedure Coding System (HCPCS), 379, 391, 392
Heart valve, 196–198; *see also* Cardiovascular system
hEGF, *see* Human epidermal growth factor
Hematoxylin and eosin (H&E), 80, 120
Hepatocyte growth factor (HGF), 223
Hepatocyte nuclear factor 1α (HNF-1α), 239
Hepatocytes, 307; *see also* Liver
hFGF-β, *see* Human fibroblast growth factor
HGF, *see* Hepatocyte growth factor
HIF-1, *see* Hypoxia inducible factor-1
High aspect ratio vessel (HARV), 39
High-temperature tetra detection gel permeation chromatography (HT-GPC), 116
hMSC, *see* Human mesenchymal stem cell
HMVEC, *see* Human microvascular endothelial cells
HNF-1α, *see* Hepatocyte nuclear factor 1α
HPOA, *see* Hypothalamic–pituitary–ovarian axis
HT-GPC, *see* High-temperature tetra detection gel permeation chromatography
Human epidermal growth factor (hEGF), 77
Human fibroblast growth factor (hFGF-β), 77
Human mammary gland, 142
Human mesenchymal stem cell (hMSC), 177
Human microvascular endothelial cells (HMVEC), 76
Hyaluronic acid, 354
Hydrodynamic forces, 41
Hydrogel, 136–137, 202, 364; *see also* Bone engineering
scaffolds, 330–331
Hydrostatic pressure bioreactor, 42–43; *see also* Bioreactor
Hydroxyapatite (HA), 130, 169
Hyperglycemia, 299
Hypothalamic–pituitary–ovarian axis (HPOA), 265
Hypoxia inducible factor-1 (HIF-1), 356

I

ICD-10-CM, *see* International Classification of Diseases, 10th Edition, Clinical Modification
ICD-10-PCS, *see* International Classification of Diseases, 10th Edition, Procedural Coding System
IFNγ, *see* Interferon gamma
IGF, *see* Insulin growth factor
IGF-1, *see* Insulin-like growth factor 1
Immune cell, 216
Induced pluripotent stem cells (iPSCs), 322
Inkjet technology, 91
Inpatient Prospective Payment System (IPPS), 392
Insulin, 299
  insulin secretion, 300
Insulin growth factor (IGF), 332
Insulin-like growth factor 1 (IGF-1), 171
Interferon gamma (IFNγ), 218
Interleukin
  IL10, 220
  IL1, 217
  IL1Ra, 220
  IL4, 220
  IL6, 218
  IL-8, 174
  IL8, 219
International Classification of Diseases, 10th Edition, Clinical Modification (ICD-10-CM), 391
International Classification of Diseases, 10th Edition, Procedural Coding System (ICD-10-PCS), 391
In vitro diagnostic (IVD), 377; *see also* 3D tissue test system
In vitro model systems, 141; *see also* Engineered composites
IPPS, *see* Inpatient Prospective Payment System
iPSCs, *see* Induced pluripotent stem cells
IVD, *see* In vitro diagnostic

J

JAK/STAT, *see* Janus kinase/signal transducers and activators of transcription
Janus kinase/signal transducers and activators of transcription (JAK/STAT), 218

L

Laboratory-developed test (LDT), 378; *see also* 3D tissue test system
Lactation, 143
Layer-by-layer fabrication, 14–15; *see also* Biofabrication

Index

with bioprinting, 25–27
LCD, *see* Local Coverage Determination
LCIS, *see* Lobular carcinoma *in situ*
LDT, *see* Laboratory-developed test
Left Heart Simulator, 65; *see also* Rice University Flow Loop System
LFA1, *see* Lymphocyte function-associated antigen 1
Liver, 306; *see also* 3D diabetic tissue models
  architectural cues within, 307–308
  hepatocytes, 307
  liver-specific diabetic cues, 308
  recapitulating proper cell signaling within, 306–307
  sinusoid, 307
  space of Disse, 307
  structure of, 307
Lobular carcinoma *in situ* (LCIS), 144
Local Coverage Determination (LCD), 383–386, 391; *see also* Coverage
LOX, *see* Lysyl oxidase
Lymphocyte function-associated antigen 1 (LFA1), 223
Lysyl oxidase (LOX), 174

M

MAC, *see* Medicare Administrative Contractor
Macula adherens, *see* Desmosomes
Malignant cellremoval, 75
Malignant tumors, 355
Mammary gland, 249, 263, 264, 278; *see also* 3D culture model
  biology, 266
  biomechanical factors in morphogenesis, 273
  biomechanical forces and hormones, 273–276
  cancer in breast, 266
  data acquisition and analysis, 276–278
  development, 264–265
  hormone impact on breast tissue properties, 276
  in vitro models for study of breast tissue, 266–267
  morphogenic processes, 267
  morphological analysis, 276
  SAMA analysis of epithelial structure morphology, 277
Mammary tissue models, 149
Mammospheres, 254–255
Manual micropipetting, 98
MAPK, *see* Mitogen activated protein kinase
Matrigel®, 176, 252
Matrix metalloproteinases (MMPs), 147, 204, 222, 355
Mature skeletal muscle, 340; *see also* Engineered skeletal muscle tissue

MEDCAC, *see* Medicare Evidence Development and Coverage Advisory Committee
Medicare, 383; *see also* Coverage; Regenerative medicine
Medicare Administrative Contractor (MAC), 383, 391
Medicare and Medicaid, 382
Medicare benefit categories, 383, 384
Medicare Evidence Development and Coverage Advisory Committee (MEDCAC), 387, 391
Medicare Modernization Act, 386
Medicare Severity Diagnosis Related Group (MS-DRG), 391, 393
Mesenchymal stem cells (MSC), 19, 77
Mesenchymal stromal cells (MSCs), 224
Metastasis, 240
Metastatic cell lines, 155
MGMT, *see* O-methylguanine-DNA methyltransferase
MHC, *see* Myosin heavy chain
Microfluidic "organ-on-a-chip" devices, 183
Microfluidics, 365; *see also* Glioblastoma multiforme
Mineralized 3D culture systems, 169, 183–184; *see also* Cell–mineral interactions
  bone affected by cancer metastasis, 175
  bone mineral, 174–176
  bone-on-a-chip models, 183
  breast cancer metastasis to bone, 170
  engineered 3D tumor models, 170
  mammary calcifications, 171–173
  mineral to "seed-and-soil" concept, 171
  site-specific metastasis, 171
Miscellaneous/Not Otherwise Classified (NOC), 391, 395
Mitogen activated protein kinase (MAPK), 223, 236
Mitral regurgitation (MR), 65
Mitral valves (MVs), 62
  holder, 67
MMPs, *see* Matrix metalloproteinases
MR, *see* Mitral regurgitation
MSC, *see* Mesenchymal stem cells
MSCs, *see* Mesenchymal stromal cells
MS-DRG, *see* Medicare Severity Diagnosis Related Group
Multicellular organisms, 234
Musculoskeletal tissues, 41
MVs, *see* Mitral valves
Myocardium, 195; *see also* Cardiovascular system
Myocytes, 288
Myofibers, 309
Myofibrils, 322
Myooids, 309
Myosin heavy chain (MHC), 326

N

NAC reconstruction, *see* Nipple areola complex reconstruction
National coverage determinations (NCDs), 387, 391; *see also* Coverage
Natural biopolymer hydrogels, 331–333
Natural killer cells (NK cells), 217
NCDs, *see* National coverage determinations
NCS, *see* Neonatal calf serum
Negatively charged polymers, 182
Neonatal calf serum (NCS), 77
Network of holes method, 69–70; *see also* Rice University Flow Loop System
New-Technology Add-On Payment (NTAP), 391, 395
Nipple and breast construction, 75, 87–88; *see also* Breast
  adipocytes in fibrin, 81
  cell culture and scaffold fabrication, 76–78
  differentiation from pre-adipocytes to adipocytes, 83
  endothelial cell channels formation, 81–83
  endothelial networks printed with fibrin gels, 83
  fibrous capsule formation, 86
  forming thick tissue-engineered constructs, 81
  histological analysis, 80–81
  immunohistochemistry of mouse explant, 86, 87
  implant scaffold and biopsies, 80
  in vitro scaffold assessment, 78–79
  in vivo assessment, 79
  in vivo studies, 84–85
  live/dead assay performed in printed gels, 82
  Masson's trichrome image, 82
  materials and methods, 76
  molding mass customized implants, 83
  NAC reconstruction, 76
  nipple areola complex, 78, 85
  nipple implant, 84
  results, 81
  vascular anastomosis, 85–87
Nipple areola complex reconstruction (NAC reconstruction), 76; *see also* Nipple and breast construction
NK cells, *see* Natural killer cells
NOC, *see* Miscellaneous/Not Otherwise Classified
Nondegradable hydrogels, 136
Nonimmune cell, 216
Nonparenchymal cells, 306
NTAP, *see* New-Technology Add-On Payment

O

OCT, *see* Optimum cutting compound
Office laser printers, 10
Office of Inspector General (OIG), 391
OI, *see* Osteogenesis imperfecta
OIG, *see* Office of Inspector General
Oil in water (O/W), 134
O-methylguanine-DNA methyltransferase (MGMT), 360
Oncogenes, 238
OPN, *see* Osteopontin
OPPS, *see* Outpatient Prospective Payment System
Optimum cutting compound (OCT), 80
Organogenesis, 382
Organs-on-chips, 312, 365; *see also* Glioblastoma multiforme
Osteoclasts, 174
Osteogenesis imperfecta (OI), 174; *see also* Mineralized 3D culture systems
Osteoinductive growth factors, 128; *see also* Bone engineering
Osteopontin (OPN), 173
Outpatient Prospective Payment System (OPPS), 392
O/W, *see* Oil in water

P

PA, *see* Preadipocytes
PA6, *see* Polyamide 6
Pancreas, 301; *see also* 3D diabetic tissue models
  architectural cues within, 305
  exocrine, 306
  pancreatic-specific diabetic cues, 305
  recapitulating proper cell signaling within, 301, 304–305
  structure of, 304
Papillary muscles (PMs), 62
  holder, 67
Parenchymal cells, 306
Paxillin, 332
PBMC, *see* Peripheral blood mononuclear cells
PBS, *see* Phosphate buffered saline
PCL, *see* Polycaprolactone
PCR, *see* Polymerase chain reaction
PDMS scaffolds, *see* Polydimethylsiloxane scaffolds
PEG, *see* Polyethylene glycol
PEGDA, *see* Poly(ethylene glycol) diacrylate
Pelvic organ prolapse (POP), 119; *see also* Polypropylene mesh
Perfusion bioreactors, 38, 40; *see also* Bioreactor
Peripheral blood mononuclear cells (PBMC), 292
Permeability, 19
PES, *see* Polyethylsulfone
PGA, *see* Poly(glycolic acid)
Phosphate buffered saline (PBS), 95
Phospho-inositide 3-kinase (PI3K), 223
PI3K, *see* Phospho-inositide 3-kinase

Index

PID, *see* Proportional-integral-derivative
PIPAAm, *see* Poly(*N*-isopropylacrylamide)
PISA, *see* Proximal isovelocity surface area
PKC, *see* Protein kinase C
PLA, *see* Poly(lactic acid)
PLAGA, *see* Poly(lactide-*co*-glycolide)
PLG, *see* Poly(lactide-*co*-glycolide)
PLLA, *see* Poly(L-lactide)
PMs, *see* Papillary muscles
Poly(ethylene glycol) diacrylate (PEGDA), 136
Poly(glycolic acid) (PGA), 135
Poly(lactic acid) (PLA), 135
Poly(lactide-*co*-glycolide) (PLAGA), 131
Poly(lactide-*co*-glycolide) (PLG), 180
Poly(L-lactide) (PLLA), 133
Poly(*N*-isopropylacrylamide) (PIPAAm), 293
Polyamide 6 (PA6), 120
Polycaprolactone (PCL), 130
Polydimethylsiloxane scaffolds (PDMS scaffolds), 202
Polyethylene glycol (PEG), 202, 333
Polyethylsulfone (PES), 157
Polymerase chain reaction (PCR), 135
Polymer fibers, 25
Polypropylene mesh (PP mesh), 107, 121
   approaches for POP implant design, 119–120
   degradation of, 118
   DSC analysis of pristine, 114
   DSC of degradation of polypropylene, 113–116
   electrospinning setup, 120
   failed vaginal mesh implant, 112
   FTIR analysis of oxidation degradation, 112–113
   FTIR spectrum of vaginal mesh, 113
   image of pristine, 111
   knitting, 109
   manufacturing, 109–112
   materials-science triad, 108
   molecular weight analyses of failed implants, 116–119
   pristine-knitted, 109
   stress–strain behavior of PP, 110
Polyvinyl alcohol (PVA), 131
Polyvinylidene fluoride (PVDF), 118
POP, *see* Pelvic organ prolapse
Porogen leaching, 129–131; *see also* Bone engineering
Porosity, 18
PP mesh, *see* Polypropylene mesh
Preadipocytes (PA), 77
Pro-and anti-inflammatory cytokines, 216, 218, 219, 225–226
   anti-inflammatory immune responses, 219–220
   bone marrow stromal cell production, 223–224
   identification of neural progenitor cells, 224–225
   IL10, 220
   IL1Ra, 220
   IL4, 220
   IL8, 219
   inflammasomes and 3D *in vitro* models, 225
   inflammatory immune responses, 217–219
   inflammatory signals, 223
   interferon gamma, 218
   signaling pathways, 220–221
   3D culture model of osteoarthritis, 222–223
   3D models of cell behaviors and cytokines, 222
   in tissue maintenance and immune responses, 221–222
   TNFα, 217
   2D *in vitro* models, 216
   2D vs. 3D models, 217
Progesterone receptors (PRs), 265
Proportional-integral-derivative (PID), 50
Protein kinase C (PKC), 236
Proximal isovelocity surface area (PISA), 66
PRs, *see* Progesterone receptors
PVA, *see* Polyvinyl alcohol
PVDF, *see* Polyvinylidene fluoride

R

R3-IGF-1, *see* R3-insulin-like growth factor-1
R3-insulin-like growth factor-1 (R3-IGF-1), 77
RANKL, *see* Receptor activator of nuclear factor kappa-B ligand
Rapid prototyping fabrication (RP fabrication), 9; *see also* Biofabrication
   advantage of, 14
   fabricated part, 10
   goal of, 10
   office laser printers, 10
Reactive oxygen species (ROS), 217, 257
Receptor activator of nuclear factor kappa-B ligand (RANKL), 174
Receptor-Interacting Protein (RIP), 220
Recombinant human bone morphogenetic protein-2 (rhBMP-2), 135
Reduction mammoplasties (RMF), 271
Regenerative engineering, 127; *see also* Bone engineering
Regenerative medicine, 381, 397; *see also* Code; Coverage
   coding, 382
   coverage, 382
   Medicare and Medicaid, 382
   organogenesis, 382
   payment, 390
Relative value unit (RVU), 390, 391
Relative Value Unit Committee (RUC), 391, 394

Relaxation modulus, 109
rhBMP-2, see Recombinant human bone morphogenetic protein-2
Rice University Flow Loop System (RUFLS), 62
 changes to mitral valve holder, 69
 control papillary muscle position, 68
 creation of system, 62
 design criteria, 68
 flow loop system, 62
 increasing regurgitation over time, 63–64
 left heart simulator, 65
 modularity, 69
 MV holder, 67
 need for modification, 62
 network of holes method, 69–70
 new mitral valve holder, 69
 new papillary muscle holders, 71
 papillary muscle geometry control, 64–68
 papillary muscle holders, 67
 platform system, 71–72
 PM positioning, 65, 70
 redesign, 66
 regurgitation, 72
 sawtooth-clamping system, 71
 slot and screw method, 70–71
 sterility, 69
RIP, see Receptor-Interacting Protein
RMF, see Reduction mammoplasties
ROS, see Reactive oxygen species
Rotating-wall bioreactors, 38–40; see also Bioreactor
Rotating wall vessel (RWV), 291
RP fabrication, see Rapid prototyping fabrication
RUC, see Relative Value Unit Committee
RUFLS, see Rice University Flow Loop System
RVU, see Relative value unit
RWV, see Rotating wall vessel

S

SAMA, see Software for Automated Morphological Analysis
Sawtooth-clamping method, 71; see also Rice University Flow Loop System
SBF, see Simulated body fluid
Scaffold, 328
Scaffoldless 3D model, 241; see also Cell–cell communications
Scanning electron microscopy (SEM), 111
SDF-1, see Stromal cell-derived factor 1
Second Harmonic Generation (SHG), 277
Selective laser sintering (SLS), 14
Self-assembly, 17–18
SEM, see Scanning electron microscopy
SFF, see Solid free-form fabrication
SHG, see Second Harmonic Generation
Simulated body fluid (SBF), 180

Single layers combination (SLC), 12, 21; see also Biofabrication
 advantages of, 12
 challenges to weaving, 24
 electrospinning, 12
 fiber-based system, 13
 weaving, 20–23
 woven 3D structures, 23–24
 using woven textiles, 20–25
Sintered microsphere scaffold methodology, 131; see also Bone engineering
Sinusoid, 307; see also Liver
Skeletal metastases, 169
Skeletal muscle, 308; see also Engineered skeletal muscle tissue; 3D diabetic tissue models
 architectural cues within, 309
 connective tissue, 309
 muscle-specific diabetic cues, 310
 myofibers, 309
 recapitulating cell signaling within, 308–309
 structure of, 309
 tissue in vivo, 322
SLC, see Single layers combination
Slot and screw method, 70–71; see also Rice University Flow Loop System
Slow-turning lateral vessel (STLV), 39
SLS, see Selective laser sintering
SMT, see Somatic mutation theory
Software for Automated Morphological Analysis (SAMA), 276, 277
Solid free-form fabrication (SFF), 14
Somatic mutation theory (SMT), 266
Space of Disse, 307
SPCL, see Starch and PCL
Spheroid/aggregate culture techniques, 91; see also 3D cancer spheroid biofabrication
Starch and PCL (SPCL), 132
Stirred-flask bioreactors, 37–38; see also Bioreactor
STLV, see Slow-turning lateral vessel
Stroma, 271
Stromal cell-derived factor 1 (SDF-1), 171, 224
Synthetic hydrogels, 333
Synthetic polymeric nanofibers, 132

T

TACE, see Tumor necrosis factor converting enzyme
TCDD (2,3,7,8-tetrachlorodibenzodioxin), 237
TDLU, see Terminal ductal lobular unit
TEBs, see Terminal end buds
Tensegrity, 18
Tensile strain bioreactor, 42; see also Bioreactor
Tensile strength, 290
Terminal ductal lobular unit (TDLU), 250

Index

Terminal end buds (TEBs), 265
TGF-beta, *see* Transforming growth factor beta
Thermal inkjet, 93; *see also* 3D cancer spheroid biofabrication
  -based biofabricator, 94
  cartridge, 93
  printing, 14
Thermally induced phase separation (TIPS), 133–134; *see also* Bone engineering
3D biofabrication, 16; *see also* Biofabrication
  biofabrication, 16–17
  design considerations, 17
  mechanical properties, 19–20
  parameters favorable to, 17
  permeability, 19
  promotion of vascularity, 19
  resolution of 3D biofabrication method, 18
  self-assembly, 17–18
  smallest block of tissue, 16
  substrate biocompatibility, 20
  surface modification, 20
  tensegrity, 18
  tissue geometry, 18–19
  tissue voxel, 16
3D biological modeling, 217; *see also* Pro-and anti-inflammatory cytokines
3D cancer spheroid biofabrication, 91, 96–100
  aggregate shape factor and growth, 95
  bioprinted cells' plots and representative bright field images, 96
  bioprinted mammalian cells, 98
  bioprinting printer setup, 93–94
  bioprinting process, 95
  cell culture and staining, 95
  data analysis, 96
  high-throughput robotic systems, 99
  manual micropipetting, 98
  materials and methods, 93
  proliferation plots of bioprinted mammalian cells, 97
  spheroid/aggregate culture techniques, 91
  thermal inkjet-based biofabricator, 94
  thermal inkjet technology, 93
  valve-based bioprinters, 93
  viability plots over time of printed spheroids, 99
3D cardiac systems, 286; *see also* Cardiovascular 3D tissue systems
3D cardiovascular tissue scaffolds, 193, 207; *see also* Cardiovascular system
  arterial tree and composition of components, 194
  biocompatible 3D scaffolds, 205
  cell-to-cell communication, 205–206
  challenges in cardiovascular *in vitro* tissue modeling, 199–201
  common scaffolds, 201
  decellularized matrices, 203
  electrospun matrices, 202–203
  mass transfer limitations in 2D vs. 3D culture, 200
  mechanical properties, 206–207
  polydimethylsiloxane, 202
  remodeling of extracellular matrix, 204–205
  scaffold considerations, 201
  scaffold microenvironment, 203
  scaffold pore size, 204
  surface properties and cellular adhesion, 203–204
  synthetic hydrogel matrices, 202
3D culture model, 267; *see also* Mammary gland
  breast, 268
  breast epithelial structures, 272–273
  collagen-based matrices, 268
  dose–response curves of breast epithelial cells, 270
  fiber maps of MCF10A epithelial structures, 274
  hormone-induced epithelial morphogenesis, 275
  mammary epithelial cell types, 268–271
  mammary gland biology and carcinogenesis, 267
  mammary stroma, 268
  MCF10A cells, 269
  primary breast cells, 270
  stroma, 271
  stromal cell types, 271–272
3D diabetic tissue models, 299, 312; *see also* Adipose; Liver; Pancreas; Skeletal muscle
  in vitro cell and tissue models, 302–303
  organ on chip models, 312
3D environment control, 62, 72; *see also* Rice University Flow Loop System
Three-dimensional printing, 14
Three-dimensional tissue test systems, 1
3DP, *see* 3D printing
3D printing (3DP), 14
3D printing bone scaffolds, 135; *see also* Bone engineering
3D tissue test system, 377
  ADLTs, 379
  Clinical Laboratory Improvement Amendments, 378
  CMS, 379
  in vitro diagnostic, 377
  laboratory-developed test, 378
  path to translation, 378
TIPS, *see* Thermally induced phase separation
Tissue
  bioreactor, 33
  engineering, 217
Tissue organization field theory (TOFT), 266

Tissue stimulation, 41; see also Bioreactor
  compression bioreactor, 42
  electrical stimulation, 43
  electromagnetic stimulation, 43
  hydrostatic pressure bioreactor, 42–43
  mechanical stimulation, 41
  tensile strain bioreactor, 42
Tissue voxel, 16
TLRs, see Toll-like receptors
TNF, see Tumor necrosis factor
TNFR-Associated Death Domain protein (TRADD), 220
TNF Receptor-Associated Factor-2 (TRAF2), 220
TOFT, see Tissue organization field theory
Toll-like receptors (TLRs), 217
TRADD, see TNFR-Associated Death Domain protein
TRAF2, see TNF Receptor-Associated Factor-2
Transcription factors, 327
Transforming growth factor beta (TGF-beta), 171
Tumor formation, 237
Tumorigenesis, 141
  stages of, 238
Tumor necrosis factor (TNF), 216
  responses elicited by, 217
Tumor necrosis factor alpha (TNFα), 217, 312
Tumor necrosis factor converting enzyme (TACE), 219
2D in vitro models, 216; see also Pro-and anti-inflammatory cytokines
TYK2, see Tyrosine Kinase-2
Type I diabetes, 300

Type II diabetes, 300
Tyrosine Kinase-2 (TYK2), 221

U

U.S. Food and Drug Administration (FDA), 107, 377, 391

V

Valve; see also Aortic valve; Mitral valves
  -based bioprinters, 93
  CryoValve® SG Pulmonary Valve, 203
  disease, 197
  heart valve 3D environment, 196
  histological slides of heart, 197
  nonregurgitant organ cultured, 66
Valve interstitial cells (VICs), 196
Vascular endothelial growth factor (VEGF), 19, 77, 135, 224, 338
Vascularization, 132–133; see also Bone engineering
VEGF, see Vascular endothelial growth factor
VICs, see Valve interstitial cells
Viscous agents, 201

W

Water/oil/water (W/O/W), 134
Weaving process, 21
Woven scaffolds, 23; see also Biofabrication
W/O/W, see Water/oil/water